DeVita, Hellman, and Rosenberg's

Cancer

Principles & Practice of Oncology Review

2nd Edition

DeVita, Hellman, and Rosenberg's

Cancer

Principles & Practice of Oncology Review

2nd Edition

Vincent T. DeVita, Jr., MD
Samuel Hellman, MD
Steven A. Rosenberg, MD, PhD

Editor

Ramaswamy Govindan, MD
Associate Professor
Department of Medicine
Division of Medical Oncology
Washington University School of Medicine
St. Louis, Missouri

Assistant Editors

Maria Q. Baggstrom, MD
Assistant Professor
Department of Medicine
Division of Oncology
Washington University School of Medicine
St. Louis, Missouri

Thomas H. Fong, MD
Department of Medicine
Divisions of Hematology and Oncology
Southern California Permanente Medical Group
Fontana, California

Janakiraman Subramanian, MBBS
Fellow of Hematology and Oncology
Department of Internal Medicine
Washington University School of Medicine
Saint Louis, Missouri

Wolters Kluwer | Lippincott Williams & Wilkins
Health

Philadelphia • Baltimore • New York • London
Buenos Aires • Hong Kong • Sydney • Tokyo

Acquisitions Editor: Jonathan Pine
Developmental Editor: Dovetail Content Solutions/Keith Donnellen
Senior Marketing Manager: Angela Panetta
Project Manager: Bridgett Dougherty
Senior Manufacturing Manager: Benjamin Rivera
Design Coordinator: Stephen Druding
Compositor: Maryland Composition/ASI

Library of Congress Cataloging-in-Publication Data

DeVita, Hellman, and Rosenberg's cancer : principles and practice of oncology review / Ramaswamy Govindan. — 2nd ed.
    p. ; cm.
  Based on: DeVita, Hellman, and Rosenberg's cancer / editors, Vincent T. DeVita Jr., Theodore S. Lawrence, Steven A. Rosenberg. 8th ed. c2008.
  Includes index.
  ISBN 978-1-60547-058-0
  1. Cancer—Examinations, questions, etc. 2. Oncology—Examinations, questions, etc. I. Govindan, Ramaswamy. II. DeVita, Hellman, and Rosenberg's cancer.
  [DNLM: 1. Neoplasms—Examination Questions. QZ 18.2 D496 2009]
  RC261.C274 2008 Suppl.
  616.99'40076—dc22

                                                            2008051304

To purchase additional copies of this book, call our customer service department at (800) 638-3030 or fax orders to (301) 824-7390. International customers should call (301) 714-2324.
Visit Lippincott Williams & Wilkins on the Internet: http://www.LWW.com. Lippincott Williams & Wilkins customer service representatives are available from 8:30 am to 6:00 pm, EST.

TO MY PARENTS
   KOLLENGODE A RAMASWAMY
   PANKAJVALLI RAMASWAMY
FOR ALL THEIR SACRIFICE, DEDICATION, AND GUIDANCE

Preface

It is always pleasurable to write the preface for a book. It signifies a formal completion of the arduous editing of countless numbers of chapters over several months and signals the imminent arrival of page proofs. Furthermore, writing a preface to the second edition tacitly acknowledges the success of the first edition. With the unprecedented explosion of knowledge over the past several years, the discipline of Oncology has become more complex and dynamic. *Cancer: Principles and Practice of Oncology (PPO)*, or simply known as the "DeVita book," has been *the* Oncology textbook for a number of years now. This companion review book, now in your hand, is an attempt to cull out the key learning points from the massive tome of "the DeVita book." While these review books are often seen as "study-aids" for last minute cramming for the board examinations, we hope this book would serve to highlight key points from each chapter of *PPO*. Each chapter in the review book corresponds to one or more chapters in the main text book just as they had in the first edition. We hope you find this book useful and informative. Please do not hesitate to contact me with comments, criticisms, and suggestions. You can reach me by email at rgovinda@im.wustl.edu.

Ramaswamy Govindan

Acknowledgments

At the outset, I want to thank the contributors for their diligence, time, and patience. My dear colleagues Dr. Maria Baggstrom, Dr. Thomas Fong, and Dr. Janakiraman Subramanian deserve special mention for their hard work, dedication, and commitment to make this project successful. As assistant editors, they worked tirelessly to procure and edit the chapters to keep our production schedule more or less on time. Keith Donnellan from Dovetail Content Solutions was truly a pleasure to work with. As always, Jonathan Pine from Lippincott Williams & Wilkins supported this idea and shepherded this to a reality by keeping a constant pressure on all of us. Embarking on a project like this takes a sizeable segment of family time away and puts more burdens on the spouse. For that, I will always be grateful to my wife Prabha and my two (still) adorable children, Ashwin and Akshay.

Ramaswamy Govindan

Contributors

Camille N. Abboud, MD
Professor
Department of Internal Medicine
Division of Oncology
Washington University School of Medicine
Saint Louis, Missouri

Douglas R. Adkins, MD
Associate Professor
Department of Internal Medicine
Washington University School of Medicine
St. Louis, Missouri

Rebecca L. Aft, MD, PhD
Associate Professor
Department of Surgery
Washington University School of Medicine
St. Louis, Missouri

Vorachart Auethavekiat, MD
Assistant Professor of Medicine
Divisions of Hematology and Oncology
Washington University at St. Louis
    Veterans Affairs Medical Center
Saint Louis, Missouri

Maria Q. Baggstrom, MD
Assistant Professor of Medicine
Division of Oncology
Washington University School of Medicine
St. Louis, Missouri

Anubha Bharthuar, MD
Fellow
Department of Medicine
Roswell Park Cancer Institute
Buffalo, New York

Sanjeev Bhalla, MD
Associate Professor of Radiology
Mallinckrodt Institute of Radiology
Barnes-Jewish Hospital
Saint Louis, Missouri

Sara K. Butler, PharmD, BCPS, BCOP
Clinical Pharmacy Specialist
Department of Pharmacy
Division of Medical Oncology
Barnes Jewish Hospital
Saint Louis, Missouri

Amanda F. Cashen, MD
Assistant Professor
Department of Medicine
Washington University School of Medicine
St. Louis, Missouri

L. Chinsoo Cho, MD, MS
Associate Professor
Department of Therapeutic Radiology
University of Minnesota Medical Center
Minneapolis, Minnesota

Alex E. Denes, MD
Associate Professor of Medicine
Department of Medical Oncology
Washington University Hospital
St. Louis, Missouri

Sarita Dubey, MD
Assistant Clinical Professor
Department of Medicine
Divisions Hematology and Oncology
University of California
San Francisco, California

Arkadiusz Z. Dudek, MD, PhD
Associate Professor
Department of Medicine
Divisions of Hematology, Oncology, and
    Transplantation
University of Minnesota Medical School
Minneapolis, Minnesota

Thomas H. Fong, MD
Department of Medicine
Divisions of Hematology and Oncology
Southern California Permanente Medical
    Group
Fontana, California

Shirish M. Gadgeel, MD
Associate Professor
Department of Internal Medicine
Karmanos Cancer Institute/Wayne State
    University
Detroit, Michigan

Becky J. Ganz, RN, BSN, MSN, ANP-BC
Adult Nurse Practitioner
Department of Medical Oncology
Siteman Cancer Center Washington
    University
St. Louis, Missouri

Boone W. Goodgame, MD
Assistant Professor
Department of Medicine
Division of Oncology
Washington University School of Medicine
St. Louis, Missouri

Mouhammed A. Habra, MD
Assistant Professor
Department of Endocrine Neoplasia and
    Hormonal Disorders
The University of Texas M.D. Anderson
    Cancer Center
Houston, Texas

Rami Y. Haddad, MD, FACP
Assistant Professor of Medicine, Acting
    Chair
Department of Internal Medicine
Divisions of Hematology and Oncology
Chicago Medical School at Rosalind
    Franklin University
North Chicago, Illinois

Jennifer L. Ivanovich, MS, MBA
Research Instructor
Department of Surgery
Washington University School of Medicine
St. Louis, Missouri

Renuka V. Iyer, MD
Assistant Professor
Department of Medicine
Roswell Park Cancer Center
Buffalo, New York

Cylen Javidan-Nejad, MD
Assistant Professor of Radiology
Mallinckrodt Institute of Radiology
Barnes-Jewish Hospital
Saint Louis, Missouri

Gregory P. Kalemkerian, MD
Professor
Department of Internal Medicine
University of Michigan
Ann Arbor, Michigan

Jason Keune, MD
Resident in Surgery
Department of Surgery
Washington University School of Medicine
St. Louis, Missouri

Nikhil I. Khushalani, MD
Assistant Professor
Department of Medicine
Division of Oncology
Roswell Park Cancer Institute
Buffalo, New York

Clint Daniel Kingsley, MD
Clinical assistant professor
Department of Internal Medicine
UAB School of Medicine
Huntsville, Alabama

Mark A. Klein, MD
Assistant Professor
Department of Medicine
University of Minnesota Medical School
Minneapolis, Minnesota

Robert A. Kratzke, MD
Associate Professor
Department of Medicine
University of Minnesota Medical School
Minneapolis, Minnesota

David I. Kuperman, MD
Instructor
Department of Medicine
Division of Oncology
Washington Unversity School of Medicine
Saint Louis, Missouri

Janessa J. Laskin, MD, FRCPC
Assistant Professor
Department of Medical Oncology
University of British Columbia
Vancouver, British Columbia

Gerald P. Linette, MD, PhD
Assistant Professor of Medicine
Division of Oncology
Washington University School of Medicine
Saint Louis, Missouri

Kathy D. Miller, MD
Associate Professor of Medicine
Divisions of Hematology and Oncology
Indiana University
Indianapolis, Indiana

Daniel Morgensztern, MD
Assistant Professor
Department of Medicine
Division of Medical Oncology
Washington University at St. Louis
    Veterans Affairs Medical Center
Saint Louis, Missouri

James C. Mosley III, MD
Fellow of Hematology and Oncology
Department of Medicine
Divisions of Hematology and Oncology
Washington University School of Medicine
Saint Louis, Missouri

Sujatha Murali, MS, MD
Instructor
Department of Hematology and Medical
    Oncology
Winship Cancer Institute
Emory University School of Medicine
Crawford Long Hospital
Atlanta, Georgia

David G. Mutch, MD
Judith and Ira Gall Professor of Obstetrics
    and Gynecology
Department of Gynecology
Washington University School of Medicine
Saint Louis, Missouri

Michael C. Perry, MD, MS, MACP
Professor of Medicine
Divisions of Hematology and Oncology
Department of Internal Medicine
Ellis Fischel Cancer Center
University of Missouri
Columbia, Missouri

Matthew A. Powell, MD
Assistant Professor
Department of Obstetrics and Gynecology
Washington University School of Medicine
Saint Louis, Missouri

Krishnan Raghavendran, MBBS
Associate Professor
Department of Surgery
University of Michigan
Ann Arbor, Michigan

Suresh S. Ramalingam, MD
Associate Professor
Department of Hematology and Medical
    Oncology
Emory University
Atlanta, Georgia

Nithya Ramnath, MD
Associate Professor
Department of Medicine
University of Michigan Comprehensive
    Cancer Center
Ann Arbor, Michigan

Lee Ratner, MD, PhD
Professor of Medicine and Molecular
    Microbiology
Department of Internal Medicine
Washington University School of Medicine
Saint Louis, Missouri

Kaunteya Reddy, MD
Resident
Department of Internal Medicine
University at Buffalo
Buffalo, New York

Ana Roshal, MD
Assistant Professor
Department of Internal Medicine
Division of Onoclogy
Washington University School of Medicine
Saint Louis, Missouri

Mark A. Schroeder, MD
Fellow in Hematology and Oncology
Department of Internal Medicine
Division of Oncology
Washington University School of Medicine
Saint Louis, Missouri

Shalini Shenoy, MD
Associate Professor
Department of Pediatrics
Washington University School of
    Medicine/St. Louis Children's Hospital
Saint Louis, Missouri

George R. Simon, MD
Member and Director, Thoracic Oncology
Department of Medical Oncology
Philadelphia, Pennsylvania

Sunit Srivastava, MD
Resident Physician
Department of Internal Medicine
University of South Florida
Tampa, Florida

Walter M. Stadler, MD, FACP
Fred C. Buffett Professor
Department of Medicine and Surgery
University of Chicago
Chicago, Illinois

Thomas F. Stinchcombe, MD
Assistant Professor
Department of Multidisciplinary Thoracic
    Oncology Program
University of North Carolina
Chapel Hill, North Carolina

Keith E. Stockerl-Goldstein, MD
Associate Professor of Medicine
Division of Oncology
Section of BMT and Leukemia
Washington University School of Medicine
Saint Louis, Missouri

Janakiraman Subramanian, MBBS
Fellow of Hematology and Oncology
Department of Internal Medicine
Washington University School of Medicine
Saint Louis, Missouri

Benjamin R. Tan, MD
Assistant Professor of Medicine
Division of Oncology
Washington University School of Medicine
Saint Louis, Missouri

David D. Tran, MD, PhD
Fellow in Oncology
Department of Internal Medicine
Divisions of Hematology and Oncology
Washington University School of Medicine
Barnes-Jewish Hospital
St. Louis, Missouri

Kathryn M. Trinkaus, PhD
Research Statistician
Division of Biostatistics
Washington University School of Medicine
Saint Louis, Missouri

Vamsidhar Velcehti, MD
Resident Intern
Department of Internal Medicine
Ochsner Clinic Foundation
New Orleans, Louisiana

Ravi Vij, MD
Associate Professor
Department of Internal Medicine
Section of BMT and Leukemia
Washington University School of Medicine
Saint Louis, Missouri

Richard Walgren, MD, PhD
Clinical Fellow
Department of Internal Medicine
Divisions of Hematology and Medical
    Oncology
Washington University School of Medicine
St. Louis, Missouri

Sunny Wang, MD
Fellow
Department of Hematology and Oncology
University of California
San Francisco, California

Andrea Wang-Gillam, MD, PhD
Assistant Professor
Department of Internal Medicine
Washington University School of Medicine
Saint Louis, Missouri

John S. Welch, MD, PhD
Fellow of Hematology and Oncology
Divisions of Hematology and Oncology
Washington University School of Medicine
Saint Louis, Missouri

Howard L. West, MD
Medical Director, Thoracic Oncology
    Program
Department of Medical Oncology
Swedish Cancer Institute
Seattle, Washington

Peter Westervelt, MD, PhD
Associate Professor
Department of Internal Medicine
Washington University School of Medicine
Saint Louis, Missouri

Megan E. Wren, MD
Associate Professor
Department of Internal Medicine
Washington University School of Medicine
Saint Louis, Missouri

Contents

1

Molecular Biology of Cancer ■ Part 1

Directions   Each of the numbered items below is followed by lettered answers. Select the ONE lettered answer that is BEST in each case unless instructed otherwise.

QUESTIONS

Question 1.1.   **Completion of the Human Genome Project has revealed that human cells have a repertoire of genes of which approximate number?**

A. 2500 genes
B. 25,000 genes
C. 250,000 genes
D. 2,500,000 genes

Question 1.2.   **One of the reasons to use cancer cell culture experiments in preclinical studies of cancers is:**

A. Allows evaluation of cancer cell interaction with the tumor microenvironment.
B. Cell cultures are amenable to easily manipulated experimental techniques.
C. Adaptation of cancer cells to growth in culture corresponds exactly to cancer cell growth in vivo.
D. Allows evaluation of cancer cell interaction with the native immune system.

Question 1.3.   **Which of the following is false with regard to genetic mutations in cancer?**

A. Gain of function mutations (oncogenes) are generally dominant at the cellular level.
B. Loss of functions mutations (tumor suppressor genes) are generally recessive at the cellular level.
C. One percent of the estimated total number of genes may contribute to some form of cancer.
D. Ninety percent of germline mutations in familial cancer syndromes are in tumor suppressor genes.

Corresponding Chapters in *Cancer: Principles & Practice of Oncology*, Eighth Edition: 1 (Cancer: A Conceptual Framework), 2 (Genomics and Proteomics), 3 (Destabilization of the Cancer Genome), 4 (Telomeres, Telomerase, and Cell Immortalization), and 5 (Cell Signaling).

Question 1.4.   Which of the following proteins has inhibitory activity in the cell cycle?

A. Cyclin D1
B. E2F
C. p16INK4a
D. Cyclin-dependent kinase 4

Question 1.5.   All of the following contribute to suppression of cancer progression, EXCEPT:

A. Autophagy
B. Apoptosis
C. Senescence
D. Angiogenesis

Question 1.6.   Which of the following does successful invasion and metastasis NOT depend on?

A. Senescence
B. Angiogenesis
C. Evasion of apoptosis
D. Self-sufficiency in growth signals

Question 1.7.   Which of the following best describes the term "protooncogene"?

A. A normal cellular gene that has been transduced by a retrovirus that is then mutated following viral replication
B. A homologue of a known oncogenic element identified in prehistoric specimens
C. A transforming viral gene that can cause malignant transformation in fibroblasts in vitro
D. The first oncogene discovered to be associated with human cancer
E. A viral oncogene that, following infection, is the direct causative agent of human cancer

Question 1.8.   Barriers to routine use of expression array technologies include:

A. Tumor specimen handling to ensure RNA stability
B. Identifying pure tumor populations in biopsy samples
C. Standardization of specimen processing and assay procedure
D. All of the above

Question 1.9.   Which of the following is a potential flaw in microarray studies?

A. Inadequate controls
B. Biased estimation of prediction accuracy
C. Correlation between clusters and clinical outcome
D. All of the above

Question 1.10.   **Which of the following about miRNAs is false?**

A. Are too small to be active inside a cell
B. Consist of RNA 19 to 24 nucleotides in length
C. Can be evaluated in array format as part of clinical studies
D. May downregulate gene expression and protein translation

Question 1.11.   **The proteome is which of the following:**

A. The set of all expressed gene products at a given time
B. The proteins expressed preferentially in malignant cells
C. The set of all proteins potentially expressed by the genome
D. The set of protonated peptides subject to matrix-assisted laser desorption ionization-time of flight (MALDI-TOF) analysis

Question 1.12.   **Information obtained for molecular profiling using gene arrays and proteomics includes the following, EXCEPT:**

A. Gene arrays can predict protein–protein interactions.
B. Protein levels and protein function do not correspond directly with gene transcript levels.
C. Polymerase chain reaction (PCR) can be used to amplify biopsy material for use in gene arrays, whereas no signal amplification technology is standard in protein arrays.
D. Proteomics can be used to investigate posttranslationally modified proteins.

Question 1.13.   **All is true about the peptidome, EXCEPT:**

A. Consists of fragments of larger proteins.
B. Included peptides must be less than 1000 daltons.
C. May be amplified in the circulation.
D. Many of the peptide fragments bind high-concentration blood proteins such as albumin.

Question 1.14.   **Which of the following methods identifies peptides with high sensitivity and in a high-throughput fashion?**

A. Surface-enhanced laser desorption/ionization time-of-flight (SELDI-TOF)
B. Hydrophobic bead capture-mass spectrometry (MS)
C. Two-dimensional (2D) polyacrylamide gel electrophoresis (PAGE)-MS
D. None of the above

Question 1.15.   **Which of the following is an example of how cDNA microarray analysis may identify genome wide profiles and regulation?**

A. Detection of amplified gene elements such as Her2/neu in breast cancer
B. Identification of expressed messenger RNA (mRNA) transcript profiles, which correlates with prognosis in adenocarcinoma of the lung
C. Measuring prostate-specific antigen (PSA) levels in prostate cancer
D. Detection of BCR-ABL fusion genes in chronic myeloid leukemia (CML) to monitor residual disease
E. Detection of ras family mutations in colon cancer

Question 1.16. **The presence of mutations in p53 has been associated with which of the following properties on cells:**

A. Loss of the G2 checkpoint following treatment with DNA-damaging agents
B. Enhanced capacity to undergo apoptosis following exposure to radiation
C. Increased capacity for DNA amplification
D. A and C

Question 1.17. **Which of the following is an example of gene amplification found in cancer?**

A. N-myc amplification in neuroblastoma
B. C-myc amplification in small cell lung cancer
C. Her2/neu amplification in breast cancer
D. All of the above

Question 1.18. **Which of the following is true regarding microsatellite instability in colon cancer?**

A. Approximately 15% of patients with hereditary nonpolyposis coli have mutations in MLH1 or MSH2.
B. There is potential resistance to 5-fluorouracil.
C. It has a less favorable prognosis.
D. Evidence is in favor of it occurring only late in sporadic colon cancer cases.

Question 1.19. **Which of the following is false about excision repair mechanisms?**

A. Reduced expression of ERCC1 in non–small cell lung cancer is associated with response to cisplatin.
B. There are two nucleotide excision repair pathways.
C. Base excision repair is involved in response to damage from chemicals and radiographs.
D. Numerous abnormalities in base excision repair machinery in multiple inherited cancers have been described.

Question 1.20. **ATR/CHK1 signaling is associated with all of the following, EXCEPT:**

A. Bone marrow failure
B. Predisposition to squamous cell carcinoma
C. Predisposition to acute leukemias
D. Decreased sensitivity to cisplatin

Question 1.21. **Breast cancer tumors that lack expression of estrogen and progesterone receptors and absence of HER2 amplification ("triple-negative") share similarities with tumors that develop in patients with germline mutations in what genes?**

A. ERCC1
B. BRCA1
C. CSA
D. CSB

Question 1.22.   **Overexpression of aurora B kinase could lead to all of the following, EXCEPT:**

    A.   Inability for sister chromatids to separate before anaphase
    B.   Rapid cell division
    C.   Aneuploidy
    D.   Increased disassembly of kinetochore proteins

Question 1.23.   **Which of the following characterizes cytogenetic abnormalities in most human cancers?**

    A.   Universal (monoclonal) population of cells containing identical cytogenetic abnormalities
    B.   Completely normal karyotype
    C.   Heterogenous complex karyotypes
    D.   Complete loss of X or Y chromosomes

Question 1.24.   **The "Hayflick phenomenon," which is the name given to the limited replicative potential of cells, is thought to arise from which of the following?**

    A.   The sequential loss of genetic material from the ends of chromosomes (telomeres) with each round of division
    B.   The gradual accumulation of uncorrected genetic defects passed on during division leading to senescence or malignancy
    C.   The activation of telomerase in aging cells leading to enzymatic loss of genetic material from telomeres
    D.   Dividing eukaryotic cells outgrowing their vascular supply

Question 1.25.   **Which of the following statements is NOT accurate regarding telomerase?**

    A.   It has both an RNA and a protein component.
    B.   It is a DNA polymerase.
    C.   Overexpression of telomerase is found in all cancer specimens.
    D.   Telomerase protects the integrity of the chromosomal ends.

Question 1.26.   **Senescence can be induced by all of the following, EXCEPT:**

    A.   Telomere shortening
    B.   Prolonged DNA damage
    C.   High-density growth
    D.   Oncogene activation

Question 1.27.   **All of the following is evidence for senescence as a tumor suppressor mechanism, EXCEPT:**

A.   Several "tumor suppressor" proteins that are involved in senescence pathways (e.g., p16INK4a) are mutated in familial cancer syndromes.
B.   Mice and humans with impaired p16INK4a and p53 function develop normally other than an age-dependent decrease in cancer and decreased susceptibility to cancer in response to carcinogen exposure.
C.   Reestablishment of p53 activity in sarcoma and hepatocellular carcinoma has led to cessation of tumor growth.
D.   Growth arrest in lung epithelium has been demonstrated in response to oncogenic events.

Question 1.28.   **All of the following are potential therapeutic strategies to induce senescence in cancer cells, EXCEPT:**

A.   Restoration of p16INK4a activity via gene therapy
B.   Restoration of p16INK4a activity via inhibition of DNA methyltransferases
C.   Inhibition of MDM2
D.   Inhibition of p16INK4a-p53 interactions

Question 1.29.   **Breakage-fusion-bridge (BFB) cycles lead to all of the following, EXCEPT:**

A.   Methylation
B.   Aneuploidy
C.   Amplifications
D.   Deletions

Question 1.30.   **Telomerase-null mice are associated with which of the following?**

A.   Decreased sensitivity to radiation
B.   Decreased sensitivity to chemotherapy that induces double-strand breaks (DSBs)
C.   Decreased genomic stability in the presence of p53 deficiency
D.   Decreased rate of spontaneous malignancy

Question 1.31.   **All of the following are receptor tyrosine kinases, EXCEPT:**

A.   Platelet-derived growth factor receptor
B.   Insulin-like growth factor receptor 1
C.   Kit
D.   Akt

Question 1.32.   **Which of the following is TRUE about receptor tyrosine kinases?**

A.   They are always monomeric.
B.   Activation always requires tyrosine phosphorylation in all classes.
C.   Different types of ligands can activate the same class of receptors.
D.   Different types of ligands induce the same receptor conformational changes on binding.

Question 1.33.   **Which of the following is FALSE about receptor phosphotyrosine phosphatases?**

    A.   No true ligands for these have been described.
    B.   They always function to antagonize tyrosine kinases.
    C.   Activation could increase intracellular phosphorylation under certain circumstances.
    D.   Most receptor phosphatases contain two catalytic domains.

Question 1.34.   **Specificity of protein kinase substrate phosphorylation is dependent on:**

    A.   Substrate structural motifs
    B.   Presence of a proline following a serine
    C.   Co-localization of substrate and kinase
    D.   A and C

Question 1.35.   **Which of the following is TRUE about GTP-binding proteins?**

    A.   GDP hydrolysis leads to a conformational change.
    B.   All are lipid-modified.
    C.   Ras-like proteins exist in trimers.
    D.   Gai stimulates adenylate cyclase.

Question 1.36.   **Which of the following are second messengers?**

    A.   Cyclic adenosine monophosphate (cAMP)
    B.   Diacylglycerol
    C.   Ras
    D.   A and B

Question 1.37.   **Regulation of protein levels can be affected by:**

    A.   Signal transduction
    B.   Translation
    C.   Proteolysis
    D.   All of the above

Question 1.38.   **Inhibition of the addition of a lipid moiety to Ras would potentially lead to:**

    A.   Increase in activation Raf
    B.   Decrease in cell proliferation
    C.   Increase in activation of MEK
    D.   A and C

ANSWERS

Answer 1.1.   **The answer is B.**

One of the surprising findings of analysis of the sequenced human genome is the presence of only approximately 25,000 expressed genes in human cells. However, only a few thousand of these seem to be expressed at any given time. Previous estimates, based on the known approximate size of human chromosomes, were that there were up to 100,000 or more individual genes expressed in human cells.

Answer 1.2.   **The answer is B.**

Preclinical and clinical studies into cancer cell pathogenesis and response to potential treatments can be guided initially with cell culture experiments because these experiments can be manipulated in a reproducible manner. However, cell culture experiments do not allow for evaluation of the interaction between cancer cells and the tumor microenvironment. Some techniques such as cellular assays that evaluate for cellular migration and invasion through a matrigel can mimic the tumor microenvironment, but they cannot replicate all of the cellular–environmental interactions. In addition, cancer cells can acquire genetic changes through multiple passages in culture such that they may not completely reflect in vivo cancer cell–host interactions.

Answer 1.3.   **The answer is D.**

Ninety percent of germline mutations in familial cancer syndromes are in tumor suppressor genes. It is thought that many dominant oncogene mutations likely cause fetal demise and therefore do not arise in familial cancer syndromes. Dominant mutations in cancer genes denote oncogenes and make up 90% of all cancer genes.

Answer 1.4.   **The answer is C.**

The cell cycle is composed of the phases G0, G1, S, G2, and M. Regulation of the cell cycle depends on an interplay of multiple proteins. Cyclin-dependent kinases (cdk) are serine/threonine kinases that are ubiquitous in the cell cycle. They generally require phosphorylation and association with cyclins for activity. Cdk4 phosphorylates retinoblastoma (Rb) protein, allowing depression of transcription factors (of which E2F is an example) essential to progression of the cell cycle. A series of inhibitors (INK4 family) act to decrease the activity of cyclins, of which p16INK4a is a member.

Answer 1.5.   **The answer is D.**

Angiogenesis encompasses a cascade of events that allow a tumor's vascular supply to be enhanced, thereby increasing cellular proliferation. Apoptosis and autophagy are two distinct mechanisms of cell death. Apoptosis is regulated via caspase cascades and mitochondrial-mediated pathways. Autophagy often is induced via nutrient starvation (as sensed by the mTor kinase) and involves autodigestion of intracellular organelles. Senescence, the permanent arrest of cell division, is regulated via the ARF-p53 and p16INK4a-Rb pathways.

Answer 1.6.   **The answer is A.**

Senescence is the permanent arrest of cell division, which would not contribute to cancer progression via invasion and metastasis. The other choices are all required for such progression. In addition, insensitivity to growth inhibitory signals and limitless replicative potential are also necessary for the complex processes of invasion and metastasis.

Answer 1.7. **The answer is A.**

It has been known for almost a century that certain viruses can cause malignant transformation. The responsible genetic elements identified in the viral genomes are called viral oncogenes (v-oncogenes). It was found that homologues of these viral oncogenes existed in the eukaryotic genome from which they had likely originated. These normal human genetic elements were given the name protooncogene. One of the first of these, src, was identified in the avian Rous sarcoma virus that had been studied as a transforming virus decades earlier. In most human cancers, mutations or aberrant expressions of oncogenes have been identified.

Answer 1.8. **The answer is D.**

Numerous barriers exist to the routine use of cDNA array technologies in clinical practice. Although techniques of RNA amplification exist, they can introduce bias in the final profile results. Samples from needle aspirates are often inadequate for expression array use. In addition, most tumor biopsies are a mixture of benign and malignant tissues. Ideally, pure tumor tissues should be used, although mixed tissues may give alternative useful information. Laser capture microscopy can potentially help this situation but is a technology not widely available in clinical practice. Finally, to obtain high-quality RNA, fresh-frozen tissue is ideal, requiring immediate freezing and storage capabilities. All of these problems will likely be solved by developing technologies but currently are keeping expression profiling as largely a research tool for molecular target and profile identification.

Answer 1.9. **The answer is D.**

Microarray technology is dependent on unbiased and rigorous statistical analysis, and as such, is susceptible to user bias. To help address the continuing need for standardization guidelines in the clinical use of microarray technology, the Minimum Information About A Microarray Experiment (MIAME) was published as a demonstration that microarray data can be independently verified, thereby reducing bias. The answers listed all may contribute to flawed interpretation of microarray data.

Answer 1.10. **The answer is A.**

MicroRNA (miRNA) consists of an RNA sequence of 19 to 24 nucleotides in length and participates in cell processes such as apoptosis and development via the effect on gene expression and protein translation. Recently, miRNA array signatures have been evaluated in clinical samples from patients with lung cancer, chronic lymphocytic leukemia, and breast cancer. In a recent lung cancer study, the miRNA profile correlated with survival.

Answer 1.11.   **The answer is C.**

The term "proteome" is generally taken to refer to all potentially expressed proteins encoded by the genome. However, many operational definitions specify only those proteins expressed at a given time or under certain conditions, so answer "A" denotes a relatively common use of the term as well. Increasingly, the term "proteome" is used in conjunction with a modifier such as "serum," cellular," or even "malignant" to denote a more limited set of conditions. Protonation is a preparative step before proteomic evaluation by current means. Most proteomic analyses require cleavage of the proteins in the samples followed by protonation of the resulting peptides before MALDI-TOF analysis.

Answer 1.12.   **The answer is A.**

Current gene array technology is focused mostly around the detection of gene transcript levels. Small quantities of nuclear material from minimal biopsy material can be amplified via PCR. However, protein–protein interactions and posttranslational processing cannot be predicted. Multiple technologies have been used to detect "proteomic signatures," which include 2D gel electrophoresis, affinity tagging, liquid chromatography coupled with mass spectrometry, and antibody arrays. Limitations of proteomic technologies include disruption of the native three-dimensional (3D) protein conformations in addition to the need for larger amounts of biopsy material needed compared with genomic arrays. This requires sensitive proteomic technology, such as antibodies in the femtomolar range.

Answer 1.13.   **The answer is B.**

The term "peptidome" refers to the low-molecular-weight range of the proteome that consists of peptides or protein fragments generally less than 50,000 daltons. It is thought that these peptide fragments are secreted from various tumors and exist in the circulation bound to carrier proteins. Studies are under way to determine if the secreted pattern of such fragments can be correlated with disease states. A confounding factor in peptidome analysis may be the susceptibility of peptides to protease degradation in the blood after secretion from the tumor. It remains to be seen if consistent patterns can be determined after protease degradation.

Answer 1.14.   **The answer is D.**

Currently, no technology is available to study the peptidome in a highly sensitive and high throughput fashion. Most of the methods in peptide detection use mass spectrometry technology. Surface-enhanced laser desorption/ionization time-of-flight (SELDI-TOF) uses chemically treated chips that peptides can "stick" to. After washing off unbound proteins and peptides, the bound peptides are ionized and analyzed. A disadvantage of this system is the inability to detect proteins less than 4 pg/mL. Hydrophobic bead capture-MS uses beads to bind peptides of interest via nonspecific hydrophobic interactions. After elution of the beads, MS is used to identify the peptides. It is a medium throughput technique with low sensitivity. Two-dimensional gel electrophoresis-MS methods cannot reliably resolve peptides less than 15 kDa and exhibit low throughput and low sensitivity. One-dimensional gel-MS methods have increased sensitivity for peptides less than 20 kDa compared with 2D gel-MS; however, it is also a slow throughput technology.

Answer 1.15.   **The answer is B.**

Profiling of cancer cells using cDNA microarray has proven to be a powerful investigational tool in cancer research. Array technology allows for genome-wide analysis of messenger RNA levels of thousands of genes in a single experiment. The results of a microarray experiment can lead to finding increased or decreased expression of specific mRNA in a wide variety of cancers. However, cDNA microarray technology will only detect alterations in gene transcript expression levels. Cancer-specific single nucleotide mutations such as ras mutations in colon cancer can be best detected with gene-specific hybridization or PCR techniques. Similarly, rearrangements or amplifications of specific genes are best detected by techniques that examine genomic DNA sequences. The measurement of secreted extracellular proteins such as PSA requires antibody directed tools, such as enzyme-linked immunosorbent assay (ELISA).

Answer 1.16.   **The answer is D.**

Mutations of p53 are among the most commonly identified in human cancers. Wild-type p53 has a function in signaling cells with damaged DNA to undergo programmed cell death (apoptosis). In the presence of an inactivating mutation of p53, commonly used genotoxic agents, such as radiation and chemotherapy, may prove less effective with the intact p53 signal. This has been demonstrated in preclinical models and correlates with some human clinical trial data. It must be noted, however, that many common malignancies harboring p53 mutations, such as small cell lung cancer and ovarian cancer, are sensitive to chemotherapy and radiation. The capacity of p53 to trigger apoptosis is associated with the cell-cycle checkpoints that have been identified as critical nodal moments at which the cell may "choose" to continue to divide or, if sufficiently damaged, progress down a path to cell death and deletion of the potentially damaged clone. Interestingly, p53 mutant transgenic mice are viable and develop normally. However, they have an accelerated rate of tumor formation under certain tumorigenic stimuli.

Answer 1.17.   **The answer is D.**

Gene amplification as a mechanism resulting in overexpression of gene products involved in tumorigenesis or tumor progression has been reported in several cancers. It is known that N-myc amplification in neuroblastoma can be a useful prognostic factor aiding in designing therapy. In small cell lung cancer, c-myc amplification has been identified in up to 10% of specimens, a percentage that may increase after treatment. Her2/neu amplification occurs in up to 30% of breast cancers and is useful in predicting response to Her2/neu targeted therapy.

Answer 1.18.   **The answer is B.**

Microsatellite instability (MIN) refers to frequent mutations in regions of simple repeat sequences. Early studies in kindreds with hereditary nonpolyposis colorectal cancer (HNPCC) demonstrated mutations in MSH2 and MLH1, which are mismatch repair genes. Approximately 85% of patients with HNPCC have mutations in MSH2 and MLH1. MIN is associated with a resistance to 5-fluorouracil treatment, more favorable prognosis, and lack of p53 mutations. The protein MSH2 complexes with MSH6 to recognize mismatched bases, and subsequent recruitment of MLH1 and PMS2 initiates the steps of repair (excision, DNA synthesis, and ligation).

Answer 1.19.   **The answer is D.**

The mismatch repair machinery of the cell includes two major pathways: nucleotide excision repair (NER) and base excision repair (BER). These pathways respond to lesions created by DNA-damaging agents, such as chemicals and radiation from numerous sources. Early discoveries in the NER pathway were made via the study of xeroderma pigmentosa, where patients exhibit extreme sun sensitivity. Two NER pathways have been described: The first involves global genome scanning for lesions, and the second detects lesions that interfere with RNA polymerases. In BER, the repair machinery responds mainly to chemical and x-ray damage and base loss by using DNA glycosylates to remove damaged bases and a complex of APEX1 endonuclease, PARP, DNA polymerase/ligase, and XRCC1 to recognize abasic sites. As of now, no inherited cancer syndromes caused by mutations in BER have been discovered.

Answer 1.20.   **The answer is D.**

DSBs can promote major cytogenetic abnormalities and are repaired via homologous recombination (HR) or nonhomologous end-joining (NHEJ). ATR/CHK1 signaling leads to activation of the Fanconi anemia repair pathway. Defects in Fanconi anemia lead to bone marrow failure, congenital abnormalities, predisposition to acute leukemias and squamous cell cancer, and increased sensitivity to DNA cross-linking agents such as cisplatin and mitomycin C.

Answer 1.21.   **The answer is B.**

Homologous recombination is one cellular mechanism for DSB repair in the cell. BRCA1 and BRCA2 are two proteins that are mutated in familial breast and ovarian cancer syndromes and play key roles in DSB repair. BRCA1 has also been linked to S phase and G2/M checkpoint control, in addition to mitotic spindle assembly. BRCA2 has been linked to cytokinesis. ERCC1 is primarily involved in nucleotide excision repair and is associated with increased response to cisplatin. CSA and CSB are also components of the NER pathway and are implicated in Cockayne syndrome.

Answer 1.22.   **The answer is A.**

The mitotic spindle is central to cell division, and Aurora kinase B is intricately involved in the process of cell division. The linking of sister chromatids before anaphase is lost partly because of the action of Aurora B kinase. Aurora B kinase also phosphorylates other kinetochore proteins to aid disassembly of kinetochore-microtubule attachments not under proper tension (as part of spindle checkpoint activation). Amplification of Aurora B kinase has been associated with sporadic tumors.

Answer 1.23.   **The answer is C.**

Human cancers are largely characterized by complex karyotypes with multiple different populations. In particular, solid tumors such as lung and colon cancer exhibit great heterogeneity that is likely the result of the high level of genomic instability found in cancers. Some less common malignancies, such as CML, are characterized by the relatively uniform presence of an abnormal karyotype, often with a limited number of detectable breakpoints and translocations. In fact, the presence of a uniform karyotypic abnormality raises the possibility of a germline cytogenetic defect that may be further evaluated by examining the karyotype of noncancerous circulating lymphocytes from the same patient. The absence of any karyotypic abnormality in cancer cell populations is less common but can occur. For example, the presence of a normal karyotype is a well-recognized observation in acute myelogenous leukemia and gives important clinical information conferring an intermediate prognosis. The loss of a single X or Y chromosome is a normal variant commonly observed in older patients. It carries little clinical significance.

Answer 1.24.   **The answer is A.**

Hayflick and Moorehead documented a landmark finding of cell biology when they observed that normal eukaryotic cells would only replicate approximately 50 to 100 times before dying. This limited replicative capacity of nontransformed cells is called the "Hayflick phenomenon." It is now known that the ends of the chromosomes, called "telomeres," gradually shorten, losing 25 to 200 base pairs with each round of division. After 50 to 100 rounds of division, the telomeres reach a critically shortened length, triggering cell senescence. Telomeres can be maintained by the enzymatic activity of telomerase, which function to restore and maintain telomeres at their full length. Activation of telomerase is a key mechanism by which some cells, such as cancer cells, evade senescence. Although gene defects occur spontaneously in cells and will lead to programmed cell death, this usually occurs in the immediate generation after the defect is established. Tumor growth does require neovascularization, but the "Hayflick phenomenon" applies to programmed senescence in nontransformed cells.

Answer 1.25.   **The answer is C.**

Telomerase is the DNA polymerase that synthesizes the repeating six base pair motif (TTAGGG) that comprises the ends of all chromosomes.

It is a nucleoprotein with both a protein and RNA component. With cell division, the telomere ends become progressively shorter until a critical length is reached and programmed cell death is initiated. Synthesizing and repairing the ends of the shortening telomeres allows cells to maintain the integrity of the chromosomal ends and is important for cells that need to divide without reaching senescence, such as cancer cells. In light of this, it is not surprising that the majority of cancer cells overexpress telomerase, but there are cancers that appear to have invoked alternative mechanisms to repair telomeres. Indeed, telomerase-deficient (deleted) mice can be induced to develop tumors.

Answer 1.26.   **The answer is C.**

Senescence refers to a state in cultured cells where growth arrest is permanent. Senescence differs from quiescence in that quiescent cells can reenter the cell cycle in response to appropriate mitogenic cues. Quiescence is generally induced by serum starvation, growth factor deprivation, high-density growth, and transient DNA damage. Senescence can be induced by prolonged DNA damage, oxidative stress, telomere shortening, and oncogene activation. Additional differences include uninducible c-fos expression in response to serum stimulation and increased PAI expression in senescence versus quiescence.

Answer 1.27.   **The answer is B.**

Cell-cycle inhibitors that lead to senescence include p16INK4a and p53, among others. It follows that mice and humans with impaired p16INK4a and p53 function develop normally other than an age-dependent increase in cancer and increased susceptibility to cancer in response to carcinogen exposure. Aside from the other correct answers listed, other evidence is supportive. Minimal residual disease data demonstrate frequent oncogenic events as evidence for a need for tumor suppression. Mice are highly susceptible to inactivation of p16INK4a and/or p53 as evidenced by experiments demonstrating development of primary tumors at 8 weeks of age (normal life span is approximately 100 weeks).

Answer 1.28.   **The answer is D.**

Knockout of INK4a and ARF loci separately and in combination leads to an increase in spontaneous tumors. Silencing of p16INK4a via hypermethylation has been well described and is associated with numerous types of cancers. Inhibition of methylation is thought to increase expression of p16INK4a. Gene therapy as a method to replace p16INK4a activity has been achieved in the laboratory. ARF leads to MDM2 activation and subsequent p53 degradation. Inhibition of MDM2 activity is thought to increase p53 levels and lead to apoptosis and senescence. p53 and p16INK4a do not interact directly.

Answer 1.29.   **The answer is A.**

Chromosomal rearrangements are thought to contribute to the malignant phenotype of many different cancers. Such rearrangements are the result of BFB cycles. Unprotected chromatids can fuse to form a dicentric chromosome. The fused chromosomes break during anaphase and create atelomeric chromosomes. Atelomeric chromosomes can fuse with other chromosomes and perpetuate the cycle. Amplification, deletions, and aneuploidy can arise this way. Methylation is an epigenetic phenomenon that is not thought to be directly related to chromosome fusion.

Answer 1.30.   **The answer is C.**

It is thought that one of the mechanisms of cancer pathogenesis is related to short telomeres that contribute to genomic instability followed by increased telomerase activity. Paradoxically, genomic instability can increase with decreased telomerase activity in the presence of concomitant p53 deficiency, suggesting that telomerase inhibition by itself is likely not sufficient as a cancer therapeutic. However, increased sensitivity to radiation and DSB-inducing chemotherapeutics is associated with decreased telomerase activity and suggests possible additive or synergistic effects.

Answer 1.31.   **The answer is D.**

Phosphorylation of tyrosine residues by tyrosine kinases is an important signal for cell stimulation and cancer growth. Each transmembrane tyrosine kinase is activated by its associated ligand. Increasingly, tyrosine kinases are an important target for novel therapeutics as well. Examples of this class of agents already in common use include both imatinib mesylate (Gleevec) and gefitinib (Iressa). All of the examples listed above are receptor tyrosine kinases except for Akt. Akt is a threonine/serine kinase and a key component of the downstream phosphatidylinositol 3 kinase-signaling pathway through which many of the tyrosine kinases transmit their signaling.

Answer 1.32.   **The answer is C.**

Receptor tyrosine kinases generally consist of an extracellular binding domain, a transmembrane domain, and an intracellular kinase domain. These receptors bind ligands that are usually peptides or proteins. Most are monomeric with the exception of the insulin-receptor family, which consists of heterodimers covalently bound by disulfide bonds. Six major classes exist. Activation of the receptor generally requires phosphorylation of a tyrosine on the receptor, but the insulin binding to the insulin receptor is an exception to this rule and activation is generated by an insulin-induced conformational change. Outside of this, most receptor tyrosine kinases are activated by oligomerization, which brings intracellular kinase domains into proximity to allow cross-phosphorylation. Ligands generally stimulate oligomerization. Although receptor classes have been defined by particular ligands, it is accepted that particular receptor classes may bind more than one class of ligand. A particular ligand may have different conformational changes in the same receptor, leading to distinct downstream signal pathway activation.

Answer 1.33.   **The answer is B.**

Receptor phosphotyrosine phosphatases (RPTPs) are similar in structure to receptor tyrosine kinases in that they consist of an extracellular domain, a single transmembrane domain, and an intracellular catalytic domain (generally two domains). Although no true ligands for RPTPs have been described, some RPTPs contain structural repeats that suggest adhesion molecule recognition. Although RPTPs act as phosphatases, they do not always function in opposition to tyrosine kinases. Particular phosphorylation events can be inhibitory to tyrosine kinases, and activation of phosphatase activity could then increase tyrosine kinase global activity.

Answer 1.34.   **The answer is D.**

Protein kinase activity is essential to many signal pathways in the cell. Although many kinases consist of the same general structure, substrate specificity plays a key role in propagate signals via different pathways. Substrate specificity relies on the combination of the protein kinase motif that binds substrates and the substrate structural motifs. In addition to this, colocalization of substrate with kinase determines which pathways are activated, and this is achieved via recruitment to the same membrane or organelle or via protein–protein interactions. Although MAP kinase substrates must contain a proline following a serine or threonine, it is not required for all kinase substrates.

Answer 1.35.   **The answer is B.**

GTP-binding proteins are well-studied mediators of signal transduction. They are organized into two main classes: (a) heterotrimeric and (b) Ras-like. These proteins act like switches and undergo conformational changes in response to the state of GTP or GDP binding. Binding of GTP induces a conformational switch that leads to increased activity. Hydrolysis of GTP to GDP leads to inactivation. All such proteins are lipid-modified, which allows membrane association that is important to its downstream pathway activation. Heterotrimeric GTP-binding proteins are divided into classes based on function; two of the classes are Gas and Gai, which stimulate and inhibit adenylate cyclase, respectively.

Answer 1.36.   **The answer is D.**

Second messengers differ from first messengers in that second messengers are generated within a cell. These are generally small molecules that exert their effect via noncovalent binding to various targets. Examples include cAMP, IP3, DAG, and eicosanoids, among others. Many such molecules induce conformational changes in the target proteins. Ras is a GTP-binding protein that plays an important role in cell growth and transcription.

Answer 1.37.   **The answer is D.**

Myriads of cellular functions are dependent on protein–protein interactions and the concentration levels of those proteins. A single stimulus received by a cell can affect the transcription levels of hundreds of genes. Regulation of histone deacetylases, histone acetylases, nuclear receptors, and phosphorylation levels all play a role. Translation of protein from mRNA can be affected by ribosomal processing. Ubiquitination results in proteasome degradation of proteins. Lysosomes contribute to protein degradation, often after receptors are endocytosed.

Answer 1.38.   **The answer is B.**

Colocalization of proteins plays an important role in signal transduction and cell signaling pathways. Ras is a GTP-binding protein that requires the addition of a lipid moiety (generally a farnesyl group) to localize it to the membrane. There, it interacts with and activates Raf, which then interacts with and interacts with MEK. Increased cell proliferation is one of the effects of signaling via this pathway, so a lack of the lipid moiety could lead to decreased cell proliferation because it is not in close proximity to the membrane and Raf. Colocalization is an important phenomenon in cell signaling and can also be achieved via protein–protein interactions (i.e., nuclear transport) and membrane localization lipid rafts.

Molecular Biology of Cancer ■ Part 2

Directions   Each of the numbered items below is followed by lettered answers. Select the ONE lettered answer that is BEST in each case unless instructed otherwise.

QUESTIONS

Question 2.1.   **The correct order of mitosis is:**

A. Prometaphase, Metaphase, Anaphase, Telophase, Prophase
B. Prometaphase, Metaphase, Prophase, Anaphase, Telophase
C. Prophase, Prometaphase, Metaphase, Anaphase, Telophase
D. Telophase, Anaphase, Prophase, Metaphase, Prometaphase

Question 2.2.   **The cyclin responsible for progressing the cell into and through mitosis is:**

A. Cyclin A
B. Cyclin B
C. Cyclin D
D. Cyclin E

Question 2.3.   **Which of the following is NOT a means of regulating cyclin-dependent kinases?**

A. Positive regulatory acetylation
B. Negative regulatory phosphorylation
C. Cdk inhibitors
D. Cyclin availability

Question 2.4.   **Which of the following is necessary for the G1/S-phase transition?**

A. Cyclin B-CDK1 complex accumulation
B. Cyclins E and A accumulation
C. Dephosphorylation of T14 and Y15
D. CDK1 activation along with binding of CDC20 to anaphase promoting complex/cyclosome (APC/C)

Corresponding Chapters in *Cancer: Principles & Practice of Oncology*, Eighth Edition: 6 (Cell Cycle), 7 (Programmed Cell Death), 8 (Angiogenesis), 9 (Invasion and Metastasis), and 10 (Cancer Stem Cells).

Question 2.5.   **Which of the following has no role in cell-cycle exit?**

A. Downregulation of CDKs and cyclins
B. Accumulation of INK4, Cip/Kip, and pRb proteins
C. Reduction of protein synthesis
D. Activation of APC/C

Question 2.6.   **A cellular signal that is NOT antimitogenic is:**

A. Interleukin (IL)-2
B. Transforming growth factor (TGF)-β
C. Interferon (IFN)-α
D. p15

Question 2.7.   **A point at which cell-cycle progression is NOT blocked is the:**

A. G1 DNA damage checkpoint
B. Pre-G1 phase DNA damage checkpoint
C. Intra-S phase DNA damage checkpoint
D. G2 DNA damage checkpoint

Question 2.8.   **DNA damage activates and stabilizes:**

A. p53
B. pRb
C. CDK4 and CDK6
D. APC/C

Question 2.9.   **Replicative senescence is initiated by means of:**

A. Downregulation of cyclins
B. p53 activation
C. Progressive telomere shortening
D. Upregulation of interferons

Question 2.10.   **Genes that encode negative regulators of growth and proliferation are:**

A. Protooncogenes
B. Oncogenes
C. S-phase genes
D. Tumor suppressor genes

Question 2.11.   **A syndrome in which the gene encoding p53 is mutated leading to early onset of cancer and multiple malignancies is:**

A. Nijmegen disease
B. Von Hippel-Landau (VHL) syndrome
C. Familial Malignant Melanoma syndrome
D. Li-Fraumeni syndrome

Question 2.12.   **Type I cell death is also known as:**

A.   Autophagy
B.   Apoptosis
C.   Necrosis
D.   Autolysis

Question 2.13.   **Apoptosis is not mediated through:**

A.   Bax/Bak
B.   BH3-only proteins
C.   Bcl-2
D.   SMAC/Diablo

Question 2.14.   **Taxanes specifically target this BH3-only Bcl-2 protein:**

A.   Nbk/Bik
B.   Bim
C.   Puma
D.   Bad

Question 2.15.   **RAF is inhibited by which of these therapeutic agents that induce apoptosis?**

A.   Sorafenib
B.   Imatinib mesylate
C.   Bortezomib
D.   Taxanes

Question 2.16.   **Bcl-2 small molecule inhibitors like ABT-737 induce apoptosis by:**

A.   Binding to the BH3 binding pocket
B.   Inhibiting tyrosine kinase activity of Bcr/Abl restoring Bim function
C.   Stimulating Bim expression
D.   Blocking proteosome degradation of Bim

Question 2.17.   **Angiogenesis inhibitors theoretically induce apoptosis by which means?**

A.   Tyrosine kinase inhibition
B.   Histone deacetylase inhibition
C.   Inhibition of antiapoptotic proteins
D.   Nutrient deprivation

Question 2.18.   **Type II programmed cell death, autophagy, is regulated by:**

A.   mTOR in the PI3-kinase/AKT pathway
B.   Bax/Bak
C.   BH3-only proteins
D.   APC/C

Question 2.19.   **Autophagy does not have a role in:**

A. Recycling of normal cellular components
B. Protection against aging
C. Cell lysis caused by surrounding inflammation
D. Innate immunity by protecting against intracellular pathogens

Question 2.20.   **Which of the following is NOT a feature of necrosis?**

A. Rapid cellular swelling
B. Lysosome activation
C. Loss of plasma membrane integrity
D. Release of intracellular components to the extracellular compartment

Question 2.21.   **The Warburg effect describes:**

A. Exponential cell growth in response to an exogenous stimulant.
B. Inefficient energy production by most cancer cells, resulting in rapid adenosine triphosphate (ATP) depletion and necrotic cell death.
C. Initiation of neoplasia requires two somatic mutations for initiation of sporadic neoplasms, and hereditary neoplasms require a genetic plus a somatic mutation.
D. Sculpting of normal human tissues as a result of cell death.

Question 2.22.   **Unless tumor cells grow an adequate blood vessel supply, they will NOT grow greater than:**

A. <1 mm^3
B. 1–2 mm^3
C. Approximately 5 mm^3
D. 1 cm^3

Question 2.23.   **Bevacizumab is:**

A. A monoclonal antibody to basic fibroblast growth factor (bFGF)
B. A monoclonal antibody to vascular endothelial growth factor (VEGF)
C. A monoclonal antibody to phospholipid lipid growth factor (PLGF)
D. A monoclonal antibody to epidermal growth factor receptor (EGFR)

Question 2.24.   **The first step in tumor angiogenesis is:**

A. A localized degradation of the surrounding basement membrane of a parental venule
B. Paracrine signaling causing increased leakiness of a parental venule's basement membrane
C. An inflammatory response causing recruitment and activation of leukocytes that mediate angiogenesis
D. Release of endothelial cell progenitors from the bone marrow

Question 2.25.   **Which of the following is NOT a function of pericytes?**

A. Paracrine signaling
B. Regulation of vessel diameter
C. Mediation of resistance to antiangiogenic therapy
D. All of the above

Question 2.26.   **Which of the following is NOT a characteristic of tumor vasculature?**

A. Increased dilation
B. Increased tortuosity
C. Increased red blood cell (RBC) flow
D. Decreased support

Question 2.27.   **Which of the following is NOT considered a primary angiogenic factor?**

A. Granulocyte-colony stimulating factor
B. VEGF
C. Angiopoietins
D. Notch-signaling receptors

Question 2.28.   **Which of the following is NOT a function of VEGF?**

A. Stimulate endothelial cell division
B. Upregulate various inhibitors of apoptosis
C. Mobilize endothelial cell progenitors
D. Create focal areas of breakdown in parental venule basement membranes

Question 2.29.   **VEGF is inducible by many factors, of which the most important may be:**

A. H1F1α
B. TSP-1
C. pVHL
D. p53

Question 2.30.   **Which of the following is NOT thought to inhibit tumor angiogenesis?**

A. TSP-1
B. IL-6, IL-8
C. DLL4
D. Vasohibin

Question 2.31.   **Metronomic low-dose chemotherapy describes:**

A. Continuous low-dose treatment with chemotherapeutics
B. Pulse dosing with low doses of chemotherapeutics
C. Continuous low-dose treatment with intermittent pulse dosings of chemotherapeutics
D. Treatment of refractory tumors with continuous low doses of chemotherapeutics in conjunction with metronidazole

Question 2.32.   **Which of the following is NOT thought to be a mechanism of antiangiogenic treatment resistance?**

A. Decreased penetration of antiangiogenic molecules into tumor cells
B. Selection of hypoxia resistant cells
C. Vascular remodeling
D. Proangiogenic growth factor redundancy

Question 2.33.   **Which of the following is NOT an associated potential toxicity of antiangiogenic therapy?**

A. Hypertension
B. Aplastic anemia
C. Bowel perforation
D. Arteriothrombotic event

Question 2.34.   **Which of the following is NOT associated with a risk of metastasis?**

A. Tumor grade
B. Depth of invasion beyond normal cellular compartments
C. Lymphovascular invasion
D. Proper immune function

Question 2.35.   **What percentage of tumor cells can give rise to metastases?**

A. <0.01%
B. 1%
C. 20%
D. >80%

Question 2.36.   **Genes that can mediate tumorigenic functions and secondarily serve metastatic-specific functions either in a general way or with particular organ selectivity are best known as:**

A. Tumorigenic genes
B. Metastasis progression genes
C. Metastasis virulence genes
D. Protooncogenes

Question 2.37.   **Cells that mediate the breakdown of the basement membrane allowing for tumor invasion are known as:**

A. Carcinoma-associated fibroblasts
B. Pericyte-derived fibroblast
C. Tumor-associated macrophages
D. Dendritic cells

Question 2.38.   **Cellular loss of this molecule leads to decreased cellular attachment and enhanced tumor invasion/motility:**

A. E-cadherin
B. β-catenin
C. α-tubulin
D. Ankrin

Question 2.39. **Which of the following is NOT a selective pressure experienced by circulating tumor cells (CTCs)?**

A. Shear stress
B. Nitric oxide
C. DARC
D. Nutrient deprivation

Question 2.40. **Which of the following molecules does NOT assist in the extravasation of CTCs?**

A. Ezrin
B. VEGF
C. $\alpha v \beta 3$ integrin
D. CXCR4

Question 2.41. **Osteoblastic bone metastases are characteristic of which type of cancer?**

A. Breast
B. Prostate
C. Lung
D. Renal cell

Question 2.42. **Which of the following does NOT typically metastasize to the liver?**

A. Colon cancer
B. Breast cancer
C. Prostate cancer
D. Melanoma

Question 2.43. **The stochastic model of tumor heterogeneity is best described as:**

A. Every cell has equal potential to initiate and sustain tumor growth, but most cells do not proliferate extensively because of the low cumulative probability of permissive events.
B. Cancer stem cells (CSCs) are biologically distinct from the bulk cell population, which does not possess tumor-initiating activity.
C. Tumors are heterogeneous secondary to random, acquired mutations.
D. Tumors are pressured into heterogeneity by variable pressures applied to the tumor.

Question 2.44. **The hierarchy model of tumor heterogeneity is best described as:**

A. Every cell has equal potential to initiate and sustain tumor growth, but most cells do not proliferate extensively because of the low cumulative probability of permissive events.
B. CSCs are biologically distinct from the bulk cell population, which does not possess tumor-initiating activity.
C. Tumors are heterogenous secondary to random, acquired mutations.
D. Tumors are pressured into heterogeneity by variable pressures applied to the tumor.

ANSWERS

Answer 2.1.   **The answer is C.**

Mitosis is divided into prophase, prometaphase, metaphase, anaphase, and telophase. Most of the internal membranous components of the cell are dissembled and dispersed in prophase. Prometaphase prepares the cell for metaphase by forming bivalent attachments to the spindle driving them to the cellular equator. Paired chromatids align along the spindle during metaphase, followed by anaphase where sister chromatids pull to opposite poles. During telophase, prophase is reversed. Mitosis is completed by daughter cells separating during cytokinesis.

Answer 2.2.   **The answer is B.**

Cyclins are the required positive regulatory subunits of cyclin-dependent kinases (CDKs). B-type cyclins, along with CDK1, are responsible for getting cells into and through mitosis. Cyclin B1 accumulates during S and G2 phase and then is degraded at the metaphase-anaphase transition.

Answer 2.3.   **The answer is A.**

After phosphorylation of the T loop, there is an increase in CDK-cyclin contacts and changes in the binding site. Proteins from the INK4 (p15, p16, p18, and p19), Cip/Kip (p21$^{\text{Cip1}}$, p27$^{\text{Kip1}}$, and p57$^{\text{Kip2}}$), and Rb (p107 and p130) families all act as inhibitors of CDKs. Function of CDKs is dependent on cellular availability of cyclins for them to have enzymatic activity. Last, nuclear import/export regulation further regulates the activity of CDKs.

Answer 2.4.   **The answer is B.**

Accumulation of cyclins E and A via transcriptional induction and interaction with CDK2 allows for entry into S phase from G1 and is regulated by proteins from the Cip/Kip family. Cyclin B-CDK1 similarly accumulates allowing for the transition into M phase from G2. Entry into M phase is signaled by the dephosphorylation of T15 and Y15 resulting in the activation of CDK1. Activation of CDK1 and binding of CDC20 to APC/C is the trigger for which sister chromatids separate and move to opposite poles during anaphase.

Answer 2.5.   **The answer is D.**

Positive cell-cycle machinery is dismantled after the reduction of CDKs and cyclins. Cell-cycle exit is also usually associated with a transient increase in the number of CDK inhibitors, such as those from the INK4, Cip/Kip, and Rb protein families. Cells in quiescence also have a reduced rate of protein synthesis. Protein synthesis is largely dependent on growth factors and mitogens activating the cell through the mitogen-activated protein kinase/extracellular signaling-regulated kinase pathway and the phosphoinositide 3 (PI3) kinase/AKT pathway.

Answer 2.6.   **The answer is A.**

TGF-β is a cytokine that binds to a class of transcription factors known as SMADs that translocate to the nucleus, where they complex with DNA-binding transcription factors and coactivators to transactivate specific genes. Interferons are another class of cytokines that have antiproliferative effects by means of upregulation of CDK inhibitors and downregulation of cyclins. INK family proteins are CDK inhibitors of which p15 specifically inhibits CDK4 and CDK6 directly and cyclin E-CDK2 and cyclin A-CDK2 indirectly.

Answer 2.7.   **The answer is B.**

Cell-cycle progression is blocked at three points: before S-phase entry (the G1-DNA damage checkpoint), during S phase (the intra-S phase-DNA damage checkpoint), and before M-phase entry (the G2-DNA damage checkpoint).

Answer 2.8.   **The answer is A.**

p53 is activated and stabilized by DNA damage. p53 primarily affects p21,GADD45, and transcriptional repression of the genes encoding cyclin B1 and CDK1. The net effect of increased activation of p53 is cell cycle arrest at G1, S, or G2 phases of the cell cycle

Answer 2.9.   **The answer is C.**

Secondary to the topology of telomeres and the requirements of DNA replication, each cell cycle causes progressive shortening of the telomeres. In most, if not all, somatic cells, when sufficient telomere attrition has been reached, cells enter into a chronic checkpoint response, which is the molecular basis of senescence. Germ-line cells forego this checkpoint by means of a special replicase, telomerase. For a somatic cell to undergo malignant transformation, the senescence barrier must be overcome allowing for unlimited proliferative capacity.

Answer 2.10.   **The answer is D.**

Tumor suppressor genes usually encode negative regulators of growth and proliferation, thereby conferring protection to cells against malignancy. Protooncogenes encode genes in which mutations may cause gain of function or an enhanced level of function leading to malignancy. Mutations of both tumor suppressor genes and protooncogenes may lead to uncontrolled proliferation and malignancy.

Answer 2.11.   **The answer is D.**

Li-Fraumeni syndrome is caused by an inherited mutation in TP53, the gene encoding the checkpoint effector p53. This disease is characterized by early onset of cancer and multiple malignancies. Nijmegen disease is caused by mutation of the gene encoding Nbs1, which is required for the activation of chk1 and chk2 kinases. VHL is caused by a mutation in the pVHL tumor suppressor gene causing development of sporadic hemangioblastomas and clear-cell renal carcinomas. Familial malignant melanoma syndrome is caused by mutation in CDKN4A, the gene encoding p16.

Answer 2.12.   **The answer is B.**

Apoptosis is a genetically programmed means of rapid and efficient killing of unnecessary or damaged cells. It is characterized by cell shrinkage, blebbing of the plasma membrane, chromatin condensation, and intranucleosomal DNA fragmentation without being followed by surrounding inflammation.

Answer 2.13.   **The answer is C.**

Bcl-2 is a protein resulting from the translocation t(14;18):(q32;q21), which is common in human follicular lymphoma. Bcl-2 localizes to the mitochondria, where it promotes cell survival and inhibits apoptosis, by different mechanisms such as oncogene activation (c-myc, E1A), activation of tumor suppressor genes (p53), growth factor and cytokine limitation, and cellular damage.

Answer 2.14.   **The answer is B.**

Taxanes specifically induce apoptosis by stimulating Bim expression. Nbk/Bik stimulates apoptosis by inhibiting protein synthesis. Puma and Noxa mediate apoptosis by p53 activation. After growth factor withdrawal, Bad stimulates apoptosis.

Answer 2.15.   **The answer is A.**

Sorafenib directly inhibits RAF, thereby causing MAP kinase inhibition and restoring apoptotic function. Imatinib mesylate, by means of blocking the constitutively active tyrosine kinase activity of the Bcr/Abl fusion gene, restores Bim and Bad apoptotic function. Bortezomib is a proteosome inhibitor that blocks Bim degradation, knowing it to induce apoptosis. Taxanes induce apoptosis by stimulating Bim expression.

Answer 2.16.   **The answer is A.**

Bcl-2 inhibitors like ABT-737 binds to the BH3 binding pocket of Bcl-2, Bcl-xL, and Bcl-w, thereby blocking the antiapoptotic effect of Bcl-2. ABT-737 exhibits some activity against some human lymphomas and small cell lung cancers in vitro. Inhibition of the tyrosine kinase activity of Bcr/Abl is accomplished through imatinib mesylate. Taxanes stimulate Bim expression, restoring apoptosis. Bortezomib blocks the proteosomal degradation of Bim.

Answer 2.17.   **The answer is D.**

Tumor cells generally have a reduced metabolic capacity that is frequently coupled with high-energy demand sustaining rapid cell growth. One means for specifically targeting tumor cells is through therapeutic nutrient deprivation. This is the basis for the use of angiogenesis inhibitors.

Answer 2.18.   **The answer is A.**

Autophagy is regulated by mTOR in the PI3-kinase/AKT pathway that functions to link nutrient availability to cellular metabolism. Defective autophagy has been implicated in carcinogenesis in certain human breast, ovarian, and prostate tumors. Type I programmed cell death, apoptosis, is regulated by Bax/Bak and BH3-only proteins. APC/C is the anaphase promoting complex/cyclosome that regulates sister chromatid separation in mitosis.

Answer 2.19.   **The answer is C.**

Autophagy is involved in recycling normal cellular constituents, damaged protein/organelle removal, innate immunity by removal of cells infected by intracellular pathogens, acquired immunity by promoting T-cell survival/proliferation, and protection against aging. Cell lysis secondary to surrounding inflammation or insult is a feature of necrosis.

Answer 2.20.   **The answer is B.**

Lysosome activation is a feature of apoptosis, as is cell shrinkage, blebbing of the plasma membrane, chromatin condensation, and intranucleosomal DNA fragmentation without being followed by surrounding inflammation. Necrosis is characterized by rapid swelling of the cell, loss of plasma membrane integrity, and release of intracellular components into the extracellular compartment resulting in an acute inflammatory response.

Answer 2.21.   **The answer is B.**

The Warburg effect describes an observation where most cancer cells produce energy by anerobic glycolycis even when oxygen is plentiful. This is an inefficient way of producing energy. Generating less ATPs per mode of glucose metabolized explaining the high glucose requirement by tumors.

Answer 2.22.   **The answer is B.**

For tumor cells to support their vast metabolic demands, they must induce and sustain a supply of new blood vessels through the process of angiogenesis. This is the basis of antiangiogenic therapy as a means of cancer treatment.

Answer 2.23.   **The answer is B.**

Bevacizumab is the first successful antiangiogenic agent that has shown activity in randomized phase III trials. It is a monoclonal antibody to VEGF. It has been shown to be effective in combination with chemotherapy for the treatment of metastatic colorectal cancer, breast cancer, renal cell carcinoma, and non–small cell lung cancer.

Answer 2.24.   **The answer is A.**

Tumor angiogenesis is first mediated by several proteolytic enzymes, such as matrix metalloproteinases and urokinase plasminogen activator, causing a focal degradation of a venule's basement membrane. This is likely a consequence of various proangiogenic growth factors secreted by the tumor cell population or reactive stromal cells.

Answer 2.25.   **The answer is D.**

The single layer of periendothelial smooth muscle cells is formed by pericytes. These cells modulate endothelial cell function and are critical for the development of a mature vessel network. In addition to regulation of vessel diameter and permeability, they provide mechanical support and survival of endothelial cells through paracrine signaling. Because of their ability to maintain endothelial cell survival, they have become an important target for antiangiogenic therapy and it is hypothesized that they may mediate resistance to this therapy.

Answer 2.26.   **The answer is C.**

The vasculature of solid tumors has several notable abnormalities. These vessels are classically much dilated with little to no basement membrane and have excessive tortuosity. A decreased number of pericytes portrays a relative lack of support and excessive vascular leakiness. These features contribute to the highly heterogeneous and often sluggish flow through solid tumors and create areas of relative nutrient deprivation and hypoxia. The increased leak from these vessels also allows for extravasation of high-molecular-weight plasma proteins, leading to areas of elevated interstitial fluid pressures.

Answer 2.27.   **The answer is D.**

VEGF promotes tumor angiogenesis is various ways, including stimulation of endothelial cell (EC) division, inducing EC locomotion/migration, enhancing EC survival by upregulating various inhibitors of apoptosis, and mobilizing endothelial progenitor cells from the bone marrow to sites of angiogenesis. Further, VEGF is approximately 50,000 times more potent than histamine in increasing vascular permeability. VEGF is expressed in most if not all of human cancers, and increased levels carry a poor prognosis.

Answer 2.28.   **The answer is D.**

There are at least four proposed mechanisms of how VEGF may promote tumor angiogenesis. VEGF can stimulate EC division, induce EC locomotion/migration, and enhance EC survival by upregulating different inhibitors of apoptosis and mobilizing endothelial progenitor cells from the bone marrow to sites of angiogenesis. The necessary breakdown of the basement membrane of a parental venule is most likely mediated by proangiogenic growth factors secreted by the tumor cells themselves.

Answer 2.29.   **The answer is A.**

H1F1α is upregulated by hypoxia. H1F1α then, in turn, activates numerous other genes, of which VEGF may be the most important.

Answer 2.30.   **The answer is B.**

IL-6/8 is thought to be secondarily angiogenic. TSP-1, DLL4, and vasohibin are all shown to inhibit angiogenesis. Embryologic studies have shown that notch/DLL4 is important in early angiogenesis; however, in the adult, it has been shown to be an inhibitor of tumor angiogenesis.

Answer 2.31.   **The answer is A.**

The effectiveness of antiangiogenic therapy is profoundly reversed during episodes of drug-free breaks. This is thought to be mediated by the rapid mobilization and homing of endothelial cells to the drug-treated tumors. This has led to the concept of metronomic low-dose chemotherapy. By reducing or eliminating altogether drug-free periods with continuous low-dose chemotherapy, the rapid reversal of antiangiogenic therapy may be prevented.

Answer 2.32.   **The answer is A.**

There are four currently proposed mechanisms by which tumors overcome antiangiogenic therapy. Tumors possess proangiogenic growth factor redundancy, so targeting one pathway of angiogenesis may not completely eliminate the ability of tumors to produce new vasculature. Decreasing the ability of the tumor to develop new vessels may also select for mutant/variant tumor subpopulations that are more resistant to hypoxia. Further, antiangiogenic therapy targets newly forming blood vessels. Tumors may exploit existing organ vasculature to obtain necessary oxygen and nutrients. Lastly, targeting newly forming blood vessels may accelerate the maturation and remodeling of blood vessels already existing blood vessels. This may produce a more stable vascularity in tumors.

Answer 2.33.   **The answer is B.**

Antiangiogenic therapy is not without side effects. Anti-VEGF therapy has been shown to lead to specific toxicities, such as hypertension, proteinuria, bowel perforation, hemorrhage, arteriothrombotic events, and others. Among these, aplastic anemia has not been documented.

Answer 2.34.   **The answer is D.**

Tumor grade, depth of invasion, and lymphovascular invasion all carry a higher risk of metastasis. Proper immune function would hinder the development of metastasis because circulating tumor cells would be targeted for destruction.

Answer 2.35. **The answer is B.**

By using radioactive nucleotides incorporated into tumor DNA, it has been shown that less than 0.01% of tumor cells can give rise to metastases.

Answer 2.36. **The answer is B.**

Metastasis progression genes promote tumor metastases among other functions. Tumorigenic genes are genes that promote primary tumor growth. Metastasis virulence genes confer protection to tumor cells in the distant environment but confer no protection to the primary tumor.

Answer 2.37. **The answer is C.**

Tumor-associated macrophages (TAMs) can comprise a large percentage of the bulk of a tumor mass. Through secretion of FGF, EGF receptor ligands, and PDGF, they can stimulate tumor cell growth and motility. Furthermore, by producing uPA, MMP7, and MMP9, TAMs help degrade basement membrane allowing tumor cells to invade and metastasize.

Answer 2.38. **The answer is A.**

Invasion starts with loss of cellular adhesion. This is largely mediated by loss of E-cadherin, the prototypic protein of the cadherin family. Cadherins are transmembrane glycoproteins that mediate cellular attachment. They anchor the cell through attachments to the actin cytoskeleton via another family of proteins called the catenins.

Answer 2.39. **The answer is D.**

CTCs experience multiple stressors in the circulation, leading to a short half-life. Of these, physical stressors such as shear forces or mechanical injury may limit CTC life span. Also, endothelial cell-mediated stressors such as nitric oxide may induce apoptosis in circulating tumor cells. DARC, a Duffy blood group glycoprotein, interacts with KAI1 expressed on circulating tumor cells causing them to undergo senescence.

Answer 2.40. **The answer is C.**

Ezrin links the cell membrane to the actin cytoskeleton and has been found to assist in extravasation of CTCs via activation of the MAPK pathway. VEGF has been shown to assist in CTC extravasation by causing disruptions in endothelial cell junctions and increased vascular permeability. CTC expression of CXCR4 interacts with CXCL12 expressed on certain organs, such as lung, liver, bone, and lymph nodes, allows for selective extravasation.

Answer 2.41. **The answer is B.**

Breast, lung, and kidney cancer typically cause osteolytic lesions on metastasizing to bone. Unlike these lesions, prostate cancer causes osteoblastic lesions on metastases to bone. In contrast with osteolytic metastasis, osteoblastic lesions results from the preferential stimulation of osteoblasts or the inhibition of osteoclasts. This is mediated through many different molecules, including bone morphogenetic proteins such as WNT, TGF-β, IGF, PDGF, FGF, and VEGF.

Answer 2.42.   **The answer is C.**

Because of the microenvironment the liver provides and the dual blood supply (from the portal vein and hepatic artery), the liver is a common site of metastasis. Colon cancer generally seeds the liver via the portal system, whereas breast, lung, and melanoma approach the liver via the systemic circulation through the hepatic artery.

Answer 2.43.   **The answer is A.**

In the stochastic model of tumor heterogeneity, every cell within the tumor has equal potential but low probability of initiating tumor growth.

Answer 2.44.   **The answer is B.**

The hierarchy model of tumor heterogeneity hypothesizes the existence of functionally distinct classes of cells within the tumor, and only those with unique self-renewal ability produce new tumor growth.

Etiology of Cancer ■ Part 1

Directions   Each of the numbered items below is followed by lettered answers. Select the ONE lettered answer that is BEST in each case unless instructed otherwise.

QUESTIONS

Question 3.1.   **All the following are true regarding cigarette smoking and cancer, EXCEPT:**

A.   Duration of smoking is the strongest determinant of lung cancer.
B.   Smoking increases the risk of squamous cell carcinoma, large cell carcinoma, and small cell carcinoma of the lung but not of adenocarcinoma of the lung.
C.   Cigarette smoking is a cause of liver cancer.
D.   Cigarette smoking is causally related to myeloid leukemia.

Question 3.2.   **The role of specific tobacco product carcinogens in specific tumors is characterized by the following, EXCEPT:**

A.   Polycyclic aromatic hydrocarbons (PAHs) are major causative factors in lung cancer.
B.   Aromatic amines are a major cause of bladder cancer.
C.   N-nitrosamines are important causative factors in esophageal cancer.
D.   Nicotine is an important carcinogen in the causation of laryngeal cancer.

Question 3.3.   **The following enzymes are involved in metabolic activation of the carcinogens in cigarette smoke:**

A.   P450 enzyme 1A1 and 1A2
B.   Glutathione-S-transferases and uridine diphosphate (UDP)-glucuronosyl transferases
C.   Nucleotide excision repair enzymes
D.   None of the above

Corresponding Chapters in *Cancer: Principles & Practice of Oncology*, Eighth Edition: 11 (Etiology of Cancer: Tobacco), 12 (Etiology of Cancer: Cancer Susceptibility Syndromes), 13 (Etiology of Cancer: Viruses), and 14 (Etiology of Cancer: Inflammation).

Question 3.4.   **Mechanisms of tumor induction by carcinogens in tobacco products include the following, EXCEPT:**

A. Bonds form between carcinogens and DNA, resulting in DNA adducts.
B. Nicotine and nitrosamines bind to cellular receptors, resulting in activation of the pathways that enhance growth and suppress apoptosis.
C. Enzymatic methylation of gene promoters, resulting in gene silencing.
D. Inhibition of DNA repair enzymes.

Question 3.5.   **Tobacco carcinogen biomarkers are characterized by the following, EXCEPT:**

A. Can be used to assess carcinogenicity of tobacco products.
B. Are not considered as good as machine measurement of smoke components in assessing tobacco products.
C. Can assess the exposure of nonsmokers to secondhand smoke.
D. Have the potential to assess individual susceptibility to cigarette smoke.

Question 3.6.   **Knudson's hypothesis regarding cancer susceptibility:**

A. Postulates that predisposition to cancer arises as the result of a heterozygous germline mutation, which then requires a second acquired mutation in the unaffected allele for tumor to develop.
B. Was validated by observations in patients with neuroblastoma.
C. Postulates that different genes are involved in familial and sporadic forms of a tumor.
D. None of the above.

Question 3.7.   **All the following are true regarding genetic changes that are involved in cancer initiation, EXCEPT:**

A. Changes in genes regulating cell cycle can be involved in cancer initiation.
B. Changes in genes that maintain DNA integrity can be involved in cancer initiation.
C. Genetic mutations involved with cancer initiation only occur in the tissue of origin.
D. Changes in genes regulating cellular functions, such as angiogenesis, can be involved in cancer initiation.

Question 3.8.   **Current American Society of Clinical Oncology (ASCO) guidelines recommend testing for cancer susceptibility syndromes in the following, EXCEPT:**

A. The general population should be tested for the common cancer susceptibility syndromes.
B. In individuals suspected to have familial syndrome.
C. Genetic test can be adequately interpreted.
D. Genetic test results will aid management of individuals undergoing the test.

Question 3.9.   **Retinoblastoma protein, Rb1 is characterized by the following, EXCEPT:**

A. Involved in maintaining the integrity of the retina
B. A central regulator of cell cycle
C. Binds to E2F transcription proteins
D. A 105-kDa protein that undergoes phosphorylation during cell cycle

Question 3.10.   **Hereditary nonpolyposis colon cancer (HNPCC) syndrome is characterized by:**

A. Mutations in genes that regulate cellular proliferation
B. Autosomal recessive inheritance
C. Greater penetrance in women
D. Mutations in genes that are involved in DNA mismatch repair

Question 3.11.   **Hereditary nonpolyposis colon cancer syndrome is associated with all the following, EXCEPT:**

A. Increased risk of stomach, ovarian, and kidney cancers
B. Presence of multiple polyps preceding the diagnosis of colon cancer
C. Younger age at diagnosis than patients with sporadic colon cancers
D. Overall incidence of 1 in 400

Question 3.12.   **Impaired activity of BRCA 1 and BRCA 2 proteins affects:**

A. Repair of double-stranded DNA breaks
B. Cell-cycle regulation
C. Microtubule stabilization
D. Angiogenesis

Question 3.13.   **Individuals with germline mutations of BRCA 1:**

A. Typically develop ER+, PR+ breast cancers.
B. Have increased risk only for breast cancer.
C. Have increased risk for pancreatic cancer.
D. Prophylactic breast surgery in these individuals is not a recognized strategy to reduce breast cancer risk.

Question 3.14.   **Neurofibromatosis Type I (NF1):**

A. Is inherited in an autosomal recessive fashion.
B. Patients have increased risk for myeloid malignancies.
C. Results from mutations in NF1 that inhibit Akt.
D. Cafe au lait spots occur in 50% of patients.

Question 3.15.   **Familial adenomatous polyposis (FAP) syndrome is characterized by the following, EXCEPT:**

A. It results from mutations in the APC gene.
B. There is an almost 100% risk of developing colon cancer by age 40 years.
C. Increased risk of desmoid tumors.
D. Nonsteroidal anti-inflammatory drugs (NSAIDs) can be recommended in place of prophylactic colectomy to reduce the risk of colon cancer.

Question 3.16.   **p53 protein is characterized by the following, EXCEPT:**

A. It is a DNA-binding transcription factor.
B. Is activated in response to cellular stress.
C. Mutations of p53 are common in hereditary cancer syndromes but rare in sporadic cancers.
D. Germline mutations of p53 are the cause of Li-Fraumeni syndrome.

Question 3.17.   **Hereditary cancer syndromes more commonly:**

A. Result from gain of function mutations
B. Result from loss of function mutations
C. Result from abnormality of genes that promote angiogenesis
D. None of the above

Question 3.18.   **Von Hippel Lindau (VHL) gene:**

A. Encodes a ubiquitin ligase to target HIF 1a and HIF 2a for degradation
B. Enhances angiogenesis
C. Is mutated in renal cell cancers in patients with VHL syndrome but not in sporadic renal cell cancers
D. None of the above

Question 3.19.   **Alteration in PTEN gene and cancer susceptibility are characterized by the following, EXCEPT:**

A. Loss of one PTEN allele can lead to cancer, but loss of both alleles is anticancer.
B. Patients inherit a mutation in the PTEN gene and then require a second hit to the normal allele to develop cancer.
C. Variations in PTEN expression rather than complete loss may lead to carcinogenesis.
D. Pharmacologic manipulation toward complete loss of PTEN expression in cancer cells may help in cancer prevention and/or therapy.

Question 3.20.   **Retroviruses are:**

A. RNA viruses that have the capacity to synthesize double-stranded DNA from single-stranded viral RNA genome
B. DNA viruses that have the capacity to synthesize double-stranded RNA from single-stranded viral DNA genome
C. Dependent on host nucleotide synthesis enzymes to replicate the viral genome
D. Viruses that cause oncogenic transformation in humans only through a direct transforming effect

Question 3.21.   **Retroviruses participate in oncogenic transformation through the following mechanisms, EXCEPT:**

A. By causing insertional mutagenesis
B. By affecting the expression of cellular growth and differentiation genes
C. Acutely transforming viruses that insert an oncogene in the infected cells
D. By inducing an inflammatory response in the tissue

Question 3.22.   **Human T-cell lymphotropic virus type I (HTLV1) is a:**

A. Retrovirus that infects CD4 T cells
B. Retrovirus that causes significant viremia
C. Retrovirus associated with adult myeloid leukemia
D. Retrovirus that is transmitted by the fecal-oral route

Question 3.23.   **Pathogenesis of adult T-cell leukemia from HTLV1 infection is related to:**

A. Insertion of the viral genome at specific locations in the T-cell genome
B. Presence of host-derived oncogene in the viral genome
C. The viral protein Tax transactivating many cellular genes, particularly interleukin (IL)-2 and IL-2 receptor
D. HTLV1 infection increasing susceptibility of T cells to other transforming viruses

Question 3.24.   **HTLV2 is a retrovirus with the following characteristics, EXCEPT:**

A. It is closely related to HTLV 1.
B. HTLV2 can also cause adult T-cell leukemia like HTLV1.
C. It is transmitted by the same routes as HTLV1, such as sexual intercourse, contaminated blood, and breastfeeding.
D. Convincing data for an etiologic role for HTLV2 in human disease are lacking.

Question 3.25.   **Pathogenesis of increased risk of cancer in human immunodeficiency virus (HIV)-infected patients is characterized by the following:**

A. HIV infection leads to the insertion of the viral genome at critical locations of the cellular genome leading to chimeric proteins that are procarcinogenic.
B. HIV genome contains oncogenes that are transcribed in the infected cells causing cancers.
C. HIV infection causes immune deficiency in infected patients, which contributes to the development of cancer.
D. HIV reverse transcriptase activates many cellular oncogenes during viral replication.

Question 3.26.   **Acquired immune deficiency syndrome (AIDS)-related Kaposi's sarcoma (KS) is characterized by the following, EXCEPT:**

A.   Immune deficiency caused by HIV is involved in the pathogenesis of KS.
B.   HHV-8 infection in HIV-infected patients is the etiologic agent of KS.
C.   Tat protein secreted by the infected HIV cells increases the level of various cytokines and contributes to the pathogenesis of KS.
D.   Mutation induced by HIV in infected endothelial cells contributes to the pathogenesis of KS.

Question 3.27.   **Pathogenesis of lymphomas in patients with HIV is linked to all the following, EXCEPT:**

A.   Epstein-Barr virus (EBV) in patients with HIV
B.   Immune deficiency caused by HIV
C.   Lymphomas that arise in the HIV-infected CD4+ T cells
D.   HIV-induced cytokine dysregulation

Question 3.28.   **Hepatitis C virus (HCV) is:**

A.   An RNA virus that is transmitted by percutaneous routes
B.   A retrovirus that is transmitted by percutaneous route
C.   A DNA virus that is transmitted by the fecal-oral route
D.   None of the above

Question 3.29.   **HCV infection is characterized by all the following, EXCEPT:**

A.   Worldwide prevalence of 170 million cases.
B.   Sixty percent of those with chronic HCV infections develop chronic hepatitis.
C.   Twenty percent of those with chronic HCV infections develop cirrhosis.
D.   Twenty percent of those with chronic HCV infections develop hepatocellular carcinoma.

Question 3.30.   **Association between HCV and hepatocellular carcinoma (HCC) includes the following, EXCEPT:**

A.   Alcohol consumption or coinfection with hepatitis B virus (HBV) in a patient with HCV increases the risk of HCC.
B.   Treatment of patients with HCV with interferon and ribavirin eliminates the risk of HCC in these patients.
C.   There is a 20- to 30-year lag period between HCV infection and the development of HCC.
D.   Inflammatory changes resulting from HCV infection are primarily responsible for development of HCC in HCV-infected patients.

Question 3.31.   **HBV has the following characteristics, EXCEPT:**

A. DNA virus that belongs to the hepadnavirus family.
B. In 95% of individuals who become infected with HBV, the infection resolves with clearance of the virus.
C. Twenty-five percent of individuals infected with HBV develop hepatocellular carcinoma.
D. HBV-infected patients who develop chronic hepatitis are at an increased risk of developing hepatocellular carcinoma.

Question 3.32.   **Human papilloma virus (HPV) has been linked with the following cancers, EXCEPT:**

A. Cervical cancer
B. Penile cancer
C. Oropharyngeal cancers
D. Esophageal cancers

Question 3.33.   **Pathogenesis of cervical cancer from HPV infection is characterized by the following, EXCEPT:**

A. E6 and E7 viral proteins are most closely related to the transforming potential of HPV.
B. Every person infected with HPV eventually develops cancer.
C. Smoking is identified as a risk factor and can increase the risk of cervical cancer in HPV-infected patients.
D. Cell-cycle regulatory proteins p53 and RB (retinoblastoma protein) are important targets of HPV oncoproteins.

Question 3.34.   **The following type of HPV has a strong association with cervical cancer:**

A. HPV-6
B. HPV-11
C. HPV-16
D. None of the above

Question 3.35.   **The recently approved HPV vaccine:**

A. Is a quadrivalent vaccine containing virus-like particles (VLPs) from four different types of HPV
B. Protects all types of HPV-causing cervical cancer
C. Is recommended for all sexually active men and women
D. Eliminates the need for routine cervical cancer screening 2 years after completing the vaccination schedule

Question 3.36.   **The role of EBV in cancer is characterized by the following, EXCEPT:**

A. EBV nuclear proteins target transcription factor RBPJk/CBF1.
B. Membrane protein LMP1 activates IKK alpha and enhances cellular proliferation and survival.
C. Involvement in minority of the gastric cancers.
D. Involvement in all Hodgkin's lymphoma.

Question 3.37.   **The risk of KS in patients with HIV is highest:**

A. In homosexual men
B. In pediatric patients with AIDS
C. In heterosexual men
D. In patients with AIDS related to blood transfusions

Question 3.38.   **Human herpes virus 8 (HHV8) infection is characterized by:**

A. HHV8 sequences are detected only in tumors of patients with KS who are HIV positive.
B. Five to seven percent of the US general population is infected with HHV8.
C. In patients with HIV, coinfection with EBV infection is necessary for development of KS.
D. HHV8 infection is transmitted only through sexual contact.

Question 3.39.   **The role of polyomaviruses in human cancers is characterized by:**

A. A double-blind study has confirmed the correlation of SV40 with human cancers.
B. SV40 DNA or antigen has been observed in some human cancers, such as osteosarcomas, mesotheliomas, and brain tumors.
C. BK and JC viruses are recognized etiologic factors in human brain tumors.
D. Epidemiologic data have confirmed the association of SV40-contaminated polio vaccines with human cancers.

Question 3.40.   **Which of the following sentences best describes immune surveillance of tumors?**

A. Innate immunity has no effective role in immune surveillance of tumors.
B. A standard mechanism of immune surveillance is involved for all tumors.
C. Immune surveillance of tumors is based on expression of appropriate tumor antigens.
D. Both innate and adaptive immune cells, along with their effector molecules, are important in immune surveillance of tumors.

Question 3.41.   **All the following statements are true regarding immune surveillance of tumors, EXCEPT:**

A. The presence of tumor-infiltrating lymphocytes in tumors, such as colon and ovarian cancer, is associated with improved prognosis.
B. In patients with paraneoplastic neurologic syndromes, the autoimmune response also controls tumor progression.
C. Among the skin cancers, melanoma risk is increased the most in immune-suppressed individuals.
D. Acute infections with bacteria could induce regressions of cancers.

Question 3.42.   **Evidence that supports the association of inflammation and cancer include the following, EXCEPT:**

A. An ulcerative lesion resulting from chronic inflammation after skin thermal injury can undergo malignant transformation.
B. Inflammatory cells are frequently present in tumor stroma.
C. Changes induced by acute bronchitis can lead to lung cancer.
D. Risk of colon cancer is increased in patients with inflammatory bowel disease.

Question 3.43.   **Infectious agents can cause cancers by:**

A. Transformation of infected cells
B. Establishing a chronic inflammatory microenvironment in the infected tissues
C. None of the above
D. Both A and B

Question 3.44.   **All statements regarding tumor necrosis factor (TNF) and cancer are true, EXCEPT:**

A. TNF can induce apoptosis of tumor and endothelial cells.
B. TNF can induce production of matrix metalloproteinase (MMP)-9 and activation of nuclear factor (NF)-kB.
C. TNF can promote carcinogenesis.
D. None of the above.

Question 3.45.   **Which of the following is TRUE regarding cyclooxygenase (COX)-2 and cancer?**

A. COX-2 inhibitors can reduce the incidence of colon cancer only in individuals with familial adenomatous polyposis.
B. COX inhibitors not only reduce colon cancers but also decrease the number of colonic polyps.
C. COX-2 inhibitors can prevent only colon cancers associated with inflammatory conditions such as ulcerative colitis.
D. None of the above.

Question 3.46.   **Cancer-associated stromal fibroblasts (CAFs) are characterized by:**

A. Lack of expression of vimentin unlike other fibroblasts
B. Consistently demonstrate genetic alterations and have undergone transformation
C. Their ability to better support tumor progression than other fibroblasts
D. Their ability to inhibit tumor progression

Question 3.47.   **Dendritic cells (DCs) are characterized by the following, EXCEPT:**

A. DCs rapidly respond to alterations in tissue homeostasis.
B. DCs secrete proinflammatory cytokines, including IL-12 and TNF.
C. DCs present antigens in the context of major histocompatibility complex class I and II to T cells.
D. DCs are activated in tumors and contribute to immune surveillance of tumors.

Question 3.48.   **Tumor-associated macrophages (TAMs):**

A. Have no role in tumor growth or tumor destruction
B. Only promote angiogenesis and tumor progression
C. Have reduced antitumor effects in the presence of IL-10
D. Produce high levels of proinflammatory cytokines and therefore are only associated with tumor destruction

Question 3.49.   **Toll-like receptors (TLRs) are:**

A. A family of at least 12 different pattern recognition receptors.
B. TLRs, along with other pattern-recognizing receptors, are important in microbial sensing.
C. TLR triggering in tumor cells may result in tumor apoptosis, but activation of TLRs in tumor infiltrating cells results in tumor promotion.
D. All the above.

ANSWERS

Answer 3.1.   **The answer is B.**

Since the 1950s, the carcinogenic potential of cigarette smoking and other tobacco products has been recognized. The cancer most commonly associated with cigarette smoking is lung cancer. The strongest determinant of lung cancer in smokers is duration of smoking. Number of cigarettes smoked is also an important factor in determining the risk. Smoking increases the risk of all subtypes of non–small cell lung cancer, including adenocarcinoma and the risk of small cell lung cancer. Some of the other cancers associated with smoking are acute myeloid leukemia, bladder cancer, stomach cancer, and pancreatic cancer. Cigarette smoking is a cause of liver cancer independently of the effects of HBV and HVC infection and alcohol consumption.

Answer 3.2.   **The answer is D.**

Cigarette smoke consists of many carcinogens. Data from carcinogenicity studies, product analyses, and biochemical and molecular biological investigations support a significant role for certain carcinogens in specific types of tobacco-induced cancers. In this regard evidence suggests a significant role for PAH and N-nitrosamines as causative factors in lung cancer. Evidence also supports the role of aromatic amines as a cause of bladder cancer and a role for N-nitrosamines as a cause for esophageal cancer. Nicotine itself is not known to initiate cancer formation, but recent evidence suggests that nicotine through nicotinic receptors may promote cellular proliferation.

Answer 3.3.   **The answer is A.**

Many cigarette smoke carcinogens are not active and require metabolic activation to transform them into active carcinogens. Cytochrome P450 enzymes convert these compounds into electrophilic entities that can covalently bind to DNA-forming DNA adducts. P-450 enzymes 1A1 and 1A2 are particularly important in the metabolic activation of some of the carcinogens in cigarette smoke. Other P450 enzymes involved in this process include 1B1, 2A13, 2E1, and 3A4. 1A1 and 1B2 are induced by compounds in cigarette smoke, and the induction of these enzymes may be a critical aspect of cancer susceptibility in smokers. The cigarette smoke carcinogens can undergo detoxification by glutathione-S-transferases and UDP-glucuronosyl transferases. Therefore, cancer susceptibility may be determined by the balance achieved between activation of the carcinogens in cigarette smoke and their detoxification. In addition, polymorphisms in genes encoding these enzymes may influence an individual's risk of cancer from these carcinogens. Cellular repair systems can remove the DNA adducts formed by smoke carcinogens and repair the DNA, but they are not involved in metabolic activation of carcinogens in cigarette smoke. Nucleotide excision repair enzymes are a component of these repair systems.

Answer 3.4. **The answer is D.**

Formation of bonds between smoke carcinogens and DNA resulting in DNA adducts is an important aspect of the carcinogenicity of cigarette smoke. DNA adducts that are not removed result in miscoding during replication leading to mutations. Mutations have been frequently observed in the KRAS oncogene in lung cancer and in the TP53 tumor suppressor gene in a variety of cigarette smoke-induced cancers. Processes, other than formation of DNA adducts, that contribute to cancer formation are activation of cellular receptors by N-nitrosamines and nicotine and the silencing of certain genes through methylation of the gene promoters. Nucleotide excision repair enzymes are part of the cellular repair systems that remove DNA adducts and repair the DNA. There are no data to suggest that carcinogens in cigarette smoke inhibit these enzymes.

Answer 3.5. **The answer is B.**

Tobacco carcinogen biomarkers are specific quantifiable substances, usually adducts or metabolites, derived from particular carcinogens in tobacco. Examples include DNA adducts, protein adducts, saliva and blood metabolites, breath compounds, and urinary metabolites. Until now, tobacco products have been evaluated mainly by machine measurement of smoke components under standard conditions. But it is now recognized that machine measurements can be misleading with respect to the health effects of tobacco products, and tobacco carcinogen biomarkers may be superior in assessing tobacco products. These products can also assess the exposure of nonsmokers to secondhand smoke and assess an individual's susceptibility to cigarette smoke.

Answer 3.6. **The answer is A.**

More than 30 years ago, Alfred Knudson postulated that predisposition to cancer arises as the result of a heterozygous germline mutation, which then requires a second acquired mutation in the unaffected allele for tumor to develop, also called the "two-hit hypothesis." The hypothesis was validated in patients with retinoblastoma. These individuals inherit a mutated Rb gene and then acquire mutation in the normal allele of the gene leading to cancer. Further studies also revealed that the genes involved in carcinogenesis of the familial form of the cancer can also be involved in the sporadic forms of that cancer.

Answer 3.7.   **The answer is C.**

For cancer to initiate, the cancerous cell has to eventually acquire the ability to proliferate or abrogate apoptosis. It is recognized that two classes of tumor suppressors may cooperate in tumor formation: (a) those that control proliferation and survival through control of the cell cycle and (b) those that are involved in the control of genomic integrity. Loss of genes involved in maintaining genomic integrity may lead to mutations in genes that control proliferation or apoptosis. Apart from alterations in genes involved with cellular functions of proliferation and survival, changes in genes involved in other cellular functions such as angiogenesis may be the driving force for carcinogenesis. In addition, even though genetic changes in tissue of origin are generally the cause of cancer initiation, in some cases the genetic changes may occur in the stromal cells resulting in aberrant stromal-parenchymal interactions, leading to carcinogenesis.

Answer 3.8.   **The answer is A.**

The ASCO guidelines state that screening for cancer susceptibility syndromes is not warranted in the general population but is recommended for individuals with a suspected familial syndrome. In addition, the guidelines recommend that the testing should be done if the results can be easily interpreted and will influence the management of the individuals being tested.

Answer 3.9.   **The answer is A.**

Rb1 protein is a central regulator of the cell cycle. It is a 105-kDa protein that undergoes phosphorylation at specific points in the cell cycle. During the G0 and G1 phases of the cell cycle, hypophosphorylated Rb1 protein binds to E2F transcription factors. Cyclin D-CDK4 phosphorylates Rb1 protein when the cell cycle transitions to the S phase. Phosphorylated RB1 protein dissociates from the E2F transcription factors, which then allows these factors to recruit and activate other cell cycle genes.

Answer 3.10.   **The answer is D.**

HNPCC, originally known as Lynch syndrome, is the most common cancer susceptibility disease and is responsible for at least 2% to 3% of total colon cancer cases in the United States. HNPCC can be caused by a germline mutation in one of five genes: MLH1, MSH2, MSH6, PMS1, or PMS2. All five genes function in DNA mismatch repair, and so mutations in these genes affect genomic integrity. HNPCC is inherited in an autosomal dominant fashion with a penetrance of approximately 90%. Men are affected at a higher penetrance, with women being less affected but at an additional risk of endometrial cancer.

Answer 3.11.   **The answer is B.**

Patients with HNPCC exhibit elevated risks for stomach, ovary, small intestine, ureter, and kidney cancers. Patients typically present with colon cancer at a younger average age than patients with sporadic colon cancer. The overall incidence of this syndrome is 1 in 400. In contrast with other familial colon cancer syndromes, patients with HNPCC rarely exhibit polyps, making early detection difficult. Family members of patients with HNPCC should be screened annually by colonoscopy starting at approximately age 20 years. This has been demonstrated to reduce both the incidence and the resultant mortality of colon cancer in patients with HNPCC. Women are also recommended to undergo yearly pelvic examinations and ultrasound examination.

Answer 3.12.   **The answer is A.**

BRCA1 and BRCA2 proteins function in DNA damage repair. BRCA1 and BRCA2 proteins are recruited to the site of double-stranded DNA breaks along with other proteins. These complexes function to repair the double-stranded break, although the precise role of BRCA1 and BRCA2 in these complexes remains unclear. These proteins have no known role in cell-cycle regulation, microtubule stabilization, or angiogenesis.

Answer 3.13.   **The answer is C.**

Patients with germline mutation in BRCA1 have an increased risk of many cancers, including breast cancer, fallopian tube cancer, prostate cancer, and pancreatic cancer. Men with BRCA1 mutation also have an increased risk of breast cancer. Cancers arising in BRCA1 mutant patients are typically high-grade invasive ductal carcinomas, negative for ER, PR, and HER2/neu. Prophylactic breast surgery does reduce the risk of breast cancer but does not completely eliminate it.

Answer 3.14.   **The answer is B.**

NF1 is inherited in an autosomal dominant fashion with a 100% penetrance for neurofibromas. Mutations in the NF1 gene are responsible for the condition. NF1 encodes the neurofibromin protein, a GTPase activating protein (GAP) for the Ras family of proteins. Ras-GAPs stimulate the GTPase activity of Ras and converts Ras-GTP to inactive RAS-GDP. Thus, loss of NF1 leads to hyperactivity of Ras and the downstream signaling pathway. Increased activity of the Ras pathway has been documented in NF1-deficient cells. NF1 is not known to have any direct effect on Akt. Patients with NF1 syndrome develop neurofibromas and have an increased risk for glioblastomas, pheochromocytomas, and myeloid leukemias. Café au lait spots are found in 100% of patients with NF1 syndrome and increase in size and frequency with age.

Answer 3.15. **The answer is D.**

FAP is caused by germline mutations in the APC gene on chromosome 5q that are inherited in an autosomal dominant fashion. The characteristic feature of FAP syndrome is the presence of numerous adenomatous polyps. Development of colon cancer by the age of 40 years is a certainty. Patients with FAP also have an increased risk of desmoids tumors and malignancies of the upper gastrointestinal tract. Prophylactic colectomy is recommended in these individuals to reduce the risk of colon cancer. NSAIDs can reduce the size and number of the polyps in patients with FAP through the inhibition of COX-2 pathway but are not recommended in place of surgery to reduce the risk of colon cancer.

Answer 3.16. **The answer is C.**

p53 protein is a labile DNA-binding transcription factor that is not expressed at high levels during normal cellular homeostasis. In response to cellular stress, including hypoxia and DNA damage, p53 protein is stabilized and activates transcription of growth arrest genes that halt the cell in G1. The G1 arrest halts the cell until damage can be repaired. If the damage persists, the cells remain in an irreversible G1 arrest or undergo apoptosis. Mutations in p53 are found in the majority of sporadic cancers, and it is hypothesized that p53 function may be compromised in some way in all cancers. p53 mutations are the cause of Li-Fraumeni syndrome. The most common cancers found in patients with Li-Fraumeni are sarcomas, breast cancer, and brain tumors.

Answer 3.17. **The answer is B.**

Hereditary cancer syndromes more commonly occur as a result of mutations that result in loss of function. Thus, Li Fraumeni syndrome, hereditary nonpolyposis colon cancer syndrome, familial adenomatous polyposis, BRCA1, and BRCA2 are caused by mutations that result in the loss of function of the gene. It is hypothesized that most oncogenic gain-of-function mutations are incompatible with embryonic development, explaining their rarity in hereditary cancer syndromes. Examples of hereditary cancer syndromes resulting from gain of function mutations are multiple endocrine neoplasia type 2 (MEN 2), which results from mutations of the receptor tyrosine kinase RET; hereditary papillary renal cancer resulting from mutations in the MET gene; and hereditary gastrointestinal stromal tumor resulting from mutations in the KIT gene. Mutations in genes that regulate angiogenesis may also lead to hereditary cancer syndromes. Von Hippel Lindau is a genetic disorder that results from loss of function mutation of the VHL gene leading to increased expression of angiogenic factors. Hereditary leiomyomatosis and renal cancer is another familial cancer syndrome that might result from genes affecting angiogenesis.

Answer 3.18. **The answer is A.**

VHL gene encodes a ubiquitin ligase to target HIF 1α and HIF 2α for degradation under normoxic conditions. In hypoxic conditions, the expression of VHL is downregulated, resulting in accumulation of HIF 1α and HIF 2α, which act as transcription factors, and the expression of angiogenic factors, such as vascular endothelial growth factor (VEGF), is upregulated. In VHL syndrome, mutations in the VHL gene result in loss of function of the VHL protein, resulting in accumulation of HIF 1α and HIF 2α even under normoxic conditions. Individuals with VHL syndrome have an increased risk of developing renal cysts, renal cancer, and hemangioblastomas of the central nervous system. VHL function is also altered in 70% to 80% of the clear cell renal carcinomas.

Answer 3.19.   **The answer is B.**

PTEN operates as a haploinsufficient tumor suppressor to oppose tumor initiation. Cancer can develop in individuals with loss of one PTEN allele resulting in cellular proliferation and survival advantages. However, complete PTEN loss is detrimental to the cancer cell because it triggers a "cellular senescence" response. This cellular senescence response to complete loss of PTEN is being evaluated for cancer chemoprevention and therapy. Many tumor suppressor genes have been found to be haploinsufficient for specific functions. The PTEN paradigm also highlights the importance of subtle incremental variations in the expression levels of tumor suppressor genes, which then can lead to devastating consequences resulting in distinct outcomes in distinct tissues. The haploinsufficient tumor suppressors contrast with the retinoblastoma paradigm or the Knudson's hypothesis. In retinoblastoma, individuals inherit a mutation in one of the alleles of the RB gene and require a "second hit" to the other allele to develop cancer.

Answer 3.20.   **The answer is A.**

Among the animal viruses, retroviruses are unique in having a RNA genome that replicates through a DNA intermediate. Once the retrovirus infects the cell, the single-stranded viral genome is converted to double-stranded DNA by an RNA-dependent DNA polymerase or reverse transcriptase. The double-stranded DNA then is integrated into a host cell chromosome. Retroviruses in animals can transform the infected cell by integrating the viral DNA close to cellular oncogenes, integrating a protooncogene in the host cell genome, or altering the cellular gene expression or function. In humans, HTLV1 is the only retrovirus that has been shown to have a direct transforming effect. HIV, the other retrovirus, is more likely to cause malignant transformation in humans through an indirect effect of immune suppression.

Answer 3.21.   **The answer is D.**

Retroviruses transform cells through either an acute process or a slow transforming process. Acutely transforming viruses insert a viral oncogene into the host cell genome leading to malignant transformation. The slowly transforming viruses cause cellular transformation either by inserting the viral DNA adjacent to a cellular protooncogene (insertional mutagenesis) or altering the expression of cellular gene expression and function by viral proteins. Inflammation and its consequences are not known to be an important cause of retrovirus-induced cellular transformation.

Answer 3.22.   **The answer is A.**

HTLV1 is a retrovirus that is endemic in different parts of the world, including the southeastern part of the United States. HTLV1, like HIV, infects CD4+ T cells, but unlike HIV, HTLV1 infection is not associated with significant viremia. HTLV1 carriers have a lifetime risk of developing adult T-cell leukemia of 3% to 5% with a latency period of 30 to 50 years between infection and development of the malignancy. The virus is not associated with acute myeloid leukemia. HTLV1 is transmitted by blood transfusions, sexual contact, needle sharing, and breastfeeding.

Answer 3.23.   **The answer is C.**

HTLV1 protein Tax activates viral gene expression by interacting with cellular transcription proteins. Subsequently through this interaction with cellular transcription proteins, Tax leads to activation of several cellular gene promoters. IL-2 and IL-2 receptor are the most relevant genes activated by Tax. Adult T cells constitutively express the alpha chain of IL-2 receptor at high levels, and this can stimulate proliferation of infected cells. The site of integration of the viral genome is random and different from patient to patient, indicating that insertional mutagenesis does not play a role in the transforming effect of HTLV1. The long latency period between the onset of the infection and the development of the malignancy suggests that HTLV1 genome does not contain an acutely transforming oncogene. Unlike HIV, HTLV1 does not have an immunosuppressive effect.

Answer 3.24.   **The answer is B.**

HTLV2 shares 70% homology at the amino acid level with HTLV1. The virus was isolated from a patient with atypical T-cell variant hairy cell leukemia, but convincing epidemiologic data for an etiologic role for HTLV2 in any human disease do not exist. HTLV2 is also transmitted by the same routes as HTLV1 and is found in 0.01% of blood donors and in a larger proportion of intravenous drug users.

Answer 3.25.   **The answer is C.**

HIV, unlike HTLV1, the other retrovirus with transforming effects in humans, does not have a direct oncogenic effect. None of the HIV proteins have a directly transforming effect, and none of the proteins are known to enhance the expression of any of the cellular oncogenes. Rarely, insertional mutagenesis resulting in T-cell lymphomas has been reported in HIV-infected patients. However, this disease does not occur disproportionately in HIV-infected patients, making the observation of insertional mutagenesis in some patients with T-cell lymphomas as a random event rather than a specific oncogenic transforming effect of the virus. Many of the malignancies observed in HIV-infected patients, including the AIDS-defining cancers such as cervical cancer or non-Hodgkin's lymphoma, are associated with coinfection by DNA viruses. Infection with these viruses and the subsequent transforming effect are facilitated by the state of immune suppression induced by the HIV infection.

Answer 3.26.   **The answer is D.**

KS tumors are histologically complex tumors. The predominant cell and the most likely candidate tumor cell of KS is the spindle cell, but the tumor also consists of inflammatory cells and angiogenic cells. A polyclonal, multicentric proliferative process seems to occur, which is reflected in the frequently observed waxing and waning clinical course of KS. HHV-8 is the primary etiologic agent of KS in HIV-infected and noninfected patients. The role of HIV in the pathogenesis of KS is related to its ability to suppress immunity. In addition to the immune suppression, secretion of Tat protein by HIV-infected cells contributes to the production of cytokines, such as vascular endothelial growth factor, and these factors enhance the proliferation of the endothelial cells. HIV does not have any direct transforming effect on endothelial cells.

Answer 3.27.   **The answer is C.**

HIV-infected patients are at an increased risk of developing non-Hodgkin's lymphoma, including Burkitt's or Burkitt's-like lymphomas. The majority of these lymphomas are B-cell lymphomas, and many are associated with EBV. In addition to the immunosuppression, it has been theorized that HIV may contribute to lymphomagenesis via dysregulation of cytokine production and subsequent alteration of B-cell growth regulation. HIV does not have a transforming effect on the infected CD4+ T cells.

Answer 3.28.   **The answer is A.**

HCV is a RNA virus that belongs to the Hepacivirus genus of the Flaviviridae family of viruses. HCV is transmitted in a majority of the cases by a percutaneous route. Before 1989, when screening for HCV began, transfusion of contaminated blood products was the most important cause of HCV infection. Use of contaminated needles by intravenous drug users remains an important source of the infection. It can also be transmitted perinatally and via sexual routes. In 10% of the cases, risk factors for transmission are not identified. The fecal–oral route is not known to be a route for infection with HCV.

Answer 3.29.   **The answer is D.**

The worldwide prevalence of HCV infection is estimated to be 170 million. HCV infection is chronic in 50% to 60% of the infected patients. Of these, 60% and 20% develop chronic hepatitis and cirrhosis, respectively. The estimated proportion of chronically HCV infected individuals who develop hepatocellular carcinoma (HCC) is 1% to 5%.

Answer 3.30.   **The answer is B.**

Alcohol consumption or co-infection with HBV greatly increases the risk of developing HCC in HCV-infected patients. The role of HCV in the pathogenesis of HCC remains to be fully clarified. The inflammatory response caused by the HCV infection leads to hepatocyte destruction, regeneration, and fibrosis. Cellular turnover as a result of the inflammatory response could have a transforming effect leading to the pathogenesis of HCC. A direct oncogenic role of HCV is unlikely, although there have been results suggesting that the HCV core protein may have an oncogenic effect. In addition, infection with different strains of the virus may pose a different level of risk for development of HCC. Treatment with interferon and ribavirin can reduce the risk of HCC from HCV infection but cannot eliminate it.

Answer 3.31.   **The answer is C.**

HBV is a small DNA virus classified as a member of the hepadnavirus family (for hepatotropic DNA viruses). HBV is the only human virus in this family. Primary HBV infection produces a subclinical infection or acute liver injury, but 95% of such infections resolve with clearance of the virus. However, 5% of patients develop persistent hepatic infection, and these individuals are at risk of developing HCC. Patients with the highest levels of HBV viremia display the highest HCC risk. Patients with persistent infection can develop chronic active hepatitis and cirrhosis. These events, through hepatocyte injury, regeneration, and inflammation, lead to increased cellular turnover and increased risk of replicative errors that could then lead to a transforming effect. A more direct oncogenic effect of HBV is suggested by the presence of integrated HBV genomes in most hepatoma cells. However, the abundance of data suggest that a direct oncogenic effect by HBV may be relevant in only a few cases.

Answer 3.32.   **The answer is D.**

Among the different human cancers, HPV has the greatest association with cervical cancer. HPV-16 and HPV-18 are associated with 70% of all cervical cancers, with other HPV strains associated with the remaining 30%. HPV is associated with penile cancers. HPV has also been linked to some head and neck cancers, and most of the HPV-associated head and neck cancers occur in the oral pharynx. Esophageal cancers in humans have not been convincingly shown to be associated with HPV.

Answer 3.33.   **The answer is B.**

Molecular studies of cervical cancer reveal that the HPV DNA is usually integrated into the cellular genome. Integration of viral DNA is generally not at specific sites. In HPV-positive cancers, there appears to be a selection for the integration of E6 and E7 coding regions and the upstream regulatory regions. This leads to E6 and E7 genes being regularly expressed in these cancers. The E6 and E7 proteins are oncoproteins and lead to cellular transformation at least partly by binding the cell-cycle regulatory proteins p53 and Rb. Only a small fraction of those individuals infected with HPV will develop cancer, and the time interval between infection and development of cervical cancer can be decades. It appears that HPV infection, though essential, is not sufficient to lead to cervical cancer, and other factors are essential for progression to invasive cancer. Epidemiologic studies suggest that smoking may be such a factor because it is associated with an increased risk of cervical cancer.

Answer 3.34.   **The answer is C.**

HPV types 16 and 18 are the two most frequent HPV types associated with cervical cancer and have been demonstrated in approximately 70% of the cervical cancers. Among the other HPV types associated with cervical cancer are HPV-31, HPV-33, HPV-39, and HPV-42. HPV-6 and HPV-11 are rarely associated with genital tract cancers.

Answer 3.35.   **The answer is A.**

Recently approved vaccine for HPV consists of virus-like proteins (VLPs) from HPV-16, HPV-18, HPV-6, and HPV-11. The expression in yeast and insect cells of the major HPV capsid protein L1, either alone or together with L2, leads to the assembly of VLPs that are morphologically identical to native virion particles. These VLPs present the epitopes that are necessary for the development of a high titer neutralizing antisera. HPV-16 and HPV-18 are associated with approximately 70% of cervical cancers and HPV-6 and HPV-11 are associated with 90% of anogenital warts. There are HPV types other than HPV-16 and 18 that can cause cervical cancer, and therefore vaccinated individuals at risk should continue to receive cervical cancer screening. In addition, the duration of protection for the specific HPV types is unknown. The vaccine has been evaluated in women and therefore for now is recommended in women only.

Answer 3.36.   **The answer is D.**

EBV is associated with many cancers. EBV nuclear proteins, particularly EBNA2, target the transcription factor RBPJk/CBF1. It is through this transcription factor that EBV nuclear proteins regulate viral LMP1 promoter and the cellular c-myc promoter. EBV viral protein LMP1 engages the TNF receptor cytoplasmic factors and the death domain proteins, including TRADD and RIP, which may activate downstream proteins inducing cellular proliferation and survival. EBV is detected in approximately 50% of Hodgkin's lymphoma. EBV is also associated with many Burkitt's lymphomas, nasopharyngeal cancers, and some gastric cancers.

Answer 3.37.   **The answer is A.**

Among patients with AIDS, KS risk is highest in homosexual men. The risk is much lower among AIDS cases related to blood transfusion and in pediatric AIDS cases. This difference in the risk of KS is a result of higher prevalence of HHV8 infection, a known cause of KS, among homosexual men. This infection could then be transmitted among homosexual patients with AIDS, placing these patients at a higher risk for KS.

The prevalence of this infection among women and prepubertal children is very low.

Answer 3.38.   **The answer is B.**

HHV8 (also KS's associated virus KSHV) sequences are found in tumors of every patient with KS, irrespective of whether the patient is HIV infected or not. The prevalence of this virus is high in countries whereas classic KS is common and ranges from 20% in Italy to 60% in sub-Saharan Africa. In the United States, which has a low incidence of classic KS, the prevalence of HHV8 infection is 5% to 7%. HHV8 is transmitted by the sexual route, particularly in homosexual men. However, in countries with a high incidence of classic KS, seroprevalence is detected in children, suggesting that other routes of transmission exist. The nonsexual routes involved in the transmission of this virus are not well defined. The rarity of KS in the United States, despite the HHV8 prevalence rate of 5%, suggests that other factors are essential for the development of KS. In patients with AIDS-KS, the HIV infection is the other factor, but the cofactors in classic KS are not yet identified. EBV is not a cofactor in the development of KS in AIDS or classic KS.

Answer 3.39.   **The answer is B.**

SV40 DNA or antigens have been detected in some human cancers, including mesotheliomas, osteosarcomas, and brain tumors. The major source for human exposure to this virus was through contaminated polio virus vaccines administered from 1955 to 1963. However, there is no epidemiologic evidence that individuals exposed to these contaminated vaccines have increased risk of cancer. In the only double-blind study conducted, there was no correlation found between SV40 and human tumors. Human polyomaviruses BK and JC are ubiquitous, and there have been occasional reports linking these viruses to human cancers. However, comprehensive analysis of the data suggests no convincing evidence of an association.

Answer 3.40.   **The answer is D.**

Both innate and adaptive immunity play a role in immune surveillance of tumors. Adaptive immune cells, T and B lymphocytes, along with their effector molecules, innate immunity cells (e.g., natural killer cells), and proinflammatory cytokines (e.g., IL-12) are all important for immune surveillance of tumors. In animal models, deficiency of different inflammatory or immune mediators leads to different tumors, suggesting that the immune surveillance mechanisms differ for tumors arising in different tissues. Immune surveillance of tumors may or may not be dependent on antigens expressed on the tumor. In addition, antigens expressed on tumor stroma or certain self antigens may be relevant for immune surveillance.

Answer 3.41.   **The answer is C.**

More than a century ago, studies showed that infection with inflammation-causing bacteria induced dramatic regressions of cancers. An important role for immune surveillance of tumors is suggested by increased incidence of certain tumors in organ transplant recipients receiving immunosuppressive therapy. Nonmelanoma skin cancers are increased 50-fold in these patients, but the risk of melanoma is increased only modestly. Immunosuppressive therapy has a differential effect on various aspects of the immune system, and different components of the immune system are relevant for surveillance of the various tumors. This differential effect may account for the differences in the risk for the various tumors in immune-suppressed patients. The presence of tumor-infiltrating lymphocytes, particularly T cells in tumors such as melanomas, colon cancers, and ovarian cancers, is associated with improved prognosis supporting the role of immune surveillance in limiting tumor progression. Tumor progression is also controlled in many patients by the autoimmune response that leads to paraneoplastic neurologic syndromes.

Answer 3.42.   **The answer is C.**

Many lines of evidence support the association of inflammation and cancer. In general, acute inflammation has a greater capacity to eradicate tumors, whereas chronic smoldering inflammatory conditions that lead to infiltration of the tissue stroma by inflammatory cells could be associated with tumor initiation and progression. Thus, in conditions such as inflammatory bowel disease or chronic inflammation associated with a nonhealing ulcer, inflammatory factors could have antiapoptotic, proangiogenic, prometastatic, and immunosuppressive effects. All these can then lead to tumor formation and tumor progression. The ability of COX-2 inhibitors to reduce human cancers, particularly colon cancers, supports this association between inflammation and cancer.

Answer 3.43.   **The answer is D.**

Approximately 15% of human cancers have an association with an infectious agent. Although some infectious agents, particularly viruses, can induce cellular transformation, many infections give rise to cancers as a result of the chronic inflammation that develops in response to these infections. Chronic hepatitis that occurs in response to HCV can result in hepatocellular carcinoma. Similarly, *Helicobacter pylori* infection results in chronic gastric inflammation that then can lead to gastric cancer.

Answer 3.44.   **The answer is D.**

Inflammatory factors could be involved in procarcinogenic or antitumor effects, and some factors could have both effects. TNF is a cytokine released by inflammatory cells in response to an inflammatory stimulus. TNF can have an apoptotic effect on tumor calls and endothelial cells. However, by activating NFkB and inducing the production of MMP-9, it can have procarcinogenic effects. The balance between these effects leads to TNF being a procarcinogenic or antitumor factor in a particular tumor.

Answer 3.45.   **The answer is B.**

The observation that COX inhibitors can reduce the incidence of cancers was one of the initial indicators of the role of inflammation in cancer formation and progression. COX-2 inhibitors can reduce the numbers of polyps and prevent cancers in individuals with FAP and patients with inflammatory bowel disease, and can reduce the number of polyps in individuals with adenomatous polyps.

Answer 3.46.   **The answer is C.**

Cancer-associated stromal fibroblasts (CAFs) are better able to support tumor progression than fibroblasts from normal tissue. CAFs have characteristics like the other fibroblasts, such as expression of vimentin. These cells have not undergone transformation, and only few studies have found genetic alterations in these cells. The protumor effects of CAFs are mediated by soluble factors released by these cells that include SDF-1/CXCL12, transforming growth factor (TGF)-β, several growth factors, and MMP-9. The soluble factors released by CAFs can induce tumor formation in adjacent epithelial cells without the presence of other carcinogenic stimuli.

Answer 3.47.   **The answer is D.**

DCs are characterized by an ability to rapidly respond to alteration of tissue homeostasis because of the presence of pattern-recognizing receptors, such as the Toll-like receptors. Once activated, these cells secrete many proinflammatory cytokines such as IL-12, TNF, and IL-6. The activated DCs migrate to the regional lymph nodes and present antigens acquired in the tissues to T cells in the context of major histocompatibility complex class I and II antigens. Thus, through the production of cytokines and activation of T cells, DCs activate both innate and adaptive immunity in response to changes in the tissue homeostasis. DCs in tumors are generally hyporesponsive because of their interaction with other inflammatory cells or the tumor cells and therefore are not involved in immune surveillance. Activation of DCs is one of the immune strategies being pursued in the treatment of some cancers.

Answer 3.48.   **The answer is C.**

TAMs are derived from monocytes and monocyte precursors from the blood. TAMs have the capacity to induce either cytotoxic and antitumor or protumor and proangiogenic effects. In most progressing tumors, TAMs mediate protumor effects They favor tumor growth by producing growth factors, angiogenic cytokines, and expression of MMPs, TGFβ, and TNF that help tumor invasion and metastasis. IL-10 produced by inflammatory cells, including the TAMs, has an immunosuppressive effect on TAMs that impairs the antitumor effects of these cells.

Answer 3.49.   **The answer is D.**

TLRs are evolutionary conserved molecules that are a family of at least 12 different pattern recognizing receptors (PRRs). TLRs are important in recognition of microbes, pathogens, and endogenous ligands that have a role in regulation of inflammation. The role of TLRs and other PRRs in tumor-associated inflammation remains to be defined. TLRs expressed on tumor cells can cause apoptosis, but activation of TLRs on tumor-infiltrating cells may promote tumor progression.

Nikhil I. Khushalani
Kaunteya Reddy

Etiology of Cancer ■ Part 2

Directions   Each of the numbered items below is followed by lettered answers. Select the ONE lettered answer that is BEST in each case unless instructed otherwise.

QUESTIONS

Question 4.1.   **Cancer in humans is:**

A. A genetically determined sequela of aging
B. A manifestation of individual exposure to carcinogens
C. A combination of a genetically susceptible individual and exposure to carcinogen
D. An unknown mechanism of development

Question 4.2.   **Which of the following has been implicated in increased cancer risk?**

A. Tobacco and alcohol
B. Diet
C. Sexual behavior
D. All of the above

Question 4.3.   **Match the following agents most commonly involved with cancer of that particular organ:**

A. Lung
B. Pleura
C. Urinary bladder
D. Liver
E. Bone marrow
F. Prostrate
G. Skin

1. Asbestos
2. Benzene
3. Tobacco
4. Cadmium
5. Ultraviolet (UV) light
6. Phenacetin
7. Aflatoxin

Corresponding Chapters in *Cancer: Principles & Practice of Oncology*, Eighth Edition: 15 (Etiology of Cancer: Chemical Factors), 16 (Etiology of Cancer: Physical Factors), 17 (Etiology of Cancer: Dietary Factors), and 18 (Etiology of Cancer: Obesity and Physical Activity).

Question 4.4.   **Which of the following statements is TRUE?**

A. Interaction of genotoxic carcinogens is random.
B. Interaction of genotoxic carcinogens is selective based on their class.
C. Genotoxic carcinogens can cause base mispairing and small deletions, but not large deletions.
D. All toxins implicated in cancers are genotoxic.

Question 4.5.   **Studies in animal models have led to which of the following conclusions?**

A. Carcinogenic agents activate oncogenes.
B. Carcinogenic agents inactivate tumor suppressor genes.
C. Carcinogenic agents cause genomic changes that are required for production of malignant phenotype.
D. All of the above.

Question 4.6.   **Which of the following statements is FALSE regarding fundamental principles of molecular epidemiology?**

A. Carcinogenesis is a multistage process.
B. Carcinogenesis involves numerous genetic events at each stage.
C. Human response to carcinogen exposure is homogeneous.
D. There is a wide range of interindividual variation to carcinogen exposure.

Question 4.7.   **Which of the following components are involved in the estimation of dose and corresponding risk in epidemiological studies?**

A. Measurement of external and internal exposure
B. Biomarkers estimating the biologically effective dose
C. Biomarkers of harm
D. All of the above

Question 4.8.   **Which of the following statements about benzene is NOT true?**

A. Benzene is metabolized in the liver by CYP2E1 (P-4502E1).
B. Benzene oxide and hydroquinone are reactive metabolites of benzene.
C. Presence of functional polymorphisms of myeloperoxidase in humans may have a protective role against toxicity of benzene to bone marrow.
D. There exists a perfect dose-response relationship of benzene in humans, and genetically susceptible individuals can be easily identified.

Question 4.9.   **Which of the following statements is TRUE?**

A. UV radiation has sufficient energy to produce ionization.
B. UV radiation does not have sufficient energy to produce ionization, but its effects are a result of molecular excitation.
C. UVC is present in sunlight that reaches the earth and has wavelengths ranging from 320 to 400 nm.
D. UV-induced damage to p53 is a late event in the development of squamous cell carcinoma of the skin.

Question 4.10.   **Which of the following is TRUE about UV light?**

A.   UVB causes direct damage to DNA with resultant pyrimidine dimer formation.
B.   UVA has deeper penetration into skin compared with UVB.
C.   Cytosine dimers are readily formed by exposure to UVB compared with thymine because it absorbs higher wavelength UV radiation.
D.   All of the above.

Question 4.11.   **Radiation was used to treat which of the following disease conditions?**

A.   Enlarged thymus glands
B.   Peptic ulcers
C.   Ankylosing spondylitis
D.   All of the above

Question 4.12.   **Which of the following statements is TRUE about radiation exposure, tissue sensitivity, and latent period?**

A.   Evidence suggests that acute and chronic myelogenous leukemias are very sensitive to induction after radiation exposure.
B.   Latent period is defined as the period of time between radiation exposure and the appearance of radiation-induced tumors.
C.   The peak incidence for the development of radiation-induced leukemia occurs between 0 and 2 years after exposure.
D.   Both A and B.

Question 4.13.   **Which of the following is TRUE regarding theoretic models of radiation interaction?**

A.   Linear and linear-quadratic models have been described.
B.   Cancer risk is directly proportional to radiation dose in the linear model.
C.   Cancer risk is directly proportional to radiation dose at low dose and a function of square of the dose at higher dose in the linear-quadratic model.
D.   All of the above.

Question 4.14.   **In regard to high linear energy transfer (LET) radiation, which of the following is NOT true?**

A.   Ionization tracks through an individual cell are few.
B.   Because of the high density of this type of exposure, the probability of producing complex effects is high.
C.   The dose response in this case is nonlinear.
D.   None of the above.

Question 4.15.   **Which of the following regarding radon is TRUE?**

A. Radon is a major source of high LET radiation to the general population.
B. Radon is chemically active and charged.
C. Radon exposure is not a risk factor for lung cancer.
D. Bystander effect is not true with radon exposure.

Question 4.16.   **Match the following:**

A. Younger age of exposure
B. Middle age at exposure
C. High penetrance genes
D. Breast cancer

1. High risk of cancer induction
2. Low risk of cancer induction
3. Ataxia-telangiectasia
4. High probability of cancer induction

Question 4.17.   **Which of the following plays a role in second cancers after radiation therapy?**

A. Age of exposure
B. Body size
C. Genetic susceptibility
D. All of the above

Question 4.18.   **Which of the following is a mechanism of radiation-induced cancer?**

A. DNA double-strand break induction
B. Telomere dysfunction and instability
C. Cytogenetic damage in progeny of irradiated cells
D. All of the above

Question 4.19.   **Which of the following influences development of skin cancer?**

A. Presence of skin pigment
B. Latitude of location on earth
C. Family history of skin cancer
D. All of the above

Question 4.20.   **Which of the following statements is TRUE regarding malignant melanoma?**

A. Malignant melanoma is more a result of chronic exposure to sunlight than acute exposure.
B. History of sunburns does not predispose one to malignant melanoma.
C. Melanoma development is independent of tumor suppressor gene pathways and mutated oncogenes.
D. Familial form of malignant melanoma involves deletions or mutations in CDKN2A.

Question 4.21.   **Which of the following is TRUE regarding asbestos?**

A. Latent period for development of mesothelioma after asbestos exposure is 30 to 40 years.
B. Asbestos fibers produce an inflammatory reaction in the lungs.
C. The majority of asbestos effects are mediated through generation of reactive oxygen species.
D. All of the above.

Question 4.22.   **Obesity is defined as a body mass index (BMI) (Quetelet's Index) greater than which of the following values?**

A. 24 kg/m^2
B. 26 kg/m^2
C. 28 kg/m^2
D. 30 kg/m^2

Question 4.23.   **Case-control studies examining the role of diet in the cause of cancer do not suffer from recall bias.**

A. True
B. False

Question 4.24.   **Which of the following instruments is the most widely used in population-based studies of dietary intake?**

A. Food-frequency questionnaire
B. 24-hour recall record
C. 7-day diet record
D. None of the above

Question 4.25.   **In the American Cancer Society Cohort Study from 1982 to 1998 examining the relation of BMI in 1982 and the risk of death from all cancers, obese individuals had a higher risk of cancer-related mortality from all of the following cancers, EXCEPT:**

A. Pancreas cancer
B. Colorectal cancer
C. Brain cancer
D. Kidney cancer

Question 4.26.   **Alcohol consumption is an etiologic factor in the development of which of the following cancers?**

A. Esophagus cancer
B. Breast cancer
C. Colorectal cancer
D. All of the above

Question 4.27.   **There is clear association between dietary fat consumption and the risk of developing breast cancer in women.**

A.   True
B.   False

Question 4.28.   **Regular consumption of red meat is associated with an increased risk of which of the following cancers?**

A.   Larynx cancer
B.   Colorectal cancer
C.   Liver cancer
D.   Esophagus cancer

Question 4.29.   **What is the relation between consumption of soy products and the risk of breast cancer?**

A.   No relation noted
B.   Increase in risk of breast cancer
C.   Decrease in risk of breast cancer

Question 4.30.   **Obesity is a risk factor for postmenopausal breast cancer.**

A.   True
B.   False

Question 4.31.   **Obesity and physical inactivity are established risk factors for which of the following cancers?**

A.   Colon cancer
B.   Postmenopausal breast cancer
C.   Both A and B
D.   Neither A or B

Question 4.32.   **Convincing evidence exists for the association between obesity and all of the following cancers, EXCEPT:**

A.   Adenocarcinoma of the esophagus
B.   Kidney cancer
C.   Ovarian cancer
D.   Endometrial cancer

ANSWERS

Answer 4.1.   **The answer is C.**

The development of cancer is a multistage process. It depends not only on genetic predispositions but is also influenced by the environment, diet, occupation, and lifestyle of an individual. Therefore, cancer results from a combination of hereditary susceptibility and individual exposure to either endogenous or exogenous factors.

Answer 4.2.　　　**The answer is D.**

All of the listed factors are implicated in cancer development. Exposure to chemicals can result in DNA damage and mutations. These genotoxic events can occur directly from exposure or indirectly through the generation of intermediate compounds that disrupt normal cellular function. Tobacco and alcohol are well known to predispose humans to numerous cancers, including cancers of the oral cavity, oropharynx, larynx, lung, and esophagus. Common examples of diet-related carcinogenesis include smoked or pickled foods (stomach cancer) and red meat (colon cancer). The relation between human papilloma virus (HPV) and cancer of the cervix is an example of cancer associated with sexual behavior.

Answer 4.3.　　　**The answers are (A) 3, (B) 1, (C) 6, (D) 7, (E) 2, (F) 4, (G) 5.**

Tobacco is the single most important risk factor in lung cancer. Although it does increase the risk of lung cancer, asbestos is a major risk factor in the development of pleural mesothelioma. Studies have shown the association between liver cancer and exposure to aflatoxins. Benzene has been well studied in the causation of leukemia. UV light exposure directly correlates to the development of skin cancer.

Answer 4.4.　　　**The answer is B.**

Genotoxic carcinogens are potent mutagens. They interact with DNA and cause base mispairing, deletions, both small and large, and are capable of causing direct chromosomal breaks. Each class of genotoxic agent reacts selectively with purine and pyrimidine targets within a nucleotide sequence. The mechanism of action of nongenotoxic carcinogens is less clear and believed to be mediated through direct cell death, deregulated hyperplasia, induction of endogenous toxic radical production, and so forth.

Answer 4.5.　　　**The answer is D.**

Studies in animal models have shown that carcinogenic agents act in a variety of different ways. They can activate oncogenes directly and inactivate tumor suppressor genes. They cause genomic changes that help propagate the malignant phenotype that manifests as unregulated growth, resistance to apoptosis, and potential for metastatic spread.

Answer 4.6.　　　**The answer is C.**

Carcinogenesis is a multistage process involving several genetic events at each stage. There is a wide interindividual variation in humans to carcinogen exposure. Herein lies the difficulty in using in vitro models to mimic human cellular response. Experimental studies that involve a single clone being exposed to a particular carcinogen to study a particular gene might not be representative of the population. It does allow the investigation of specific mechanisms that may be involved in carcinogenesis.

Answer 4.7.   **The answer is D.**

There are four components in the estimation of dose and effect in epidemiologic studies. Measurements of internal and external exposure, markers of the biologically effective dose, and markers of damage are all important, and these components help quantify the exposure at the cellular level. When assessing these surrogate markers, their sensitivity and specificity, reproducibility, and general applicability for human use should be taken into appropriate consideration.

Answer 4.8.   **The answer is D.**

Benzene is metabolized in the liver by CYP2E1 into active metabolites. These metabolites are known to bind to DNA in the bone marrow cells. Myeloperoxidase is involved in the production of active metabolites of benzene (benzoquinone). Functional polymorphisms in myeloperoxidase might play a protective role by reduced enzyme expression in some individuals. Currently, the dose response of benzene needs further evaluation.

Answer 4.9.   **The answer is B.**

UV light is one of the forms of nonionizing radiation. Although it does not have sufficient energy to produce ionization, its effect is mediated by molecular excitation, interaction with the host tissue, and eventual DNA damage. UVA, UVB, and UVC are present in solar energy, although UVC (wavelength 240 to 290 nm) does not reach the earth because it is absorbed by the atmosphere. Squamous cell carcinoma and basal cell carcinoma of the skin are typically a result of chronic sun exposure. At the molecular level, p53 damage appears to be an early event in carcinogenesis. UVB appears to be the primary mediator, although there is accumulating evidence that UVA may also be contributory.

Answer 4.10.   **The answer is D.**

UV light can be classified into UVA, UVB, and UVC. Among these, UVA has the highest wavelength and UVC has the lowest. UVA and UVB are present in sunlight eventually reaching the earth, with UVC being absent secondary to atmospheric absorption. All three wavelengths can cause damage to DNA. UVA is not absorbed by the atmosphere and has the greatest penetration into tissue among the three. It can result in the production of reactive oxygen radicals that can cause molecular damage and death. Following the interaction of UVB with DNA, several biologically important products are obtained, including the cyclobutane dimer and 6-4 photoproduct, of which the former appears more important in causing mutagenic effects.

Answer 4.11.   **The answer is D.**

All the disease conditions listed above were treated with radiation in the past. Other examples include tinea capitis, tonsillar enlargement, benign breast, and gynecologic disease. Studies in these cohorts have contributed toward the understanding of radiation-related acute and chronic toxicity, as well as the development of radiation-related cancers such as thyroid cancer and breast cancer.

Answer 4.12.   **The answer is D.**

The latent period is defined as the time between the radiation exposure and the development of a radiation-induced tumor. Acute and chronic myelogenous leukemias are sensitive to induction and their peak latent period is usually around 4 to 8 years, although cases as early as 2 years have also been reported. For solid tumors, the latent period is typically longer and can even exceed two decades.

Answer 4.13.   **The answer is D.**

Studies at the molecular and cellular levels and epidemiological data have helped derive two dose-response models of radiation interaction. First is the linear model wherein cancer risk is directly proportional to radiation dose. In the linear quadratic model, the risk is proportional to dose at low dose and rapidly increases with high doses.

Answer 4.14.   **The answer is C.**

High LET results in few energy tracks in the cell. Although few, they have a high density that is sufficient to produce complex effects. The dose–response relationship in this case is linear because of the higher effectiveness of this type of radiation. Radon exposure (e.g., in uranium mines) is an example of high LET.

Answer 4.15.   **The answer is B.**

Radon is a naturally occurring high LET radiation found in rocks and soil. It is chemically inert and uncharged, but spontaneous decay results in its progeny, which are radioactive and electrically charged. The latter can attach to ambient dust particles, which when inhaled can result in lung irradiation. This is a well-defined etiologic factor in the development of lung cancer. Bystander effect is an interesting feature observed with radon wherein the cells exposed to radon send out signals to adjacent cells, which are not exposed. These signals result in mutagenic and oncogenic changes.

Answer 4.16.   **The answers are (A) 1, (B) 2, (C) 4, (D) 3.**

The age at time of exposure plays a critical role in cancer induction. Younger age at exposure increases the risk substantially when compared with middle age of exposure. Good examples are breast cancer and thyroid cancer. When compared with middle-aged women, young children and adolescents have a higher risk of developing breast cancer after exposure to radiation. The defects involved in ataxia-telangiectasia may be involved in radiation-induced breast cancer secondary to increased radiation sensitivity.

Answer 4.17.   **The answer is D.**

Age plays an important role in induction second cancers because children are more susceptible to radiation. Because children have a smaller body size, multiple organs may be exposed, as the area exposed to radiation is large. Genetic susceptibility is an important factor in induction of second cancers. Common second cancers after radiation include those of the breast, thyroid, esophagus, and lung, as well as leukemia.

Answer 4.18.   **The answer is D.**

Induction of DNA double-strand breaks, telomere instability, and dysfunction are all effects of radiation exposure. It was initially believed that the mutagenic and cytogenetic effects of ionizing radiation occurred in the first few cell divisions after exposure, but it is now thought that this kind of damage can occur in several generations in progeny of radiation-exposed cells.

Answer 4.19.   **The answer is D.**

Individuals who lack skin pigment, have a history of sunburn, have a family history of skin cancer, and live closer to the equator have a higher risk of developing skin cancer. The development of malignant melanoma is less dependent on the total exposure of sunlight; rather, acute exposures causing sunburn is of greater concern. A history of five or more sunburns in adolescence doubles the risk of developing melanoma. In addition, the site of development does not seem to be related to the site of chronic exposure in melanoma.

Answer 4.20.   **The answer is D.**

In the familial form of malignant melanoma, deletions and mutations of CDKN2A are most often seen. CDKN2A encodes p16INK4A and p14ARF, both tumor suppressors. Oncogene activation involving the RAS pathway is also seen in melanoma. Clinically, its development seems to be related to acute, repeated sunburn rather than chronic exposure.

Answer 4.21.   **The answer is D.**

It is well known that the most common form of cancer after asbestos exposure is malignant mesothelioma. Occupational exposure can be linked in approximately 50% to 80% of patients. The latent period is typically long, approximately 30 to 40 years. There are two main types of asbestos fibers, amphibole and chrysolite; the former is more commonly linked to mesothelioma. These fibers induce an inflammatory response, resulting in the development of reactive oxygen species that mediate the cytotoxic and genotoxic effects of asbestos. Asbestos can directly affect mitosis and chromosomal segregation with resultant aneuploidy. Loss of a copy of chromosome 22 is one of the most commonly seen abnormalities in this malignancy.

Answer 4.22.   **The answer is D.**

Quetelet's Index (or BMI) is calculated as the weight (in kilograms) divided by the square of the height (in meters). Being overweight is defined as a BMI of 25.0 to 29.9 kg/m^2, whereas a BMI greater than 30 kg/m^2 constitutes being obese. Approximately one third of the US population in 2000 met this definition of obesity with physical inactivity being the likely cause.

Answer 4.23.   **The answer is B.**

Recall bias is commonly encountered in case-control studies examining the effect of dietary factors in causing cancer. Another type of bias seen is control selection bias. Individuals under study (cases) may overemphasize their consumption of foods traditionally considered unhealthy, which may skew the results observed.

Answer 4.24.   **The answer is A.**

The food frequency questionnaire requests subjects to recall and report their average intake of a variety of food over the preceding year. Although this instrument tends to overrepresent foods considered healthy (vegetables and fruits, so-called social desirability bias), it is the most widely used in large studies of dietary pattern reporting in large studies. The 24-hour recall method offers too narrow a window to accurately reflect dietary patterns, and the 7-day diary record is cumbersome for data transfer and extraction.

Answer 4.25.   **The answer is C.**

In this study of more than 900,000 individuals who were cancer-free at enrollment in 1982, an increased BMI was associated with an increased risk of cancer-related death. Cancers of the esophagus, pancreas, liver, gall bladder, colorectum, kidney, breast, uterus, and cervix were among those in which this association was noted, whereas no such relation was found for cancers of the brain and bladder and for melanoma. The relative risk of death from cancer was 1.52 and 1.62 in men and women, respectively, who had a BMI greater than 40, compared with individuals of normal weight. Elevated levels of endogenous estrogen, insulin, and proinflammatory factors, and decreased levels of sex hormone binding proteins and insulin-like growth factor are believed to contribute to the increased risk of cancer in overweight individuals.

Answer 4.26.   **The answer is D.**

The International Agency for Research on Cancer categorizes alcohol as a carcinogen. Cancers of the head and neck region (oral cavity, pharynx, larynx), esophagus, liver, breast, and colorectum are linked to alcohol consumption in a dose-dependent manner. For some of these cancers, smoking in addition to alcohol consumption increases the risk in a synergistic fashion.

Answer 4.27.   **The answer is B.**

Initial case-control studies examining the relation of breast cancer in women to the consumption of dietary fat suggested a positive correlation with a pooled relative risk of 1.35 in a meta-analysis of 12 studies. This risk was greater in postmenopausal women. However, cohort studies have failed to confirm these findings, including the large Nurses' Health Study and the Women's Health Initiative Randomized Controlled Dietary Modification Trial.

Answer 4.28.   **The answer is B.**

Several studies have demonstrated an increased risk of colorectal cancer with the regular consumption of red meat, with a stronger association with processed meat. A meta-analysis of prospective studies examining this subject confirms these findings with a relative risk of 1.24.

Answer 4.29.   **The answer is C.**

Available evidence suggests that there is a decreased risk of breast cancer associated with consumption of soy products. This hypothesis was borne from initial observations of lower incidences of breast cancer in women in Asia, where soy consumption is high. Soybeans contain genistein and daidzein, whose metabolites have several biologic effects, including inhibition of the epidermal growth factor receptor tyrosine kinase activity and competition with estrogen for the estrogen receptor. In a meta-analysis of 18 studies, a modest decrease (odds ratio, 0.86) in the risk of breast cancer was noted with high soy intake.

Answer 4.30.   **The answer is A.**

Adult obesity and adult weight gain are associated with an increased risk (relative risk 1.5 to 2.0) for developing breast cancer in postmenopausal women. This risk approximates 18% per 5 kg/m^2 increase in BMI. There is a higher circulating level of estrone derived from androstenedione in women who are obese because adipose tissue serves as the primary source of endogenous estrogen in the postmenopausal state. Physical inactivity is also an established risk factor in postmenopausal breast cancer.

Answer 4.31.   **The answer is C.**

There is good evidence suggesting an increased risk of colon cancer and postmenopausal breast cancer in individuals who are obese or physically inactive. This relation has not been established for rectal cancer. In colon cancer, postulated mechanisms of obesity-related carcinogenesis include insulin resistance, elevated levels of insulin and insulin-like growth factor (IGF), and inflammation. These contribute to cellular proliferation, DNA damage, and tumor growth. Improved colonic transit time in subjects who are physically active is another possible mechanism contributing to decreased risk of colon cancer in this cohort. The effects of obesity and physical inactivity have been more pronounced in men compared with women.

Please refer to question 30 for a more detailed discussion on the relation between these factors and postmenopausal breast cancer.

Answer 4.32.   **The answer is C.**

An etiologic association exists between high BMI and cancers of the esophagus (adenocarcinoma), endometrium, kidney, colon, and breast (postmenopausal), whereas such evidence in ovarian cancer is inconclusive. Obesity increases gastroesophageal reflux disease, which is a known risk factor for esophageal adenocarcinoma. The obesity epidemic in North America may, in part, be responsible for the dramatic increase in the incidence of this cancer during the past two decades. There is a linear risk between increasing weight and endometrial cancer, which, like breast cancer, is hormonally dependent. The mechanisms are believed to be similar as well, with an increase in circulating estrogen levels in overweight or obese women. In kidney cancer, there is a 7% increase in risk for every unit increase in the BMI. The data in ovarian cancer at this time are inconclusive, and a positive association, if any, is weak.

Epidemiology of Cancer

Directions   Each of the numbered items below is followed by lettered answers. Select the ONE lettered answer that is BEST in each case unless instructed otherwise.

QUESTIONS

Question 5.1.   **All the following are true about prevalence and incidence, EXCEPT:**

A. Prevalence is calculated by dividing the number of existing cases by the total population.

B. Cumulative incidence is the proportion of people who develop the disease during a specified period of time.

C. Prevalence is considered a more relevant measure of disease frequency for etiologic evaluation, and incidence reflects the public health burden of the disease.

D. The quality of incidence data varies substantially depending on the accuracy of the population numbers, the completeness of reporting the diagnosis, and the degree with which the diagnosis is pursued.

Question 5.2.   **Surveillance, Epidemiology, and End Results (SEER) program of the National Cancer Institute provides data on new cancer cases and cancer survival within the United States. All the following are true about the SEER database, EXCEPT:**

A. Geographic areas are selected for their ability to operate high-quality data reporting systems and their epidemiologically significant population subgroups.

B. The population covered by the SEER database is comparable to the US population in regard to poverty and education.

C. SEER data provide information on the demographic characteristics of cancer cases and cancer characteristics (site, morphology, and stage).

D. The SEER database includes approximately 1% of the US population.

Corresponding Chapter in *Cancer: Principles & Practice of Oncology,* Eighth Edition: 19 (Epidemiology of Cancer).

Question 5.3.   **Which of the following are potential types of bias associated with case-control studies?**

A. Selection bias
B. Recall bias
C. Misclassification bias
D. All of the above

Question 5.4.   **All the following are differences between molecular epidemiology and genetic epidemiology, EXCEPT:**

A. Molecular epidemiology assesses genetic involvement, whereas genetic epidemiology focuses mainly on heredity.
B. Molecular epidemiology studies unrelated individuals, whereas genetic epidemiology investigates family members in the format of pedigrees.
C. Molecular epidemiology usually studies low penetrance markers that are commonly present in the general population, whereas genetic epidemiology research is often designed to identify markers with high penetrance but low prevalence in the general population.
D. Molecular epidemiology uses linkage analysis, whereas genetic epidemiology often calculates relative risks or odds ratios.

Question 5.5.   **For all the following analytical studies, the individual is the unit of analysis, EXCEPT:**

A. Ecological
B. Cross-sectional
C. Cohort
D. Case-control

Question 5.6.   **Dr. Bush wants to study the relationship between diet soda consumption and the development of gastrointestinal cancer. He selects the controls from patients who have been referred to the gastroenterology clinic. This is as an example of:**

A. Information bias
B. Selection bias
C. Misclassification bias
D. All of the above

Question 5.7.   **The probability that an individual will develop or die of cancer in a lifetime is frequently reported in the media. For example, it is reported that lung cancer will affect 1 in 13 men over a lifetime. Although this statistic provides some valuable information, the problem(s) with this statistic is:**

A. It underestimates the risk for individuals with certain risk factors.
B. It overestimates the risk for individuals without certain risk factors.
C. It underestimates and overestimates the risk for individuals depending on the age.
D. All of the above.

Question 5.8. **To accurately portray the incidence of various cancers, the data require standardization, particularly when comparing data from different countries. The reasons why this is required are the following:**

A. Different age structures between separate countries
B. Different numbers of men and women between the separate countries
C. Cohort effects
D. All the above

Question 5.9. **Cancers that are more common in women than in men include all the following, EXCEPT:**

A. Gallbladder cancer
B. Breast cancer
C. Thyroid cancer
D. Lung cancer

Question 5.10. **Socioeconomic status (SES) affects the incidence and death rate from cancers. All of the following are true, EXCEPT:**

A. The incidence of prostate cancer is higher in middle and higher SES groups than in lower SES groups.
B. In economically developing countries, major cancer risk factors such as cigarette smoking, obesity, and physical inactivity are more common among higher SES groups than among the power SES groups.
C. The death rate from all cancers combined is inversely related to SES.
D. In white women in the United States, the death rate from all cancers is equivalent for women with less than 12 years education and women who are college graduates.

Question 5.11. **Migrant studies have helped differentiate whether variations in cancer rates across countries and among different racial and ethnic groups are caused by environmental factors or inherited genetic factors. An example of this is the difference in death rates from selected cancers comparing Japanese in Japan with first- and second-generation Japanese in California with native California whites. All the following are true, EXCEPT:**

A. Mortality from cancers of the stomach and liver are higher among Japanese in Japan.
B. Among first-generation Japanese who migrated to California, the mortality from stomach and liver cancer is substantially lower than in Japanese in Japan and higher than in California whites.
C. The mortality from colon cancer approximately doubled among first-generation Japanese who moved to California and approached the rates of California whites by the second generation.
D. The mortality from colorectal cancer is higher among Japanese in both the United States and Japan than in California whites.
E. All of the above are true.

Question 5.12.   **There has been increasing interest in the use of computed tomography (CT) screening for lung cancer. Potential problems with CT screening for lung cancer include:**

    A.   Lead-time bias
    B.   Length-time bias
    C.   Neither
    D.   Both

Question 5.13.   **The recent development of molecular and molecular biomarkers has changed the development of epidemiology studies and clinical trials. The further investigation of molecular markers, especially phenotypic markers, will require which of the following issues to be addressed:**

    A.   Reproducibility of assays
    B.   Versatile assays
    C.   Sensitive and specific assays
    D.   Quality assurance procedures
    E.   All of the above

Question 5.14.   **Statistical methods are required to evaluate the role of chance. An usual way to calculate chance is to establish the upper and lower limits of a 95% confidence interval around a point estimate for relative risk (risk ratio, rate ratio, or odds ratio). All are true about confidence intervals, EXCEPT:**

    A.   If the confidence interval does not include 1, the observed association is statistically significant.
    B.   The width of the confidence interval is not inversely related to the number of participates in a study or sample size.
    C.   The calculation of the confidence interval assumes the only thing that would differ in hypothetical replications of the study would be statistical or chance element in the data.
    D.   The calculation of the confidence interval assumes that the variability in the data can be described adequately by statistical methods and that biases are nonexistent.
    E.   The choice of 95% is almost default in the upper and lower limits of the interval (e.g., 90% or 99%) and can be calculated and interpreted accordingly.

Question 5.15.   **All of the following are true about lung cancer prevalence, EXCEPT:**

    A.   The number of lung cancer cases in economically developing countries now exceeds the number in developed countries.
    B.   Globally, an estimated 85% of lung cancers in men and 47% of lung cancers in women are attributable to tobacco smoking.
    C.   The lung cancer incidence rate in 2002 in Chinese women is higher than that among women in France and Germany despite the low prevalence of smoking.
    D.   The highest rates of lung cancer are among men in eastern Europe, North America, and the rest of Europe, reflecting differences in historical patterns of smoking.
    E.   All of the above are true.

ANSWERS

Answer 5.1.   **The answer is C.**

Prevalence reflects the public health burden of the disease (i.e., how many patients need to be treated and/or followed by the health system), and incidence is considered a more relevant measure of disease frequency for etiologic evaluation. An example would be breast cancer in women and prostate cancer in men are more prevalent, whereas lung cancer compromises only a small fraction of the prevalent cases but is the most common fatal cancer. The incidence of a disease can vary depending on the reporting to the cancer diagnosis and the presence of screening tests such as prostate-specific antigen (PSA).

Answer 5.2.   **The answer is D.**

The SEER database covers approximately 26% of the US population.

Answer 5.3.   **The answer is D.**

Case-control studies can optimize the speed, efficiency, and cost of studies but are susceptible to biases. Specific biases include recall (the status of the subject, case, or control may influence how he/she recalls and reports previous exposures), selection (individuals in the study, as cases or controls, are different from the target population), and misclassification (occurs if the ascertainment of disease by the observer is influenced by the exposure status; e.g., a physician may examine the subject if he/she knows the subject has been exposed and likely at a higher risk, and the exposed subject visits the doctor more often if he/she thinks they are at higher risk related to an exposure).

Answer 5.4.   **The answer is D.**

Both molecular epidemiology and genetic epidemiology have an emphasis on molecular analysis, but linkage analysis is usually performed in genetic epidemiology studies because participants are genetically related family members.

Answer 5.5.   **The answer is A.**

Ecological studies use groups of people as the unit and are performed when the level measures of exposure and/or outcome are available. An example would be the relationship between dietary fat intake and the incidence of a type of cancer by country.

Answer 5.6.   **The answer is B.**

The patient population that has been referred to the gastroenterology clinic may be significantly different than the general population in terms of the incidence of cancers of the gastrointestinal tract and/or soda consumption.

Answer 5.7.   **The answer is D.**

Although this figure is popular and useful, it significantly overestimates the risk in the never-smoking population and underestimates the risk on the smoking population. The incidence of lung cancer also increases with age, so this number overestimates the risk in younger people and underestimates the risk in older people.

Answer 5.8.   **The answer is D.**

Age standardization eliminates differences in the age structure, which is important because cancer has a higher incidence in older people, and a country with an older or younger population may have a different incidence of a cancer related to the age distribution. Gender similarly influences the incidence of cancer. A cohort effect typically results from the introduction of a risk factor that becomes established at a young age in people born in the same time period. An example would be lung cancer death rates peaked in cohorts born around the late 1920s and early 1930s, and cigarette smoking also peaked during this time period.

Answer 5.9.   **The answer is D.**

Although the number of deaths from lung cancer is increasing in women and decreasing in men, reflecting changes in the prevalence of smoking a generation ago, lung cancer remains more common in men.

Answer 5.10.   **The answer is D.**

SES influences the incidence of cancer when screening diagnostic tests are available (e.g., PSA), most likely because of differences in access to care. Patients with higher SES are more likely to undergo screening tests and have a higher incidence of disease. The mortality from all cancers is inversely related to SES. In many economically developing countries, major cancer risk factors are more common among the educated, higher SES groups than the poor. In the United States white women with less than 12 years of education have twice the death rate from all cancers combined as college graduates.

Answer 5.11.   **The answer is E.**

Migrant studies have helped to differentiate whether variation in cancer rates across countries and among different racial and ethnic groups is due to environmental factors or inherited factors. In this study, the increase in the mortality from colorectal cancer among Japanese migrants was presumably reflecting the changing dietary and physical activity patterns among migrants, and the rate of colorectal cancer in Japan has increased dramatically since World War II, most likely reflecting changes in lifestyle in the Japanese population. The higher rate of stomach and liver cancer among Japanese in Japan and the decline in first-generation Japanese, and the fact that the risk among second-generation Japanese and whites is similar most likely reflect the influence of an environmental exposure.

Answer 5.12.   **The answer is D.**

Lead-time bias reflects when earlier detection (lead time) did not change outcome. For example, a person receives the diagnosis of lung cancer on screening CT scan in 2008 and subsequently dies of lung cancer in 2010, whereas a person who does not undergo CT screening receives the diagnosis in 2010 and dies of lung cancer in 2010. The outcome is the same, but it would appear that the survival time has increased from 1 to 3 years. Length-time bias refers to the detection of indolent cancers by screening at a higher rate than the more aggressive cancers, resulting in an apparent survival advantage to screening.

Answer 5.13.   **The answer is E.**

The analysis of phenotypic markers, such as proteins, requires a reliable laboratory method of being quantitative (a wide range of measurable concentration), sensitive (able to detect a small amount of the analyte), specific (able to detect only the molecule of interest, no other molecules), reproducible (high precision and low variation), and versatile (easy to use). In addition, appropriate quality assurance procedures during sample processing and testing, as well as control samples in specimen analysis, will be required.

Answer 5.14.   **The answer is B.**

A larger sample size leads to less variability in the data, a tighter confidence interval, and a higher possibility in finding a statistically significant relationship.

Answer 5.15.   **The answer is E.**

The number of lung cancers cases in economically developing countries now exceeds the number in developed countries, but the proportion of all cancer deaths attributable to lung cancer is higher (22%) in developed countries than in developing countries (15%). The percentage of lung cancer cases caused by smoking among men in Europe and North American is higher (90% to 95%), where cigarette smoking has been entrenched for decades. Environmental factors such as exposure to coal smoke, indoor emissions from burning other fuels, exposure to fumes from frying foods at high temperatures, and secondhand smoke are all thought to contribute to the high rate of lung cancer among Chinese women.

Rebecca L. Aft
Jason Keune

Principles of Surgical Oncology

Directions   Each of the numbered items below is followed by lettered answers. Select the ONE lettered answer that is BEST in each case unless instructed otherwise.

QUESTIONS

Question 6.1.   **Bupivacaine, when injected as a local anesthetic, has an expected duration of action of:**

A.   15 to 30 minutes
B.   30 to 90 minutes
C.   120 to 240 minutes
D.   120 to 480 minutes

Question 6.2.   **Epidural anesthesia involves the injection of a local anesthetic agent:**

A.   Into the cerebrospinal fluid, by puncturing the dura between L2 and L4
B.   Into the extradural space within the spinal canal
C.   Into the space outside of the spinal canal, superficial to the ligamentum flavum
D.   Into the subarachnoid space

Question 6.3.   **Which of the following is NOT one of the benefits of inhaled isoflurane compared with its predecessor halothane?**

A.   It is well tolerated as an agent of inhalational induction.
B.   Reduction in cardiac output is minimized.
C.   There is less sensitization to the effects of endogenous catecholamines.
D.   There is lower risk of severe hepatotoxicity.

Corresponding Chapter in *Cancer: Principles & Practice of Oncology*, Eighth Edition: 20 (Principles of Surgical Oncology).

Question 6.4.   An 83-year-old man presents for colon resection after evaluation for microcytic anemia revealed a 3-cm villous adenoma in his cecum. Colonoscopy was performed, and the adenoma was not able to be resected. Biopsy revealed dysplastic changes. No evidence of metastatic disease was seen on computed tomography (CT) of the chest, abdomen, and pelvis. Which of the following statements is TRUE?

    A.   Surgery should be avoided in this patient because of the prohibitive morbidity and mortality in this octogenarian.

    B.   The patient's medical history and physical examination are the best determinants of preoperative risk.

    C.   The patient requires a cardiac stress test and possible cardiac catheterization before surgical resection.

    D.   No additional testing besides routine laboratory testing is required.

Question 6.5.   A 67-year-old man with poorly controlled diabetes, congestive heart failure (CHF) with an ejection fraction of 14%, and Stage III chronic kidney disease is scheduled to undergo pancreaticoduodenectomy. He should be categorized as American Society of Anesthesiologists Class:

    A.   II

    B.   III

    C.   IV

    D.   V

Question 6.6.   A 42-year-old woman presents with a 4-year history of a lump on her right lateral thigh. On examination, she has a firm nodule in her right thigh, approximately 5 cm in size. The mass appears to be in the subcutaneous tissue but is not freely mobile. The patient has no associated neurologic findings. The next appropriate step in management is:

    A.   Perform fine-needle aspiration

    B.   Perform core biopsy

    C.   Perform excisional biopsy

    D.   Obtain magnetic resonance imaging (MRI)

Question 6.7.   A 45-year-old woman with a body mass index (BMI) of 34 is scheduled to undergo Ivor Lewis esophagectomy for a T2N0M0 adenocarcinoma of the distal esophagus. Her relative risk of pulmonary complications after surgery compared with a nonobese patient is approximately:

    A.   0.8 to 1.7

    B.   1.5 to 2.0

    C.   1.7 to 3.0

    D.   2.0 to 4.5

Question 6.8.   The same patient presents to a center regarded as very experienced in minimally invasive surgery. Her esophagectomy is performed laparoscopically. Compared with open esophagectomy, she is expected to have:

    A.   No difference in either lymph node retrieval or 3-year survival

    B.   No difference in lymph node retrieval but a decreased 3-year survival

    C.   Decreased lymph node retrieval but no difference in 3-year survival

    D.   Decreased lymph node retrieval and 3-year survival

Question 6.9.   **The decreased venous return and increased transmitted intrathoracic pressure inherent in laparoscopic surgery are thought to cause which of the following physiologic changes during laparoscopic procedures?**

A. Increased heart rate
B. Decreased cardiac index
C. Decreased systemic vascular resistance
D. Decreased central venous pressure

Question 6.10.   **Retrospective analyses of colon resection for colon cancer have demonstrated that the difference in the rate of recurrence at laparoscopic port sites compared with the rate of recurrence in analogous open procedures is approximately:**

A. 0
B. Greater by 10%
C. Greater by 20%
D. Not known

Question 6.11.   **A 55-year-old man with a several-month history of hemoccult positive stools has recently been diagnosed with gastric cancer by upper endoscopy. Staging CT demonstrates no evidence of intra-abdominal disease. You recommend a staging laparoscopy before definitive resection because:**

A. CT has a high false-negative rate in the staging of most cancers.
B. Carcinomatosis and peritoneal seeding are more accurately diagnosed with laparoscopy.
C. Nontherapeutic laparotomies can be avoided in more than 20% of patients after staging laparoscopy.
D. All of the above.

Question 6.12.   **The benefits of laparoscopy are:**

A. Reduction in postoperative pain
B. Decreased healing time
C. Decreased adhesion formation
D. All of the above

ANSWERS

Answer 6.1.   **The answer is C.**

The duration of action of bupivacaine is 120 to 240 minutes. The duration of action of a local anesthetic is directly related to its vasodilatory capabilities. The addition of epinephrine to a local anesthetic causes localized vasoconstriction, thereby prolonging the duration of the anesthetic effect. Topical anesthesia refers to the application of local anesthetics to the skin or mucous membranes. Local anesthesia involves injecting anesthetic agents directly into the operative field. Peripheral nerve block results from the deposition of a local anesthetic surrounding major nerve trunks.

Answer 6.2.   **The answer is B.**

Epidural anesthesia refers to injection of local anesthetic into the epidural or peridural space. This potential space is bounded by the dura
anteriorly and the ligamentum flavum posteriorly and includes the lymphatics, areolar tissue, and epidural venous plexus. The primary site of
action of the local anesthetic is on the spinal nerve roots that traverse
the space.

Answer 6.3.   **The answer is A.**

Isoflurane, which appeared in 1979, replaced the earlier inhalational
agent halothane. Isoflurane minimized the cardiac depressive effects
known to be caused by fluorinated hydrocarbons, as well as decreased
the arrhythmogenic effect of catecholamines. The incidence of hepatotoxicity is lower with isoflurane. Both isoflurane and halothane have
a foul odor and are therefore poor choices for agents of inhalational
induction.

Answer 6.4.   **The answer is B.**

Surgery in the elderly population is decided on a case-by-case basis. Physiologic age does not always correlate with chronologic age. Approximately
half of surgical morbidity is attributed to perioperative cardiac events.
The American College of Cardiology has defined an algorithm to estimate risk and the need for preoperative testing. Risk is stratified on the
basis of the intrinsic risk of the procedure, the patient's cardiac history,
and the exercise tolerance of the patient. High-risk procedures carry a
risk of cardiac morbidity greater than 4% (noncarotid vascular surgery,
thoracic procedures, abdominal procedures, major head and neck procedures, and emergent procedures). Intermediate-risk procedures (1%
to 4% risk of cardiac morbidity) include carotid surgery, radical prostatectomy, and orthopedic procedures. Low-risk procedures (<1% risk)
include breast surgery and soft tissue biopsies. Patient risk factors include
history of CHF, diabetes, prior myocardial infarction (MI), angina, and
ventricular arrhythmia. These patients should undergo some form of
preoperative risk assessment with cardiac stress testing before high-risk
surgery.

Answer 6.5.   **The answer is C.**

This patient should be classified as American Society of Anesthesiologists
Class IV. A patient with Class IV has an incapacitating systemic disease
that is not correctable by operation, such as organic heart disease with
marked signs of cardiac insufficiency.

Answer 6.6.   **The answer is D.**

Sarcoma must be considered in the differential diagnosis of soft tissue
masses. Imaging by MRI can provide information on size, tumor characteristics, and relationship to adjacent structures. Subsequent tissue sampling is essential to obtain a diagnosis.

Answer 6.7.　　**The answer is A.**

Several prospective cohort studies have contributed to the development of a risk index for postoperative pulmonary complications after surgical procedures. The American Society of Anesthesiologists has summarized these data. The relative risk of pulmonary complications in an obese patient undergoing a thoracic procedure is 0.8 to 1.7.

Answer 6.8.　　**The answer is A.**

A prospective study of 483 patients conducted by Smithers et al (Smithers BM, Cotley DC, Martin I, et al. Comparison of the outcomes between open and minimally invasive esophagectomy. Ann Surg 2007;245(2): 232–240) revealed no differences in lymph node retrieval and 3-year survival between open and laparoscopic procedures.

Answer 6.9.　　**The answer is B.**

A recent study of patients undergoing laparoscopic colectomy for carcinoma demonstrated increased mean arterial pressure, central venous pressure, mean pulmonary artery pressure, pulmonary capillary wedge pressure, and systemic vascular resistance. Cardiac index and ejection fraction decreased significantly, although heart rate remained unchanged.

Answer 6.10.　　**The answer is A.**

Retrospective reviews have demonstrated a wound site recurrence rate of less than 1% in patients undergoing surgery for colon cancer. Port site recurrence rates for a similar population of patients have been reported to be approximately 1%. Port site metastases have been associated with aerosolization caused by the pneumoperitoneum, tumor manipulation, and degree of tumor burden.

Answer 6.11.　　**The answer is D.**

One of the most important aspects of laparoscopic staging is the exclusion of patients from undergoing a major operation by identifying metastatic or unresectable disease (e.g., carcinomatosis), which is easily missed on imaging studies. Undetected metastatic disease has been found in 13% to 57% of patients initially staged with having no metastatic disease by conventional imaging. However, laparoscopy is not yet performed as a routine procedure because many patients are often symptomatic and require palliative resection.

Answer 6.12.　　**The answer is D.**

All of the above are the beneficial effects of laparoscopy. This is attributed to the use of small incisions and lack of retractors holding the incision open. In addition, exposure to CO_2 contributes to a diminished acute phase systemic response, which likely leads to decreased inflammation and pain.

7

Principles of Radiation Oncology

Directions   Each of the numbered items below is followed by lettered answers. Select the ONE lettered answer that is BEST in each case unless instructed otherwise.

QUESTIONS

Question 7.1.   **Which of the following describes the specific pathways for the repair of double-strand DNA breaks?**

A.   The repair may be by homologous recombination (HR) or nonhomologous end-joining (NHEJ) pathway.

B.   The HR repair pathway functions by degrading the single strand at each side of the break and then annealing the two ends.

C.   The NHEJ pathway functions by replicating the missing genetic information from the homologous DNA template.

D.   NHEJ is a minor component of mechanism for repair of double-stranded DNA breaks in mammalian cells.

Question 7.2.   **Which of the following is NOT true about ionizing events in tissues caused by x-rays?**

A.   Radiation dose describes the quantity of energy deposited per mass of tissue.

B.   The fast electrons produced by high-energy x-ray photons can damage deoxyribonucleic acid (DNA) by a direct action.

C.   The relative biological effectiveness (RBE) describes the ratio of doses required to yield an equivalent biologic event.

D.   Indirect action of ionizing radiation where hydroxyl radicals damage target tissues is not commonly seen.

Corresponding Chapter in *Cancer: Principles & Practice of Oncology*, Eighth Edition: 21 (Principles of Radiation Oncology).

Question 7.3.   **Which of the following statements describes the DNA damage from ionizing radiation?**

A. Single-stranded breaks of the DNA are thought to represent the lethal event.
B. The majority of radiation-induced, double-stranded breaks are rejoined in cells within 2 hours.
C. There is essentially no difference between double-stranded rejoining and DNA repair.
D. The efficiency of DNA rejoining is not related to the cell's ability to survive the standard radiotherapy (2 Gy).

Question 7.4.   **Which of the following statements describes the dose-related cellular response to radiation?**

A. In mammalian cells, there is generally a linear relationship between the cell killing and the dose given.
B. The term "D_0" describes the slope of the exponential survival curve and represents a dose required to reduce the surviving fraction to 37%.
C. Both mammalian cells and bacterial cells display "shoulder" in the low-dose region.
D. In general, postirradiation conditions that accelerate the cell division are the ones most favorable to repair of potentially lethal damage.

Question 7.5.   **Which of the following statements is FALSE regarding independent events (4 R's) that occur during fractionated radiotherapy?**

A. Repopulation refers to spontaneous repopulation and induced cell proliferation or recruitment of cells after irradiation.
B. Repair explains the shoulder of the radiation survival curve showing that cells can repair some of the radiation damage.
C. Redistribution explains migration of cells away from an irradiation source.
D. Reoxygenation explains how the proportion of hypoxic cells present in a tumor return to preradiation level.

Question 7.6.   **Which of the following statements is NOT true regarding molecular responses to radiation-induced cellular injury?**

A. The protein p53 appears to have a minor role in activation of apoptosis and cell-cycle arrest after DNA damage.
B. The signaling/surveillance proteins ATM and ATR appear to have central roles in the response pathways.
C. Phosphorylation of p53 is predominantly ATM-dependent after radiation damage, whereas ATR performs it after ultraviolet (UV)-induced damage.
D. Ionizing radiation damage activates several signaling pathways that may contribute to lethality independently of DNA damage.
E. Irradiation leads to induction of tumor necrosis factor (TNF), a protein expression.

Question 7.7. **Nonirradiated cells can express all of the following responses after radiation damage to neighboring cells, EXCEPT:**

A. Gene induction
B. Induction of genomic instability
C. Differentiation
D. Changes in apoptotic potential
E. Double-stranded breaks in DNA

Question 7.8. **Which of the following best describes the modern linear accelerator?**

A. A modern linear accelerator (LINAC) can deliver energies up to 1 MeV.
B. The ^{60}Cobalt teletherapy unit is a megavoltage machine that relies on radioactive cobalt to produce an electron beam.
C. Unlike LINAC, the ^{60}Cobalt unit is always "on" and must be kept in a shielded position until the beam is needed for treatment.
D. The focal point of the gantry's rotation is called the field edge.

Question 7.9. **Which of the following statements describes the role of oxygen in radiation effects?**

A. A greater dose of radiation is required for cell killing in an oxic condition compared with a hypoxic condition.
B. A randomized trial showed that epoetin b improved survival in patients with head and neck cancer.
C. Oxygen need not be present at the time of irradiation for oxygen enhancement of radiotherapy to occur.
D. Hyperbaric oxygen often shows a dramatic increase in curability with standard fractionated radiotherapy.
E. The oxygen enhancement ratio (OER) has more relevance on the exponential portion of the cell survival curve.

Question 7.10. **Which of the following best describes the concept of altered fractionation?**

A. Accelerated fractionation does not reduce the overall treatment time.
B. Hyperfractionation refers to a radiotherapy schedule that uses multiple daily treatments more than 6 hours apart with reduced fraction size and increased number of fractions.
C. A Radiation Therapy Oncology Group (RTOG) 9003 randomized trial showed that standard fractionation treatment was superior to hyperfractionation and accelerated fractionation with concomitant boost used for advanced head and neck squamous cell carcinomas.
D. Continuous hyperfractionated accelerated radiation therapy (CHART) gives a higher total dose than the standard fractionated treatment.

Question 7.11. **Which of the following statements describing interaction of chemother-apy and radiotherapy is FALSE?**

A. Hydroxyurea preferentially kills cells in the radio-resistant phase of the cell cycle (M phase).
B. Radiation appears to increase the cellular uptake of platinum drugs and the number of platinum intermediates.
C. Paclitaxel is thought to synchronize tumor cells in the G2/M phase.
D. Some chemotherapy can recall irradiated volumes by erythema on the skin or by production of pulmonary reactions.

Question 7.12. **Which of the following statements is NOT true regarding modulation of radiation by hyperthermia?**

A. Localized heat treatment can be delivered with microwaves, ultra-sound, or radiofrequency sources of energy.
B. The lethality of hyperthermia is thought to be in part from denatur-ation of proteins.
C. Similar to radiation-induced kill, lethality from heat is most pro-nounced when cells are in the G2/M phase.
D. The temperature 42.5°C seems to be critical, with small increments above this temperature leading to a steep increase in lethality.

Question 7.13. **Which of the following statements best describes the tissue effects from radiation?**

A. Early or acute effects typically occur within months after irradiation.
B. Large a/b ratio has a small "shoulder" in the low-dose portion.
C. The frequencies of late effects depend strongly on radiation fraction size.
D. Typical human tumors and early-responding normal tissues have a small a/b ratio.

Question 7.14. **Which of the following statements is an INCORRECT description of the interaction of x-rays with biologic material?**

A. In modern treatment with greater than 4 MeV photons, photoelec-tric effect dominates the interaction.
B. In photoelectric effect, an incoming x-ray transfers all its energy to an inner orbit electron, which is ejected from the atom. A photon is produced as an outer shell electron fills the vacant hole.
C. In Compton scattering, energy from the x-ray is both absorbed and scattered. The photon emerges with reduced energy and a change in direction.
D. In pair production, an electron and a positron are produced.

Question 7.15. **Which of the following statements describes the depth dose characteristics of radiation?**

A. Higher energy photons deposit more dose to the skin surface.
B. For a given energy, electrons generally penetrate deeper in tissue compared with photons.
C. Electron beams deposit less dose to the skin surface as the incident electron energy increases.
D. Depth of maximum dose increases as the energy of the incident beam increases.

Question 7.16. **Which of the following statements is NOT true regarding brachytherapy?**

A. Isotopes with properties of long half-lives and high energy are used for permanent implants.
B. Relative to external beam energies, the emitted spectra are of low energy.
C. High doses can be delivered within a few centimeters of the source.
D. Half-life is the time required for half of the initial number of nuclei to decay.

Question 7.17. **The following statements describe proton beams and neutron beams used for therapy, EXCEPT:**

A. Charged particles such as protons can be accelerated by an electric field.
B. Neutrons have no charge and interact in matter mainly by generating recoil protons.
C. Proton beams in the range of 50 to 500 MeV have been used.
D. A neutron beam is notable for its characteristic Bragg peak.

Question 7.18. **Which of the following best describes the treatment planning process?**

A. At the time of image acquisition for planning, tumor motion caused by respiration must be determined.
B. Immobilization is not important because it does not add to accuracy.
C. Three-dimensional dose distribution in each patient is easily measured.
D. Intensity-modulated radiation therapy (IMRT) cannot control the shaping of the dose distribution.

ANSWERS

Answer 7.1.   **The answer is A.**

There are two generally accepted mechanisms of repair. They are broadly known as the HR or NHEJ. HR functions by replicating the missing genetic information from the homologous DNA template. NHEJ functions by degrading the single strand at each side of the break and then annealing the two ends in a region of microhomology. The NHEJ may result in loss or gain in genetic information and is mutation prone. Some have suggested that HR and NHEJ have overlapping complementary roles. NHEJ is a dominant mechanism for repairing double-stranded DNA breaks in mammalian cells. Several investigators have demonstrated enhanced radiosensitivity of human cell lines by inhibiting the proteins required for NHEJ.

Answer 7.2.   **The answer is D.**

All other statements are true. The indirect effects of x-rays predominate the biologic effects seen with x-rays. The photons cause ejection of fast electrons. The ejected fast electrons can directly damage the DNA (direct action) or, more commonly, the fast electrons interact with plentiful water molecules to produce hydroxyl radicals ($OH-$), which in turn can damage the biologic target (indirect action).

Answer 7.3.   **The answer is C.**

Although single-stranded and double-stranded breaks are observed from ionizing radiation, it is the double-stranded breaks that are thought to represent the lethal event. Although the majority of the radiation-induced, double-stranded breaks are rejoined in cells within 2 hours after exposure, the process can continue for 24 hours. The DNA repair refers to the correction of the DNA to the original genetic codes, whereas the double-stranded rejoining refers to the joining of the DNA without regard to the original genetic sequence. The efficiency of rejoining of DNA after radiation exposure has been correlated with the portion of cells surviving treatment with 2 Gy.

Answer 7.4.   **The answer is B.**

D_0 is related to the slope of the exponential survival curve and represents a dose that is required to reduce the surviving fraction to 0.37% or 37% of the original population. The smaller D_0 represents more radiosensitivity. Mammalian cell lines display a "shoulder" in the low-dose region and the exponential relation at higher doses. The "shoulder" represents a reduced efficiency of cell killing. The linear quadratic model rather than the linear model best describes the cellular response to radiation. The postirradiation conditions that suppress the cell division are the ones most favorable to potentially lethal damage repair.

Answer 7.5.   **The answer is C.**

Repair explains the shoulder of the radiation survival curve showing that cells can repair some of the radiation damage. The majority of sublethal damage repair occurs within 6 hours after irradiation. Redistribution explains differences in cell-cycle radiation sensitivity, with the mitotic (M) phase being the most sensitive. Cells gradually increase in resistance as they proceed through the late G1 and S phases. Repopulation refers to spontaneous repopulation and induced cell proliferation or recruitment of cells after irradiation. This may occur in some tumors but occurs less than that in normal tissues. Reoxygenation explains how a proportion of hypoxic cells present in a tumor return to preradiation level. Some tumor cells may reoxygenate after radiotherapy, and the proportion of the hypoxic cells that was present before irradiation may be seen.

Answer 7.6.   **The answer is A.**

Phosphorylation of p53 is predominantly ATM-dependent after radiation damage, whereas ATR performs it after UV-induced damage. The protein p53 appears to have a key role in activation of apoptosis and cell-cycle arrest after DNA damage. The chemical inhibitor of p53, a-pifithrin, has been shown to protect mice from lethal doses of total body radiation. Ionizing radiation damage activates several signaling pathways that may contribute to lethality independently of DNA damage. An example includes activation of sphingomyelinase, which hydrolyzes plasma membrane-derived sphingomyelin and produces ceramide. Ceramide can promote apoptosis. Radio resistance can be seen in cells that are sphingomyelinase deficient. Irradiation leads to a rapid activation of the TNF-α receptor and induction of TNF-α protein expression.

Answer 7.7.   **The answer is E.**

The responses of nonirradiated cells appear to be cell-type dependent. This may be mediated by diffusible substances or by cell–cell contact. The double-stranded breaks are seen after cells are directly irradiated.

Answer 7.8.   **The answer is C.**

A modern LINAC can deliver energies up to 25 MeV. The focal point of the gantry's rotation is called the isocenter. The 6^{60}Cobalt teletherapy unit is a megavoltage machine that relies on radioactive cobalt to produce a photon beam. Unlike the LINAC, the ^{60}Cobalt unit is always "on" and must be kept in shielded position until the beam is needed for treatment.

Answer 7.9.   **The answer is E.**

Greater doses of radiation are required for cell killing in hypoxic conditions. The oxygen enhancement is seen more readily during the exponential portion of the survival curve because of the reduced capacity for cells to repair sublethal damage under hypoxic conditions. Tumor cells growing in a physiologic hypoxic condition have reduced capacity to repair sublethal damage. The OER is the ratio of dose required for equivalent cell killing in the absence of oxygen compared with the dose required in the presence of oxygen. The range of OER varies from 2.5 to 3.5. Oxygen must be present at the time of irradiation for oxygen enhancement of radiotherapy to occur. OER is more important for radiation that damages cells via hydroxyl radical intermediates. Hyperbaric oxygen often does not show a dramatic increase in curability with standard fractionated radiotherapy. However, hyperbaric oxygen appears to increase curability in a small number of fractions. A meta-analysis showed that hyperbaric oxygen improves the local control of solid tumors by approximately 10%. Unfortunately, a randomized trial published recently showed that epoetin b did not improve cancer control or survival in patients with head and neck cancer.

Answer 7.10.   **The answer is B.**

Hyperfractionation refers to a radiotherapy schedule that uses multiple daily treatments more than 6 hours apart with reduced fraction size and increased number of fractions. A randomized trial performed by the European Organization for Research and Treatment of Cancer (EORTC) showed that a hyperfractionated regimen was significantly better than standard fractionation in improving local control. Accelerated fractionation reduces the overall treatment time. It delivers the same dose with the same fraction size but in a shorter overall treatment time. An RTOG 9003 randomized trial showed that standard fractionation treatment was inferior to hyperfractionation and accelerated fractionation with concomitant boost used for advanced head and neck squamous cell carcinomas. CHART, as developed at Mt. Vernon Hospital in the United Kingdom, gave a 54 Gy total dose, which is significantly lower than the standard fractionated treatment dose for lung cancer.

Answer 7.11.   **The answer is A.**

Radiation appears to increase the cellular uptake of platinum drugs and increase the number of platinum intermediates. Hydroxyurea preferentially kills cells in the radio-resistant phase of the cell cycle (S phase). The G2/M phase of the cell cycle is the most radiosensitive portion of the cell cycle. Paclitaxel is thought to synchronize tumor cells in the G2/M phase, which is relatively radiosensitive. Some chemotherapy can recall irradiated volumes by erythema on the skin or by the production of pulmonary reactions.

Answer 7.12.   **The answer is C.**

Localized heat treatment can be delivered with microwaves, ultrasound, or radiofrequency sources of energy. The temperature 42.5°C appears to be critical, with small increments above this temperature leading to a steep increase in lethality. The lethality of hyperthermia is thought to be in part from denaturation of proteins. Unlike radiation-induced kill, lethality from heat is most pronounced when cells are in the radio-resistant S phase. When hyperthermia and radiation are combined in vitro, the net effect is greater than additive lethal effect. However, in a clinical setting, the effect appears to be additive or independent.

Answer 7.13. **The answer is C.**

Early or acute effects typically occur within weeks after irradiation. They often occur in tissues that have rapid turnover, and it is thought to result from the depletion of the clonogenic or stem cells within that tissue. The frequencies of late effects depend strongly on radiation fraction size. There are fewer late effects with smaller fraction size. Large a/b ratio has a large "shoulder" in the low-dose portion. The a/b ratio represents the dose at which the quadratic (b) and linear a components of cell kill are equivalent. The dose response to radiation can be described by the formula $S = \exp(-aD - bD2)$, where S is surviving fraction and D represents dose. Typical human tumors and early-responding normal tissues have large a/b ratios (9 to 13 Gy).

Answer 7.14. **The answer is A.**

The relative probabilities of photoelectric, Compton, and pair production interaction depend on the photon energy and the atomic number of the irradiated material. In modern treatment machines with greater than 4 MeV photons, the Compton interactions and pair productions are commonly seen. At diagnostic equipment energy range (25 kvp), photoelectric effect predominates. In photoelectric effect, an incoming x-ray transfers all its energy to an inner orbit electron, which is ejected from the atom. A photon is produced as an outer shell electron fills the vacant hole. In Compton scattering, energy from the x-ray is both absorbed and scattered. The photon emerges with reduced energy and a change in direction. In pair production, an electron and a positron are produced, which then deposit energy through collisions with other electrons. The threshold energy for pair production is 1.02 MeV.

Answer 7.15. **The answer is D.**

Higher energy photons deposit less dose to the skin surface. Thus, it is called the skin-sparing effect of high-energy photons. Depth of maximum dose increases as the energy of the incident beam increases. It is often desirable to use high-energy photons (>10 MeV) to reach deeply located tumors. For a given energy, electrons do not penetrate deeper in tissue compared with photons. It is for this reason that electron beams are often used to treat superficially located tumors such as skin cancer. Electron beams, unlike photons, deposit more dose to the skin surface as the incident electron energy increases.

Answer 7.16. **The answer is A.**

Relative to external beam energies, the emitted spectra are of low energy, but high doses can be delivered within a few centimeters of the source. Isotopes with properties of very short half-lives and low energy are used for permanent implants, such as for prostate cancer treatment with iodine-125 with a half-life of 59.4 days and an x-ray energy of 27 to 35 keV.

Half-life is the time required for half of the initial number of nuclei to decay.

Answer 7.17.   **The answer is D.**

A proton beam is notable for its characteristic Bragg peak. This describes a sharp increase in energy deposition at the end of the proton beam track. Charged particles such as protons can be accelerated by an electric field in the gap between the magnets. Neutrons have no charge and interact in matter mainly by generating recoil protons from hydrogen atoms and nuclear disintegrations. Proton beams in the range of 50 to 500 MeV have been used to treat cancer. The energy of the proton beam can be modulated so that the Bragg peak occurs at a specified depth.

Answer 7.18.   **The answer is A.**

Immobilization is critically important because it adds to the accuracy of daily setup and treatment. A planning computed tomography (CT) scan is obtained after immobilization has been completed. At the time of image acquisition for planning, tumor motion caused by respiration must be determined. The planning volume must account for respiratory movement and uncertainty of tumor position. Three-dimensional dose distribution in each patient is not easily measured, and it must be predicted from computer calculation. IMRT can have a high degree of control on the shaping of the dose distribution. The computer determines the intensity profiles to achieve the desired dose distribution.

Sujatha Murali
Suresh S. Ramalingam

CHAPTER

8

Principles of Medical Oncology

Directions   Each of the numbered items below is followed by lettered answers. Select the ONE lettered answer that is BEST in each case unless instructed otherwise.

QUESTIONS

Question 8.1.   **Historically, the first chemotherapeutic drugs used in the clinical setting were:**

A. Anthracyclines
B. Epidermal growth factor receptor inhibitors
C. Antimetabolites
D. Alkylating agents

Question 8.2.   **In children with lymphoblastic leukemia, folic acid was observed to:**

A. Cause disease proliferation
B. Cause disease regression
C. Have no effect
D. Improve survival

Question 8.3.   **Antimetabolite chemotherapeutic agents include all of the following, EXCEPT:**

A. Gemcitabine
B. Fluoropyrimidines
C. Mitoxantrone
D. Cytarabine

Question 8.4.   **In a subset of patients with advanced or metastatic disease, which of the following has curative potential with primary induction chemotherapy?**

A. Germ cell cancer
B. Non–small cell lung cancer
C. Gastric cancer
D. Colorectal cancer

Corresponding Chapter in *Cancer: Principles & Practice of Oncology*, Eighth Edition: 22 (Principles of Medical Oncology).

Question 8.5.   **The goals of therapy in incurable, advanced, metastatic disease include all of the following, EXCEPT:**

A.   Palliate tumor-related symptoms
B.   Eradicate all evidence of cancer
C.   Improve quality of life
D.   Prolong time to tumor progression

Question 8.6.   **Neoadjuvant chemotherapy is commonly used in patients with:**

A.   Metastatic disease
B.   Localized cancers for which other treatment modalities exist and may be curative
C.   Hematologic malignancies
D.   Pancreatic cancer

Question 8.7.   **All of the following are true concerning the role of adjuvant chemotherapy, EXCEPT:**

A.   Risk reduction of local recurrence
B.   Risk reduction of distant recurrence
C.   Primary therapy instead of surgery and/or radiation
D.   Prolongation of disease-free and overall survival in osteogenic sarcoma

Question 8.8.   **In patients with hormone-sensitive breast cancer, adjuvant Tamoxifen is administered for:**

A.   5 years
B.   3 years
C.   2 years
D.   1 year

Question 8.9.   **The most important indicator of the effectiveness of chemotherapy is:**

A.   Achievement of a minor response
B.   Achievement of a partial response
C.   Achievement of a complete response
D.   Achievement of stable disease

Question 8.10.   **A partial response is defined as:**

A.   At least a 50% reduction in measurable tumor mass
B.   At least a 10% reduction in measurable tumor mass
C.   Improvement in quality of life
D.   Improvement in survival

Question 8.11.   **All of the following are true concerning neoadjuvant chemotherapy, EXCEPT:**

A.   The tumor mass can act as a biologic marker for chemosensitivity.
B.   Surgical resection may be able to spare vital organs.
C.   It may be effective in treating micrometastatic disease.
D.   It does not affect lymph node staging at the time of resection.

Question 8.12. **In early-stage colon cancer treated with adjuvant chemotherapy, the majority of relapses occur:**

A. Within the first 5 years
B. Within the first 3 years
C. Within the first 2 years
D. Within the first year

Question 8.13. **Gompertzian kinetics are characterized by:**

A. Clinically undetectable tumors are at their lowest growth fraction.
B. The growth fraction is stable over time.
C. The growth fraction increases exponentially with time.
D. The growth fraction decreases exponentially with time.

Question 8.14. **Combination chemotherapy was initially developed to treat:**

A. Lung cancer
B. Breast cancer
C. Hematologic malignancies
D. Sarcoma

Question 8.15. **All of the following are true regarding an intermittent treatment approach, EXCEPT:**

A. Salvage therapies should show a good response.
B. Sufficient time is needed between the termination of induction chemotherapy and progressive disease.
C. A majority of responses should be achieved during the induction chemotherapy period.
D. Reinitiation of the induction chemotherapy is not indicated.

Question 8.16. **The importance of dose intensity in the adjuvant setting has been confirmed in which of the following:**

A. Breast cancer
B. Pancreatic cancer
C. Non-Hodgkin's lymphoma
D. Multiple myeloma

Question 8.17. **Dose-dense chemotherapy was developed after the observation that:**

A. The growth of cells is significantly lower in the early part of the growth curve.
B. The log cell kill is higher in smaller volume tumors, resulting in more rapid growth between chemotherapy cycles.
C. Growth between chemotherapy cycles is halted.
D. More frequent administration of chemotherapy led to less toxicity.

Question 8.18.   In most cases, normal bone marrow and gastrointestinal (GI) precursor cells are able to counteract the effects of cytotoxic chemotherapy because:

A.   They are not exposed to the chemotherapeutic agent.
B.   They have intact mechanisms for apoptosis and cell-cycle arrest.
C.   They have rapid turnover.
D.   They possess resistance mechanisms.

Question 8.19.   All of the following are true concerning p53, EXCEPT:

A.   It is a tumor suppressor gene.
B.   It is a potent inducer of apoptosis.
C.   It causes S phase arrest in the cell cycle.
D.   It can be protective against chemotherapy cytotoxicity.

Question 8.20.   Drug resistance in advanced tumors is thought to be due to:

A.   Mutations in important genes in cell-cycle regulation
B.   Drug-specific spontaneous mutations
C.   Wild-type p53
D.   Low tumor growth rate

Question 8.21.   The final stage of the programmed cell death pathway is mediated by:

A.   Bcl-2
B.   p53
C.   Tumor necrosis factor (TNF)
D.   Caspase cascade

Question 8.22.   Imatinib inhibits all of the following, EXCEPT:

A.   Epidermal growth factor receptor (EGFR)
B.   C-kit
C.   Platelet-derived growth factor
D.   Bcr-abl

Question 8.23.   Cetuximab use in colorectal cancer is characterized by:

A.   Approval in the first-line setting
B.   Limited utility as monotherapy
C.   High toxicity
D.   Response rates of 21% to 23% when used with irinotecan

Question 8.24.   In multiple myeloma, bortezomib causes all of the following, EXCEPT:

A.   Cell-cycle arrest
B.   Apoptosis
C.   Restoration of chemosensitivity
D.   Increased adherence of myeloma cells to bone marrow stroma

Question 8.25. **Cyclin-dependent kinases are inhibited by:**

A. Bortezomib
B. Cetuximab
C. Flavopiridol
D. Trastuzumab

Question 8.26. **All of the following are limitations of the RECIST criteria, EXCEPT:**

A. Bone only disease is difficult to measure.
B. Partial responses are not taken into account.
C. Tumor necrosis after therapy may actually increase the size of a mass.
D. There may be several nonmeasurable sites of tumor involvement.

Question 8.27. **Computed tomography (CT) contrast perfusion and dynamic contrast magnetic resonance imaging (MRI) may be useful in evaluating:**

A. Response to alkylating agents
B. Response to antiangiogenic agents
C. Degree of tumor necrosis
D. Overall survival

Question 8.28. **Which of the following is true regarding the use of time to progression as an end point in clinical trials?**

A. Uses a smaller sample size when compared with using overall survival as an end point.
B. Not confounded by subsequent therapies.
C. The study can be completed in a shorter amount of time.
D. All of the above.

ANSWERS

Answer 8.1. **The answer is D.**

Alkylating agents were first used as antineoplastic agents after observing bone marrow and lymphoid hypoplasia in soldiers exposed to nitrogen mustard in World War II.

Answer 8.2. **The answer is A.**

Folic acid has been observed to have a significant proliferative effect in children with lymphoblastic leukemia. This led to the development of folic acid analogues as antineoplastic agents.

Answer 8.3. **The answer is C.**

Fluoropyrimidines, gemcitabine, and cytarabine are considered antimetabolites because of their ability to inhibit the normal pathways involved in purine and pyrimidine synthesis. They are the first examples of "targeted" therapy. Mitoxantrone is an anthracycline.

Answer 8.4.   **The answer is A.**

Germ cell cancers are curable with primary induction chemotherapy in a subset of patients presenting with advanced or metastatic disease. In the metastatic setting, non–small cell lung cancer, gastric cancer, and colorectal cancer are not considered curable with conventional chemotherapy alone.

Answer 8.5.   **The answer is B.**

In most cases, the goals of chemotherapy in patients with advanced or metastatic malignancies include palliation of tumor-related symptoms, improvement in quality of life, and prolongation of time to tumor progression. Eradication of all evidence of disease, although it may occur, is not generally the goal of therapy in this setting.

Answer 8.6.   **The answer is B.**

Neoadjuvant chemotherapy is used in a variety of locally advanced solid tumors in an effort to confer possible future surgical resectability. Chemotherapy is typically not used in the neoadjuvant setting in hematologic malignancies, metastatic disease, or pancreatic cancer.

Answer 8.7.   **The answer is C.**

Adjuvant chemotherapy is used as an adjunct to surgery and/or radiation to reduce the risk of local or distant recurrence from occult micrometastatic disease. Randomized Phase III data support the use of adjuvant chemotherapy in breast cancer, colorectal cancer, non–small cell lung cancer, gastric cancer, Wilms' tumor, and osteogenic sarcoma.

Answer 8.8.   **The answer is A.**

The standard length of therapy for adjuvant tamoxifen is 5 years. Tamoxifen is cytostatic rather than cytocidal, so long-term therapy should be given.

Answer 8.9.   **The answer is C.**

The most important indicator of the effectiveness of chemotherapy is the rate of complete response. Despite improvements in response rates and overall survival in certain metastatic diseases, unless a complete response is achieved with chemotherapy, the patient is not considered cured.

Answer 8.10.   **The answer is A.**

A partial response is defined as at least a 50% improvement in measurable tumor mass. Although there are data to suggest that quality of life and survival may improve when a partial response is achieved, these are qualitative measures.

Answer 8.11.   **The answer is D.**

Complete extent of disease may not be evident at the time of surgery when chemotherapy is used in the neoadjuvant setting. Because chemotherapy may treat micrometastatic disease, lymph node status at surgery may not be reflective of prechemotherapy involvement with tumor.

Answer 8.12.   **The answer is B.**

The majority of relapses in early-stage colon cancer treated with adjuvant chemotherapy occur within the first 3 years. Therefore, adjuvant trials may use 3-year disease-free survival as the primary end point.

Answer 8.13.   **The answer is D.**

Gompertzian kinetics provides a model of tumor growth whereby the growth fraction of a tumor decreases exponentially over time. Clinically undetectable tumors are at their highest growth fraction. Therefore, chemotherapy would result in a significantly higher fractional cell kill.

Answer 8.14.   **The answer is C.**

Combination chemotherapy was initially used to treat hematologic malignancies. After success with leukemias and lymphomas, combinations began to be used to treat solid tumors.

Answer 8.15.   **The answer is D.**

Reinitiation of the original induction chemotherapeutic agent is possible if there is a good response.

Answer 8.16.   **The answer is A.**

In stage II node-positive breast cancer, a large study confirmed the importance of increased dose intensity and impact on survival. Conversely, dose reduction in the adjuvant setting for breast cancer resulted in decreased relapse-free survival in one study.

Answer 8.17.   **The answer is B.**

The growth of cells is significantly faster in the early part of the growth curve enabling chemotherapy to cause a greater log cell kill. Dose-dense chemotherapy, by administering cytotoxic drugs more frequently, can produce greater effects on smaller volume tumors.

Answer 8.18.   **The answer is B.**

Normal bone marrow and GI precursor cells possess intact genetic machinery to undergo apoptosis, repair DNA damage, and halt cell-cycle progression. Therefore, cells that have been damaged by chemotherapy undergo programmed cell death and are not allowed to continue on through the cell cycle.

Answer 8.19.   **The answer is C.**

p53 is a tumor suppressor gene that mediates apoptosis in cells with DNA damage. It plays a role in G1 and G2 arrest of the cell cycle after exposure to cytotoxic agents.

Answer 8.20.   **The answer is A.**

Recent evidence has suggested that mechanisms of drug resistance are due to gene mutations in cell-cycle regulatory pathways rather than drug-specific mutations. Wild-type p53 acts as a tumor suppressor of the mdr-1 gene. Increasing growth rates may lead to increased drug resistance as the result of more rapid entry of cells into the cell cycle.

Answer 8.21.   **The answer is D.**

Caspase activation occurs through the activity of the intrinsic and extrinsic pathways of apoptosis. Bcl-2 is involved in the intrinsic pathway, and TNF mediates the extrinsic pathway. p53 is a tumor suppressor gene involved in the early activation of the programmed cell death pathway.

Answer 8.22.   **The answer is A.**

Imatinib inhibits bcr-abl, platelet-derived growth factor (PDGF), and c-kit. It is used to treat chronic myeloid leukemia (CML) and GI stromal tumors that express the c-kit tyrosine kinase.

Answer 8.23.   **The answer is D.**

Cetuximab is a chimeric antibody with promising activity in colorectal cancer and other solid tumors. Currently, it is used in the second or third-line setting, either alone or in combination with chemotherapy. In irinotecan-resistant patients, reported overall response rates with the cetuximab/irinotecan combination are 21% to 23%. Toxicity is usually manageable and is mostly related to rash.

Answer 8.24.   **The answer is D.**

Bortezomib is a proteosome inhibitor approved for use in multiple myeloma. Mechanisms of action include cell-cycle arrest, apoptosis induction, and restoration of chemosensitivity. It also causes decreased adherence of myeloma cells to the bone marrow stroma.

Answer 8.25.   **The answer is C.**

Overexpression of cyclin-dependent kinases can lead to inhibition of the Rb gene, a key tumor suppressor. Flavopiridol acts as a cyclin-dependent kinase inhibitor and may also have antiangiogenic properties.

Answer 8.26.   **The answer is B.**

The RECIST criteria use evaluation of tumor size to define a response. Limitations include the inability to measure the extent of response in sites with unmeasurable tumor, such as pleural and ascitic fluid, bone only disease, and leptomeningeal disease.

Answer 8.27.   **The answer is B.**

CT contrast perfusion has been studied in assessing blood flow to rectal tumors treated with bevacizumab. The functionality of vascular endothelial growth factor receptor blockers has also been studied using dynamic-contrast MRI. The utility of these tests in assessing response to alkylating agents, tumor necrosis, or effect on overall survival is not known.

Answer 8.28.   **The answer is D.**

Time to tumor progression as an end point for studies involving meta-static cancer has several advantages over using overall survival: Sample size may be smaller, subsequent therapies do not confound the data, and the study may be able to be completed in a shorter amount of time.

Principles of Immunotherapy

Directions	Each of the numbered items below is followed by lettered answers. Select the ONE lettered answer that is BEST in each case unless instructed otherwise.

QUESTIONS

Question 9.1.   **Which of the following types of immunity is most responsible for the host response to tumor development?**

A.   Humoral immunity
B.   B-cell–mediated immunity
C.   T-cell–mediated immunity
D.   Antibody-mediated immunity

Question 9.2.   **Currently, what is the proposed mechanism for using immunotherapy to destroy cancer cells?**

A.   Develop antibodies to target growth factors on cancer cells
B.   Increase levels of immune lymphocytes
C.   Develop antibodies to directly destroy the cancer cells
D.   Increase levels of antigen-presenting cells

Question 9.3.   **Which of the following is NOT an approach to identify antigens involved on tumor cells?**

A.   Developing antibodies to identified peptides and assessing presentation on the cancer cell surface
B.   Developing tumor-reactive T cells to detect identified peptides on cancer cell surface
C.   Using T cells to assess cytokine release or lysis when present with cancer cells
D.   Using antisera from patients with cancer to screen cancer DNA libraries

Corresponding Chapter in *Cancer: Principles & Practice of Oncology,* Eighth Edition: 23 (Principles of Immunotherapy).

Question 9.4.   **Which of the following is an example of a nonmutated testis antigen?**

A. gp100
B. PRAME
C. CDK4
D. NY-ESO-1

Question 9.5.   **Which of the following has NOT been a target for the development of reactive T cells?**

A. Prostate-specific antigen (PSA)
B. Carcinoembryonic antigen (CEA)
C. p53
D. Epidermal growth factor receptor (EGFR)

Question 9.6.   **Which of the following types of cancers is most associated with a viral exposure?**

A. Colon cancer
B. Acute myelogenous leukemia
C. Hepatocellular carcinoma
D. Lung cancer

Question 9.7.   **Which of the following best describes the role of the human papilloma virus (HPV) vaccine in cervical cancer?**

A. Prevents the development of cervical cancer in all patients
B. Induces regression of cervical cancer tumors
C. Prevents the development of HPV16 and 18
D. Prevents the development of cervical cancer in patients with HPV infections

Question 9.8.   **Which of the following is the proposed mechanism for development of hepatocellular carcinoma secondary to hepatitis B or C?**

A. Hepatitis B virus (HBV) produces oncogenic proteins that result in transformation into malignancy.
B. Increases in the number of somatic mutations in normal hepatocytes.
C. Inhibition of normal immune responses to hepatitis infections.
D. HBV or hepatitis C virus (HCV) infections lead to cirrhosis, which develops into hepatocellular carcinoma.

Question 9.9.   **Which of the following is TRUE of the tumor microenvironment?**

A. T cells in the peripheral blood have functional impairment.
B. Expression of lysine is found in myeloid cells, which results in downregulation of T-cell receptor (TCR) zeta-chain expression.
C. Monocytes express Gr-1 molecules, leading to upregulation of T cells.
D. Tumors secrete granulocyte-macrophage colony-stimulating factor (GM-CSF), leading to an accumulation of CD34+ suppressor cells.

Question 9.10.   **Which of the following is NOT an approach to cancer immunotherapy?**

A.   Passive transfer of activated immune cells with antitumor activity
B.   Active immunization
C.   Active transfer of activated immune cells
D.   Nonspecific stimulation of immune reactions

Question 9.11.   **Which of the following results in inhibition of T cells?**

A.   CTLA-4
B.   CD28
C.   B7-1
D.   B7-2

Question 9.12.   **Of 1306 vaccine treatments, what is the overall objective response rate to vaccine treatment?**

A.   3.3%
B.   10.6%
C.   20.4%
D.   49.2%

Question 9.13.   **Which of the following is NOT an example of active immunization?**

A.   Whole cell vaccines
B.   Heat shock proteins
C.   Natural killer (NK) cell vaccines
D.   Dendritic cell vaccines

Question 9.14.   **What is the purpose of adoptive cell transfer (ACT) therapies?**

A.   Decreasing the number of reactive T-cells ex vivo and transfer back to the patient
B.   Increasing the number of cytokines ex vivo and transfer back to the patient
C.   Activating and expanding self/tumor-reactive T cells and transfer back to the patient
D.   Modulating CD4+ tumor-specific T cells before transferring back to the patient

Question 9.15.   **What is the main mechanism of the graft-versus-leukemia effect demonstrated after a donor lymphocyte infusion?**

A.   T cells within the lymphocytes recognize target antigens on residual tumor cells.
B.   Enhancing the presence of killer inhibitory receptors (KIRs) recognized by donor NK cells.
C.   Lack of recognition of minor histocompatibility antigens within hematopoietic cells.
D.   Increases in CD8+ cells that recognize target antigens on tumor cells.

Question 9.16.   **What is the major limitation of using antibody-based therapies against tumors that overexpress CEA?**

A.   Delivery of the antibody to the tumor
B.   Penetration of the tumor tissue
C.   Invasion of normal CEA-expressing tissue
D.   Stabilization of the antibody

Question 9.17.   **Which of the following most correctly defines immunoediting?**

A.   Observation by the immune system for development of outgrowth of tumors.
B.   Selective pressure by immune systems leads to outgrowth of mutated tumor variants.
C.   Development of mechanisms by the tumor to prevent recognition by the immune system.
D.   Use of cytokine release to inhibit response by T cells.

ANSWERS

Answer 9.1.   **The answer is C.**

Initially it was thought that the action of antibodies or humoral immunity was mainly responsible for the response to malignant cell development. However, it has been discovered that malignant cell development is closely related to the cellular arm of the immune response, specifically a response to T cells. B cells do not play a major role in the immune response to tumor cells.

Answer 9.2.   **The answer is B.**

For existing malignancies, the main mechanism for immunotherapy is to try to increase the level of immune lymphocytes. These immune lymphocytes would be responsible for recognizing the cancer antigens and destroying the cancer cells. Although the development of antibodies that target growth factors on cancer cells may help in reducing the overall tumor burden, this does not work on directly destroying the cancer cells.

Answer 9.3.   **The answer is A.**

There are three methodologies for identifying tumor antigens that are present on the surface of the cancer cells. The first approach is using T cells that have a known ability to recognize intact cancer cells and assessing this by cytokine release or lysis in culture. The second approach is using a "reverse immunology" technique where T cells are generated by sensitization with peptides from proteins previously described. These T cells are then used to test the ability to detect intact cancer cells and to determine if the peptides are found on the surface of the cancer cell. The final approach is to use antisera from patients with known cancer and compare them with cancer DNA libraries already constructed. The development of antibodies has not been used to detect antigens on the cell surface.

Answer 9.4.   **The answer is D.**

Cancer testis antigens are expressed in the testes, placenta, or both, but are not usually found in other tissues. There are two main gene families that make up the cancer testis antigens: MAGE and NY-ESO. These antigens are found in many tumor expression patterns.

Answer 9.5.   **The answer is D.**

Reverse immunology has been used to develop reactive T cells to commonly overexpressed gene products found in certain types of cancer. Targets of this technique have been CEA, PSA, and Her-2/neu. p53 is often overexpressed in many cancer types. One of the difficulties in using p53 is the common mutations that are found and the wide expression of p53 in normal cellular tissues. Although EGFR has been used in the development of some tyrosine kinase inhibitors, it has not been used in the development of reactive T cells.

Answer 9.6.   **The answer is C.**

Genital and hepatic cancers are most commonly associated with viral exposure and infection. Cervical cancer is associated with HPV infections, whereas hepatitis is a risk factor for the development of hepatocellular carcinoma.

Answer 9.7.   **The answer is C.**

The HPV vaccines that have been developed protect women from contracting the strands of HPV that are commonly associated with the development of cervical cancer: HPV 16 and 18. This vaccine will not prevent cervical cancer in everyone, because only 70% of cervical cancer is related to HPV. If a patient already has cervical cancer, it will not provide a tumor response, and if the patient has already contracted HPV16 or 18, it will not offer any additional protection to the patient.

Answer 9.8.   **The answer is B.**

Unlike HPV infections, HBV and HCV infections do not seem to produce oncogenic proteins that lead to transformation into carcinoma. It is thought that the majority of the liver damage results from immune responses directed against HBV-infected cells and inflammation. There is an increased cell turnover in chronic hepatitis infections that could lead to an increase in the amount of somatic mutations in the normal hepatocytes, thus leading to an increased risk of carcinoma.

Answer 9.9.   **The answer is D.**

Several models have demonstrated impairment of the immune system within the tumor microenvironment. Although the T cells within the tumor show impairment, it has been shown that peripheral T cells do not have the same dysfunctionality. Expression of arginase within myeloid cells has been shown to downregulate TCR zeta-chain expression and lead to T-cell function impairment. Myeloid suppressor cells have been discovered to secrete GM-CSF, resulting in an accumulation of CD34+ suppressor cells.

Answer 9.10.   **The answer is C.**

The main approaches to cancer immunotherapy involve stimulation of effector cells, inhibition of regulatory cells, active immunization, and passive transfer of activated immune cells with antitumor activity.

Answer 9.11.   **The answer is A.**

When CTLA-4 is engaged on the T cell, the T-cell function is impaired. This is an example of a nonantigen specific therapy. When CD28 is engaged, T cells are stimulated. B7-1 and B7-2 are ligands that are costimulatory on the T cells.

Answer 9.12.   **The answer is A.**

The results of treatment with cancer vaccines have been very low. Of 1306 vaccine treatments, the objective response rate is only 3.3%. The objective response rate used has been criticized by many, suggesting that the response rate may be even lower than 3.3%.

Answer 9.13.   **The answer is C.**

There are multiple active immunization approaches that have been explored for cancer therapy, such as whole cell vaccines, dendritic cell vaccines, and heat shock proteins. NK cell therapy has been explored as a passive immunological therapy.

Answer 9.14.   **The answer is C.**

Adoptive cell transfer (ACT) therapies function by stimulating T cells ex vivo by activating and expanding self/tumor-reactive T cells before transfer back to the patient. CD8+ T cells have been subject to much research because they are potent effectors of the adaptive tumor response. CD4+ T cells are more controversial, because they can either help or hinder antitumor immune responses.

Answer 9.15.   **The answer is A.**

The graft-versus-leukemia effect from donor lymphocyte infusions is thought to be due to the increase in recognition of target antigens on the residual tumor cells. This will result in ultimate tumor cell kill. Lack of presence of KIRs recognized by donor NK cells confers a better response and more graft-versus-leukemia effect.

Answer 9.16.   **The answer is B.**

Antibodies directed at the glycoprotein CEA have not been successful in the treatment of solid tumors. This is mainly because of the lack of penetration of the antibody into the tumor tissue in vivo.

Answer 9.17. **The answer is C.**

Immunoediting is a mechanism where the tumor develops mechanisms that prevent the immune system from recognizing the tumor and responding appropriately. Immunosurveillance is the process of the immune system observing for the development of malignancies. Immune escape is the process of exerting selective pressure by the immune system that leads to outgrowth of mutated tumor variants, ultimately leading to the loss of recognition by the immune system.

Principles of Health Services Research

Directions   Each of the numbered items below is followed by lettered answers. Select the ONE lettered answer that is BEST in each case unless instructed otherwise.

QUESTIONS

Question 10.1.   **Health services research focuses on "effectiveness" of care, rather than "efficacy." Which of the following is TRUE regarding "effectiveness"?**

A. Effectiveness will vary geographically.
B. Effectiveness can be measured by the results of randomized clinical trials.
C. Effectiveness research cannot be funded by the National Institutes of Health.
D. Effectiveness of care increases with cost of care.

Question 10.2.   **Which of the following is NOT a common difficulty in conducting health services research?**

A. Grouping patients on the basis of site or mechanism of care delivery introduces selection bias.
B. It is difficult to identify confounders, patient characteristics that cannot be measured but correlate with both the outcome and the primary predictor.
C. Obtaining informed consent increases the cost of studies.
D. Groups to which patients are assigned are heterogeneous.

Question 10.3.   **Which of the following is NOT true regarding the Surveillance, Epidemiology, and End Results (SEER) registry?**

A. Initial patient and disease characteristics from the time of cancer diagnosis are obtained from qualified hospital registries.
B. Subsequent treatments and clinical outcomes are integrated into the SEER registry.
C. SEER data can be linked with Medicare claims to provide additional details regarding patients' treatments.
D. SEER data are correlated with population bases to allow for estimates of incidence rates.

Corresponding Chapter in *Cancer: Principles & Practice of Oncology*, Eighth Edition: 24 (Principles of Health Services Research).

Question 10.4.   The quality care of health care is most frequently measured by all of the following, EXCEPT:

A. Practice according to established guidelines
B. Appropriate certifications and credentialing of personnel
C. Availability of specific services or technologies
D. Clinical outcomes, such as survival or quality of life

Question 10.5.   Which of the following is NOT true regarding the association between outcomes and high-volume centers?

A. The strongest association between cancer surgery and outcomes is with high-risk procedures such as pancreatectomy and esophagectomy.
B. Medicare outcomes data do not substantiate improved outcomes for lower-risk cancer surgeries at high-volume centers.
C. Differences in 30-day mortality between hospitals approach 10% for some procedures.
D. Suggestions of improved outcomes at high-volume centers are subject to confounders, such as patient selection.

Question 10.6.   Why are patient-reported outcomes an important end point in oncology research?

A. Cancer treatments often have a large impact on overall survival.
B. Cancer treatment decisions are often straightforward.
C. Cancer treatments that are curative need to be advanced.
D. Cancer treatments often have significant toxicity.

Question 10.7.   Studies of patient-recorded outcomes require "instruments," such as surveys and symptom diaries. A good instrument should show all of the following, EXCEPT:

A. Subjectivity: Allows patients to elaborate on symptoms.
B. Variability: A broad range of responses.
C. Internal consistency: Answers to questions regarding similar symptoms correlate well with each other.
D. Reliability: Repeat administration on the same patient gives similar results.

Question 10.8.   Which of the following is NOT true regarding "health-related quality of life" (HRQOL) instruments?

A. They are limited because they are not cancer specific.
B. They are broad measures that incorporate several different domains.
C. The most common domains include physical, psychologic, and social functioning.
D. They evaluate the impact of illness AND treatment on these domains.

Question 10.9. **The burden of symptoms on a patient can be quantified by measures of "utility." Which of the following is TRUE regarding "utility" in this sense?**

A. It measures the impact of disease on a patient's independence.
B. It compares a patient's preference for a specific disease state compared with perfect health.
C. It measures the burden of relieving the symptoms on the health care system.
D. It specifically refers to a patient's evaluation of his/her own disease.

Question 10.10. **Which of the following is NOT true regarding the costs of healthcare in the United States?**

A. Total annual healthcare expenditures are approximately $2 trillion, or $7000 per person.
B. Approximately 30% of healthcare expenses occur in the last year of life.
C. The costs associated with cancer care are estimated to be 15% of overall medical expenses and 30% of Medicare expenses.
D. Cancer pharmaceuticals account for 40% of all Medicare pharmaceutical spending.

Question 10.11. **Newer, targeted biologic agents are most likely to have what effect on the cost of cancer care?**

A. Decrease costs by postponing death and more expensive medical interventions
B. Decrease costs by reducing toxicities and turning cancer into a "chronic disease"
C. Increase costs by turning cancer into a "chronic disease"
D. Increase costs by increasing toxicities

Question 10.12. **Which of the following is NOT true regarding methods of assessing the economic impact of medical treatments?**

A. Cost-minimization analysis takes into account the indirect costs that patients experience (e.g., changes in quality of life) and seeks to minimize these.
B. Cost-effectiveness analysis compares cost with a relevant clinical variable, such as cost per year of life.
C. Cost-utility analysis compares cost with quality-adjusted-life-years (QALYs) such that the toxicities of therapies and the quality of life in the setting of a chronic illness can be weighed along with the benefit.
D. Cost-benefit analysis assigns a dollar amount to a QALY, so that two costs may be compared directly. This requires assigning a monetary value to a quality-adjusted year of life.

Question 10.13.   **Assume a new drug for metastatic breast cancer is expensive but claims to reduce overall costs. Which of the following is NOT true regarding comparing the costs of a new drug with a current standard?**

A. Fixed costs may be higher with the new drug.
B. Indirect costs for the patient may be lower if the infusion time is less, and therefore patients have to pay less for parking or have fewer premedications to purchase.
C. Costs will vary on the basis of perspective, for example, the infusion center may experience fewer costs, but home-health costs may increase.
D. Late toxicities must be compared with gain, a true comparison of the costs.

Question 10.14.   **Cost-benefit is frequently modeled as dollars per QALY. Which is NOT true regarding this method of modeling?**

A. The cost of hemodialysis ($50,000 per QALY) is frequently used as a standard for what society in the United States is willing to fund.
B. In less affluent countries, the threshold of society support is often correlated with per capita gross domestic product (GDP).
C. The legislation that established Medicare prohibits the consideration of cost in determining coverage.
D. Insurers frequently incorporate these types of modeling in determining coverage.

ANSWERS

Answer 10.1.   **The answer is A.**

"Effectiveness" is the real-world measure of the delivery of health care. Although results of clinical trials can show the potential "efficacy" of therapies, delivery systems limit the real-world effectiveness of any intervention. Effectiveness varies on the basis of multiple social and societal factors and is the subject of extensive federally funded research.

Answer 10.2.   **The answer is C.**

Although health services research is usually observational, and not prospective or randomized, this does not imply that a hypothesis cannot be tested to determine causal relationships. Any grouping of subjects will introduce selection bias and confounders. As much as possible, factors can be controlled by multivariate analyses, but confounders are by definition not measured. Although rare health services studies are prospective and require informed consent, more often they sample established datasets and do not require additional informed consent.

Answer 10.3.   **The answer is B.**

SEER provides adequate baseline information for most observational studies and is valuable in that it can be linked to Medicare claims data for treatment details and correlated to populations to allow for estimates of incidence rates. However, one limitation of SEER is that limited longitudinal follow-up information is available in the registry.

Answer 10.4.   **The answer is D.**

Quality can be measured by "structural" metrics, which include characteristics of organizations and providers, as well as by "process" metrics,
which are usually defined as adherence to established clinical guidelines.
Only rarely are clinical measures used to evaluate quality of care delivery.

Answer 10.5.   **The answer is B.**

Medicare data have been used to substantiate better outcomes for most
cancer-related surgeries at high-volume centers compared with lower
volume centers. This association is strongest for the highest-risk procedures, in which 30-day mortality differences sometimes approach 10%.
Such data are confounded by patient selection, in that healthier patients
may be more likely to travel to tertiary or higher-volume centers.

Answer 10.6.   **The answer is D.**

Because many cancer treatments often have significant toxicity with only
modest impact on overall survival, outcomes of interest to patients, including symptoms and quality of life, are an important end point for
clinical research. Increasing knowledge in this area can facilitate what
are often complex and not straightforward treatment decisions. In areas
of cancer treatment where cure is possible or clinical benefit is striking,
patient-reported outcomes may play less of a role.

Answer 10.7.   **The answer is A.**

A useful instrument is sufficiently variable, internally consistent, and reliable. Subjectivity is not a desirable characteristic.

Answer 10.8.   **The answer is A.**

Health-related quality of life instruments are a particular type of patient-
reported outcome measure that incorporates a variety of domains. They
evaluate how disease and its treatment affect areas such as physical, psychologic, and social functioning. A variety of instruments can be used,
several of which are specific for cancer.

Answer 10.9.   **The answer is B.**

"Utility" as used in health services research is synonymous with "preference" and enables comparisons between specific disease states. For example, living with chronic cancer pain can be compared with living in
perfect health and assigned a numeric score. These rankings can be
assessed by patients, families, healthcare workers, or healthy "jurors,"
with varying usefulness.

Answer 10.10.   **The answer is C.**

Healthcare expenditures in all areas have rapidly increased in the past
15 years, much faster than inflation, such that health insurance premi-
ums are no longer affordable for many parties. The rapid accumulation

of costs in the last year of life has generated considerable concern regarding the benefit of many expensive treatments. Cancer treatments costs in particular have increased, although they currently account for 5%, not 15% of overall medical expenditures, and 10%, not 30% of Medicare treatments. However, these numbers are expected to escalate as Medicare assumes more pharmaceutical costs and the cost of cancer care and the number of Medicare patients with cancer increases in concert with the aging population.

Answer 10.11.   **The answer is C.**

Although newer targeted agents do have the potential to prolong life and turn cancer into a "chronic disease," the significant financial repercussions of long-term treatment with costly medications have not been effectively measured but are likely to place considerable strain on the current healthcare system.

Answer 10.12.   **The answer is A.**

The various methods of comparing the benefits and costs of medical treatments have subtle but important differences. The most straightforward analysis, cost minimization, assumes equivalent outcomes, and therefore the least expensive intervention is preferred. Cost-effectiveness analysis compares cost with a relevant clinical variable, such as cost per year of life. These analyses are usually more intuitive but difficult to generalize across treatment types. Cost-utility analysis is similar but compares cost with QALYs such that the toxicities of therapies and the quality of life in the setting of a chronic illness can be weighed along with the benefit. This method has been adopted by the US Preventive Health Service Panel as the best way to account for outcomes compared with cost. Cost-benefit analysis goes one step further by assigning a dollar amount to a QALY, so that two costs may be compared directly. Because this requires assigning a monetary value to a person's life, these analyses are used less often.

Answer 10.13.   **The answer is B.**

All associated costs must be considered to accurately compare medical interventions. Fixed costs to patients or providers are relatively easy to estimate; however, these rates may still vary depending on the volume or the number of times a cost recurs. Specific monetary expenses incurred by patients, such as parking or prescription co-pays, are direct costs and not indirect costs. Indirect costs would include time off from work or even time from lost leisure opportunities for those who are not currently working.

Answer 10.14.   **The answer is D.**

Although there are multiple methods of estimating cost-effectiveness, actually implementing these analyses for decision making is problematic. One example of the application of a cost-benefit analysis is that when Congress made the decision to fund hemodialysis, the cost was considered to be approximately $50,000 per QALY. This value subsequently became an accepted standard for society's willingness to fund a particular intervention. This principle can be generalized to other countries on the basis of their annual per capita GDP. Consideration of economic factors is further complicated by the fact that the original Medicare charter actually prohibits such analysis in decisions regarding coverage. Insurers are rarely inclined to consider cost-effectiveness because they are unlikely to benefit from long-term improvements in outcomes and are more concerned with current cost controls. Although cost-effectiveness analyses can be informative, practical utility of the results is rarely realized.

Systemic Therapy for Cancer

Directions   Each of the numbered items below is followed by lettered answers. Select the ONE lettered answer that is BEST in each case unless instructed otherwise.

QUESTIONS

Question 11.1.   **Which of the following statements is NOT true of the cancer chemotherapy drug development process?**

    A.   Phase I trials have generally not been disease or target specific.

    B.   Phase II study design end points often include symptom reduction, tumor regression, progression-free survival, and overall survival.

    C.   In general, the primary end points of Phase III trials include improvement in survival and/or reduction in tumor-related symptoms.

    D.   In contrast with other areas of drug development, Phase IV studies are rarely used in the development of chemotherapy.

Question 11.2.   **Several genetic polymorphisms have been found to be associated with chemotherapy response and outcome. Which of the following associations is INCORRECT?**

    A.   The expression of thymidylate synthase is linked to the presence of two or three tandem repeats in the 5′-untranslated region of the gene. Homozygosity for the two repeat variant is associated with a longer median survival time in patients with metastatic colorectal cancer treated with 5-fluorouracil.

    B.   A coding single nucleotide polymorphism (SNP) or mutation in the tyrosine kinase domain of epidermal growth factor receptor (EGFR) can alter the sensitivity of the receptor's kinase function to gefitinib.

    C.   Although rare, DPD deficiency, a result of one of several molecular variations in dihydropyrimidine dehydrogenase, can contribute to a life-threatening toxic response to administration of 5-fluorouracil in an otherwise healthy patient with cancer.

    D.   SNPs in the nucleotide excision repair pathways (e.g., ERCC1, XRCC1, and XPD), but not in GSTP1, modulate beneficial effects of oxaliplatin therapy.

Corresponding Chapters in *Cancer: Principles & Practice of Oncology,* Eighth Edition: 25 (Pharmacology of Cancer Chemotherapy), 26 (Pharmacology of Cancer Biotherapeutics), and 27 (Pharmacology of Endocrine Manipulation).

Question 11.3.   **A 58-year-old man with colon cancer received his first dose of irinotecan. Which of the following is MOST correct regarding predictable side effects of this therapy?**

    A. Cholinergic effects resulting from inhibition of acetylcholinesterase by irinotecan are responsible for diarrhea and abdominal cramping occurring 24 hours after drug administration.

    B. Mucosal toxicity of irinotecan therapy leads to diarrhea in the first 24 hours of therapy.

    C. Diarrhea and myelosuppression would be anticipated to be worse in individuals who are homozygous for UGT1A1*28, have biliary obstruction, or have hepatic dysfunction.

    D. Early gastrointestinal (GI) toxicity can be managed with loperamide, whereas atropine should be reserved for management of late-developing diarrhea.

Question 11.4.   **A 50-year-old man with a squamous cell carcinoma of the oropharynx is evaluated for postoperative systemic therapy with concurrent radiation therapy. Clinical staging was T3, N0, and major adverse features were noted on his surgical specimen. His medical history is also significant for complete unilateral hearing loss. In addition to monitoring the patient for changes in hearing, which of the following should be chosen to optimize his curative therapy and preserve hearing?**

    A. Initiate treatment with intravenous (IV) cisplatin 100 mg/m^2 on days 1, 22, and 43 concurrent with radiation therapy of 60 Gy in 30 fractions over a period of 6 weeks.

    B. Initiate concurrent radiation and platinum therapy, but substitute carboplatin for the cisplatin.

    C. Initiate concurrent radiation and cisplatin therapy, but prehydrate the patient with at least 2 L of normal saline.

    D. Initiate concurrent radiation and cisplatin therapy, and add IV thiosulfate therapy.

Question 11.5.   **Which of the following statements regarding the platinum analogs is CORRECT?**

    A. Carboplatin has the same range of clinical activity as cisplatin but is less nephrotoxic, less emetogenic, and less myelosuppressive.

    B. Cisplatin and satraplatin are usually dosed in mg/m^2, whereas carboplatin and oxaliplatin are usually dosed in mg/m^2/min.

    C. Cisplatin is effective in upper GI malignancies, whereas oxaliplatin is more effective in colorectal cancer.

    D. Oral dosing regimens for satraplatin eliminate renal toxicity caused by inadequate pretreatment hydration.

Question 11.6.   A 19-year-old man is beginning dose-intensive chemotherapy for extraosseous Ewing's sarcoma consisting of 3-week cycles of ifosfamide 2 g/m^2/d × 3 days, etoposide 150 mg/m^2/d × 3 days, cyclophosphamide 1.5 g/m^2 on day 5, and doxorubicin 45 mg/m^2 on day 5. Which of the following is TRUE?

A. Like melphalan, an amino acid transporter is responsible for the uptake of the alkylating agents cyclophosphamide and ifosfamide.
B. This regimen is commonly given via peripheral IV access.
C. Efficacy of ifosfamide and cyclophosphamide is likely to increase in the presence of a cytochrome P450 inhibitor.
D. The major route of degradation of the alkylating agents is spontaneous hydrolysis.
E. The combined use of cyclophosphamide and ifosfamide obviates the need for mesna.

Question 11.7.   A 48-year-old female patient with a history of rheumatoid arthritis managed with nonsteroidal anti-inflammatory agents (NSAIDs) was recently diagnosed with a high-grade lymphoma notable for extensive intra-abdominal disease. She is scheduled to begin high-dose methotrexate (MTX). Pretreatment evaluation demonstrates a significant volume of ascites and impaired renal function (creatinine clearance of 58 mL/min). Select the one best response:

A. Ascitic fluid is unlikely to have any effect on cumulative MTX exposure and will likely reaccumulate if it is evacuated before starting MTX.
B. High-dose methotrexate therapy is contraindicated with a creatinine of less than 60 mL/min, and alternative therapy should be offered.
C. The ascetic fluid should be drained, the NSAID should be discontinued, and renal function should be re-evaluated before selecting therapy.
D. High-dose MTX therapy can be safely started in this patient if careful attention is paid to hydration and urinary alkalinization.
E. Given the patient's mild renal insufficiency, probenecid should be given to promote renal excretion of MTX.

Question 11.8.   Which of the following statements regarding complication of high-dose methotrexate therapy is FALSE?

A. Fever, cough, and interstitial pulmonary infiltrates may represent a self-limited pneumonitis.
B. Up to 15% of patients receiving high-dose MTX develop seizures.
C. Acute transient paresis, aphasia, and behavioral changes may occur within the first week of treatment and generally resolve within 72 hours.
D. Chronic neurotoxicity presenting with dementia and motor paresis may develop in the second or third month of treatment.
E. Leucovorin reverses neurotoxicity when it develops.

Question 11.9. **The spectrum of activity and toxicity observed with 5-fluorouracil therapy demonstrates dose and schedule dependency. Which of the following is correctly paired?**

A. Overall response rates are significantly higher with bolus 5-FU than those seen with infusional schedules of 5-FU.

B. The overall response rate is lower with 5-FU/leucovorin than it is with single-agent 5-FU.

C. Toxicity of the weekly Roswell Park regimen consists primarily of neutropenia, whereas toxicities associated with continuous infusion include diarrhea and the hand–foot syndrome.

D. Bolus dosing would be expected to increase the number of cancer cells exposed to drug during the S-phase.

Question 11.10. **A 38-year-old woman with HER2-positive metastatic breast cancer progressed after receiving doxorubicin and cyclophosphamide followed by paclitaxel plus trastuzumab and is started on capecitabine and laptinib. Which is TRUE?**

A. Capecitabine is rapidly absorbed from the gut and has approximately 80% oral bioavailability except in individuals with inherited dihydropyrimidine dehydrogenase deficiency.

B. The activity of capecitabine is independent of liver function and unlikely to be affected by extensive liver metastatic disease because bioactivation of 5'deoxyfluorouridine to 5-FU occurs in tumor tissues.

C. Circulating HER2 extracellular domains are predictive of resistance to laptinib.

D. The benefits of using lapatinib may stem, in part, from its inhibition of heterodimerized receptors.

Question 11.11. **Cytarabine (Ara-C) and gemcitabine are structurally related analogues of deoxycytidine. This structural resemblance confers similarities in metabolism and mechanism of action. However, these agents differ in the following manner:**

A. Myelosuppression is dose-limiting with Ara-C but not with gemcitabine.

B. Gemcitabine is active in both hematologic and solid tumor malignancies, whereas Ara-C is not active in solid tumors.

C. Defects in nucleoside transport render cells resistant to Ara-C but not gemcitabine.

D. In rare but potentially life-threatening side effects, Ara-C is associated with hemolytic-uremic syndrome.

E. Gemcitabine is associated with conjunctivitis and hand–foot syndrome.

Question 11.12.   **A 54-year-old woman with chronic lymphocytic leukemia (CLL) was previously treated with fludarabine. Which of the following treatment-related toxicities is associated with multiple courses of therapy?**

A. Interstitial pneumonitis
B. Immunosuppression associated with decreases in B cells
C. Reactivation of latent varicella-zoster infection
D. *Pneumocystis jirovecii* pneumonia (previously termed *Pneumocystis carinii* pneumonia)
E. Tumor lysis syndrome

Question 11.13.   **A 56-year-old Caucasian man presents with a relapse of his hairy cell leukemia 4 years after his initial treatment. Which of the following statements can you correctly tell him?**

A. Some 65% to 91% of subjects achieve a durable complete remission (CR) after a single treatment of cladribine, but the CR rate with salvage therapy is poor.
B. The CR rate of salvage therapy with cladribine in patients who were previously treated with interferon-α is less effective than if cladribine was used as initial therapy.
C. Salvage therapy with cladribine is less effective and of shorter duration in hairy cell leukemia than it is in non-Hodgkin's lymphoma.
D. Retreatment with cladribine results in a CR in 60% of patients who relapse.
E. The CR rate with cladribine is inferior in patients treated with salvage therapy with a history of splenectomy.

Question 11.14.   **The patient in Question 13 is treated with cladribine salvage therapy. Which of the following infectious complications is MOST typically observed?**

A. Aspergillus pneumonia
B. Cryptococcal meningitis
C. Sepsis with *Pseudomonas aeruginosa*
D. *Pneumocystis jirovecii* pneumonia
E. Herpes zoster

Question 11.15.   **A previously healthy 32-year-old woman with HER2 overexpressing meta-static breast cancer is receiving trastuzumab, carboplatin, and docetaxel. Pretreatment medications include ranitidine, diphenhydramine, lorazepam, and palonosetron. She returns to your office the next day with swollen legs. On examination she has gained 2 kg and has 3+ bilateral lower-extremity edema, and her lung examination results were clear. Which of the following is MOST correct?**

A. The addition of dexamethasone to her pretreatment medications would have prevented her new symptoms.
B. She is likely having an allergic reaction to her docetaxel.
C. She has new-onset cardiomyopathy related to her treatment with trastuzumab.
D. Her lower-extremity edema is an acute manifestation of docetaxel-induced neurotoxicity.
E. Her fluid retention is likely to be transient and will not return with subsequent therapy.

Question 11.16.   **The vinca alkaloids are highly bound to plasma proteins, substrates for cytochrome P-450 metabolism, and substrates of the ABC transporters. As a result of these features, the vinca alkaloids participate in several drug interactions. All of the following are examples, EXCEPT:**

A. Vincristine may precipitate seizures by reducing plasma phenytoin levels for up to 10 days after treatment with vincristine.
B. Concurrent use of azithromycin and vincristine may result in severe toxicity.
C. When used in combination, L-asparaginase should be given at least 12 hours before vincristine to avoid delayed hepatic clearance of vincristine.
D. Pulmonary toxicity may result from the combined use of vinca alkaloids and mitomycin C.
E. Vinblastine antagonizes transporter-mediated efflux of methotrexate.

Question 11.17.   **Which of the following increase EGFR-mediated signaling?**

A. High expression levels of EGFR
B. Formation of heterodimer duplexes with other members of this receptor family
C. Increased paracrine ligand expression
D. Dysregulation of downstream signal transduction pathway
E. All of the above

Question 11.18.   **Adverse events with sunitinib are generally mild to moderate. Which of the following is NOT a reported toxicity of sunitinib?**

A. Hypertension
B. Mucositis
C. Yellow skin discoloration
D. Interstitial lung disease
E. Congestive heart failure

Question 11.19.   **Several new and developing agents target EGFR. Which of the following statements regarding anti-EGFR therapy is INCORRECT?**

A. Cell-surface expression of EGFR is downregulated on binding of cetuximab.
B. Antibody-dependent cellular cytotoxicity is induced by binding of the immunoglobulin (Ig)G1 molecule cetuximab.
C. Rash is a class effect of EGFR inhibitors, regardless of whether the inhibitor is a small molecule or antibody.
D. Hypomagnesemia is a class effect of EGFR inhibitors.
E. In comparison with cetuximab, the structure of panitumumab would predict that fewer infusion reactions are likely to occur because panitumumab is an IgG2 antibody.

Question 11.20.   **In your outpatient clinic you see a 77-year-old woman with myelodysplastic syndrome. By World Health Organization criteria, she has refractory anemia with excess blasts (RAEB-2) and an International Prognostic Scoring System (IPSS) score of 1.5. You offer to treat her with 5-azacytidine. She is interested in the therapy and asks you how long she will need to be treated to determine if she will respond to therapy:**

A. Even in the absence of an overt response or failure, therapy should be continued for at least 4 to 6 months before determining that she is not responding to treatment.
B. Improvements in peripheral blood counts and bone marrow results occur within the first treatment cycle.
C. If no improvement in peripheral blood counts and bone marrow results is observed by the end of the second cycle, then therapy should be discontinued.
D. A response to therapy can be predicted by the development of a rash within the first cycle of therapy.
E. In clinical studies, 90% of patients responded within three cycles of therapy.

Question 11.21.   **You have been caring for a 72-year-old man with multiple myeloma. At his most recent appointment, he informs you that he has been reading on the Internet, and as a result he is interested in starting treatment with bortezomib. Which of the following facts that he provides you with is INCORRECT?**

A. In heavily pretreated patients, a phase II study demonstrated a single agent objective response rate (ORR) of 28%.
B. Common side effects include nausea, vomiting, diarrhea, constipation, neutropenia, and anemia.
C. When neuropathic pain develops, it is reversible when treated with vitamin supplementation.
D. When combined with pegylated doxorubicin, the ORR was 79% in relapsed patients.
E. Bortezomib is typically given on days 1, 4, 8, and 11 of a 3-week cycle.

Question 11.22. **In comparing the pharmacology of thalidomide and lenalidomide, which of the following is TRUE?**

    A. Thalidomide is more potent with less nonhematologic toxicities.

    B. Lenalidomide is better tolerated, but myelosuppression can be dose-limiting.

    C. Thalidomide is associated with less sedation, constipation, and neuropathy.

    D. Adding dexamethasone to lenalidomide therapy reduces the incidence of thromboembolic events.

    E. When using lenalidomide, no dose adjustments are required for patients with multiple myeloma and renal failure.

Question 11.23. **An otherwise healthy 35-year-old woman with metastatic melanoma is scheduled to begin therapy with interleukin (IL)-2 720,000 IU/kg IV every 8 hours up to a total of 14 doses, twice over a 3-week course. Appropriate management would NOT require:**

    A. Cardiac stress testing and exclusion from therapy if exercise-induced ischemia is found

    B. Scheduled administration of acetaminophen and indomethacin concurrent with IL-2 dosing

    C. Avoidance of dexamethasone and other steroids during administration of IL-2

    D. Supplementation of IV fluids with sodium bicarbonate to prevent acidosis

    E. Pretreatment screening for symptoms of depression, as well as renal, hepatic, and pulmonary function

Question 11.24. **Shortly after beginning therapy, this patient develops nausea, chills, fever, and erythroderma. She is supported through these symptoms and completes 12 of the first 14 doses. She returned for the second round of treatment in this 3-week course. After receiving her eighth dose, her examination reveals the following: blood pressure of 98/64 mm Hg, heart rate of 105 beats/min, and temperature of 37.9°C. Her blood gas reveals development of a mild respiratory acidosis, and her husband reports that she is becoming more irritable but not confused. The BEST response is to:**

    A. Hold the IL-2 infusions until symptoms resolve and then restart therapy.

    B. Reduce the dose of IL-2 by 25%.

    C. Stop the IL-2, order blood cultures from peripheral and central venous access sites, and broaden empiric antibiotic coverage.

    D. Evaluate volume status, increase fluids if indicated, and continue IL-2 therapy.

    E. Discontinue therapy and discharge the patient in the morning.

Question 11.25. While you are attending a local high school sporting event you become engaged in a discussion with a couple of your neighbors who you know have teenage daughters. One of your neighbors asks you about your opinion on the use of human papillomavirus (HPV) vaccines. You can correctly tell them all of the following, **EXCEPT:**

A. The vaccines contain virus-like particles (VLP) composed primarily of the L1 major structural protein, and the intact virus is not present. Thus, the vaccine cannot directly cause an HPV infection.
B. On the basis of the HPV types selected for inclusion in the vaccine, the current vaccines are expected to eliminate the need for cervical cancer screening.
C. Because Gardasil contains VLPs from HPV-6, 11, 16, and 18, it will also target genital warts.
D. In clinical studies, vaccination resulted in near complete protection against persistent infection and cervical disease from the targeted HPV types.
E. Although the divalent vaccine has shown some cross-protection toward other viral serotypes, protection seems to be mainly type specific.

Question 11.26. For routine follow-up, you see a 35-year-old woman who is currently taking tamoxifen as treatment for her surgically resected premenopausal estrogen receptor (ER)-positive breast cancer. She was first diagnosed with depression 15 years ago and has previously had improvement in her symptoms with paroxetine. She discontinued her treatment when her depression improved 5 years ago, but recently she has been experiencing insomnia, anhedonia, weight gain, and blunted affect. She recognizes the symptoms of her depression and asks you to prescribe therapy for her. For treatment of her depression, you select:

A. Venlafaxine
B. Bupropion
C. Fluoxetine
D. Imipramine
E. Paroxetine

ANSWERS

Answer 11.1. **The answer is D.**

For most anticancer agents, development continues and broadens after initial market approval. Phase IV studies are undertaken to further examine and optimize drug regimens, and explore the utility of new agents in combinations with other agents that are known to be active in a given disease.

Answer 11.2. **The answer is D.**

Polymorphisms in several genes (ERCC1, XRCC1, XPD, GSTP1, and TS) have been shown to potentially modulate the response of cancer cells to oxaliplatin therapy. Favorable genotypes for codon 751 of XPD, codon 118 of ERCC1, codon 105 of GSTP1, and a polymorphism in the 3′UTR of TS have been identified. Combination analysis of these four polymorphisms in patients with metastatic colorectal cancer who received FOL-FOX revealed that individuals with favorable genotypes at two or more polymorphic sites survived a median of 17.4 months compared with 10.2 months in patients who harbored only one favorable genotype, and the overall survival was 5.4 months in patients with no favorable genotype ($p <.001$).

Answer 11.3.   **The answer is C.**

Approximately 75% of the irinotecan dose undergoes hepatic metabolism and biliary excretion. Glucuronidation of the active metabolite of irinotecan, SN-38, by UGT1A1 demonstrates polymorphic variation. Homozygosity for UGT1A1*28 is associated with delayed drug clearance. Predictable toxicities of irinotecan include myelosuppression, mucositis, and diarrhea. Diarrhea occurring within the first 24 hours of irinotecan exposure is associated with the anticholinergic properties of the agent. In contrast, diarrhea occurring later than 24 hours is associated with mucosal cytotoxicity. Both late-phase diarrhea and myelosuppression are exacerbated when hepatobiliary clearance is reduced.

Answer 11.4.   **The answer is C.**

Concurrent chemoradiation therapy using cisplatin is indicated in this patient because of the high-risk features identified on surgical pathology. However, cisplatin therapy is associated with a real risk of ototoxicity. Approximately 25% of administered cisplatin is excreted in the urine in the first 24 hours, representing the major route of elimination of cisplatin in this interval. Maintenance of renal clearance by prehydration can help to minimize renal injury, preserving the timely clearance of this drug and aiding in the prevention of ototoxicity.

Answer 11.5.   **The answer is C.**

DNA lesions are similar for all four clinically active platinum agents, and the range of epithelial malignancies that are sensitive to cisplatin and carboplatin is similar (but not identical). Oxaliplatin-containing regimens are standards of care in advanced colorectal cancer, but oxaliplatin has not been as extensively studied in other malignancies. Cisplatin is effective in esophageal and stomach cancer, and the effectiveness of oxaliplatin outside of the colon is not fully known. Differences in the range of clinical effects of the various platinum agents are suspected to be due to structural differences in the carrier ligands and leaving groups.

Answer 11.6.   **The answer is D.**

The major inactivation pathway for most alkylating agents is via spontaneous hydrolysis. Enzymatic conversion does occur, and Phase II metabolism is responsible for the formation of mercapturates that undergo renal elimination. Enzymatic processes can also play a role in activation of the alkylators, such as the CYP2B6-mediated activation of the prodrug cyclophosphamide.

Answer 11.7.   **The answer is C.**

The use of NSAIDs and the accumulation of "third-space" fluids can have a negative impact on renal function, and renal function should be reevaluated. In addition, MTX can accumulate in ascites or pleural effusions altering clearance kinetics, and it is advisable to evacuate these fluid collections before treatment and to monitor drug levels closely.

Answer 11.8.   **The answer is E.**

There is no evidence to support the therapeutic use of leucovorin in the management of neurotoxicity.

Answer 11.9.   **The answer is C.**

The overall response rates are significantly higher, and the overall safety profile is improved with infusional regimens. The main toxicity of 5-FU treatment administered per the Roswell Park regimen is neutropenia, but when given via continuous infusion, the main toxicities are diarrhea and the hand–foot syndrome.

Answer 11.10.   **The answer is D.**

Lapatinib is an orally bioavailable, reversible inhibitor of EGFR and HER2 that halts receptor-mediated tyrosine kinase activity. HER2 expression in breast cancer is correlated with shortened disease-free survival and resistance to both chemotherapy and endocrine therapy. EGFR-HER2 and HER2-HER3 heterodimers have longer and greater proliferative signals than the corresponding homodimers. The rationale for targeting both EGFR and HER2 is to silence homodimers of both receptors and to mute the additive effects of the heterodimer complexes.

Answer 11.11.   **The answer is B.**

The structural similarities of gemcitabine and cytarabine result in similarities in mechanism of action and metabolism. However, gemcitabine has shown significant clinical activity in multiple human solid tumors (i.e., pancreatic, small cell and non–small cell lung, bladder, ovarian, and breast cancers) and has activity in hematologic malignancies such as non-Hodgkin's lymphoma.

Answer 11.12.   **The answer is A.**

Myelosuppression and immunosuppression are anticipated toxicities associated with using fludarabine in the first and subsequent cycles of treatment and result in the decline of CD4+ T cells. In contrast, pulmonary toxicity occurring as interstitial pneumonitis occurs less predictably and is associated with multiple courses of treatment.

Answer 11.13.   **The answer is D.**

Cladribine is the current drug of choice for hairy cell leukemia and is associated with a durable CR rate of 65% to 91% after a single course. Management of relapsed disease with cladribine retains similar efficacy with a response rate of up to 60%. In addition, salvage with cladribine in patients previously treated with interferon-α or splenectomy is as effective as first-line therapy.

Answer 11.14.   **The answer is E.**

A variety of pathogens are responsible for infections seen with cladribine-induced immunosuppression, and herpes zoster is the most typical.

Answer 11.15.   **The answer is A.**

Docetaxel induces a fluid retention syndrome consisting of weight gain, edema, and third-space fluid accumulation. This syndrome and hypersensitivity reactions can be prevented by administering dexamethasone 8 mg orally starting 1 to 2 days before docetaxel and continuing this therapy for a total of 3 to 5 days.

Answer 11.16.   **The answer is C.**

Hepatic clearance of the vinca alkaloids is reduced in the presence of L-asparaginase. To minimize this potential interaction, the vinca alkaloids should be given 12 to 24 hours before L-asparaginase.

Answer 11.17.   **The answer is E.**

Each of these mechanisms can play a role in amplification of the EGFR signaling pathway.

Answer 11.18.   **The answer is D.**

Interstitial lung disease is not an adverse reaction reported to be observed in patients treated with sunitinib.

Answer 11.19.   **The answer is E.**

Panitumumab is a humanized antibody made up of murine hypervariable amino acid domains grafted into a human antibody. Cetuximab is a chimeric antibody composed of murine variable regions with human constant regions. The predominantly human antibody structure of panitumumab confers a reduced potential for transfusion reactions. Activation of antibody-dependent cellular cytotoxicity is dependent on IgG class structure (i.e., IgG1 vs. IgG2), but IgG class structure is not responsible for the difference in the rate of transfusion reactions.

Answer 11.20.   **The answer is A.**

Hematologic improvements in myelodysplasia syndrome may require prolonged treatment with the azacitidine analogues. In the Cancer and Leukemia Group B (CALGB) studies of 5-azacitidine, 90% of subjects who responded to therapy did so by the sixth cycle, but the median time to development of first clinical response was three cycles. Thus, to maximize the ability to detect whether a patient will respond to therapy and to maximize the number of patients who will respond, it is important to commit to treatment for four to six cycles. Of course, therapy can be deemed ineffective if a patient demonstrates disease progression at an earlier time point.

Answer 11.21.   **The answer is C.**

In a phase II study, bortezomib therapy was associated with neuropathic pain in 12% of subjects and required prompt dose reduction or discontinuation of therapy to prevent irreversible damage.

Answer 11.22.   **The answer is B.**

Therapy with lenalidomide is generally better tolerated than therapy with thalidomide and is associated with less sedation, constipation, and peripheral neuropathy. Lenalidomide therapy can be dose-limited by myelosuppression manifested as neutropenia and thrombocytopenia.

Answer 11.23.   **The answer is A.**

The safe administration of high-dose IL-2 requires careful selection of patients because of the inherent toxicity of treatment (e.g., fever, hypotension, and edema). Candidates for therapy should be considered only in the absence of a history of cardiac disease, and patients older than 40 years of age should have stress testing. The finding of exercise-induced ischemia would exclude a patient from therapy. On the basis of her age, this patient would not be directed to stress testing in the absence of any cardiac symptoms, personal history of cardiac disease, or family history of early heart disease.

Answer 11.24.   **The answer is D.**

When administering IL-2 therapy it can be challenging to differentiate between tolerable side effects and true risks to a patient's health. Common side effects of IL-2 therapy include fever, chills, lethargy, diarrhea, nausea, anemia, thrombocytopenia, eosinophilia, erythroderma, hepatic dysfunction, confusion, and acidosis. Myocarditis can be seen in approximately 5% of subjects as well. Capillary leak syndrome can present with fluid retention, hypotension, respiratory distress, and prerenal azotemia. Treatment also predisposes patients to infections with gram-positive and less frequently gram-negative bacteria. As presented, this patient is demonstrating predictable but tolerable side effects that should allow continuation of therapy with monitoring.

Answer 11.25.   **The answer is B.**

The high-risk HPV types are associated with cervical and anal cancer. HPV-16 is the most common, accounting for more than half of the cervical cancer cases worldwide, and HPV-18 accounts for the next highest frequency. Collectively these two types account for approximately 70% of cervical cancer cases and a higher proportion of other HPV-associated cancers. Unfortunately, even if the vaccine was 100% effective, the type-restrictive nature of this protection results in vaccination having little or no effect on the other 30% of HPV-associated cervical cancer cases. Thus, although the costs and frequency of screening may change, it remains important to continue screening for cervical cancer.

Answer 11.26.   **The answer is A.**

Tamoxifen is a prodrug that is activated through oxidation by CYP2D6 to biologically active metabolites, including endoxifen. In humans, this enzyme is highly polymorphic resulting in variations in the levels of the active metabolites. Potent inhibitors of CYP2D6 can also result in marked reduction in the circulating levels of active metabolites. With the exception of venlafaxine, all of the antidepressants included as possible choices are known to inhibit CYP2D6.

Feng Gao
Kathryn Trinkaus

CHAPTER

12

Design and Analysis of Clinical Trials

Directions

Each of the numbered items below is followed by lettered answers. Select the ONE lettered answer that is BEST in each case unless instructed otherwise.

QUESTIONS

Question 12.1. **Which of the following is NOT true concerning a clinical trial?**

A. The sample size of a clinical trial is fixed and determined before the trial begins.
B. Clinical trials are prospectively planned experiments involving human subjects.
C. A well-chosen control group provides a baseline against which to measure effects of experimental treatment.
D. Clinical trials test a clearly stated hypothesis using a predefined analysis plan.

Question 12.2. **Phase I trials on cytotoxic agents are designed to determine a dose that is appropriate for use in Phase II trials. Which of the following statements is TRUE of Phase I trials?**

A. Phase I trials involve the first use of a drug, device, or procedure in humans in a new disease setting or a new combination of therapies.
B. Patients for Phase I trials are usually not chosen on the basis of their likelihood of having a favorable response to the experimental treatment.
C. Phase I trials do not require statistical justification because the sample sizes are usually small.
D. A and B.

Corresponding Chapter in *Cancer: Principles & Practice of Oncology,* Eighth Edition: 28 (Design and Analysis of Clinical Trials).

Question 12.3. **Which of the following regarding the conventional 3 + 3 Phase I designs is NOT true?**

 A. Participants are often those with end-stage disease whose treatment options have been exhausted.

 B. Dose levels are usually prespecified and based on a modified Fibonacci series.

 C. Cohorts of three to six patients are treated at each dose level, and the initial dose is chosen to cause little or no toxicity.

 D. The optimal dose recommended for Phase II is chosen using a dose-toxicity curve generated from a statistical model fitted to the full data.

Question 12.4. **Although simple and easy to implement, the conventional 3 + 3 Phase I design is known to suffer from some major limitations. Accelerated titration designs, among others, have been proposed to address these problems. Which of the following is NOT an element in an accelerated titration design?**

 A. Permitting within-patients dose escalation

 B. Using a dose-toxicity model to guide the dose escalation

 C. Treating one patient per dose level before any grade 2 or greater toxicity is seen

 D. Fitting a statistical model to the full data in data analysis

Question 12.5. **A drug, device, or other treatment may be considered for Phase II testing when:**

 A. The maximum tolerable dose is known but there is genuine doubt about efficacy, and patients with the condition of interest and a likely favorable outcome can be recruited as study participants.

 B. A standard treatment exists for comparison.

 C. Accrual is rapid enough to allow recruitment of 20 to 30 patients.

 D. An appropriate control group can be recruited at the same time as the experimental group.

Question 12.6. **Which of the following statements regarding the patient selection for a Phase II trial is NOT true?**

 A. Participants for a Phase II trial should be those who are most likely to benefit from the experimental treatment.

 B. Initial Phase II trials should be performed on patients with a minimum amount of prior chemotherapy, and a "window-of-opportunity design" can be used to allow previous untreated patients to receive one or two courses of the experimental drug before they are switched to a standard treatment.

 C. The "uncertainty principle," which states that a patient is eligible if the treating physician is genuinely uncertain about the best treatment for that patient, should be followed to ensure the generalizability of the conclusion from a Phase II trial.

 D. For trials on molecularly targeted drugs, the study can be conducted more efficiently by focusing on patients whose tumors express the target, and the techniques of genome-wide expression profiling may facilitate the patient selection.

Question 12.7.   **Phase II trials of a single agent are designed to determine whether the experimental drug has any antitumor activity against a given type of tumor, and the antitumor effect is often measured as an objective response based on tumor shrinkage. However, such a trial is not appropriate for the question of patient welfare because:**

A.   The welfare of patients with cancer is often measured by survival or symptom control, but there is no necessary relation between such beneficial end points and tumor response.

B.   Survival is inherently a comparative end point that should be assessed in a prognostically comparable set of patients. Unfortunately, Phase II trials are often conducted without concurrent controls.

C.   Comparing the survival times of responders and nonresponders is not a valid means of showing a treatment is beneficial to patients because responders may have more favorable prognostic factors than nonresponders.

D.   All of the above.

Question 12.8.   **Patients in a Phase II trial are often recruited in a two-stage manner that allows a potential early stopping, thus saving patients from unnecessary exposure to inactive agents. Which of the following is NOT true of a two-stage design?**

A.   The optimal two-stage design minimizes the average sample size and thus optimizes the protection of patients given an inactive agent.

B.   Simon's two-stage designs are often applied in Phase II trials on molecularly targeted drugs and therapeutic cancer vaccines.

C.   The minimax design minimizes the total sample size. Compared with the optimal design, the minimax design usually enrolls more patients in the first stage and fewer patients in total sample size.

D.   With $p0 = 0.10$, $p1 = 0.25$, a type I error of 0.05, and 80% power, for example, a Simon's minimax design will enroll 22 patients in the first stage. If three or more responses are observed, 18 more patients will be enrolled in the second stage. If eight or more responses are observed at the end of study, the treatment will be claimed as showing preliminary evidence of efficacy.

Question 12.9.   **Unlike cytotoxic agents that work by killing tumor cells, cytostatic agents work via biologic effects that modify the environment of tumor growth; that is, inhibition of a molecular target. Which of the following is NOT true regarding early-phase trials on cytostatic agents such as molecularly targeted drugs and cancer therapeutic vaccines?**

A. Because cytostatic agents usually have a good safety profile, Phase I trials on such drugs are often designed to identify a biologically active dose rather than maximum tolerated dose (MTD).

B. Because therapeutic cancer vaccines work via stimulation of tumor-reactive T cells, heavily treated patients with end-stage disease are less likely to benefit from a cancer vaccine.

C. The response rate based on tumor shrinkage is the best primary end point measuring treatment efficacy in Phase II trials on cytostatic agents.

D. Because of the nature of low toxicity profiles in cytostatic agents, factorial designs and randomized studies have appealing features and are used to evaluate multiple drugs in a single trial.

Question 12.10.   **Which of the following best describes Simon's Phase 2.5 design on molecularly targeted drugs and cancer therapeutic vaccines?**

A. The design compares progression-free survival times of the same patient from the current trial with his/her previous trial.

B. The design first treats all eligible patients with two to four courses of the experimental drugs. Patients are then evaluated, and the experimental drug is either continued or discontinued, depending on their response to the initial treatment.

C. The design is similar to a Phase III trial except that it allows a relatively large type I (false positive) error and targets for a relatively large difference, thus requiring fewer patients.

D. The design will compare time to progression of patients in the study with a prospectively identified and prognostically comparable historical control.

Question 12.11.   **Which of the following is NOT true of Phase III trials?**

A. The primary end points should be demonstrably related to patient benefit.

B. Eligibility criteria should be broad to enhance generalizability of results.

C. Conditions of treatment should be suited to community patient care.

D. A quality-of-life measure should be included to measure benefit to patients.

Question 12.12.   **Which of the following is TRUE of randomized treatment assignment?**

A.   Trial participants are a representative sample of patients with the disease of interest.

B.   Randomization may fail to balance unknown prognostic factors in small studies.

C.   Randomization is unnecessary if controls can be matched closely enough to trial participants.

D.   Randomization is ineffective unless patients and treating physicians are unaware of treatment assignment for the duration of the study.

Question 12.13.   **Randomization is generally NOT necessary in which of the following scenarios?**

A.   Study of patients with a disease that will uniformly and rapidly progress to an end stage

B.   Phase III trial

C.   Screening study on multiple cytostatic agents, such as molecularly targeted drugs or cancer therapeutic vaccines

D.   Phase II trial on cytotoxic agents using time to progression as the primary efficacy end point

Question 12.14.   **Which of the following is NOT true of power and hypothesis testing in clinical trials?**

A.   Statistical power mainly depends on the anticipated size of treatment effect. Trials designed to detect a small effect will demand large sample sizes.

B.   Statistical power is also heavily influenced by the prespecified type I error (probability of erroneously claiming a "positive" result), and a two-sided type I error of 0.05 has been widely accepted, especially in Phase III trials.

C.   Because a confidence interval provides information about the size and direction of treatment effect, it is more informative than significance testing, especially for "negative" trials.

D.   Because data from small randomized trials can be pooled for meta-analysis, the calculation of sample size for a randomized clinical trial is no longer as critical as it was.

Question 12.15. **Which of the following is NOT true for therapeutic equivalence (or noninferiority) trials?**

A. Therapeutic equivalence trials are designed to test similarity, as measured by a clinical end point, between the experimental drugs and the standard treatment.

B. Because it is impossible to prove equivalence in true sense, in practice therapeutic equivalence will be accepted if the difference in efficacy is within a prespecified level (δ).

C. The traditional superiority trials cannot be used to prove equivalence because a "negative" finding may be simply due to inadequate sample size.

D. A trial designed to demonstrate therapeutic equivalence requires fewer patients because it usually allows a relatively large type I error.

Question 12.16. **Therapeutic equivalence trials often express results as an estimate of difference between two treatments with a 95% confidence interval. Which of the following statements about the 95% confidence interval is NOT correct?**

A. The confidence interval is a range of values consistent with the observed difference, given the precision with which the trial can measure that difference.

B. The trial estimates that in 5 of 100 cases the true difference will fall outside the 95% confidence interval.

C. It is unlikely that the true difference is smaller than the lower limit or larger than the upper limit of the confidence interval.

D. If the confidence interval includes 0, then the trial has shown that the two treatments do not differ.

Question 12.17. **Which one of the following describing the pros and cons of Bayesian methods in planning clinical trials is NOT true?**

A. In the traditional statistical (frequentist) methods, the treatment effect is regarded as a fixed but unknown parameter, and the likelihood of the parameter is described using a probability derived from observed frequencies in a defined distribution. In contrast, a Bayesian statistical method assumes that the treatment effect itself is a random quantity drawn from a prior distribution.

B. Bayesian methods are widely applied in planning Phase III trials.

C. Because Bayesian methods can incorporate information from preclinical studies and sources outside of the trial, many designs for Phase I and II trials have been developed within a Bayesian framework.

D. The prior distribution of parameters heavily influences the meaningfulness and interpretation of Bayesian-based clinical trials.

Question 12.18. **The intention-to-treat analysis is considered the primary analysis of data from a clinical trial. Which of the following describes an intention-to-treat analysis?**

   A. An ineligible patient is not included in an intention-to-treat analysis because the study treatment is not appropriate for that patient.

   B. All patients who give consent and are randomized are included in the intention-to-treat analysis in the study arm to which they were randomized.

   C. Data from patients who are ineligible or who die or withdraw from the study before completion should be analyzed separately from data from eligible patients who complete the trial.

   D. Lack of compliance can distort the results from patients who fail to complete the trial, so these data should be dropped from an intention-to-treat analysis.

Question 12.19. **An interim analysis is any assessment of data performed during patient enrollment or follow-up period of a trial. Which of the following is NOT true for planning clinical trials with interim analyses?**

   A. Multiple looks at outcome data over the course of a trial will alter type I and II errors. Unless they are included in the design, multiple looks will cause the operating characteristics of the trial to deviate from the planned values.

   B. A variety of group-sequential designs have been proposed to guide the statistical significance testing of a fixed number of interim analyses that are usually specified from the outset.

   C. The method of stochastic curtailment is designed to calculate conditional power (the projected probability of rejecting the null hypothesis at the end of study), conditional on the accumulated information and to stop the trial if the conditional power is small (e.g., 0.2). In such a "futility" analysis, the number of interim analyses does not need to be fixed in advance.

   D. A data-safety committee is usually put in charge of the interpretation of interim analyses. The committee also includes the study leaders to notify the patients and medical community in a timely manner.

Question 12.20. **One of the most important features that makes survival data different from other kinds of data is the presence of censoring. That is, the actual survival times for some patients cannot be observed during study. Which of the following is NOT true for the analysis of survival data?**

A. Survival (or disease-free survival) curves provide a superior tool for summarizing survival data.

B. Two methods are most frequently used for the estimation of survival curves. The life table method requires relatively large sample size, and the Kaplan-Meier product limit method is appropriate for any sample size.

C. Traditional summary statistics, such as means and standard deviations, can provide a sufficient summary for survival data without censoring.

D. The statistical power of clinical trials using survival as a primary end point will be mainly determined by the actual number of events (i.e., death or progression) rather than the total number of patients.

Question 12.21. **An important assumption in the analysis of survival data is noninformative censoring. That is, censoring is not related to the outcome of interest. For a clinical trial with cancer-specific survival as the primary end point, which of the following patients is more likely to suffer from informative censoring?**

A. Alive at the time of study closeout
B. Withdrawal from the trial because of disease progression
C. Died of accident
D. Moving out of the region

ANSWERS

Answer 12.1. **The answer is A.**

Sample size may be altered during the course of a trial of any phase on the basis of outcomes observed during the trial.

Answer 12.2. **The answer is D.**

Statistical power is not the focus of Phase I trial design, but the issues (e.g., patient safety) are major, and long-term consequences (e.g., loss of patient benefit and waste of resources) are severe if resources are incorrectly directed toward ineffective treatments or away from effective treatments. Therefore, careful statistical design is needed if sound and sufficient information is to be drawn from small and often heterogeneous patient samples.

Answer 12.3. **The answer is D.**

The conventional $3 + 3$ Phase I design is totally algorithm based, and the dose recommended for Phase II trials is chosen among the fixed and prespecified levels. The recommended dose, commonly referred to as the maximum tolerated dose (MTD), is usually taken as the highest level for which the dose-limiting toxicity (DLT) rate is less than 33%.

Answer 12.4. **The answer is B.**

The accelerated titration design permits within-patient dose escalation and treats only one patient per dose level until grade 2 or greater toxicity is seen. Data analysis in an accelerated titration design takes a model-based approach that considers the information from all participants. Its dose escalation is totally algorithm-based, rather than model-based.

Answer 12.5. **The answer is A.**

Phase II trials may be single-arm trials testing a single treatment, so no direct comparison of treatments may be involved. The ideal sample size depends on many factors, including the nature and variability of the primary outcome, the expected effect size, and the procedures to be used to test hypotheses. An appropriate primary outcome is determined by the nature of the treatment being tested and the goals of the study.

Answer 12.6. **The answer is C.**

Phase II trials should be performed on patients with a well-defined type of tumor and preferably on those without any prior chemotherapy. For studies of cytostatic agents, selecting patients on the basis of their molecular target can significantly increase the efficiency of the study, as well as sparing patients who do not express the target exposure to an ineffective treatment. However, generalizability of a trial is usually a major consideration for planning Phase III rather than Phase II trials.

Answer 12.7. **The answer is D.**

There is no biologically inherent relationship between response and survival. For example, a meta-analysis on randomized clinical trials by Torri et al. showed that a large improvement in response rate only corresponded to a minor increase in survival. In addition, survival end points are comparative in nature and require taking the distribution of potential prognostic factors into consideration.

Answer 12.8. **The answer is B.**

Trials of cytostatic agents often choose time to progression as the primary end points. When testing cytotoxic agents, the use of Simon's two-stage designs is limited to situations where outcome assessment can be made shortly after patients are treated. These designs usually are not practical for end points requiring a long period of follow-up.

Answer 12.9. **The answer is C.**

Cytostatic agents, such as antiangiogenesis factors, growth modulators, or cancer vaccines, usually selectively work on molecular targets to modulate tumor environment. They may prolong patient survival without causing tumor shrinkage. Therefore, time to progression is often used as the primary end point for such trials.

Answer 12.10. **The answer is C.**

Option A represents a design that used growth modulation index for the assessment of efficacy, option B describes a randomized discontinuation design, and option D is frequently used for trials on the combination of cytotoxic agents. Simon's Phase 2.5 designs are similar to Phase III trials except that they allow a relatively large type I error and are able to identify only a relatively large difference.

Answer 12.11. **The answer is D.**

Validated quality of life instruments are useful parts of Phase III trials, especially if they are directly related to areas of concern to patients. Many areas of patient benefit (e.g., longer survival, lower risk of relapse, accessibility, or lower cost) may not be readily measured by these instruments.

Answer 12.12. **The answer is B.**

A random sample helps to provide a fair, unbiased comparison of the treatments within the population of patients from whom participants are recruited, although this population may not be representative of all patients with the disease. Randomization may not result in equal, or nearly equal, numbers of patients with a particular characteristic in each treatment group, but it does distribute biasing characteristics according to a known probability distribution so that they do not obscure identification of treatment effects, if any, by statistical tests. Matching is not a substitute for randomization; in fact, matching too closely can mask real treatment effects. Blinding of participants or treating physicians to treatment assignment can reduce bias introduced in the process of treatment, whereas randomization reduces bias in patient selection. Randomized assignment to treatment can be used with or without blinding.

Answer 12.13. **The answer is A.**

Randomization is not necessary for patients with a disease that will uniformly and rapidly progress to an end stage. In such a setting of homogeneity, a historical control usually is sufficient.

Answer 12.14. **The answer is D.**

It is true that meta-analysis can combine the results of small randomized studies and may address questions that cannot be answered by any individual study alone. However, by no means can meta-analyses replace carefully designed and adequately powered randomized trials. This is because different trials can be heterogeneous in terms of diagnostic and staging procedures, supportive care, and methods of patient evaluation and follow-up. Such heterogeneity may obscure small to moderate therapeutic effects and undermine the ground for any pooled analyses.

Answer 12.15. **The answer is D.**

This claim may be true for bioequivalence studies but not for therapeutic equivalence trials. In the former, for example, the objective is to show biological equivalence of two proprietary preparations of a drug, and a relatively large type I error or large tolerable difference (δ) is acceptable. For trials targeting equivalence in therapeutic effect (e.g., mortality rate), however, usually a much smaller δ is of interest, and this will require a very large sample size.

Answer 12.16. **The answer is D.**

The trial has shown that 0 is a plausible value for the difference but not that the difference equals zero.

Answer 12.17. **The answer is B.**

Because Bayesian methods can incorporate information from preclinical studies and sources outside of the trial, they are appealing in planning Phase I and II trials. In these trials, information regarding the experimental treatment is sparse, and study design is based on a variety of (usually subjective) assumptions. However, Phase III trials intend to provide reliable and objective guidance for decision making in a given disease, so the subjective nature of prior distributions in Bayesian methods limits their popularity in planning Phase III trials.

Answer 12.18. **The answer is B.**

Omitting patients who die or withdraw without completing the study is a serious source of bias, as is dropping patients for noncompliance or deviation from protocol. These may be patients for whom the treatment does not work or has serious adverse consequences. There is no sound way to identify and eliminate this bias in the context of the trial, so the intention-to-treat analysis includes all consenting, randomized patients in the study arm to which they were randomized.

Answer 12.19. **The answer is D.**

For Phase III trials, it is mandatory to have an independent data safety committee that has the power to recommend termination of the study based on safety concerns, outstanding benefit, or futility. Because the study leaders have a conflict of interest with respect to the decision to continue the study, they are not part of the committee.

Answer 12.20. **The answer is C.**

Even if survival data have no censoring, a survival curve still provides a better approach for data summary because it takes the length of follow-up time into consideration. In addition, survival times are usually skewed to the right, and the conventional means and standard deviations may not be adequate for data description.

Answer 12.21. **The answer is B.**

For this study, noninformative censoring means that the probability distributions of cancer-specific survival are similar for both censored and noncensored patients. However, patients who have experienced disease progression are more likely to have a poor prognosis.

Cancer Prevention

Directions   Each of the number items below is followed by lettered answers. Select the ONE lettered answer that is BEST in each case unless instructed otherwise.

QUESTIONS

Question 13.1.   **Continued smoking after the diagnosis of cancer has been associated with the following effects in patients undergoing surgery:**

A. Increased risk of infection
B. Poor wound healing
C. Respiratory complications
D. All the above

Question 13.2.   **Adverse effects of smoking in patients undergoing cancer therapy include the following, EXCEPT:**

A. Clinical radiation pneumonitis from thoracic radiotherapy
B. Decreased survival in patients with localized prostate cancer treated with radiotherapy
C. Increased rates of neutropenia from irinotecan
D. Decreased efficacy from erlotinib

Question 13.3.   **Which of the following may be classified as nonsmoker?**

A. An 82-year-old man who smoked for 10 years and quit 50 years ago
B. A 25-year-old woman who never smoked cigarettes
C. A 38-year-old man who smoked approximately 75 cigarettes in his lifetime
D. B and C

Corresponding Chapters in *Cancer: Principles & Practice of Oncology*, Eighth Edition: 29 (Cancer Prevention: Tobacco Dependence and Its Treatment), 30 (Cancer Prevention: Chemoprevention), and 31 (Cancer Prevention: Role of Surgery in Cancer Prevention).

Question 13.4. **What is the best measurement for nicotine dependence?**

A. Number of cigarettes smoked per day
B. Age of smoking initiation
C. Time from waking up to the first cigarette smoking
D. All the above

Question 13.5. **What is the mechanism of action for varenicline?**

A. α2 agonist
B. α2β4 partial agonist and antagonist
C. Antidepressant
D. None of the above

Question 13.6. **Which of the following neoplasias is NOT an intraepithelial marker for invasive cancer?**

A. Colorectal adenoma
B. Junctional nevus
C. Actinic keratosis
D. Bronchial dysplasia

Question 13.7. **In clinical trials, systemic retinoids and beta-carotene were shown to reduce cancer incidence in this group of high-risk individuals:**

A. Skin cancer in patients with xeroderma pigmentosum
B. Lung cancer in heavy smokers
C. Cervical cancer in patients with cervical dysplasia
D. Colorectal cancer in patients with adenoma

Question 13.8. **Which of the statements is/are TRUE regarding nonsteroidal anti-inflammatory drugs (NSAIDs) in the prevention of colorectal cancer?**

A. Chemopreventive effects of low-dose aspirin on colorectal cancer development were demonstrated in clinical trials, and its overall benefits outweigh the risks in adults at average risks of developing colorectal cancer.
B. High-dose sulindac prevents the development of new polyps, although it does not cause the regression of established polyps.
C. In randomized trials, both rofecoxib and celecoxib were shown to reduce the risk of metachronous colorectal adenomas and colorectal cancer.
D. Considering the risks associated with these agents, screening strategy alone seems to be sufficient in average-risk adults.

Question 13.9. **The risk of which of the following toxicities is increased in patients treated with raloxifene?**

A. Endometrial cancer
B. Vertebral fracture
C. Venous thromboembolism
D. Coronary artery heart disease

Question 13.10.   **Which of the following statements regarding BRCA mutations is false?**

A. The lifetime risk of ovarian cancer increases to 25% to 40% in BRCA1 mutation carriers.
B. Prophylactic bilateral salpingo-oophorectomy (BSO) is strongly recommended in women with BRCA mutations because of the lack of effective screening methods.
C. BSO decreases the risk of breast cancer in patients with BRCA1 or BRCA2 mutations.
D. Both BRCA1 and BRCA2 mutations are autosomal recessive.

Question 13.11.   **Which of the following statements regarding familial adenomatous polyposis (FAP) is FALSE?**

A. The development of colorectal cancer is inevitable in the absence of colectomy.
B. It is characterized by the presence of 100 or more adenomatous polyps in the colorectum.
C. It accounts for approximately 5% of the colorectal cancer cases.
D. It is an autosomal dominant disorder.

Question 13.12.   **What is the best treatment for a patient with FAP presenting with approximately 300 colorectal polyps and 15 rectal adenomas?**

A. Observation
B. Total proctocolectomy with permanent ileostomy (TPC)
C. Proctocolectomy with ileal pouch-anal anastomosis (IPAA)
D. Total colectomy with ileorectal anastomosis (IRA)

Question 13.13.   **Which of the following does not represent an indication for microsatellite instability (MSI) testing in patients with suspected hereditary nonpolyposis colorectal cancer (HNPCC) according to the revised Bethesda guidelines?**

A. Colorectal cancer in a patient aged less than 50 years
B. Presence of synchronous colorectal cancer regardless of age
C. Colorectal cancer with MSI histology regardless of age
D. Colorectal cancer diagnosed in two or more first-degree relatives with HNPCC-related tumor regardless of age

Question 13.14.   **Which of the following does NOT represent a HNPCC-related tumor?**

A. Gastric cancer
B. Carcinoma of the small bowel
C. Pancreatic cancer
D. Breast cancer

Question 13.15.   **Which of the following statements regarding multiple endocrine neoplasia (MEN)2A is false?**

A.   It is an autosomal recessive disorder characterized by mutations in the RET protooncogene.
B.   All patients with MEN2A develop medullary thyroid carcinoma (MTC).
C.   Patients with MEN2A mutation should undergo thyroidectomy before age 6 years.
D.   Hyperparathyroidism may develop in up to 35% of patients.

ANSWERS

Answer 13.1.   **The answer is D.**

Continued smoking is associated with several complications after surgery, including increased risk of infection in general, flap necrosis in patients undergoing mastectomy with transverse rectus abdominis myocutaneous (TRAM), and respiratory complications after thoracotomy for lung cancer. Proposed mechanisms for these complications include tissue hypoxia by higher levels of carboxyhemoglobin and nicotine-induced vasoconstriction, and higher levels of sputum production under general anesthesia.

Answer 13.2.   **The answer is C.**

Cigarette smoking has significant adverse effects in patients undergoing radiation or chemotherapy. Patients with lung cancer are more likely to develop clinical radiation pneumonitis, and those with prostate cancer have decreased survival from definitive radiation in the treatment of localized prostate cancer, perhaps as the result of tissue hypoxia or aberrant methylation of promoter genes in smokers. Several studies have shown decreased benefit from epithelial growth factor receptor (EGFR) tyrosine kinase inhibitors, including gefitinib and erlotinib, in never-smokers compared with current or former smokers. Smokers have decreased incidence of neutropenia, presumably by inducing drug-metabolizing enzymes in an accelerated metabolism that may decrease its efficacy.

Answer 13.3.   **The answer is D.**

The standard definition of nonsmokers includes patients who smoked less than 100 cigarettes in their lifetime. In contrast, patients who smoked more than five packs of cigarettes and already quit are classified as former smokers.

Answer 13.4.   **The answer is C.**

The number of cigarettes smoked per day and age of initiation, subtracted from the current age, reflect the total dose of cigarette consumption. The best measurement of nicotine dependence is the time from waking up to the first cigarette smoking. Patients who smoke the first cigarette within 30 minutes from waking up have high level of dependence and will likely need more intensive cessation therapy.

Answer 13.5.   **The answer is B.**

Several pharmacological agents have been used for the treatment of nicotine dependence, including the α2-agonist clonidine and the antidepressants nortriptyline and bupropion. Varenicline is a partial agonist and antagonist of the α2β4 nicotinic acetylcholine receptor that received Food and Drug Administration (FDA) approval for the treatment of tobacco dependence in 2006. In a recent study, varenicline was more effective than placebo or sustained-release bupropion for smoking cessation.

Answer 13.6.   **The answer is B.**

In chemopreventive studies, intraepithelial neoplasias could be used as surrogate end points, allowing cancer diagnosis at an early stage, identification of high-risk individuals, and reduction in the size and duration of chemoprevention trials. Colorectal adenoma, actinic keratosis, and bronchial dysplasia are neoplastic surrogates for colorectal carcinoma, squamous cell carcinoma of the skin, and lung carcinoma, respectively. Unlike dysplastic nevus, which is a premalignant pigmented skin lesion, junctional nevi is not a premalignant lesion.

Answer 13.7.   **The answer is A.**

In smokers, however, the Alpha-Tocopherol, Beta-Carotene Trial (ATBC) and the Carotene and Retinol Efficacy Trial (CARET) showed increased risk of lung cancer in patients receiving beta-carotene with or without retinol. Although topical all-trans retinoic acid (ATRA) might cause regression of cervical dysplasia, this effect was not seen in studies involving systemic retinoids or beta-carotene. Prospective studies found no protective effect of beta-carotene supplementation. Retinoids and beta-carotene have been studied extensively in both clinical and epidemiologic trials. Systemic retinoids were initially shown to reduce skin cancer incidence by 63% during therapy in patients with xeroderma pigmentosum. However, the protective effect was lost after discontinuing the treatment.

Answer 13.8.   **The answer is D.**

Several studies have shown protective effects from NSAIDs in patients with colorectal cancer. Although regular use of aspirin was associated with protective effects in population base studies, the benefit of low-dose aspirin was not yet clear in randomized clinical trials. The limited benefit of NSAIDS, including low-dose aspirin, in preventing colorectal cancer, does not justify their use in average risk individuals. Sulindac, at high dose, was associated with both regression of existing polyps and prevention of new polyps in patients with familial adenomatous polyposis, but the protection was transient and incomplete. Although the cyclooxygenase (COX)-2 inhibitors rofecoxib and celecoxib were shown to reduce the risks of metachronous adenoma, the studies were terminated early because of their side effects, being unable to detect the reduction of colorectal cancer incidence. Although NSAIDs reduce the risk of colorectal adenoma and colorectal cancer, these agents are associated with significant gastrointestinal and cardiovascular toxicities, which outweigh the benefits. Therefore, the best strategy for the general population remains effective screening.

Answer 13.9. **The answer is C.**

Raloxifene is a nonsteroidal selective estrogen receptor modulator that binds to estrogen receptor leading to estrogen agonist effects in some tissues and estrogen antagonist effects in others. Raloxifene has estrogen agonist activity in the bone but is less active than tamoxifen in the uterus. Unlike tamoxifen, raloxifene was not associated with increased risk of uterine cancer. Because of raloxifene's agonist activity in bone, it reduced the risk of vertebral fracture. Raloxifene does not increase the risk of coronary artery heart disease, but studies showed increased risk of venous thromboembolism and fatal stroke.

Answer 13.10. **The answer is D.**

The lifetime risk of ovarian cancer increases from the baseline of 1.5% in the general population to 15% to 25% in BRCA2 mutation carriers and to 25% to 40% in BRCA1 carriers. BSO significantly decreases the incidence and mortality for ovarian cancer in this population. An additional benefit from this procedure is the decreased risk of breast cancer development in patients with BRCA mutations, presumably through lowering hormonal exposure at younger age. Both BRCA1 and BRCA2 are inherited as autosomal dominant.

Answer 13.11. **The answer is C.**

FAP is an autosomal dominant disorder characterized by at least 100 colorectal adenomatous polyps, and virtually all patients develop colorectal cancer in the absence of surgery. This disease, however, is uncommon, representing less than 1% of the total number of colorectal cancer cases.

Answer 13.12. **The answer is D.**

Because of the virtually universal risk of developing cancer by the age of 40 years in the absence of therapy, patients with FAP should undergo surgery, with the timing depending on the extent of disease. Among the surgical options, TPC is rarely used and most patients will be treated with IRA or IPAA. On of the main factors in deciding whether to remove the rectum is the risk of rectal cancer. Therefore, IRA may be considered in patients with less than 1000 colorectal polyps and less than 20 rectal adenomas. In contrast, patients with a higher number of rectal adenomas, adenomas larger than 3 cm, or severe dysplasia should undergo proctectomy in addition to colectomy, through IPAA.

Answer 13.13. **The answer is C.**

The revised Bethesda criteria are used to identify individuals and families at high risk for HNPCC, where the MSI testing is indicated. The five criteria include (a) colorectal cancer in a patient aged less than 50 years; (b) presence of synchronous or metachronous HNPCC cancer regardless of age; (c) colorectal cancer with MSI histology in patients aged less than 60 years; (d) colorectal cancer diagnosed in one or more first-degree relatives with an HNPCC-related tumor with one of the cancers being diagnosed at age less than 50 years old; and (e) colorectal cancer diagnosed in two or more first-degree or second-degree relatives with HNPCC-related tumor regardless of age. Therefore, answer C is incorrect because only patients aged less than 60 years with MSI histology should be screened. MSI histology includes the presence of tumor-infiltrating lymphocytes, Crohn's-like lymphocytic reaction, signet ring differentiation, and medullary growth pattern.

Answer 13.14. **The answer is D.**

HNPCC is associated with several extracolonic malignancies, including endometrial cancer, ovarian cancer, urothelial tumors, biliary and pancreatic cancers, carcinomas of the small bowel, and brain tumors. Breast cancer, although commonly associated with multiple familiary disorders, is not considered one of the HNPCC-related tumors.

Answer 13.15. **The answer is A.**

MEN2A is a syndrome characterized by the presence of MTC in virtually all patients and hyperparathyroidism in up to 35% of patients. Because the best chance of cure in familial MTC is surgical resection before malignant transformation, thyroidectomy is indicated early in the course of the MEN syndromes, being recommended preferably within the first month of life in patients with MEN2B and before the age of 6 years in patients with MEN2A. The pattern of inheritance is autosomal dominant.

14

Genetic Counseling

Directions   Each of the numbered items below is followed by lettered answers. Select the ONE lettered answer that is BEST in each case unless instructed otherwise.

QUESTIONS

Refer to the following pedigree for Questions 1 to 4.

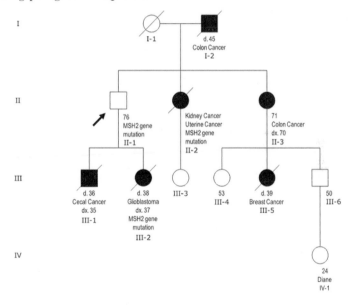

Corresponding Chapter in *Cancer: Principles & Practice of Oncology*, Eighth Edition: 32 (Genetic Counseling).

Question 14.1.   The family depicted has hereditary nonpolyposis colon cancer (HNPCC) syndrome. This syndrome is characterized by a high risk to develop colon and endometrial cancer and an increased risk to develop a variety of other tumor types. Before her death, individual III-2 had genetic testing of the MLH1 and MSH2 genes, and an MSH2 gene mutation was identified. Specifically, the mutation is c.942 + 3A>T. MLH1, and MSH2 gene mutations account for 80% to 90% of families with HNPCC. Individual II-1, depicted with the arrow, has not been diagnosed with cancer. He has undergone frequent colonoscopy screening. He has also had genetic testing and was found to carry the family MSH2 gene mutation. The finding that individual II-1 has not been diagnosed with cancer can be explained by which of the following concepts?

    A.   Genetic testing laboratory error
    B.   Clinical variability
    C.   Genetic heterogeneity
    D.   Reduced penetrance

Question 14.2.   Assuming individual II-3 has the family MSH2 gene mutation, what is the calculated probability Diane (individual IV-1) has inherited the MSH2 gene mutation?

    A.   0%
    B.   12.5%
    C.   25%
    D.   50%

Question 14.3.   Diane (individual IV-1) is 24 years of age. She approaches her primary care physician about her medical management, given her family history of HNPCC syndrome. She has a healthy body weight and does not smoke. Both her paternal grandmother (II-3) and her father (III-6) refuse to have genetic testing. In addition to her annual PAP smear, which of the following cancer screening is most appropriate for Diane?

    A.   Colonoscopy screening to begin at 50 years of age
    B.   Sigmoidoscopy screening to begin by 25 years of age
    C.   Colonoscopy screening to begin by 25 years of age
    D.   Colonoscopy and mammography screening to begin by 25 years of age

Question 14.4.   Diane (individual IV-1) decides to pursue genetic testing to aid in her medical management. She states her father will not undergo genetic testing. What specific genetic test should be ordered?

    A.   Full sequencing of the MSH2 gene
    B.   Full sequencing of the MSH2 and MLH1 genes
    C.   Site-specific targeted mutation analysis of the MSH2 gene
    D.   Deletion analysis using multiplex ligation-dependent probe amplification (MLPA)

Question 14.5.   **Samuel is a 42-year-old man who presents for routine evaluation. He carries a diagnosis of Von Hippel-Lindau disease (VHL). He was previously treated for three retinal hemangioblastomas. His father died of kidney cancer at 57 years of age. Samuel's daughter, Rachel, is 18 years of age and recently underwent an abdominal computed tomography (CT) scan for acute right lower abdominal quadrant pain. She was found to have a hemorrhagic ovarian cyst and a small adrenal nodule reported by the radiologist to be consistent with a pheochromocytoma. Which of the following statements is the best explanation for the difference in clinical presentation in this family?**

A.   VHL has variable expressivity.
B.   VHL has incomplete penetrance.
C.   VHL has gender-dependent expression.
D.   VHL is a multigene disorder.

Question 14.6.   **Consider the screening recommendations for the family listed in Question 5. What cancer screening is most appropriate for Rachel given her age and family history of VHL?**

A.   No screening is appropriate until Rachel is 25 years old.
B.   Urinary catecholamine metabolite screening.
C.   Urinary catecholamine metabolite screening and abdominal ultrasound or CT scan.
D.   Urinary catecholamine metabolite screening, abdominal ultrasound or CT scan, and ophthalmologic examination.

Refer to the following pedigree for Questions 7 to 9.

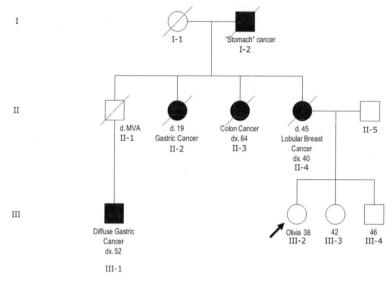

Question 14.7.   **Olivia is a 38-year-old healthy woman who presents to her primary care physician concerned about her family history of cancer. She has no chronic health concerns. Both her mother's and father's family are of Ashkenazi Jewish ancestry. Olivia pursues an evaluation with a clinical geneticist for assessment and genetic testing. The clinical geneticist diagnoses the family with which cancer predisposition syndrome?**

    A.   HNPCC syndrome
    B.   Hereditary breast cancer 1 (BRCA1) syndrome
    C.   Li-Fraumeni syndrome
    D.   Hereditary breast cancer 2 (BRCA2) syndrome
    E.   None of the above

Question 14.8.   **Which of the following features is NOT consistent with hereditary cancer in the family depicted?**

    A.   Multiple affected family members
    B.   Lobular breast cancer and diffuse gastric cancer pathology
    C.   Ashkenazi Jewish heritage
    D.   Affected family member diagnosed at a young age

Question 14.9.   **Which of the following concepts best describes the finding of multiple genes leading to the same phenotype?**

    A.   Genetic heterogeneity
    B.   Clinical variability
    C.   Allelic heterogeneity
    D.   Genetic pleiotropy

Question 14.10. Jennifer is a 38-year-old woman who was diagnosed with stage IIA ductal carcinoma at 30 years of age. She undergoes direct genetic testing of the BRCA1 and BRCA2 genes and is found to have a BRCA2 gene variant. Specifically the variant is Q713L (2366A>T), which results in the substitution of leucine for glutamine at amino acid 713 of the BRCA2 protein. The functional significance is unknown. Jennifer's sister, Angela, is 40 years of age and has no personal history of cancer. Which is the most appropriate genetic testing approach for Angela?

A. Genetic testing is recommended for Angela because it will clarify her breast cancer risk.
B. Genetic testing is not recommended for Angela because it will not clarify her breast cancer risk.
C. Genetic testing is recommended for Angela because it will help clarify Jennifer's genetic test results.
D. A and C.

Question 14.11. Genetic testing of what cancer syndrome is considered to be ethically appropriate to perform during childhood?

A. Familial adenomatous polyposis
B. Hereditary BRCA1 or hereditary BRCA2
C. Li-Fraumeni syndrome
D. Cowden syndrome
E. A and C

Refer to the following pedigree for Questions 12 and 13.

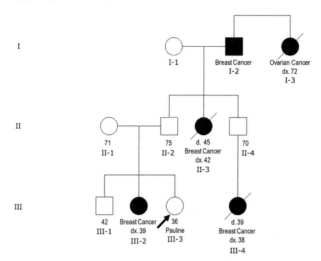

Question 14.12.	**Pauline, depicted by the arrow, is a healthy 36-year-old woman who presents to her gynecologist concerned about her breast cancer risk. She requests genetic testing. No other family member has undergone genetic testing. The gynecologist orders BRCA1 and BRCA2 gene testing. No mutation is identified. Which of the following statements is the correct interpretation of Pauline's testing?**

A. Pauline's test result is a true negative.
B. Pauline's test result is an unknown variant.
C. Pauline's test result is uninformative.
D. Pauline's test result is positive. |
| *Question 14.13.* | **Pauline's sister, individual III-2, is currently undergoing neoadjuvant chemotherapy for an aggressive ductal carcinoma of the breast. She is not interested in pursuing genetic testing at this time given the demands of her treatment. What breast health screening recommendations do you make for Pauline given her negative genetic testing?**

A. Mammography beginning at age 40 years
B. Mammography and breast ultrasound beginning at age 40 years
C. Mammography and breast ultrasound beginning now
D. Mammography and breast magnetic resonance imaging (MRI) beginning now |

Question 14.14.   Henry is an 18-year-old man who presents to the gastroenterologist with a 2-week history of rectal bleeding. He has had multiple bowel movements a day for as long as he can remember. His father is healthy and well and recently had his first colonoscopy at 53 years of age with no abnormality identified. Henry's mother also has had a colonoscopy performed, and two polyps were removed. Henry does not know the type of polyps. Henry has two older siblings who are healthy and well. There is no maternal or paternal family history of colon cancer. On colonoscopy, Henry is found to have numerous (~50) colonic polyps found throughout the colon, consistent with the clinical diagnosis of familial adenomatous polyposis (FAP). Which of the following statements best explains Henry's clinical history?

A. Henry has developed numerous polyps caused by an APC gene mutation.
B. Henry has developed numerous polyps caused by MYH gene mutations.
C. Henry has developed numerous polyps caused by a either a MLH1 or MSH2 gene mutation.
D. Henry has developed numerous polyps caused by a p53 gene mutation.
E. A or B.

Question 14.15.   A 28-year-old woman with bilateral ductal cancer presents to the medical oncologist for assessment and treatment. Her medical history is notable for intussusception at 6 years of age. The medicine resident notices small blue/black hyperpigmented macules on her lips, buccal mucosa, and fingertips on her physical examination. What is her syndrome diagnosis?

A. Hereditary BRCA1 syndrome
B. Hereditary BRCA2 syndrome
C. Li-Fraumeni syndrome
D. Peutz-Jeghers syndrome
E. Cowden syndrome

ANSWERS

Answer 14.1.   **The answer is D.**

Penetrance may be defined as the proportion of individuals with a mutant genotype who show any manifestation of the given disorder. A disorder that is expressed in less than 100% of individuals with the mutant genotype is said to have reduced penetrance. For example, if only 60% of individuals with the genotype express clinical features, the disease is considered to be 60% penetrant. Expression in hereditary cancer syndromes occurs when an individual is diagnosed with one of the associated malignancies or associated benign lesions. Almost all cancer syndromes show reduced penetrance. This concept is important to understand because many families believe if a family member has not developed a specific cancer, he/she cannot pass on the gene mutation to a child.

Answer 14.2.   **The answer is C.**

HNPCC syndrome is an autosomal dominant disease. Calculation of Diane's probability to have inherited the gene mutation is based on straightforward autosomal dominant inheritance. By assuming individual II-3 has the MSH2 gene mutation, the calculated probability Diane's father (III-6) has inherited the mutation is 50%. The probability Diane has inherited it from her father is 50%. Thus, Diane's calculated probability to have inherited the MSH2 gene mutation is 25% (50% × 50%). Most hereditary cancer syndromes identified to date are inherited in an autosomal dominant manner with reduced penetrance. In a clinical setting it would be important not to assume individual II-3 has the mutation. Although she has been diagnosed with colon cancer, the cardinal feature of HNPCC syndrome, individuals may be diagnosed with an associated cancer type and not have the causal gene mutation. That is, an individual may develop a sporadic cancer that does not result from the underlying family gene mutation. If individual II-3 does not have the MSH2 gene mutation, her sporadic colon cancer would be a phenocopy, a mimic of the syndrome phenotype. II-3's daughter, who died of breast cancer at 39 years of age, does not provide any insight as to whether II-3 has the gene mutation. Breast cancer has been reported in some families with HNPCC; however, an association in larger studies has not consistently been demonstrated.

Answer 14.3.   **The answer is C.**

HNPCC syndrome is associated with a 70% to 80% lifetime risk for colon cancer and a 20% to 60% risk for endometrial cancer. There are also increased risks for gastric (intestinal type), ovarian, urinary tract, and central nervous system (CNS) tumors with the level of risk varying for each cancer type. Colonoscopy screening is recommended to begin by 20 to 25 years of age or 10 years before the youngest age of cancer diagnosis and repeated every 1 to 2 years. Sigmoidoscopy is not recommended because of the predominance of right-sided colon cancers. Approximately two thirds of all colon cancers in HNPCC occur in the ascending colon. Consensus recommendations also include endometrial cancer surveillance with transvaginal ultrasound and endometrial biopsy; however, the efficacy of this screening regimen is unknown. Although Diane's (IV-1) paternal aunt (III-5) died of breast cancer at a young age, there are insufficient data to prove breast cancer is one of the associated cancers in HNPCC syndrome. As such, intensified mammography screening is not warranted. Intensified surveillance recommendations are available for many hereditary cancer syndromes. Limited data exist to prove the efficacy of these screening protocols. However, until larger datasets are developed, consensus recommendations are issued to help guide clinicians in the care of high-risk families.

Answer 14.4.   **The answer is C.**

The MSH2 gene mutation, c.942 + 3A>T, identified in an affected family member, results in an A>T change at the third nucleotide of the splicedonor site of intron 5 and causes an in-frame deletion of exon 5. The mutation can be detected using sequencing.

As such, site-specific sequencing, also known as targeted mutation analysis, is the only test that is needed. Full sequencing of the MSH2 gene is unnecessary and may result in excess cost to the individual pursuing genetic testing. Approximately 20% of MSH2 gene mutations are large deletions or gene rearrangements. These mutations cannot be detected using sequencing. Southern blot analysis and multiplex ligation-dependent probe amplification (MLPA) are techniques used to detect large deletions. A working knowledge of the types of mutations that have been described for a given gene, as well as an understanding of the limitations of the techniques used by a given laboratory, is crucial in overseeing the clinical genetic testing of a family.

Diane (IV-1) has the right to pursue clinical genetic testing to aid in her medical management. If her testing is positive for the MSH2 gene mutation, then her father and paternal grandmother may gain information they have previously chosen not to obtain. In advance of ordering the testing it is crucial to discuss if and how Diane is going to communicate her test results with her family and their potential reactions. By facilitating this discussion, the clinician is acknowledging some of the psychosocial implications associated with hereditary disease and providing anticipatory guidance as to how Diane may address potential reactions from her family.

Answer 14.5.   **The answer is A.**

VHL disease is an autosomal-dominant cancer predisposition syndrome associated with retinal hemangioblastoma, clear cell renal cell cancer, pheochromocytoma, brain and spinal hemangioblastomas, and endolymphatic sac tumors. Benign renal and pancreatic cysts, as well as epididymal cystadenomas, are also common. All individuals with VHL disease have a VHL gene mutation. VHL is a highly penetrant disease, with approximately 100% of gene carriers showing some manifestation. However, VHL is also characterized by variable expressivity that refers to the finding that individuals with the same genetic disease may have different clinical manifestations. This variability may be seen within a family or among families. In this family, the three family members have the same genetic disease, but each expresses a different feature. The severity and age of onset may also vary. For example, some individuals may develop a single retinal hemangioblastoma while a different family member develops develop multiple retinal lesions and/or other clinical features of VHL. The age of onset for a given generation does not predict the age of onset for future generations.

Recognizing the variable expressivity of the known hereditary cancer syndromes is an essential clinical skill in the identification and medical management of individuals with hereditary disease. Families often focus on a specific cancer type and may not understand the potential genetic link between two seemingly disparate malignancies. This singular focus may act as a barrier for complete reporting of the family cancer history or result in individuals failing to pursue the recommended surveillance because they do not appreciate the genetic link among different cancer types.

Answer 14.6.   **The answer is D.**

Rachel has an adrenal nodule that is believed to be consistent with a pheochromocytoma, a cardinal feature of the VHL syndrome. Regardless of this finding, Rachel has a 50% probability to have inherited the gene mutation, and as such, intensified surveillance is recommended. Direct genetic testing could be used to confirm the presence of a VHL gene mutation. Current medical recommendations for individuals with, or at risk to inherit, a VHL gene mutation include the following:

- annual physical examination with thorough neurologic examination and blood pressure check;
- urinary catecholamine metabolite screening by 5 years of age for families with pheochromocytoma;
- annual ophthalmology examination by 5 years of age;
- abdominal ultrasound by 16 years of age with CT/MRI screening for any suspicious lesion; and
- brain/spine MRI examination may be considered, but the efficacy in asymptomatic individuals is unknown.

The intensified surveillance recommendations reflect two key clinical parameters of hereditary cancer: Benign and malignant lesions tend to develop at a younger age than the average age of onset in the general population; and cancer predisposition syndromes are associated with diverse malignancies necessitating extensive and coordinated cancer surveillance and follow-up. The medical care of families with hereditary disease is complex and requires the coordinated efforts of multiple providers to ensure individuals with the highest cancer risks benefit from intensified surveillance or medical intervention. Clinicians need to consider what role they will serve in the medical management of families with hereditary disease.

Answer 14.7.   **The answer is E.**

The family cancer history meets the diagnostic criteria for the hereditary diffuse gastric cancer syndrome (HDGC). HDGC is an autosomal-dominant, highly penetrant cancer predisposition syndrome that results from mutations in the e-cadherin gene (CDH1). This syndrome is associated with a 70% cumulative lifetime risk for diffuse gastric cancer, an adenocarcinoma that causes thickening of the gastric wall (linitis plastica) without a distinct mass. There is also a 40% lifetime risk for lobular breast cancer. The youngest reported case of gastric cancer is 14 years with a median age at diagnosis of 38 years. Intensified surveillance with upper endoscopy and breast mammography with MRI is recommended. Prophylactic gastrectomy may also be considered given the limitation in detecting diffuse lesions. Precancerous lesions have been detected in a small series of "prophylactic" gastrectomy specimens.

It is a challenge for healthcare providers to stay well informed of their own medical discipline, let alone to maintain a working knowledge of the advances for other specialties and rare syndromes. Working collaboratively with a clinical geneticist and genetic counselor may help to facilitate the identification of families with hereditary cancer. Although these syndromes may be considered "rare," they often go unrecognized and the opportunity for positive medical intervention for a family is lost. The first step in the identification of hereditary cancer begins with a thorough collection and evaluation of the family cancer history. Detailed reviews of many hereditary cancer syndromes can be found at http://www.gene tests.org.

Answer 14.8. **The answer is C.**

Most hereditary cancer syndromes identified to date are characterized by their highly penetrant, autosomal dominant (AD) inheritance. As such, the features of hereditary cancer are the same as other highly penetrant AD diseases. The characteristics include young age of onset, multiple primary cancers in one individual, multiple affected family members in at least two generations, diverse cancer types that are part of a known cancer syndrome, and specific pathology known to be associated with a given syndrome. A family's ethnic and religious background is important to consider. As with any genetic disease, the frequency of cancer predisposition gene mutations may vary among ethnic groups. Knowing a family's ethnic background may provide a helpful clue in deciding to pursue a given diagnosis over another. In the family presented, the Ashkenazi Jewish ancestry was not a feature or clue to their diagnosis. Although BRCA1 and BRCA2 gene mutations occur more commonly among Jewish families, e-cadherin gene mutations do not. In contrast, the pathology of the breast and gastric cancers proved invaluable in the syndrome identification of this family. The hereditary diffuse gastric cancer syndrome is associated with lobular breast cancer and diffuse gastric cancer. Consider if the family had only reported a history of breast and gastric cancer with no specific pathology details. The differential diagnoses would have expanded to include BRCA1 and BRCA2 cancer syndromes and HNPCC syndrome. Knowing the histopathologic features allowed for a direct diagnosis to be made in this family. The use of tumor pathology to identify hereditary disease is quickly evolving.

Answer 14.9. **The answer is A.**

Genetic heterogeneity is the presence of mutations in more than one gene resulting in the same phenotype or disease. Allelic heterogeneity refers to different mutations in the same gene that cause similar phenotypes. Genetic heterogeneity exists for the hereditary diffuse gastric cancer (HDGC) syndrome because mutations in the e-cadherin gene account for only one third of families with this syndrome. Mutations in other genes have not been identified. HNPCC syndrome is another example of genetic heterogeneity because mutations in MLH1, MSH2, MSH6, or PMS2 result in the syndrome phenotype. In contrast, RET protooncogene mutations represent allelic heterogeneity. Germline mutations in exon 10 or 11 of the RET gene result in the multiple endocrine neoplasia (MEN) syndrome type 2A. Mutations in exon 16 result in MEN type 2B, which is distinct from type 2A by its early onset, aggressive medullary thyroid cancer, mucosal neuromas, and distinctive body habitus.

Understanding if genetic heterogeneity exists for a given syndrome is crucial in the genetic testing of a family. If individual III-1 undergoes e-cadherin gene testing and no mutation is identified, the genetic basis for the cancer predisposition in this family remains unknown. The negative test result does not exclude the working diagnosis, rather it indicates clinical genetic testing is not informative for this family at this time.

Answer 14.10.   **The answer is B.**

Missense variants result in the substitution of one amino acid for another. These variants occur frequently in the BRCA1 and BRCA2 genes. The functional significance cannot be determined with gene sequencing alone. Functional analysis of the BRCA1 and BRCA2 proteins is not available. Angela has a 50% probability to have the BRCA2 gene variant, but because the functional significance is unknown, testing Angela does not provide any clinically relevant information for her. Furthermore, because Angela has not been diagnosed with cancer, genetic analysis does not provide any new information to clarify Jennifer's test results. If Angela had been diagnosed with early-onset breast cancer, then analysis for the BRCA2 gene variant would have been offered for research purposes only to help determine if the variant is tracking with disease in the family.

For this family, genetic testing did not provide any new information to facilitate their medical decision making. Individuals with these types of gene variants are often left intellectually and emotionally frustrated by the testing. Imagine deciding to pursue expensive genetic testing with the intention of using the results to guide your personal and family medical care only to learn the testing provides no clear answer. As clinical genetic testing quickly becomes available following gene discovery, clinicians must contend with the identification of variants of unknown functional significance. The development of functional, rather than descriptive, testing will help to address this challenging clinical issue. Until such techniques are developed, it is important to inform individuals of the possibility of identifying these types of variants of unknown before the initiation of genetic testing.

Answer 14.11.   **The answer is E.**

Predictive genetic testing is considered appropriate to perform in children if the condition occurs during childhood and useful medical surveillance or medical interventions are available. When considering the use of predictive genetic testing during childhood, both the American College of Medical Genetics and The American Society of Human Genetics argue "timely medical benefit to the child should be the primary justification for genetic testing in children and adolescents." The classic presentation of familial adenomatous polyposis is characterized by the development of hundreds to thousands of polyps found throughout the colon. Colonoscopy screening is recommended to begin by 10 years of age because the average age of polyp formation is 16 years with the earliest report case to be 7 years. The Li-Fraumeni syndrome is a rare cancer syndrome associated with increased risks to develop a variety of malignancies, including, but not limited to, sarcoma, breast, brain, leukemia, adrenocortical carcinoma, and gonadal germ cell tumors. At-risk children are recommended to undergo frequent surveillance with abdominal ultrasound. Both of these syndromes develop in children, and children may benefit from the early identification of precancerous or cancerous lesions.

Predictive testing for adult-onset disorders is not recommended for children if there is no evidence for childhood onset and there are no acceptable medical interventions available. The BRCA1 cancer syndrome represents one such disorder. Delaying genetic testing until adulthood for adult-onset disorders allows individuals to make an autonomous decision about whether or not to pursue testing. Furthermore, this approach protects their confidentiality, allows individuals to evaluate the potential impact on their medical care, and allows them to process the emotional and psychological implications of hereditary disease.

Answer 14.12. **The answer is C.**

Pauline's testing is uninformative because the underlying genetic basis for cancer predisposition has not yet been identified in her family. When possible, genetic testing should always begin with an affected family member. In essence, when evaluating a family with genetic disease, testing should begin with the person who expresses features of the inherited condition. In the case of hereditary cancer syndromes, expression is defined as a person who is diagnosed with one of the associated malignancies or benign lesions. If Pauline's sister undergoes clinical BRCA1 and BRCA2 genetic testing, then these results may change the interpretation of Pauline's testing. For example, if Pauline's sister's testing is positive for a mutation, then Pauline's testing would be interpreted as a true negative. If Pauline's sister's testing is negative, then Pauline's testing was of no clinical value because the basis for disease remains unknown. Without prior knowledge of the family's gene mutation, Pauline's negative testing may have provided a false and dangerous sense of security.

Answer 14.13. **The answer is D.**

The underlying genetic basis for cancer predisposition remains unknown. Even though Pauline had negative genetic testing, it is not known if she inherited the disease causing gene mutation. As such, Pauline, and her paternal family members, should continue to be considered at high risk and followed accordingly. The clinician must return to the family cancer history to determine her medical follow-up. The family history is consistent with the clinical diagnosis of either the hereditary BRCA1 or BRCA2 syndrome. Pauline should follow the same recommendations as families with a confirmed diagnosis of one of these syndromes, until genetic testing proves informative for her family. Intensified surveillance with mammography and breast MRI screening, beginning by 25 years of age, is recommended. In studies of individuals with an increased breast cancer risk, the combination of mammography and breast MRI proved to be more effective in identifying abnormal breast lesions than mammography alone. The combination of mammography and breast ultrasound for women with an increased breast cancer risk is still under investigation.

In a 1997 study published by Giradello and colleagues in the *New England Journal of Medicine,* approximately one third of all ordering physicians misinterpreted the results of APC gene testing. The majority of errors arose as physicians misinterpreted a negative test result when the genetic basis for disease had not previously been established in a given family. Ongoing genetics education is needed for practitioners who assume the genetics care and testing of families with hereditary disease.

Answer 14.14.   **The answer is E.**

In the classic presentation, FAP is characterized by hundreds to thousands of polyps found throughout the colon. Gastric fundic gland polyps and duodenal polyps also occur. Attenuated familial polyposis is associated with fewer colonic polyps (generally defined as <100) with a later average age of colon cancer diagnosis than identified among individuals with the classic presentation. Familial polyposis is an autosomal dominant cancer syndrome resulting from mutations in the APC gene. Approximately 15% to 20% of individuals with FAP have no affected parent, meaning they have a new mutation in the APC gene. The frequency of new mutations varies among genes. Some genes have a very low, if any, frequency of new mutations (e.g., BRCA1), whereas others have a high rate of new mutations (e.g., NF1).

In 2002, biallelic mutations in the MYH gene were found to cause a similar phenotype to FAP. MYH is a DNA glycosylase in the base excision repair pathway. Two mutations (biallelic) are necessary for expression of the phenotype. As such, MYH-associated polyposis follows an autosomal recessive pattern of inheritance. Two mutations, Y165C and G382D, occur in the majority of individuals identified to date. As a result, many molecular diagnostic laboratories will only screen for these two mutations, rather than performing full analysis of the MYH gene.

Henry has no family history of colon cancer, and both of his parents have undergone colonoscopy screening. He may have developed multiple colonic polyps as a result of a new mutation in the APC gene. If this were true, Henry's siblings would not be at risk to have inherited the APC gene mutation. Henry's children, however, would each have a 50% probability to have the APC gene. It is also possible Henry has biallelic MYH gene mutations. If this were true, Henry's siblings would each have a 25% probability to inherit both MYH gene mutations. Clinical genetic testing is available for both the APC and MYH genes. For individuals with multiple colonic polyps with no family history of disease, APC gene testing is typically performed first and then followed by MYH gene testing if the initial testing is negative.

Answer 14.15.   **The answer is D.**

Peutz-Jeghers syndrome is characterized by the association of hyperpigmented macules, increased cancer risk, and gastrointestinal polyposis. Blue/black macules may be found around the mouth, buccal mucosa, nostrils, eyes, and fingertips. These lesions may fade over time. Hamartomatous polyps (Peutz-Jeghers type) most commonly occur in the small bowel but can also develop in the colon or stomach. Recurrent obstruction and intussusception may occur. Individuals with Peutz-Jeghers syndrome are at increased risk for a variety of tumors, including breast, colorectal, ovarian, gastric, and pancreatic cancers. Affected females are also at increased risk for adenoma malignum of the cervix and a benign ovarian tumor, sex cords tumors with annular tubules (SCTAT). Peutz-Jeghers syndrome results from mutations in the STK11 gene found on chromosome 19. The Peutz-Jeghers syndrome serves as an example of the importance of a detailed physical examination, in combination with the family cancer history, to identify individuals with a hereditary cancer syndrome. Other physical features that provide important diagnostic clues include the mucosal neuromas of the lips and tongue in the multiple endocrine neoplasia syndrome type 2B; trichilemmomas or papillomatous lesions in the Cowden syndrome; and sebaceous adenomas in the Muir-Torre syndrome.

Cancer Screening

Directions   Each of the numbered items below is followed by lettered answers. Select the ONE lettered answer that is BEST in each case unless instructed otherwise.

QUESTIONS

Question 15.1.   **Studies of screening for cancer are subject to several types of bias. If screening detects a cancer earlier (before it becomes symptomatic), but treatment has no effect on the course of the disease, then the subject will seem to live longer than if he or she had presented symptomatically. (That is, the cancer is known for a longer period of time, but the time of death is not altered.) This type of bias is known as:**

A.   Lead-time bias
B.   Length bias
C.   Volunteer bias
D.   Overdiagnosis bias

Question 15.2.   **A healthy 13-year-old girl received a vaccine against human papilloma (HPV) virus. This is an example of:**

A.   Primary prevention
B.   Secondary prevention
C.   Tertiary prevention
D.   Case finding

Question 15.3.   **A healthy 48-year-old woman went to see her primary care physician because she found a breast lump. The workup found a 1-cm invasive ductal carcinoma. This is an example of:**

A.   Primary prevention
B.   Secondary prevention
C.   Tertiary prevention
D.   Case finding

Corresponding Chapter in *Cancer: Principles & Practice of Oncology,* Eighth Edition: 33 (Cancer Screening).

Question 15.4.   A healthy 85-year-old man was found to have an elevated prostate-specific antigen (PSA) level. He had no urologic symptoms. Evaluation and biopsy revealed a localized prostate cancer with a low Gleason score. This is an example of:

A. Primary prevention
B. Secondary prevention
C. Tertiary prevention
D. Case finding

Question 15.5.   In the preceding case (Question 5), you might be concerned about:

A. Lead-time bias
B. Length bias
C. Volunteer bias
D. Overdiagnosis bias

Question 15.6.   A new screening test for ovarian cancer was developed. It was tested in a tertiary care academic medical center in a group of women with breast cancer (BRCA) mutations and was found to have a sensitivity of 70%, specificity of 90%, and positive predictive value of 10%. If a woman in the study population is found to have a positive (abnormal) test result, how would you interpret it?

A. There is a 30% chance that this represents a false-positive result.
B. There is a 10% chance that this represents a false-positive result.
C. There is a 9 in 10 chance that this represents a false-positive result.
D. You can be 90% sure that your patient has the disease.

Question 15.7.   If the use of this test (from Question 7) is expanded to the general population, it is expected that:

A. The test sensitivity will be lower.
B. The test specificity will be lower.
C. The positive predictive value will be lower.
D. The test specificity will be higher.

Question 15.8.   Which one or more of the following screening tests for colorectal cancer have been proven effective in randomized controlled trials?

A. Fecal occult blood testing
B. Flexible sigmoidoscopy
C. Air-contrast barium enema
D. Colonoscopy

Question 15.9.   A patient's family history should influence recommendations for colorectal cancer screening:

A. True because a positive family history indicates a need for earlier and/or more frequent screening.
B. False because the generally recommended screening protocols are adequate regardless of family history.
C. False because a family history of colorectal cancer has no significant effect on an individual's risk of disease.

Question 15.10.   **Almost all cervical cancers are associated with infection by sexually transmitted HPV. Of the following statements about HPV infection in young women (in their teens and 20s), which one is INCORRECT?**

A.   HPV infection is common in young, sexually active women.

B.   HPV infection is often transient in young women.

C.   In young women, most cases of low-grade squamous intraepithelial lesion (LSIL) will regress without treatment.

D.   HPV infection and LSIL are the earliest stages in the development of cervical cancer and require aggressive treatment.

Question 15.11.   **Regarding population screening for ovarian cancer, which of the following tests have been proven effective? Choose one or more:**

A.   Annual pelvic examination

B.   Annual measurement of serum CA 125

C.   Two-stage screening: annual CA 125 then transvaginal ultrasound if elevated CA 125

D.   None of the above

Question 15.12.   **The United States Preventive Services Task Force, the American College of Obstetricians and Gynecologists, and the American College of Physicians agree on which one of the following recommendations for ovarian cancer screening?**

A.   Annual pelvic examination for women ages 20 to 70 years.

B.   No population-based screening is recommended.

C.   Transvaginal ultrasound every 5 years.

D.   Annual serum CA 125 measurement.

Question 15.13.   **Women are at increased risk of breast cancer if they have:**

A.   Lobular carcinoma in situ (LCIS)

B.   Atypical ductal hyperplasia (ADH)

C.   A history of mantle radiation for Hodgkin's lymphoma

D.   All of the above

Question 15.14.   **For women who have had a hysterectomy, which one of the following is the most appropriate practice for screening for cervical cancer with PAP smears?**

A.   PAP smears should be performed every 1 to 3 years indefinitely.

B.   PAP smears should be performed every 1 to 3 years until age 65 years.

C.   Women who have a history of cervical cancer can discontinue screening after a total abdominal hysterectomy.

D.   Women who have had a total hysterectomy for benign conditions no longer need PAP smears.

Question 15.15. **Which one statement regarding screening for breast cancer is MOST true?**

A. Teaching women to perform a thorough breast self-examination (BSE) has been shown to have a small but measurable impact on breast cancer mortality rates.
B. The monthly BSE is a crucial component of breast cancer screening programs.
C. The BSE has been shown to be ineffective for breast cancer screening.
D. There have been no studies examining the impact of BSE on breast cancer detection.

ANSWERS

Answer 15.1. **The answer is A.**

Lead-time bias is the interval between the diagnosis of disease at screening and when it would have been detected because of the development of symptoms. Length bias is the overrepresentation among screen-detected cases of those with a long preclinical period (thus, less rapidly fatal), leading to the incorrect conclusion that screening was beneficial. Volunteers who choose to participate in screening programs are likely to be different from the general population in ways that affect survival. They may be more compliant or may have healthier habits. Conversely, they may volunteer because they think they are at higher risk for disease.

Answer 15.2. **The answer is A.**

Primary prevention refers to the prevention of disease, such as the removal of colon polyps to prevent the development of colon cancer. Secondary prevention refers to the identification of disease at an early asymptomatic stage through screening. Case finding occurs when a patient with symptomatic disease presents to a physician for evaluation.

Answer 15.3. **The answer is D.**

Primary prevention refers to the prevention of disease, such as the removal of colon polyps to prevent the development of colon cancer. Secondary prevention refers to the identification of disease at an early asymptomatic stage through screening. Case finding occurs when a patient with symptomatic disease presents to a physician for evaluation.

Answer 15.4. **The answer is B.**

Primary prevention refers to the prevention of disease, such as the removal of colon polyps to prevent the development of colon cancer. Secondary prevention refers to the identification of disease at an early asymptomatic stage through screening. Case finding occurs when a patient with symptomatic disease presents to a physician for evaluation.

Answer 15.5.   **The answer is D.**

Overdiagnosis is the detection of a cancer that would not have progressed to become symptomatic in the person's lifetime. A low-grade tumor in an 85-year-old man may never have become clinically apparent without screening. Diagnosis of the cancer may subject him to unnecessary tests and treatments.

Answer 15.6.   **The answer is C.**

The sensitivity of a test reflects its ability to detect a known disease, and the specificity reflects the ability of a test to give a normal result when the disease is known to be absent. From the point of view of the clinician, the presence or absence of a disease is unknown, and the pertinent question is the accuracy of the test result. The positive predictive value (PPV or PV+) is an estimate of the accuracy of the test in predicting the presence of disease; the negative predictive value (NPV or PV−) is an estimate of the accuracy of the test in predicting the absence of disease. The PPV represents the proportion of all positive tests that are true positives: $TP/(TP+FP)$. A PPV of 10% means that 10% of positive test results are true positives, so 90% are false positives.

Answer 15.7.   **The answer is C.**

The sensitivity and specificity are characteristics of the test itself and are not affected by the population characteristics. On the other hand, the PPV and NPV values are influenced by the disease prevalence in the population being tested.

Answer 15.8.   **The answer is A.**

Fecal occult blood testing has been proven effective in replicated randomized controlled trials. For the other screening modalities the only published data are from observational and case-control studies. There are ongoing randomized controlled trials of endoscopy, but no data are yet available.

Answer 15.9.   **The answer is A.**

A family history of colorectal cancer (CRC) or adenomatous polyps in one first-degree relative or two or more second-degree relatives confers a significantly increased risk of colonic neoplasia, and earlier or more frequent screening is needed. The risk is not significantly increased for individuals with CRC in just one second-degree relative or any third-degree relatives.

Answer 15.10.   **The answer is D.**

HPV infection is common in young, sexually active women but is often transient. Up to 70% of high-risk HPV infections will resolve spontaneously. Similarly, up to 90% of low-grade squamous intraepithelial lesions will regress without treatment. Concerns have been raised that screening young women could lead to overdiagnosis, aggressive treatment, and unnecessary harm from ablative surgical procedures.

Answer 15.11.   **The answer is D.**

No screening strategies have been shown to be effective for screening for ovarian cancer for several reasons. Ovarian cancer has a low prevalence in the population, thus lowering the positive predictive values of any tests. CA 125 has limited sensitivity (it misses many early-stage cancers) and limited specificity (many false positives). Transvaginal ultrasound has inadequate specificity.

Answer 15.12.   **The answer is B.**

The United States Preventive Services Task Force, the American College of Obstetricians and Gynecologists, and the American College of Physicians all discourage routine screening for ovarian cancer in the general population. The currently available screening tests do not have adequate sensitivity and specificity, especially considering the relatively low prevalence in the population.

Answer 15.13.   **The answer is D.**

LCIS is associated with an annual risk of developing breast cancer of up to 1% per year. Screening with mammography and physical examination can reduce breast cancer mortality in women with LCIS to the same level as that of the general population. ADH or ductal atypia increases cancer risk four- to fivefold, or even higher in women with a family history of breast cancer or those with ADH at ages less than 30 years. A personal history of mantle radiation (especially between the ages of 10 and 30 years) has also been shown to elevate breast cancer risk. Cases of breast cancer have been reported as early as 8 years after treatment, so screening of these women as early as 8 years posttreatment has been recommended.

Answer 15.14.   **The answer is D.**

Women without a cervix are not at risk for cervical cancer unless there was a history of cervical cancer (then PAP smears are for follow-up of the cancer, not for screening). Vaginal cuff smears are unnecessary; they have an extremely low likelihood of detecting vaginal dysplasia, and the false-positive rate is high.

Answer 15.15.   **The answer is C.**

Large trials of careful BSE instruction have failed to show any mortality benefit, so BSE is no longer a standard component of breast cancer screening programs (the American Cancer Society lists BSE as an option).

Sanjeev Bhalla
Cylen Javidan-Nejad

16

Advances in Diagnostics

Directions   Each of the numbered items below is followed by lettered answers. Select the ONE lettered answer that is BEST in each case unless instructed otherwise.

QUESTIONS

Question 16.1.   **Regarding external nontunneled venous catheters placed into the subclavian or jugular veins, which is TRUE?**

A.   The best alternative for routine long-term or outpatient use
B.   Highest risk of infection
C.   Low rate of migration
D.   Routinely use a subcutaneous cuff

Question 16.2.   **Which best explains the Groshong catheter tip?**

A.   Slit valve stays open to allow passive reflux of blood.
B.   Opens only with positive pressure so blood cannot be aspirated from a catheter with a Groshong tip.
C.   Opens only with negative pressure so that infusions cannot take place through a catheter with a Groshong tip.
D.   Does not obviate the need for a heparin flush.

Question 16.3.   **Which is NOT true regarding implantable port devices?**

A.   The catheter and port are entirely beneath the skin.
B.   The reservoir (port) may be accessed repeatedly.
C.   Devices are not computed tomography (CT) or magnetic resonance (MR) compatible.
D.   May be placed in the interventional radiology suite.

Corresponding Chapters in *Cancer: Principles & Practice of Oncology,* Eighth Edition: 34 (Specialized Techniques in Cancer Management) and 35 (Role of Endoscopy in Cancer Management).

Question 16.4.   **Regarding percutaneous needle biopsy, which is NOT true?**

A. Needle biopsy may be useful in distinguishing infection versus tumor.
B. Core biopsies are often required in the diagnosis of lymphoma, thymoma, and sarcoma.
C. If lymphoma is suspected, cells are sent in Roswell Park Memorial Institute (RPMI) solution.
D. Intravenous contrast is necessary.
E. Even though procedures are image guided, prebiopsy imaging is key to procedural planning.

Question 16.5.   **Regarding percutaneous lung needle biopsy, which is TRUE?**

A. CT is faster than fluoroscopy.
B. Fluoroscopy is better for central (mediastinal) lesions.
C. Most common complications are pneumothorax and hemoptysis.
D. With appropriate image guidance, pneumothorax rates are less than 10%.

Question 16.6.   **Regarding percutaneous ablation of pulmonary tumors, which is NOT true?**

A. Currently reserved for patients whose operative risk is too high.
B. Performed under conscious sedation.
C. Efficacy is based on size and location of the lesion.
D. Most common complication is pulmonary hemorrhage.

Question 16.7.   **Regarding percutaneous abdominal and pelvic biopsies, which is NOT true?**

A. Pneumothorax is a well-known potential complication of adrenal biopsies.
B. Liver biopsies may need a core biopsy to distinguish well-differentiated neoplasms from benign lesions.
C. Fewer complications are sustained from crossing the transverse colon than the inferior vena cava when performing pancreatic biopsies.
D. Pelvic percutaneous biopsies are the preferred technique when ovarian cancer leads the differential diagnosis.
E. Pelvic sarcomas often require core biopsies.

Question 16.8.   **Regarding percutaneous gastrostomy tubes, which is NOT true?**

A. Requires less sedation than endoscopy-placed feeding tube.
B. May be placed for feeding or decompression.
C. Contraindicated in patients with prior gastrectomy.
D. Contraindicated in patients with ascites.
E. If in place more than 4 weeks, no imaging guidance is required to reinsert the tube if it falls out.

Question 16.9.   **Regarding percutaneous nephrostomy, which is NOT true?**

A. Treatment for pyonephrosis
B. Useful for diverting urine proximally from a genitourinary fistula
C. Requires preprocedural antibiotics
D. Requires CT guidance to access the kidneys

Question 16.10.   **Regarding biliary procedures, which is NOT true?**

A. High strictures are usually treated by interventional radiology, and low strictures are usually treated by gastroenterology.
B. The right biliary system is more likely to have isolated dilated segments from a central mass.
C. Biliary dilatation is the major indication for intervention.
D. Pruritus can be cured by draining just one segment.
E. Cholangitis may require multiple catheters to cure sepsis.

Question 16.11.   **Regarding percutaneous transhepatic biliary drainage, which is NOT true?**

A. Preprocedural antibiotics are required.
B. Drainage is usually via a two-staged procedure: external drainage then internal drainage.
C. High biliary outputs warrant nutritional replenishment.
D. Contrast is usually used.
E. Liver function usually takes weeks to return to normal.

Question 16.12.   **Regarding percutaneous cholecystostomy, which is NOT true?**

A. May be a diagnostic tool in unexplained sepsis.
B. May be a therapeutic tool in acute cholecystitis.
C. A transhepatic approach is preferred.
D. Distension of the gallbladder during cholecystography is avoided in the acute setting.
E. It usually avoids a future cholecystectomy.

Question 16.13.   **Regarding malignant pleural effusions, which is TRUE?**

A. Surgical pleurodesis offers a higher success rate in their management than chemical pleurodesis.
B. Usually transudates from tumor obstruction.
C. Usually asymptomatic.
D. Thoracentesis is the definitive treatment.
E. Large-bore tubes are better than small-bore catheters in their management.

Question 16.14.   **Regarding superior vena cava obstruction, which is NOT true?**

A.   Occlusion is a common consequence of thoracic malignancy.
B.   Collateral vessels predispose to hemorrhage and require embolization.
C.   Radiographic occlusion may be asymptomatic.
D.   Angioplasty with stenting is better than radiation therapy for immediate symptomatic relief.
E.   Recurrent obstruction may be treated with thrombolysis, balloon angioplasty, or repeat stenting.

Question 16.15.   **Which is NOT an indication for an inferior vena cava filter?**

A.   History of recurrent gastrointestinal hemorrhage
B.   Recurrent venous thrombus despite anticoagulation
C.   Propagating lower-extremity thrombus
D.   Eccentric mural thrombus in inferior vena cava
E.   Planned surgery

Question 16.16.   **Regarding inferior vena cava filters, which is TRUE?**

A.   Femoral approach is preferred for their deployment.
B.   Symptomatic caval thrombosis is fairly rare complication.
C.   It is permanent.
D.   Jugular approach requires the patient to lie flat for 6 hours.
E.   There is no role for inferior vena cavogram before deployment.

Question 16.17.   **With respect to recurrent ascites, which is NOT true?**

A.   Transjugular intrahepatic portosystemic shunt (TIPS) has been used to control ascites from portal hypertension.
B.   TIPS is contraindicated in patients with hepatic encephalopathy.
C.   Peritoneovenous shunting is an effective method of dealing with malignant ascites.
D.   TIPS is more beneficial in dealing with ascites from portal hypertension than medical management alone.
E.   Large-volume paracentesis is an effective method for obtaining symptomatic relief from malignant ascites.

Question 16.18.   **Regarding percutaneous abscess drainage, which is TRUE?**

A.   Urinomas are readily distinguished from abscesses with routine imaging.
B.   Transbowel approach is an acceptable route of drainage.
C.   Bilomas do not require drainage because they are sterile.
D.   Pancreatic leaks may be suspected because of high amylase.
E.   Small bowel leaks require surgical intervention.

Question 16.19.   **Regarding concepts of hepatic embolization, which is NOT true?**

   A. Coils provide an effective hepatic embolization technique.
   B. The hepatic artery provides greater blood supply to hepatic tumors than the portal vein.
   C. Hypervascular lesions are more sensitive to ischemia than hypovascular lesions.
   D. For neuroendocrine tumors, therapy is often aimed at symptomatic relief.
   E. Postembolization symptoms are often self-limited.

Question 16.20.   **Regarding hepatic tumor ablation, which is NOT true?**

   A. Percutaneous ethanol injection (PEI) is not as useful for metastatic disease as it is for hepatocellular carcinoma (HCC).
   B. Radiofrequency ablation (RFA) is limited when the tumor is near a vessel.
   C. Acetic acid is an alternative to ethanol.
   D. Combination therapy refers to a combination of intra-arterial and percutaneous therapies.
   E. RFA and PEI are usually reserved for larger tumors (>7 cm).

Question 16.21.   **Regarding the variety of imaging modalities, which is NOT true?**

   A. Bone magnetic resonance imaging (MRI) has essentially replaced radiography for the evaluation of osseous lesions.
   B. Sonography may be used for the evaluation of chest lesions.
   C. Multidetector computed tomography (MDCT) has resulted in improved temporal resolution in cross-sectional imaging.
   D. MRI has the advantage of functional analysis.
   E. Both MDCT and MRI allow for high-quality multiplanar imaging.

Question 16.22.   **Regarding nuclear medicine studies, which is TRUE?**

   A. Increased number of images results in increased radiation dose.
   B. Bone scintigraphy is a good screening for bone metastases from prostate cancer when the prostate-specific antigen (PSA) is less than 5.
   C. Sentinel node mapping is of no value in the staging of melanoma.
   D. Positron emission tomography (PET)/CT relies on spiral CT for its attenuation correction.
   E. Single photon emission computed tomography (SPECT) relies on injection of fluorodeoxyglucose (FDG) for diagnosis.

Question 16.23. **Regarding therapeutic response assessment, which is TRUE?**

A. There are three categories of response: complete response, partial response, and disease progression.

B. Response Evaluation Criteria in Solid Tumors (RECIST) rely on bidirectional measurements.

C. Partial response represents less than 25% reduction in the sum of the tumor cross-products.

D. One shortcoming of the RECIST is the lack of inclusion of bone marrow involvement by neoplasm.

E. There is no role in using perfusion techniques to assess tumor response.

Question 16.24. **Regarding brain neoplasms, which is TRUE?**

A. Cross-sectional imaging is a highly specific way to distinguish recurrent tumor from radiation change.

B. MRI with contrast is superior to CT for the evaluation of sellar lesions.

C. CT plays no role in the presurgical evaluation when high-quality MRI is used.

D. Because of high spatial resolution, MRI does not require contrast to detect cerebral lesions.

E. Functional MRI is a great way to look at the behavior of small nodules and avoid overstaging a patient.

Question 16.25. **Regarding head and neck cancers, which is TRUE?**

A. MRI is favored over CT when the lesion is in the upper aerodigestive tract near the skull base.

B. Neck CT with intravenous contrast is better than endoscopy in the evaluation of small mucosal lesions of the aerodigestive tract.

C. There is no role for PET/CT in head and neck cancers because intravenous contrast material is not used.

D. CT does not delineate bone involvement in paranasal sinus tumors.

Question 16.26. **Regarding lung cancer, which is TRUE?**

A. Chest radiography screening results in improved mortality.

B. CT screening further improves mortality because smaller lesions are detected.

C. MDCT can accurately predict chest wall or mediastinal invasion in greater than 95% of patients.

D. MRI is useful in the evaluation of superior sulcus tumors.

E. PET/CT obviates the need for any additional imaging in the staging of clinically suspected metastatic non–small cell lung cancer (NSCLC).

Question 16.27.   **Regarding lung cancer treatment planning, which is TRUE?**

A. Adrenal lesion biopsy is no longer needed in the era of MRI and MDCT.
B. Routine imaging of the brain and bone in the absence of clinical suspicion of metastases is unwarranted.
C. CT of the chest requires intravenous contrast to exclude adrenal metastases.
D. Liver should be imaged in its entirety on an initial staging CT because of the high incidence of liver metastases.

Question 16.28.   **Regarding lymphoma, which is TRUE?**

A. Lymphangiography remains a highly sensitive and specific way to evaluate portal and mesenteric lymphadenopathy.
B. CT is an effective way to evaluate bone marrow involvement.
C. Routine MRI is equally as sensitive as CT for detection of lymphadenopathy in the chest, abdomen, or pelvis.
D. Gallium scintigraphy is better than PET in the detection of lymphadenopathy from lymphoma.
E. The added sensitivity of PET is its ability to adequately characterize bone marrow involvement by lymphoma.

Question 16.29.   **Regarding breast cancer, which is TRUE?**

A. Annual screening mammography should begin at age 50 years.
B. There is no role for early screening in high-risk patients.
C. Calcium is an indication of benign disease.
D. Final assessment on mammography is based on likelihood of malignancy.
E. Percutaneous biopsy of a potential cancer is contraindicated for fear of seeding the needle tract.

Question 16.30.   **Regarding nonmammographic breast imaging, which is TRUE?**

A. Sonography is not useful for the evaluation of dense breasts.
B. To distinguish cysts from solid masses, sonography should be used as a first-line tool.
C. Because of breast geometry, sonography cannot be used for needle biopsy guidance.
D. MRI is limited because of the inability to have MRI-guided biopsies.

Question 16.31.   **Regarding breast cancer staging, which is NOT true?**

A. Lymphoscintigraphy is useful for the staging of large breast cancers (>5 cm).
B. Disease greater than one quadrant is known as multicentric disease.
C. More than one focus of disease in the same quadrant is known as multifocal disease.
D. Sonography is limited in the detection of depicting carcinoma in situ (DCIS).
E. MRI is useful in the detection of infiltrating lobular cancer.

Question 16.32. **Regarding breast MRI, which is TRUE?**

A. Not useful in the postoperative breast.
B. More specific than sensitive in neoplasm detection.
C. Intravenous contrast is not needed.
D. Obviates need for biopsy.
E. Impact on mortality has yet to be determined.

Question 16.33. **Regarding colorectal cancer, which is TRUE?**

A. CT colography is limited by reliance on intravenous contrast.
B. Transrectal ultrasound (TRUS) is a useful way of evaluating the entire colon.
C. MDCT is an accurate way to evaluate the bowel wall tumor extension.
D. MRI is better than CT in the evaluation of distant metastasis.
E. MRI is a more sensitive way to assess localized disease extension than MDCT.

Question 16.34. **Regarding gynecologic malignancies, which is TRUE?**

A. Transabdominal ultrasound is the first step in staging endometrial cancer.
B. CT is limited in the assessment of localized extension of cervical cancer.
C. MRI is more sensitive than MDCT for detecting myometrial invasion of cervical cancer.
D. MRI is much better than MDCT in detecting lymphadenopathy from gynecologic malignancies.

Question 16.35. **Regarding cervical cancer, which is TRUE?**

A. Ultrasound is a highly effective way to stage cervical cancer.
B. MRI is a more effective technique for evaluating parametrial invasion than CT.
C. CT is an effective staging tool for localized disease.
D. No role for PET in the staging of cervical cancer.

Question 16.36. **Regarding ovarian cancer, which is NOT true?**

A. Ultrasound is an effective method for distinguishing ovarian from uterine lesions.
B. MRI is superior to ultrasound in determining whether an adnexal lesion is malignant.
C. CT and MRI are better than ultrasound for the detection of peritoneal disease.
D. MRI is better than CT for detection of lymphadenopathy from ovarian cancer.

Question 16.37.   **Regarding prostate cancer, which is TRUE?**

A. Imaging is key in its early detection.
B. MDCT is a useful way to localize a biopsy site.
C. CT is not useful for the detection of distant nodal disease.
D. The role of MRI is to determine whether the cancer is confined to the prostate.
E. The main role of MR spectroscopy is to determine whether a prostate nodule is malignant.

ANSWERS

Answer 16.1.   **The answer is B.**

External nontunneled catheters are routinely placed into the internal jugular, subclavian, or femoral veins. These catheters may be single or multiple lumens. When placed under sterile conditions, these catheters are safely used for 1 to 2 weeks. Because of their short subcutaneous length, these catheters may easily migrate. The absence of an external cuff makes these catheters more prone to infection.

Answer 16.2.   **The answer is D.**

One of the more unique features of some catheters is the presence of a Groshong tip. This slit-like opening along the side of the distal catheter is designed to stay closed. It may be opened with negative or positive pressure. The goal is to prevent passive reflux of blood into the catheter and minimize infection or thrombus formation. Because of frequent valve incompetence, heparin flushes are still required.

Answer 16.3.   **The answer is C.**

The implantable port device has simplified care of the patient requiring long-term nutritional support or intravenous access. These single or double-lumen catheters are attached to a reservoir (port) containing 3 to 5 mL of heparin and covered by a diaphragm that enables repeat access using a noncoring needle. The entire apparatus sits beneath the skin and is attached to the fascia of the pectoralis muscle. These may be placed in the operating room and, more recently, in an interventional suite. Patients often prefer these devices because they enable an active lifestyle and guarantee venous access. This latter point is important in patients needing frequent blood draws or in whom frequent contrast-enhanced imaging is required. Ports may be used for intravenous contrast and are both CT and MR compatible. Of note, rapid injection rates more than 1.5 mL/sec cannot be administered through a regular port.

Answer 16.4.   **The answer is D.**

Percutaneous needle biopsy has become an important tool in diagnosing new masses. Radiologists and referring physicians must be aware of the general technique for appropriate patients to be referred for this minimally invasive procedure. All of the choices given for this question are correct except the need for intravenous contrast. In fact, contrast is often not needed as it exits the bloodstream long before the biopsy ends. On occasion, contrast is administered to plan the part of the lesion that is most likely to yield a diagnosis (least necrotic and, therefore, most enhancing). Oftentimes, a contrast-enhanced scan has already been performed and so a repeat is not needed. The biopsy physician must review the preprocedural studies to determine the best route to the lesion and the lesion or part that will be biopsied. The differential will determine whether core biopsies must be performed (as in lymphoma, sarcoma, mesothelioma, thymoma), the solution must be in RPMI (lymphoma), or cultures must be sent (infection a consideration). As treatments based on molecular analysis of tumors continue to improve, percutaneous tissue sampling will surely increase. The physician's job is to make sure the correct patients are selected.

Answer 16.5. **The answer is C.**

Although many centers have converted all chest needle biopsies to CT guidance, fluoroscopy continues to be a safe and preferred method for lung needle biopsies. This comes, in part, because it is faster than CT because real-time visualization of the needle tip can be part of the procedure. Conventional fluoroscopy also has a significantly lower radiation dose than the newer CT fluoroscopy. The advantage of CT is that it allows for better resolution of smaller lung lesions and central lesions. Despite the use of small needles and appropriate planning, hemoptysis and pneumothorax remain fairly common complications of this procedure. Oftentimes they are self-limiting. In most centers, pneumothorax rates approach one third of all patients undergoing lung biopsies. Less than 10% require chest tube placement.

Answer 16.6. **The answer is D.**

Percutaneous thermal ablation of lung cancer is a relatively new technique that uses CT guidance to place a probe within a lung neoplasm. This probe is then used to deliver targeted thermal therapy. Studies are under way to determine how this technique compares with more well-established therapies. The procedure is performed under conscious sedation and can usually be completed within 1 hour. Efficacy is predominantly based on the volume of the lesion and the location. Accessible lesions less than 3 cm are likely to completely respond. Complications include hemorrhage, infection, and pneumothorax. The first two are unusual if sterile technique is used and any coagulopathy is corrected before beginning. Pneumothorax may be seen in 25% to 40% of patients undergoing ablation.

Answer 16.7. **The answer is C.**

As with lung biopsies, preprocedural imaging is important in determining the route of approach and type of needles to be used for percutaneous abdominal and pelvic biopsies. Certain organs, because of their most common locations, are associated with certain complications. The adrenal gland is one such organ. Because of its cranial location in the retroperitoneum, percutaneous biopsy may lead to pneumothorax. The pancreas is another such organ. It is often surrounded by bowel, precluding an unobstructed approach to a pancreatic mass. In such cases, a transcaval approach is preferred. The differential diagnosis from any preprocedural imaging will also dictate biopsy technique. Although liver masses may represent well-differentiated neoplasm (e.g., fibrolamellar HCC), core biopsies are required to distinguish them from normal liver or benign lesions, such as focal nodular hyperplasia. Core biopsies are also valuable in diagnosing histology or retroperitoneal and pelvic masses that may be sarcomas. When ovarian cancer heads the differential diagnosis, alternatives to percutaneous biopsy should be sought. High risk of tract and peritoneal seeding make an open procedure the favored route of tissue sampling.

Answer 16.8.   **The answer is D.**

Percutaneous gastrostomy (also known as g-tube) is an alternative to an endoscopically placed gastrostomy tube that is beginning to gain acceptance as a method of providing nutrition or gastric decompression. It can be placed quickly with less sedation than required for its endoscopic counterpart. Percutaneous placement can be via a pull technique, where the catheter is advanced into the stomach and a snare is used to retrieve it through the skin, and in a push technique, where the catheter is pushed externally into the stomach via a tract that is serially dilated. The former method may allow for larger catheters to be placed, but the latter method may result in less seeding of the tract in aerodigestive malignancies. Contraindications to the percutaneous technique include uncorrectable coagulopathy, gastric varices, and previous gastrectomy. Ascites may hinder endoscopic placement because of the increased distance from stomach to skin and therefore decreased effectiveness of gastric translumination. It is not a contraindication for percutaneous placement. The presence of ascites may require gastropexy, whereby the stomach is affixed to the abdominal wall. When gastropexy has been performed or after a tract has been established (usually after 4 weeks of a gastrostomy tube in place), catheter replacement may be performed without image guidance.

Answer 16.9.   **The answer is D.**

Percutaneous nephrostomy (referred to informally as a "perc" or "PCN") is a way of percutaneously draining a kidney that is usually hydronephrotic. Preprocedural imaging is key to identifying the site of obstruction and relevant information regarding the collecting system. It is performed as a way to treat an infected, hydronephrotic kidney (pyonephrosis), divert urine away from a fistula, or preserve renal function if the obstruction is temporary or treatable. Percutaneous nephrostomies are usually performed from a posterior or flank approach with fluoroscopic or ultrasound guidance and do not require CT guidance. Preprocedural antibiotics are used that target skin organisms to prevent infection from the procedure itself. Postprocedural antibiotics depend on the quality of the urine aspirated at the time of the procedure.

Answer 16.10.   **The answer is C.**

Hepatobiliary drainage is one of the main procedures in most interventional radiology suites today. Bile duct obstructions can be divided into high and low obstructions—an important distinction because the former are usually referred to interventional radiologists and the latter are usually treated endoscopically by gastroenterologists. Isolated segments or isolated bile ducts occur when the duct is obstructed and no longer is communicating with the other ducts. These, too, usually fall to interventional radiologists for treatment. Because the right duct is shorter than the left, isolated right segments are more common than isolated left segments from a central mass. Percutaneous drains can only drain a portion of the liver, but that may be all that is required to cure pruritus. For an infected biliary tree (cholangitis), multiple catheters may be required to cure sepsis. Because catheters may be in place for a long time and the remainder of a terminally ill patient's life, percutaneous drainage should be reserved for patients who are symptomatic or in whom clear benefit will be obtained. Biliary dilatation on its own is not an indication for drainage.

Answer 16.11.   **The answer is E.**

Patients who are scheduled to undergo percutaneous biliary drainage receive prophylactic antibiotics targeting skin flora to avoid infection from the procedure. First, percutaneous transhepatic cholangiography (PTC) is performed to provide information about the biliary tree. This step provides invaluable information regarding the nature of an obstruction. Drainage is usually done as a two-step procedure. First, an external drain is used to cross a level of obstruction. If the patient can tolerate this catheter with side holes proximal and distal to the obstruction without any external drainage, the catheter is converted to an internal one. When external outputs are high, oral replenishment of electrolytes may be required. In a majority of patients, drainage can result in rapid recovery of hepatic function with decrease in liver enzymes and bilirubin.

Answer 16.12.   **The answer is E.**

Percutaneous cholecystostomy is a safe procedure in the treatment of acute cholecystitis (calculus or acalculous) in patients who are unable to undergo cholecystectomy. Because of its few complications, percutaneous cholecystostomy can be a useful diagnostic tool in patients with sepsis of unknown cause. Ultrasound or CT is used for needle guidance. A transhepatic route is usually preferred to minimize intraperitoneal leakage and subsequent bile peritonitis. Although cholecystography can be a useful diagnostic tool, distension of the gallbladder in the acute setting is avoided to prevent rupture. In a majority of patients, the catheter will be left in place until the patient's condition improves, the tract is established (2 to 4 weeks), and the tube can be removed. In others, the tube will be left in place until the time of definitive treatment, which is usually a cholecystectomy. In certain high-risk patients, percutaneous stone removal can be performed via the cholecystostomy. Recurrent disease may be found in up to 50% of these patients within 5 years. This conservative approach is often reserved for patients with limited life expectancy. Most patients will undergo a future cholecystectomy after the acute illness has resolved because of the high incidence of recurrence of cholecystitis.

Answer 16.13.   **The answer is A.**

Malignant pleural effusions are a common cause of chest pain, dyspnea, and cough in patients with metastatic cancer, usually breast carcinoma, lung carcinoma, and lymphoma. These effusions are usually symptomatic and exudates. Thoracentesis will result in immediate relief of symptoms, but the majority of these effusions will recur. Definitive treatment requires tube drainage at first, which may be better accomplished via image guidance so that the tube rests in the location of the majority of the fluid. This is particularly true when the amount of fluid is small or the effusion is loculated. Although surgical teaching suggests large-bore catheters are required for successful drainage, recent data suggest that smaller bore catheters are equally as effective and may be associated with less pain and restriction of mobility. A majority of patients will not be adequately treated with chest tube drainage alone. In these patients, pleurodesis is performed to give better long-term results. Mechanical pleurodesis can be performed at surgery (usually video-assisted thoracoscopic surgery [VATS]) and offers a slightly higher success rate than chemical pleurodesis (which relies on a sclerosing agent such as talc, doxycycline, or bleomycin). Although hospital stays are shorter with surgical pleurodesis, chemical pleurodesis is less invasive and expensive, and has a lower morbidity. Another approach currently under investigation is the use of a long-term tunneled chest tube drainage catheter. Drainage can be performed in an outpatient setting. In this group, mechanical pleurodesis may be achieved in up to 50% of patients in 30 days.

Answer 16.14.   **The answer is B.**

Superior vena cava (SVC) obstruction is a fairly common consequence of thoracic malignancy, usually lung cancer. Radiographic SVC occlusion is often asymptomatic secondary to collateral formation throughout the mediastinum with diversion of blood to the azygous or inferior vena cava systems. These patients do not warrant any treatment. In others, no collateral vessels have formed, resulting in symptoms of head and neck swelling, headache, and mental status changes. In these symptomatic patients, radiation may be beneficial when the tumors are radiosensitive. This form of therapy usually works but may require therapy over weeks with symptomatic relief over days. An alternative therapy is balloon angioplasty with stent deployment. This technique (if the obstruction can be crossed intravascularly) results in immediate symptomatic relief. Recurrent symptoms may follow stent deployment and are usually related to tumor overgrowth, neointimal hyperplasia, and rarely stent migration.

Recurrent occlusion may be treated with thrombolysis, angioplasty, or repeat stenting.

Answer 16.15.   **The answer is D.**

The incidence of pulmonary embolism in cancer is three times that in the general population. The first-line treatment for pulmonary embolism or deep venous thrombosis is systemic anticoagulation. In patients in whom anticoagulation is contraindicated (brain metastases, gastrointestinal hemorrhage), an inferior vena cava (IVC) interruption filter should be considered. An IVC filter is also warranted when a deep venous thrombus continues to propagate or emboli continue to be observed despite anticoagulation or if surgery is planned. Free-floating clots within the inferior vena cava or a deep vein is also another relative indication for a filter because these types of thrombi tend to embolize. Eccentric, mural thrombi are usually chronic and less likely to embolize. Their presence alone would initially warrant systemic anticoagulation.

Answer 16.16.   **The answer is B.**

IVC filters can be deployed by a femoral or jugular approach. The latter is preferred because of a decreased chance of dislodging a clot in a deep femoral vein or the inferior vena cava, the ability to place a simultaneous venous line if needed, and the ability of the patient to sit upright in bed after the procedure. A femoral approach requires the patient to lie flat in bed for 4 hours after the procedure, which is less comfortable. The predeployment cavogram is important in excluding any congenital anomalies or IVC thrombus that may alter the site of deployment. Therefore, intravenous contrast is usually used for IVC filter placement. Complications of IVC filter placement are fairly uncommon and include symptomatic IVC thrombosis. Recent work suggests that this may be seen in less than 3% of patients with IVC filters. A retrievable filter was recently approved for use in the United States. This filter can be left in place, however, if the need for it persists.

Answer 16.17.   **The answer is C.**

Ascites is a common association with malignancy, from either malignant peritoneal deposits or end-stage liver disease. In the latter group, refractory ascites may be managed by a portal vein bypass in the form of a percutaneous shunt known as a transjugular intrahepatic portosystemic shunt (TIPS). In this procedure, a stent is placed in the liver from the portal vein to the hepatic vein. Portal pressures are reduced and ascites resolves. Although TIPS has gained in its use in patients with portal hypertension, certain patients are not TIPS candidates: Those with congestive heart failure and pre-existing hepatic encephalopathy, because the TIPS can exacerbate these underlying conditions. TIPS has been shown to be superior to medical therapy alone in patients with ascites. In patients with malignant ascites, large-volume paracentesis is the most common means of managing their condition. Although this technique allows for immediate, symptomatic relief, it is rarely definitive, and repeat treatments with all their associated risks are often required. Long-term catheters have been used with some degree of success. Another alternative is a peritoneovenous shunt (e.g., a Denver shunt). Their role in the management of malignant ascites remains unclear.

Answer 16.18. **The answer is D.**

Percutaneous techniques have dramatically changed the way postoperative abdominal fluid collections are managed. A majority can be drained without the need for reoperation. Postoperative leaks may result from urine leaks, bile leaks, bowel leaks, pancreatic leaks, or lymphatic obstruction. These may warrant drainage if infection is suspected, leak is suspected, mass effect is symptomatic, or the fluid requires further characterization. Cross-sectional imaging has made tremendous strides with recent advances in CT but does not always allow for adequate characterization of fluid collections with standard protocols. An example is a urinoma, which may be overlooked unless delayed images are obtained, and small bowel leaks, which may be confused with ascites if oral contrast is not administered. Bilomas can be another confusing fluid collection, which may be suspected in patients with a history of hepatobiliary surgery. Because of communication with the bowel via the bile ducts, these fluid collections can lead to peritonitis and should be drained. Pancreatic leaks should be suspected when the amylase is elevated (three to five times serum levels).

Answer 16.19. **The answer is A.**

Hepatic tumor embolotherapy is a promising tool for the treatment of hepatic lesions. This therapy relies on the increased reliance of tumors on hepatic arterial perfusion compared with normal liver. The result is that a variety of agents can be used intraarterially to cause in situ tumor death. Hypervascular tumors are known to be sensitive to ischemia, which has given rise to hepatic particle embolization with very small particles. Because of their larger size, coils are not used for hepatic embolotherapy. In patients with HCC, the goal of embolization is to prolong survival. In patients with neuroendocrine tumor, the control of symptoms is the more common end point. When tumors are bulky, pain control may be the main goal of treatment. Occasionally, postembolization syndrome may be witnessed and is marked by pain, fever, nausea, and vomiting; its course is usually self-limited.

Answer 16.20. **The answer is E.**

An alternative to embolotherapy is percutaneous tumor ablation. This is usually reserved for patients who are not surgical candidates. Whereby embolotherapy is the mainstay for patients with high-volume disease, percutaneous ablation may be used in patients with limited disease (one to three lesions). PEI and percutaneous acetic acid injection have been used in cirrhotic patients with HCC. The hard surrounding cirrhotic liver contains the injected material within the tumor and allows for uniform distribution of material within it. This therapy is reserved for tumors less than 5 cm because larger lesions preclude effective uniform distribution of ethanol and may cause ethanol toxicity from the increased volume of ethanol needed. More recently, RFA has been used for small HCCs. RFA uses heat to cause cell death and requires a larger tract than PEI. Not all lesions are amenable to RFA, although it has been shown to be slightly more effective than PEI for treatment of small lesions. Like PEI, RFA is limited in larger lesions. When a lesion is near a vessel, the vessel can act as a "heat sink," precluding temperatures sufficient to cause cell death. In certain lesions, combination therapy may be warranted, which combines embolotherapy and percutaneous ablation.

Answer 16.21. **The answer is A.**

Recent years have seen great advances in anatomic imaging. Among these is faster scanning techniques with MRI and faster CT. The advent of MDCT has resulted in improved temporal resolution and the ability to scan a targeted region in many phases of enhancement. The improved spatial resolution of MDCT has resulted in improved reconstructions in both coronal and sagittal plains. Although acquired axially, these images can rival MRI in their depiction of complex nonaxial anatomy. MRI remains superior to CT in its ability to create functional images (spectroscopy, perfusion, and cine images). Ultrasound also has seen dramatic improvements with better probes and more sophisticated techniques of scanning (tissue harmonics, extended field of view). Although not traditionally used for thoracic imaging because of the air interface with normal lung, sonography may be useful for needle guidance in thoracentesis and peripheral lung lesion biopsy. Occasionally, a mass can be characterized by sonography by use of color Doppler. With all of the recent advances, it would be tempting to discount the role of conventional radiography. One area in which plain films are still of great value is bone radiography. The high spatial resolution of bone films allows for lesion characterization that is complementary to MRI. At Washington University, no bone MRI is interpreted without a comparison radiograph. Lack of a comparison bone film may result in benign disease being confused with malignancy.

Answer 16.22. **The answer is D.**

Nuclear medicine studies are a form of molecular imaging that have been around for a while but continue to occupy an important role in staging and diagnosis. This has become even more true in the era of PET and PET/CT. Nuclear medicine studies rely on the administration of biologically active material (usually injected). Images are then obtained to document the biodistribution of the material. Although resolution of the images is somewhat limited, when viewed in conjunction with anatomic imaging, the studies can be enormously powerful. Because radioactivity is with the agent that is administered, radiation dose is completely independent of the number of images obtained, unlike CT, which increases the radiation dose with increased number of images. Bone scintigraphy represents one of the older techniques in which a tracer is injected that is taken up by osteoblasts. Tumors with a predisposition to osseous metastases are well imaged by this technique. However, it is very sensitive but not very specific, because any process resulting in increased bone turnover will result in increased tracer uptake. As a result, bone scintigraphy should be reserved for instances in which there is a reasonable likelihood of osseous metastasis. For example, in prostate cancer, a bone scan is recommended when serum PSA levels are greater than 10. Another technique that has been in use for a few years is sentinel node mapping. In this technique, radiotracer is injected into a tumor and the lymph node drainage pattern is mapped. The first or sentinel node that is seen can then be biopsied. This technique is useful when lymph node drainage patterns are unpredictable, such as melanoma or breast cancer. A recent major advance in nuclear medicine has been the increased use of PET in the diagnosis and staging of a variety of tumors. PET relies on the injection of a radiotracer (currently, usually FDG), which is taken up by metabolically active tissues. These tissues may represent infection, inflammation, or neoplasm. When combined with CT (PET/CT), this has become a powerful tool in neoplasm detection and characterization. A major pitfall of anatomic imaging is that it relies on an abnormal mass or abnormal size of a normal structure before pathology is appreciated. PET/CT allows for normal-sized structures (e.g., lymph nodes) with disease to be imaged before they become enlarged. This has been helpful in accurately staging many different types of tumors. The advantage of using a simultaneous CT for attenuation correction is that areas of increased uptake can be more accurately localized. Another major advantage is that by using spiral CT for the transmission scan for attenuation correction, the entire process has become faster, which has resulted in improved patient satisfaction and throughput.

Answer 16.23.   **The answer is D.**

A major role of imaging in oncology is to determine the effect of therapy on the clinical behavior of a tumor. To that end, a new study may show complete response to therapy, partial response (defined as >50% reduction in the sum of tumor cross products), and stability or progression (defined as 25% increase in the sum of one or more of the tumor deposits). In 1994, an attempt was made to create a more reliable method of assessing tumor response. These principles were published as the RECIST guidelines. These RECIST principles relied on the same four categories of tumor response assessment and used unidimensional measurements to quantify tumor size. RECIST also more strictly defined disease progression. Major criticism of RECIST rests on the lack of universal application of one measurement to all tumors, which may vary in shape, and the lack of inclusion of bone or marrow involvement. Newer techniques may make measurement less important in assessing tumor response to therapy. These include PET, where altered FDG metabolism may be seen as a sign of response, and rapid perfusion techniques that may measure altered tissue perfusion, which may be another early sign of tissue response.

Answer 16.24. **The answer is B.**

Neuroimaging continues to be on the forefront of modern anatomic imaging. MRI with contrast has become the standard method for detecting and characterizing intracerebral masses. It is very helpful in diagnosing and planning surgery for brain masses, especially those near the brainstem, posterior fossa, pituitary region, and cerebellopontine angle. CT is limited in these regions secondary to beam hardening from adjacent bone. Although spatial resolution of MRI is higher than CT, intravenous contrast is still used. It can be helpful in the detection of small lesions and meningeal lesions. CT with contrast is usually reserved for patients unable to undergo MRI or in some cases in which it may help in refining a differential diagnosis by showing calcium or osseous destruction. Both techniques are limited in their ability to differentiate between tumor recurrence and radiation change. Newer techniques have recently been developed that may allow for improved performance in the MRI detection and characterization of brain lesions and in the presurgical planning. These include MR spectroscopy, perfusion, and diffusion-weighted imaging. Spectroscopy, which relies on noninvasive measurements of brain tumor metabolites, is useful in guiding biopsy. It is limited, however, in small lesions (<2 cm) and in those adjacent to bone, fat, or cerebrospinal fluid (CSF).

Answer 16.25. **The answer is A.**

Head and neck cancers can be challenging to detect on imaging. Usually, CT or MRI is reserved once a lesion is detected by endoscopy. Endoscopy is far better than imaging for the detection of small mucosal lesions. The role of imaging is to evaluate any extension of disease. Both CT with contrast and MRI with contrast are used for staging of head and neck cancers. The preference seems to vary by institution. For upper aerodigestive malignancies, MRI is the favored technique because of less artifact from the skull base. PET/CT has become a valuable tool in the staging of head and neck cancer. Although CT with intravenous contrast is usually used initially, PET/CT with FDG but no intravenous contrast allows for a nice complement. This is particularly true in the postoperative neck, which can be confusing on routine CT or MRI. CT is usually favored when early cortical base erosion is suspected or if invasion of the orbital walls or paranasal sinus walls is the clinical question.

Answer 16.26. **The answer is D.**

Lung cancer is the most common cancer in both men and women, and its incidence is increasing. Screening, therefore, has been a topic of a great deal of discussion. Unfortunately, studies have not demonstrated any improvement in mortality from chest radiograph screening, although lesions were detected at more favorable stages. Studies are currently under way to determine whether CT with its ability to detect smaller lesions will be any better. It is still too early to tell whether detecting smaller lesions will affect mortality from this dreaded disease. Another role of imaging lung cancer is in the staging of disease. Despite improvements in spatial resolution, CT is still limited in its ability to detect chest wall and mediastinal invasion. MRI has shown greater promise in the evaluation of tumor extension because of its improved multiplanar capability and soft-tissue resolution. This is particularly true in the superior sulcus or lung apex where MRI can delineate tumor involvement of the subclavian vessels and brachial plexus better than CT. PET/CT is also useful in the staging of lung cancer. It is better than CT alone in the detection of mediastinal lymphadenopathy and sensitive for adrenal and bone metastases. Because of its high sensitivity, PET/CT may overstage patients with NSCLC. Because of the high glucose uptake of normal brain, PET/CT with FDG is limited for the evaluation of brain metastases. If these are suspected clinically, further imaging with MRI may be indicated.

Answer 16.27.   **The answer is B.**

Adrenal glands represent the most common site of abdominal metastases from lung cancer. For this reason, a routine chest CT should include the adrenal glands. Most adrenal nodules in patients with lung cancer will be adrenal adenomas. Because of their high lipid content, many (but not all) will be low attenuating on non-contrast CT examinations. If intravenous contrast is given, adenomas will enhance and may not be distinguishable from metastases. Many adrenal adenomas will show signal dropout on opposed phase gradient recalled echo imaging. PET may also be helpful in adrenal imaging in that metastases should have increased uptake when they are larger than 1 cm. Because of false positives with CT, PET, and MRI, any patient with isolated suspected adrenal metastasis should be biopsied to prevent false overstaging. Routine imaging of the brain, liver, and bone is not warranted in patients with lung cancer unless suspected metastasis has a clinical basis because likelihood of disease is low.

Answer 16.28.   **The answer is C.**

Lymphoma is a fairly common neoplasm that has seen dramatic change in its imaging in the era of cross-sectional imaging. In the past, lymphangiography was used for evaluation of paraaortic lymphadenopathy, but its role in lymphoma imaging has been replaced by CT, MRI, and PET. CT is an efficient way to evaluate nodal and solid-organ involvement by lymphoma but is limited in the evaluation of bone marrow involvement. MRI is equally as effective as CT in the evaluation of nodal and solid-organ involvement. MRI tends to take longer, is more expensive, and often is performed in patients unable to undergo CT or who cannot receive intravenous iodinated contrast. MRI is also useful in depicting bone marrow involvement. PET is highly accurate in the staging of lymphoma and with CT fusion is better than gallium scintigraphy for the staging of lymphoma. PET is limited in evaluating bone marrow involvement by lymphoma because increased uptake can be seen diffusely in reactive bone marrow, especially after chemotherapy and marrow-stimulating drugs.

Answer 16.29.   **The answer is D.**

Mammography remains the standard of care for breast cancer screening. Annual screening is recommended beginning at 40 years. High-risk patients (those with personal or strong family history of breast cancer) should consult their physician regarding initiation of screening at an earlier age. In these patients, there may be a role for screening sonography or MRI. On mammography, screening is based on the detection of a spiculated mass, architectural distortion, or microcalcifications that may be indicative of in situ carcinoma. Each mammogram has a final assessment category defined by the American College of Radiology breast imaging reporting and data system (BI-RADS) lexicon based on the likelihood of malignancy (1 = normal; 5 = highly suggestive of malignancy). This standardized reporting format has gained wide acceptance and serves as a model for other screening imaging modalities. Imaging can provide guidance for biopsy of any suspicious lesion (by ultrasound, mammography, and, most recently, MRI). Unlike with ovarian cancer, there is no fear of seeding the needle tract. Percutaneous needle biopsy is faster, safer, and less expensive than surgical biopsy. Patients undergoing percutaneous needle biopsy are more likely to be treated with a single, definitive surgery than patients undergoing surgical biopsy.

Answer 16.30.   **The answer is B.**

Breast sonography is an important adjunct to mammography in the detection of breast cancer. It is especially useful in patients with dense breasts but is not standard of care in breast cancer screening. It is a great first-line tool in the evaluation of a mass to determine whether it is cystic or solid and to guide intervention. It is faster and cheaper than breast MRI. The role of MRI of the breast is currently under study. Until recently, the role of MRI in screening has been limited because of the inability to biopsy lesions that were not palpable and only seen on MRI. MRI-compatible biopsy devices have recently been developed. Studies are under way to determine the makeup of these mammographically occult, sonographically occult, nonpalpable lesions.

Answer 16.31.   **The answer is A.**

Understanding breast cancer staging and potential therapy requires one to realize that more than one focus of breast cancer in one quadrant (multifocal disease) may warrant a wider excision and that disease in more than one quadrant (multicentric disease) may warrant mastectomy. Sonography is useful in depicting axillary adenopathy, which also affects staging, but sonography is limited in DCIS. MRI is sensitive in evaluating ipsilateral and contralateral breasts in women with cancer. It is particularly useful in depicting invasive lobular carcinoma and finding an occult primary tumor in patients presenting with axillary lymphadenopathy. Nuclear medicine techniques may also be used for breast cancer staging. PET may play a role in depicting metastases and showing tumor response to therapy. Lymphoscintigraphy also has become useful for lesions less than 5 cm and in some centers is considered the standard of care. For larger lesions, the results of lymphoscintigraphy may not be reliable for sentinel node mapping.

Answer 16.32.   **The answer is E.**

As useful as breast MRI may be on a case-by-case basis, its impact on breast cancer mortality has yet to be determined. MRI is a sensitive technique that is not as specific; consequently, biopsy of detected lesions may be needed. For this reason, MRI-compatible biopsy instruments have been devised. MRI is still expensive and requires intravenous contrast for dynamic enhancement. In the postoperative breast, however, MRI can be useful in separating recurrent tumor from postoperative change.

Answer 16.33.   **The answer is E.**

Colorectal cancer is the most common gastrointestinal malignancy. As a result, many studies have been performed to determine an effective way of screening for this malignancy. MDCT has recently allowed for the propagation of CT colography, which shows early promise. This technique is relatively noninvasive and does not require intravenous contrast. In the initial staging of colorectal cancer, CT, MRI, and TRUS are all commonly used. TRUS allows for clear visualization of the layers of the bowel wall and can allow for accurate depiction of tumor penetration. TRUS does not allow for visualization of the entire colon. CT is best used for assessing metastases and lymphadenopathy. Even MDCT does not allow for differentiation of the layers of the bowel wall. MRI, because of its better soft-tissue resolution, is better than CT for localized staging. High-resolution sequences may allow for clearer depiction of extension into adjacent fat and organs. CT and MRI have similar sensitivity and specificity for assessing nodal involvement.

Answer 16.34.   **The answer is C.**

Imaging in endometrial and cervical cancer is usually performed after a diagnosis is clinically made. The main role of imaging is to determine the depth of myometrial invasion, endocervical tumor extension and lymphadenopathy with endometrial cancer, and the extent of parametrial extension and lymphadenopathy with cervical cancer. Imaging is also performed to evaluate for distant metastases. MRI is better than CT in delineating localized invasion of both tumors. CT is limited in depicting the extent of myometrial invasion from endometrial carcinoma and the extent of parametrial invasion from cervical cancer. MRI is approximately equal to CT in delineating lymphadenopathy from gynecologic malignancy. Although transabdominal sonography is often used to investigate the pelvis, it should not be routinely performed in endometrial cancer staging. Even transvaginal ultrasound is limited because of its limited field of view and lack of soft-tissue resolution.

Answer 16.35.   **The answer is B.**

Imaging in cervical cancer is usually performed after a positive biopsy or PAP smear. The main role of imaging is to determine the extent of parametrial extension and lymphadenopathy. MRI is better than CT in delineating localized invasion. CT is limited in depicting the extent of parametrial invasion from cervical cancer. MRI is slightly better than CT in delineating lymphadenopathy from cervical cancer. Although transabdominal sonography is often used to investigate the pelvis, it should not be routinely performed in cervical cancer staging. Even transvaginal ultrasound is limited because of its limited field of view and lack of soft-tissue resolution.

Answer 16.36. **The answer is D.**

Imaging in adnexal masses is aimed at delineating the origin of the mass (ovarian or uterine), whether a mass is malignant, and whether distant metastases are present. Ultrasound is effective at identifying the location of an adnexal tumor (bowel, ovarian, or uterine) and in distinguishing benign from malignant disease. When ultrasound is inconclusive, CT or MRI may be used. MRI is more accurate in separating malignant from benign ovarian pathology. Staging accuracy for MRI equals that of CT. Both are thought to be slightly more accurate than ultrasound, especially in the evaluation of peritoneal disease. CT is slightly better than MRI for the evaluation of lymphadenopathy. Both are equal in their depiction of hepatic metastases.

Answer 16.37. **The answer is D.**

Digital rectal examination and serum PSA are effective means for screening for prostate cancer. Imaging plays no role in prostate cancer detection. It is useful (usually by ultrasound) for guiding biopsy. CT does not allow adequate prostate resolution for cancer detection in an abnormal prostate. It is useful, however, for detection of metastases. MRI, especially with an endorectal coil, provides high-quality imaging of the zones of the prostate. Its role is to determine whether the cancer is confined to the prostate. Spectroscopy is a relatively new technique that may improve tumor localization and detection of extracapsular spread. The role of spectroscopy is not in the characterization of a prostate nodule.

Cancer of the Head and Neck

Directions   Each of the numbered items below is followed by lettered answers. Select the ONE lettered answer that is BEST in each case unless instructed otherwise.

QUESTIONS

Question 17.1.   **In the progressive development of squamous cell cancer of the head and neck (SCCHN), which of the following is the latest event?**

A.   Loss of 9p
B.   Loss of 3p
C.   Loss of 17p
D.   Loss of 11q

Question 17.2.   **Which of the following statements about the epidermal growth factor receptor (EGFR) in squamous cell cancers of the head and neck is TRUE?**

A.   EGFR does not play an important role in these tumors.
B.   EGFR can activate cell signaling pathways that lead to the cell growth and division.
C.   EGFR overexpression downregulates angiogenesis.
D.   All of the above.

Question 17.3.   **Which of the following are risk factors for SCCHN?**

A.   Tobacco use
B.   Alcohol use
C.   Fanconi's anemia
D.   All of the above

Corresponding Chapter in *Cancer: Principles & Practice of Oncology*, Eighth Edition: 36 (Cancer of the Head and Neck).

Question 17.4.   **A 55-year-old man presents to an otolaryngologist with the symptoms of left-sided otalgia for 3 months and a left-sided neck mass. On examination, he has a 2-cm lymph node below his left sternocleidomastoid and a left-sided tonsil mass. A biopsy is performed that shows a poorly differentiated squamous cell carcinoma with basal cell-like features. He has no history of tobacco use and only drinks alcohol rarely. What is the most likely cause of his tumor?**

    A. Epstein-Barr virus (EBV)
    B. Human herpes virus 6 (HHV-6)
    C. Human papilloma virus (HPV)
    D. Human immunodeficiency virus (HIV)

Question 17.5.   **A 56-year-old man presents to his primary care physician with a 3-month history of right ear pain and two masses on the right side of his neck. On examination, he is found to have a 3-cm right tonsil mass and two separate right-sided lymph nodes below the sternocleidomastoid. One lymph node is 2 cm, and the other is 1 cm in diameter. He has a fine-needle aspiration (FNA) of one of the neck lymph nodes, and it is consistent with a squamous cell carcinoma. A neck and chest computed tomography (CT) show no additional lymphadenopathy or distant metastasis. What is the stage of his disease?**

    A. Stage II
    B. Stage III
    C. Stage IVA
    D. Stage IVC

Question 17.6.   **Which of the following statements is TRUE?**

    A. Only classic radical neck dissections should be performed for the management of SCCHN.
    B. Complications from neck dissections include hematoma; seroma; lymphedema; wound infections and dehiscence; damage to the VII, X, XI, and XII cranial nerves; carotid exposure; and carotid rupture.
    C. In a surgically treated tumor without radiographic evidence of lymph node metastasis, an elective neck dissection should only be performed if the risk of occult metastasis to the neck is greater than 50%.
    D. For patients who have had a neck dissection for SCCHN, there is no benefit for postoperative radiation.

Question 17.7.   **Which of the following statements is TRUE?**

    A. The combination of cisplatin and 5-FU has been clearly shown to improve survival over single-agent methotrexate in the treatment of metastatic SCCHN.
    B. Cetuximab has no activity in metastatic or recurrent SCCHN.
    C. The combination of cisplatin and 5-FU has a higher response rate than single-agent methotrexate in the treatment of metastatic SCCHN.
    D. Higher doses of chemotherapy have led to improved survival.

Question 17.8.   A 66-year-old man presents to his otolaryngologist with a 4-cm left floor of mouth squamous cell cancer. He has a left-sided 3-cm lymph node felt on examination and seen on CT. Magnetic resonance imaging (MRI) shows that the primary tumor is invading into the mandible. He has no evidence of distant metastasis on CT of his chest. What is the most appropriate primary therapy for this patient?

    A. Surgery
    B. Radiation
    C. Chemoradiation

Question 17.9.   A 54-year-old woman recently had a resection of a squamous cell cancer of the supraglottis with bilateral neck dissections. The pathology shows a T2 lesion, which was completely excised with negative margins but perivascular and perineural invasion. There are 2 of 28 positive lymph nodes with extracapsular extension on the right and no positive lymph nodes. What is the most appropriate primary therapy for this patient?

    A. Observation
    B. Radiation
    C. Chemoradiation

Question 17.10.   True or false: The addition of cetuximab to definitive radiation has been shown to improve overall survival for patients with SCCHN?

    A. True
    B. False

Question 17.11.   Which of the following statements is FALSE?

    A. Radiation therapy alone for locally advanced squamous cell cancer of the larynx has a lower overall survival than concurrent chemoradiation.
    B. Concurrent chemoradiation allows for better local control than radiation alone for squamous cell cancer of the larynx.
    C. A total laryngectomy may not be necessary for the treatment of laryngeal cancer.
    D. Large-volume laryngeal tumors are best treated with surgery.

Question 17.12.   True or False: There is an overall survival benefit for adjuvant chemotherapy after resection of a squamous cell cancer of the larynx.

    A. True
    B. False

Question 17.13. **Which of the following statements is FALSE?**

A. The three subtypes of nasopharyngeal carcinoma are World Health Organization (WHO) type I, squamous cell carcinoma; WHO type II, nonkeratinizing carcinoma; and WHO type III, undifferentiated carcinoma or lymphoepithelioma.

B. Most nasopharyngeal carcinomas are treated with surgery.

C. Common presenting symptoms of nasopharyngeal carcinomas include painless upper neck mass, nasal stuffiness, facial pain, and headache.

D. The majority of nasopharyngeal carcinomas are metastatic to neck lymph nodes at presentation.

Question 17.14. **A 56-year-old woman presents to her primary care physician with left-sided facial swelling and facial drooping. The patient has weakness of the lower portion of her facial nerve and a palpable parotid mass. A biopsy is performed showing a high-grade mucoepidermoid carcinoma. There are no palpable neck lymph nodes. What is the best treatment for this patient?**

A. Radiation

B. Chemoradiation

C. Surgery

D. Surgery followed by adjuvant radiation

Question 17.15. **Which of the following statements is FALSE?**

A. Treatment of head and neck cancer requires a multidisciplinary team, including medical oncologists, otorhinolaryngologists, radiation oncologists, nurses, speech therapists, nutritionists, and social workers.

B. Once the patient is able to get nutrition via a g-tube, there is no benefit to having the patient continue to swallow during radiation.

C. Intensity-modulated radiation therapy (IMRT) can decrease xerostomia in patients treated with radiation for head and neck cancer.

D. The severity of the side effects of radiation depends on the radiation field, the radiation dose, and the concomitant chemotherapy agents.

ANSWERS

Answer 17.1. **The answer is D.**

Dr. Sriranski has proposed a molecular progression model of the development of SCCHN based on analysis of the 10 most common allelic changes found in these malignancies. The earliest events appear to be the loss of 9p and 3p given that these are found in preinvasive lesions. This is to be followed soon afterward by the loss of 17p. The loss of 11q, 13q, 14q, and p53 mutation is not typically found in preinvasive lesions and therefore must be a later event.

Answer 17.2.   **The answer is B.**

The EGFR plays a key role in the development of squamous cell cancers of the head and neck. There is often a moderate increase in the number of copies of this gene. The overexpression leads to activation of multiple signaling pathways that lead to cell growth and resistance to apoptosis. Evidence suggests that EGFR overexpression can lead to an increase in vascular endothelial growth factor production, leading to angiogenesis.

Answer 17.3.   **The answer is D.**

Several risk factors for development of SCCHN have been identified. The two most important are tobacco and alcohol use. They seem to be synergistic. Other risk factors include occupational exposure to chemicals and irritants, such as aromatic hydrocarbons and wood dust, and viruses, such as HPV and EBV. In addition, patients with Fanconi's anemia are at increased risk.

Answer 17.4.   **The answer is C.**

It has been recognized recently that HPV is the primary cause of many squamous cell cancers of the oropharynx. HPV DNA can be found in approximately 50% of tonsil and base of tongue tumors. These tumors are often described as having a basal cell-like appearance and are frequently nonkeratinizing. These tumors are more commonly found in never smokers. In general, these tumors carry a better prognosis than other tumors of the head and neck. The overall survival and disease-free survival are improved, and the risk of second primaries is lower compared with non-HPV–associated tumors.

Answer 17.5.   **The answer is C.**

The patient has a tonsil mass that is between 2 and 4 cm. This makes his primary tumor T2. He has multiple ipsilateral regional lymph nodes with the largest lymph node being smaller than 6 cm, which is N2b disease. His tumor shows no evidence of distant metastasis. The patient's disease is T2N2bM0, which is stage IVA.

Answer 17.6.   **The answer is B.**

Control of neck disease is very important in the management of SCCHN. Both surgery and radiation can be used. When a tumor is treated surgically, a neck dissection is recommended even in a clinically negative neck if the risk of occult metastasis exceeds 10% to 15%. Modified neck dissections that can preserve structures such as the cranial nerve XI, internal jugular vein, and sternocleidomastoid can often be performed without compromise of disease control. Patients with positive neck lymph nodes clearly have a benefit from postoperative radiation if multiple lymph nodes are involved or N3 disease and sometimes chemoradiation depending on the pathologic findings. Complications from neck dissections include hematoma; seroma; lymphedema; wound infections and dehiscence; damage to the VII, X, XI, and XII cranial nerves; carotid exposure; and carotid rupture.

Answer 17.7.   **The answer is C.**

The treatment of metastatic squamous cell cancer is challenging. Many chemotherapeutic agents, including cisplatin, carboplatin, 5-FU, taxanes, ifosfamide, and methotrexate, have activity against metastatic SCCHN. Combinations of chemotherapy and higher doses of chemotherapy have a higher response rate but more toxicity. Combination chemotherapy has not shown a clear survival benefit over single-agent chemotherapy. Cetuximab has shown activity alone or in combination with a platinum in the treatment of metastatic SCCHN. Currently, the EXTREME trial, a randomized study examining the addition of cetuximab to combination chemotherapy, is ongoing.

Answer 17.8.   **The answer is A.**

This patient has a stage IVA (T4aN1M0) squamous cell cancer of the oral cavity. The therapy that has the most experience in this situation is surgery. Radiation and chemoradiation as primary therapy will be of little utility here, particularly with invasion of the mandible. He will most likely require radiation or chemoradiation after surgery depending on the findings.

Answer 17.9.   **The answer is C.**

After gross tumor resection, adjuvant therapy with radiation or chemoradiation is recommended for locally advanced SCCHN. The decision on what adjuvant therapy is to be recommended is based on operative findings. Major risk factors for local recurrence are positive margins or lymph node disease with extracapsular extension. Minor risk factors include primary tumors that are T3 or T4, N2, or N3 disease, perineural invasion, and vascular embolism. If the patient has any major risk factor or two or more minor risk factors, adjuvant chemoradiation is recommended. If the patient has a minor risk factor, adjuvant radiation is recommended. If the patient has no adverse risk factors, observation is recommended.

Answer 17.10.   **The answer is A.**

Cetuximab is an EGFR antibody that has been used to treat SCCHN. It has been used alone or combined with chemotherapy for treatment of metastatic disease, as well as with radiation, to treat locally advanced SCCHN. In a multicenter, randomized phase III trial comparing chemoradiation with cetuximab with radiation alone for SCCHN of the oropharynx, larynx, and hypopharynx, cetuximab improved both local control and overall survival.

Answer 17.11.   **The answer is D.**

The treatment of larynx cancers has changed significantly over the last 20 years. The traditional approach to locally advanced tumors of the larynx was a total laryngectomy often followed by adjuvant radiation. With improvements in surgical techniques and chemoradiation, it is often possible to preserve the larynx. For low-volume disease, a hemilaryngectomy can be performed saving the voice. Nonsurgical treatments can also be good options. Both radiation alone and concurrent chemoradiation for locally advanced tumors of the larynx have equal chance of cure. Concurrent chemoradiation, however, gives the best local control; therefore, it is the standard of care. Unfortunately, large-volume tumors of the larynx may not be curable by chemoradiation or larynx-preserving surgery and should be treated with a total laryngectomy.

Answer 17.12. **The answer is B.**

Adjuvant chemotherapy has been tested in several trials to improve the survival of patients with SCCHN. Unfortunately, it has not been shown to improve survival. Currently, adjuvant chemotherapy is only used in the treatment of locally advanced nasopharyngeal cancer. Even its benefit is unclear.

Answer 17.13. **The answer is B.**

Nasopharyngeal carcinomas are unusual in the United States but are much more common in China and Southeast Asia. On the basis of pathology, there are three subtypes of nasopharyngeal carcinoma: WHO type I, squamous cell carcinoma; WHO type II, nonkeratinizing carcinoma; and WHO type III, undifferentiated carcinoma or lymphoepithelioma. The WHO type III is associated with EBV. These tumors typically present with a painless upper neck mass, nasal stuffiness, facial pain, and headache. Cranial nerve involvement occurs in approximately 25% of patients. Cranial nerves II, III, IV, V, and VI can be affected by the tumor extending into the cavernous sinus. Lateral pharyngeal space extension of the tumor affects cranial nerves IX through XII. Approximately 80% to 90% of patients have neck lymph node involvement at presentation with half of patients having bilateral neck disease. These tumors are almost exclusively treated with radiation because it is very difficult to obtain a complete resection. For more locally advanced tumors (node positive or T3-4N0), chemoradiation with concurrent cisplatin followed by adjuvant cisplatin-5-FU is used.

Answer 17.14. **The answer is D.**

The treatment of choice for both benign and malignant tumors is primarily surgical. Inoperable malignancies are treated by radiation therapy with occasional success. Radiation therapy is given postoperatively for nearly all high-grade lesions. Radiation therapy is advised for low-grade malignant lesions that are recurrent and those with positive margins or narrow margins on the facial nerve. Postoperative radiation therapy is advised for selected benign mixed tumors when there is microscopic residual disease after operation and for nearly all patients after surgery for recurrent disease.

Answer 17.15. **The answer is B.**

The treatment of head and neck cancer requires a multidisciplinary approach. This is because treatment will often require several different modalities (e.g., surgery followed by chemoradiation) to support the patient through treatment and recovery from the side effects. Radiation to the head and neck has many short and long-term toxicities. Short-term side effects include severe mucositis with pain and inability to swallow and burns. The long-term effects include xerostomia, dental caries, and fibrosis resulting in trismus and difficulty swallowing. The degree of toxicity from radiation varies from patient to patient and depends on the dose of radiation, the radiation port, the radiation technique, and whether chemotherapy is used concurrently. IMRT is a radiation technique that allows varying doses of radiation to be given to different parts of a radiation field. This allows a parotid gland to be spared resulting in less long-term xerostomia. To decrease the risk of long-term swallowing dysfunction, patients should be strongly encouraged to continue to swallow to exercise the pharyngeal muscles even if they are receiving the majority of nutrition via a g-tube.

Janessa J. Laskin

Cancer of the Lung

Directions   Each of the numbered items below is followed by lettered answers. Select the ONE lettered answer that is BEST in each case unless instructed otherwise.

QUESTIONS

Question 18.1.   **A 67-year-old man with a 40 pack-year smoking history presents to his primary care physician with a bacterial pneumonia clearly visible on a chest radiograph with dense consolidation in the left lower lobe (LLL). After antibiotic therapy, he improves, but when the chest radiograph is repeated 3 months later, there is a residual opacity noted. A chest computed tomography (CT) scan demonstrates a 3-cm spiculated mass in the LLL and enlarged left hilar lymph nodes. He feels well and has no respiratory symptoms. The MOST appropriate course of action would be:**

A.   Referral to a thoracic surgeon for immediate left lower lobectomy.
B.   Bronchoscopy with brushings and washings for diagnostic tissue.
C.   Thoracentesis. Although there is no visible fluid on CT, there is always some fluid in the chest cavity that can be used for diagnosis.
D.   Given his age and smoking history, this is so likely to be a non–small cell lung cancer (NSCLC) that he should begin empiric therapy with radiation and chemotherapy.

Question 18.2.   **Which of the following is the MOST true about staging for NSCLC?**

A.   It is based on the size and location of the primary tumor, the presence or absence and location of cancer-involved lymph nodes, and the presence or absence of distant metastatic disease.
B.   It is not helpful for estimating survival rates or curability of NSCLC because these rates are based on very small patient numbers, and each individual with NSCLC has an unpredictable outcome.
C.   It is a two-stage system introduced by the Veterans' Administration Lung Study Group that is based on the feasibility of encompassing all of the known cancer within a radiation field.
D.   The tumor, node, and metastasis (TNM) staging system is an antiquated classification system because molecular profiling can now provide more accurate prognostic information.

Corresponding Chapter in *Cancer: Principles & Practice of Oncology*, Eighth Edition: 37 (Cancer of the Lung).

Question 18.3. **A 65-year-old woman with a persistent cough is found to have a 3-cm right lower lobe mass on CT scan. She is otherwise well, her pulmonary function is excellent, and she has no significant medical history. There is no obvious metastatic disease, but there are enlarged (2-cm) hilar lymph nodes present on CT scan. A mediastinoscopy is negative, and she proceeds to a right upper and middle lobectomy. The pathology identifies a 3.6-cm moderately differentiated adenocarcinoma; three of five hilar nodes are positive for cancer, but the full mediastinal node dissection is clear of metastasis. She had no surgical complications; she lost 5 lbs, but otherwise she has made a good postoperative recovery. What stage is her cancer, and what is the MOST appropriate next step?**

A. Stage II: Because of her hilar nodes, adjuvant radiation is suggested for local control and overall survival benefit.

B. Stage IB: Adjuvant chemotherapy with four cycles of carboplatin and paclitaxel.

C. Stage II: There is no evidence to support additional therapy, but because of the chance of recurrence she should be followed closely for 5 years.

D. Stage II: Adjuvant chemotherapy with four cycles of a platinum-based doublet regimen.

Question 18.4. **A 63-year-old man with a 3-cm left upper lobe mass is evaluated by an experienced thoracic surgeon. He undergoes a positron emission tomography (PET)-CT scan, and no local nodes or distant metastases are detected. He has a bronchoscopy, and a squamous cell carcinoma is detected on brushings from the left upper lobe (LUL) area. Because of the patient's extensive comorbidities, the surgeon sends him for a preoperative assessment; after much deliberation, the surgical team decides that he will not survive a surgery. His performance status is 1, he has not lost any weight, and his pulmonary function tests are 66% of predicted. What is his best option?**

A. Because he cannot have surgery, his cancer is not curable and therefore no further treatment is indicated.

B. High-dose chemotherapy with curative intent.

C. High-dose radiation therapy with curative intent.

D. He should be started on a maintenance regimen of an epidermal growth factor receptor (EGFR) inhibitor to keep the cancer under control.

Question 18.5.   A 58-year-old woman, ex-smoker (40 pack-years, quit 5 years ago), sees her primary care physician because of increasingly frequent episodes of hemoptysis. She is having these nearly every day, sometimes more often, and coughs up white sputum with streaks of bright red blood on almost every occasion. She is still working full time as a court reporter, but she is noticing increasing shortness of breath on exertion (performance status [PS] 1). On examination, the physician palpates a hard, nontender 2-cm right supraclavicular node. A fine-needle aspirate of the node identifies a mixed adenosquamous carcinoma. A PET-CT detects a centrally located 4-cm right upper lobe (RUL) primary lung lesion and several right paratracheal nodes. No distant metastases are detected. She is anxious to have "everything possible" done to treat her cancer. What is her clinical disease stage, and what is the MOST appropriate course of therapy for this patient?

A. Stage IIIB: concurrent platinum-based chemotherapy with high-dose radiation

B. Stage IIIB: neoadjuvant radiation therapy followed by surgical resection and possibly chemotherapy depending on the final pathology

C. Stage IIIA: concurrent platinum-based chemotherapy with high-dose radiation, followed by surgical resection if there is at least a partial response to the chemoradiation

D. Stage IIIA: two cycles of cisplatin-based doublet chemotherapy followed by high-dose radiation, followed by two cycles of docetaxel

Question 18.6.   A 65-year-old woman, lifelong never-smoker, has an increasing cough and pleuritic chest pain. A CT scan of her chest and upper abdomen shows multiple bilateral pulmonary nodules (the largest measuring 3 cm extending to the pleura), three liver metastases (the largest being 4 cm), and a 3-cm left adrenal metastasis. Her Eastern Cooperative Oncology Group (ECOG) PS is 1, she has no weight loss, and her only medical history is gestational diabetes. A CT-guided biopsy of one of the lung nodules identifies it as an adenocarcinoma consistent with a lung primary. Which of the following would be an appropriate course of action?

A. Because she is a lifelong never-smoker, it would be rare for her to have a primary lung cancer; therefore the biopsy must be repeated before any treatment is begun.

B. Palliative chemotherapy with four to six cycles of a platinum-based doublet chemotherapy regimen.

C. Supportive care for her pleuritic pain, but because chemotherapy has never been demonstrated to improve quality of life, she will likely not want to take it.

D. Palliative chemotherapy with a single agent such as gemcitabine or vinorelbine.

Question 18.7. **The woman from Question 6 receives six cycles of cisplatin and gemcitabine; she tolerates it well, and her pain improves after the first cycle. She has some mild peripheral neuropathy and her creatinine is slightly higher than at baseline, but not significantly. Her CT scan after two cycles demonstrates a 40% shrinkage of the masses, and a repeat CT scan after four cycles is stable (no growth or further shrinkage). She asks about continuing the chemotherapy because she is feeling so much better. What should you advise her?**

A. Given that her creatinine is slightly higher, it would be appropriate to switch to carboplatin and continue this combination for another six cycles.

B. Although her cancer is not likely to shrink any more, studies have demonstrated that continuing the chemotherapy will provide her with a survival advantage.

C. There is no survival advantage to continuing the chemotherapy beyond six cycles.

D. Because she continues to feel so well, it is appropriate to continue this combination until her cancer progresses.

Question 18.8. **A physically fit, PS 0, 61-year-old man is seen by a thoracic surgeon for consideration of a left upper lobectomy for a newly diagnosed adenocarcinoma of the lung. The PET-CT does not identify any hilar, mediastinal, or distant metastatic disease. The surgeon also orders a CT scan of the head, and a 2-cm solitary brain metastasis is identified in the right frontal cortex. The patient is entirely asymptomatic from this brain lesion. What course of action is MOST appropriate?**

A. He can proceed with the surgical resection of the lung and either a resection of the brain metastasis or stereotactic radiosurgery, with either procedure followed by whole brain radiation.

B. Because this is metastatic, it is not curable and he should receive palliative brain and lung radiation.

C. He should be referred to a medical oncologist for palliative chemotherapy.

D. He should have whole brain radiation followed by palliative chemotherapy; because this has metastasized, it is inevitable that it will grow elsewhere, and thus a systemic approach is most appropriate.

Question 18.9.   **A 54-year-old man presents to the emergency department with an episode of hemoptysis. He was feeling otherwise well but had an increased cough for the preceding 4 months that did not resolve with antibiotics from a walk-in clinic. The morning he presented, he started to cough and could not seem to stop, and then suddenly he began to cough up blood. In total, approximately one third of a cup came up, and his wife called the ambulance. He has been working full time as a forklift operator, started smoking at age 17 years, and smokes approximately 20 cigarettes per day. He has mild hypertension and diabetes both controlled with diet. The bleeding stops spontaneously, and the brushings from a bronchoscopy identify poorly differentiated adenocarcinoma. The CT scan identifies a 5-cm central spiculated right lung mass, large mediastinal nodes (2 to 3 cm), and several areas of bone metastases in his ribs. Two weeks later, he is evaluated for consideration of palliative chemotherapy. He has been looking up treatment options on the Internet and demands the "best" chemotherapy available, which from his reading he thinks is carboplatin-paclitaxel plus bevacizumab. What should you advise him?**

   A.   Because he is a smoker, he probably has squamous carcinoma and bevacizumab does not work for this histology, so he should receive carboplatin-paclitaxel alone.

   B.   Carboplatin-paclitaxel plus bevacizumab is the standard of care for first-line metastatic disease, and that is the best chemotherapy for him.

   C.   Chemotherapy is likely going to cause more bleeding in the lung, and so he should receive best supportive care alone.

   D.   In the original phase II clinical trial of chemotherapy plus bevacizumab, there were several cases of fatal hemoptysis, and therefore patients with significant hemoptysis should probably not receive this combination.

Question 18.10.   **The man in Question 10 receives four cycles of carboplatin-paclitaxel with good effect and no further hemoptysis. Four months after completing the chemotherapy, he has a repeat CT scan that shows a 15% growth in his original lung mass, three new liver metastases, the largest measuring 3 cm, and a large right pleural effusion. He feels reasonably well, ECOG PS 1 from fatigue, and his weight is down 10 lbs from a gradually decreasing appetite. What treatment options are appropriate?**

   A.   There is no evidence that further chemotherapy is of benefit, and therefore he should receive best supportive care including pain management and steroids to stimulate his appetite.

   B.   Single-agent pemetrexed or docetaxel.

   C.   Repeat administration of carboplatin-paclitaxel for another four cycles.

   D.   Palliative drainage of the pleural effusion and a repeat CT scan in 6 months.

Question 18.11. A 48-year-old woman with a metastatic adenocarcinoma of the lung (liver and bone metastasis) develops progressive disease 5 months after completing four cycles of carboplatin-gemcitabine. During her initial chemotherapy, she had to be hospitalized twice for febrile neutropenia, and she is hesitant to start another chemotherapy regimen. However, with the progression of her cancer, she is now short of breath and her ECOG PS is 2. She has a minimal smoking history (5 pack-years, quit 20 years ago), and both of her parents were born in Japan. What chemotherapy is the MOST appropriate?

A. With an ECOG PS of 2, there is no evidence to start any chemotherapy, and she should receive supportive care and be considered for home oxygen.

B. An oral EGFR inhibitor (erlotinib or gefitinib).

C. An oral EGFR inhibitor (erlotinib or gefitinib) might be appropriate, but because she has some smoking history and does not have bronchioloalveolar carcinoma, her chance of responding is less than 5%.

D. Docetaxel, but not pemetrexed, because docetaxel has the lowest incidence of febrile neutropenia.

Question 18.12. A 67-year-old retired elementary school teacher and long-time smoker is found to have extensive-stage small cell lung cancer (SCLC) with liver metastasis and a large central right-sided chest mass (7 cm). She completes four cycles of cisplatin-etoposide chemotherapy and feels much better. Her thoracic mass decreases to 3 cm, and her liver metastases are also smaller. What is the next step for her care?

A. She should be offered prophylactic cranial irradiation (PCI).

B. PCI is only beneficial in patients with limited stage disease.

C. She should be switched to a maintenance chemotherapy regimen with topotecan.

D. Because she had a good response, the cancer is probably cured and she can be discharged from follow-up.

Question 18.13. A 65-year-old man with a cough is found to have a large central mass on CT scan. A biopsy under bronchoscopy identifies a typical carcinoid tumor. Other than the cough, he is well with ECOG PS 0, no weight loss, and no significant medical history. Which of the following is the MOST appropriate statement?

A. Approximately 30% of patients with bronchial carcinoids present with the typical syndrome, including facial flushing, diarrhea, and wheezing.

B. The survival is significantly better for patients who have atypical carcinoids compared with typical carcinoids.

C. When possible, surgical resection is the best treatment; adjuvant radiation and/or chemotherapy can be added if high-risk features are present.

D. Because this disease is similar to SCLC, a systemic approach is necessary and surgery is rarely used.

Question 18.14.   **Which of the following statements is NOT true?**

A. In a retrospective analysis of a subgroup of patients receiving adjuvant chemotherapy for resected NSCLC, only those who had a low level of ERCC1 benefited from cisplatin-based chemotherapy.
B. ERCC1 is primarily inhibited by oral tyrosine kinase inhibitors of EGFR, such as erlotinib.
C. A small study of patients with resected stage I lung cancers suggested that patients with high RRM1 expression had a longer than expected median survival.
D. Gene expression profiles and proteomic techniques have been able to identify signatures that predict for survival and disease recurrence patterns, and with some enhancements these will likely enter the clinical arena in the near future.

Question 18.15.   **Which of the following statements is NOT true?**

A. KRAS mutations are more common in SCLC than in NSCLC.
B. Chromosome 3p allele loss is one of the most common events in lung cancer pathogenesis.
C. EGFR is another name for HER1.
D. Although the overexpression of c-KIT is common in SCLC, imatinib was not associated with a high response rate in phase II trials in SCLC.

ANSWERS

Answer 18.1.   **The answer is B.**

It is critical to obtain a tissue diagnosis for any cancer whenever possible. Although it is likely he has NSCLC, it could easily be an SCLC or a metastasis from elsewhere, and the prognosis and treatments would vary substantially. The diagnostic yield from a fiberoptic bronchoscopic procedure for a patient with a visible lung lesion is at least 90%, and this can be readily performed with minimal morbidity and risk. Although a thoracic surgeon may need to become involved, or could even perform the bronchoscopy, even if he had an NSCLC, this patient would require further staging investigations to rule out locally advanced or distant metastatic disease. Thoracentesis, needle aspiration, or drainage of a known pleural effusion can often provide a diagnosis; however, this procedure is not without risk (primarily of a pneumothorax) and should only be performed if there is a clearly visible and moderately sized effusion on chest radiography or CT scan. A CT or fluoroscopic-guided fine-needle biopsy would be another diagnostic option for this patient.

Answer 18.2.   **The answer is A.**

The current standard staging system in use of NSCLC is based on the TNM criteria accepted by the American Joint Committee on Cancer and the Union International Contre le Cancer. The current TNM system provides general prognostic information that is based on large historical cohorts. The newest version, to be implemented in 2009, is based on data accrued from more than 100,000 patients. Unfortunately, accurate biological profiling is not yet available. Staging for SCLC is based on the Veterans' Administration Lung Study Group definition of the high-dose radiation that can potentially be delivered to "limited" stage disease. When tumor size or metastasis makes this impossible, a patient is staged as "extensive."

Answer 18.3. **The answer is D.**

This cancer is a stage T2N1M0 or stage II (stage IIB to be complete). Postoperative radiation therapy (PORT) is somewhat controversial, but it is not considered to be the standard of care and is generally not recommended outside of a clinical trial. Although there is some evidence to suggest that PORT may improve local control, there is no definitive evidence it prolongs overall survival. A meta-analysis suggested PORT may even have a detrimental effect on survival (although this was based on studies using older radiotherapy techniques). In recent years, several randomized phase III studies have demonstrated a significant survival benefit associated with adjuvant chemotherapy. These studies include the International Adjuvant Lung Cancer (IALT) study, the BR.10 study led by the National Cancer Institute of Canada involving the North American Intergroup sites, and the Adjuvant Navelbine International Trialist Association (ANITA) study. The weight of the evidence suggests that four cycles of a cisplatin-based doublet regimen is associated with this survival advantage, and this would be the standard of care for patients who make a good postoperative recovery and have adequate baseline kidney and liver function.

Answer 18.4. **The answer is C.**

As radiation therapy techniques have evolved over time, it is entirely appropriate to treat this medically inoperable patient with high-dose, curative-intent radiation therapy. Chemotherapy would not cure this cancer. EGFR inhibitors can be used with palliative intent in a second- or third-line setting for patients with advanced NSCLC, but they would not be appropriate for this patient.

Answer 18.5. **The answer is A.**

On the basis of imaging and the positive supraclavicular node biopsy, this is a stage IIIB cancer (T2N3). The N3 node renders this an inoperable locally advanced cancer; even with neoadjuvant therapy, a surgical approach would not be considered the standard of care. In randomized phase III clinical trials, concurrent chemoradiotherapy has consistently demonstrated superior survival results compared with sequential chemotherapy and radiation schedules, albeit at the expense of increased toxicity for the concurrent approach. Because this patient is relatively well and wants aggressive management, two to four cycles of a cisplatin-based chemotherapy concurrent with curative doses of radiation (at least 60

Gy) would be the most appropriate suggestion. In clinical trials, this regimen is associated with a 20% to 30% risk of grade 3 esophagitis, but a median survival of approximately 17 months and a 5-year overall survival of 15% to 20%.

Answer 18.6. **The answer is B.**

The standard of care for palliative chemotherapy in NSCLC is four to six cycles of cisplatin or carboplatin plus another chemotherapy agent, such as gemcitabine, vinorelbine, paclitaxel, or docetaxel. Randomized phase III clinical trials have been unable to clearly discriminate a clinically significant difference between these combinations, and therefore any of the regimens can be chosen on the basis of cost, convenience, and toxicities. In patients with a good PS, combination chemotherapy has been shown to prolong survival and improve quality of life over best supportive care alone. Single-agent chemotherapy is generally less toxic and can be used in patients with a poor PS (ECOG 2) or in an elderly patient (>70 or 75 years old), although age alone should not preclude the administration of a doublet chemotherapy. The combination of two chemotherapy agents has been shown to produce an increased chance of response and a longer median survival compared with a single-agent therapy. An increasing number of lifelong never-smokers are being diagnosed with primary lung cancer. If the pathologist is unsure of the diagnosis or there is a clinical reason to suspect another primary, then a repeat biopsy might be warranted. There are numerous immunohistochemical markers that can be done to help identify the primary cancer or at least rule out other possible primaries, such as breast or colorectal cancers.

Answer 18.7. **The answer is C.**

The goal of chemotherapy is to improve overall survival and palliate symptoms. Randomized studies have demonstrated that there is no survival advantage to continuing chemotherapy beyond four to six cycles, but there is additive toxicity. In most cases, there is no further disease response between the second and fourth cycles, and thus for most patients four cycles of chemotherapy is sufficient. In addition, in multiple large randomized phase III studies comparing a variety of platinum-based doublet regimens, the average number of cycles patients received was four, suggesting that this is the limit of tolerability. These studies demonstrated the survival advantage statistics we quote for patients.

Answer 18.8. **The answer is A.**

Synchronous brain metastases are relatively common in NSCLC and should be screened for preoperatively even in asymptomatic patients. Although this does represent a metastatic event, long-term survivals in the range of 10% to 20% have been reported after resection or stereotactic radiosurgery for a solitary brain metastasis. Therefore, if a patient has a good PS and is otherwise fit for a curative thoracic surgery, then it should be performed along with definitive brain treatment with the possibility of long-term survival.

Answer 18.9.   **The answer is D.**

There were four episodes of fatal hemoptysis in the original randomized phase II clinical trial of carboplatin-paclitaxel plus two different doses of bevacizumab in patients with advanced NSCLC of all histologies. In retrospect, it was the patients who had central squamous cell carcinomas who developed cavitations on the chemotherapy combination. Therefore, in the subsequent randomized phase 3 studies testing bevacizumab in combination with chemotherapy, patients with squamous cell carcinoma, brain metastasis, or a history of significant hemoptysis (>1/2 teaspoon) were excluded because of the risk of bleeding. It is possible that bevacizumab works well in squamous cell carcinomas, as evidenced by the rapid cavitations; however, this approach should not be used outside of a clinical trial. Although the myelosuppression of a chemotherapy regimen could lead to more bleeding, it is rare and should not prevent a trial of palliative chemotherapy.

Answer 18.10.   **The answer is B.**

In patients fit enough to receive second-line chemotherapy, a randomized phase III clinical trial clearly demonstrated a survival and quality of life advantage associated with second-line docetaxel compared with best supportive care (BSC) alone. A more recent phase III study demonstrated that pemetrexed seemed to have a similar efficacy to docetaxel and was associated with less systemic toxicity, such as alopecia, fewer episodes of febrile neutropenia, and fewer hospitalizations in general. Thus, either docetaxel or pemetrexed would be reasonable choices for this patient, and the choice can be made on the basis of toxicities and cost considerations. Recycling the original chemotherapy is unlikely to be advantageous because it has only been 4 months since he originally had this chemotherapy, and it is most likely that his cancer cells will be resistant to these drugs.

Answer 18.11.   **The answer is B.**

A large randomized phase III study (BR.21) conducted by the National Cancer Institute of Canada randomized patients who had received two prior rounds of chemotherapy or one round if they were not candidates for a taxane. Patients with an ECOG PS less than 2 were included in this trial, and they received erlotinib or best support care in a 2:1 randomization. There was a clear survival advantage to receiving the erlotinib regardless of the ECOG PS. Although there does seem to be some correlation with response and clinical factors such as sex, never smoking status, adenocarcinoma, bronchioloalveolar cancer, and an east Asian ethnicity, the absence of these factors does not preclude a response, and the presence of all of them does not guarantee a benefit. In an unselected clinical population, such as BR.21, the response rate was 8.9%, which is similar to the response rate with docetaxel or pemetrexed. In a randomized trial comparing docetaxel with pemetrexed in a second-line setting, the rate of febrile neutropenia was higher in the docetaxel arm.

Answer 18.12.   **The answer is A.**

Approximately 10% of people with SCLC have central nervous system metastasis at the time of diagnosis, but the risk of developing brain metastasis after diagnosis is in the range of 20% to 25%. Because this is usually a devastating and fatal event, radiation therapy has been introduced to try to diminish this risk. Historically, PCI has been demonstrated to reduce the incidence of brain metastasis in both limited and extensive SCLC. Up until recently, there were studies demonstrating a survival benefit in limited stage only. However, a recent randomized phase III trial demonstrated a survival advantage for PCI in patients with extensive-stage disease, as long as they had some response to their initial chemotherapy. As with NSCLC, multiple randomized studies have compared four to six cycles of chemotherapy with longer schedules or other maintenance chemotherapies such as topotecan, and no overall survival advantage has been identified with prolonged administration of chemotherapy.

Answer 18.13.   **The answer is C.**

Patients with primary bronchial carcinoids rarely present with carcinoid syndrome (2%), whereas this is seen in 30% of those with a primary gastrointestinal carcinoid. Patients with typical carcinoids have a significantly better prognosis with 5-year survival rates of more than 80%, compared with approximately 50% for those with atypical carcinoid tumors. Surgery is the primary treatment for carcinoids, particularly for the typical subset. Adjuvant chemotherapy or radiation is sometimes added in those thought to have more high-risk disease, such as residual positive surgical margins, or atypical carcinoids with nodal involvement. Atypical carcinoid shares some similarities to SCLC, although usually the mitotic rate and proliferative index (e.g., using Ki67 staining) is lower for carcinoids. Chemotherapy can be used for metastatic or unresectable disease, but the expected response rate is lower than for SCLC.

Answer 18.14.   **The answer is B.**

ERCC1 is a component of the nucleotide excision-repair pathway that is involved in the recognition and elimination of DNA adducts, such as those formed by cisplatin. The EGFR pathway is the target of the oral tyrosine kinase inhibitors, such as erlotinib. These are entirely separate cellular pathways and targets. In recent years, there has been a huge influx of powerful molecular profiling data, and through these kinds of studies, lung cancer will ultimately be subdivided into groups with particular prognostic and predictive patterns to guide clinical practice. As of now, these techniques require further validation before they are universally applied.

Answer 18.15.   **The answer is A.**

KRAS mutations, which are commonly point mutations, are only rarely seen in SCLC but are common in NSCLC. Chromosome 3p allele loss is indeed one of the most common events in lung cancer pathogenesis, noted to occur in 90% of SCLC and 80% of NSCLC. The family of EGFRs has four well-described receptors. This family is also referred to as the ERB or HER family, of which the receptor commonly referred to as EGFR is also known as ERB1 or HER1. HER2, or ERB2, is another receptor in this HER family and is targeted in breast cancer by the monoclonal antibody trastuzumab (Herceptin). Although c-KIT is highly expressed in SCLC and imatinib (a c-KIT tyrosine kinase inhibitor) was active against SCLC lines, it failed to demonstrate a single response in a phase II study including 19 patients with SCLC.

Gregory P. Kalemkerian

Neoplasms of the Mediastinum

Directions   Each of the numbered items below is followed by lettered answers. Select the ONE lettered answer that is BEST in each case unless instructed otherwise.

QUESTIONS

Question 19.1.   **A 51-year-old woman presents with dull anterior chest pain. She is a lifelong nonsmoker. Her medical history is significant for Hashimoto's thyroiditis, for which she has been taking levothyroxine for 1 year. Examination is unremarkable. Laboratory studies show normal blood counts, lactate dehydrogenase (LDH), α-fetoprotein, and beta-human chorionic gonadotropin (β-hCG). Chest radiograph reveals clear lung fields with a retrosternal density. Computed tomography (CT) scan shows a 4-cm, smooth, anterior mediastinal mass. What is the most likely diagnosis?**

A. Small cell lung cancer
B. Pericardial cyst
C. Nonseminomatous germ cell tumor (NSGCT)
D. Thymoma

Question 19.2.   **A 5-year-old boy has been experiencing left upper back pain that radiates around his left chest wall for 2 months. Examination reveals a healthy-appearing boy with no spinal or chest wall tenderness or masses. He is neurologically intact. A chest radiograph suggests a left paravertebral mass adjacent to T5. A magnetic resonance imaging (MRI) scan shows a 2-cm, smooth, fusiform mass abutting the T5-6 neural foramen without bony erosion. What is the most likely diagnosis?**

A. Non-Hodgkin's lymphoma
B. Neurogenic tumor
C. Thymoma
D. Mediastinal germ cell tumor

Corresponding Chapter in *Cancer: Principles & Practice of Oncology*, Eighth Edition: 38 (Neoplasms of the Mediastinum).

Question 19.3. A 63-year-old woman presents with substernal chest pain, cough, and intermittent diplopia that have progressed over the past 6 months. She has a 30 pack-year smoking history. Her medical history is significant for diet-controlled diabetes mellitus. Examination reveals bilateral ptosis, downward drift of the eyes on prolonged upward gaze, and ocular divergence on extreme lateral gaze. Motor strength is normal in the upper and lower extremities. A chest radiograph shows widening of the mediastinum and filling of the retrosternal space. CT scan shows a 6-cm, smooth, anterior mediastinal mass abutting the superior pericardium, sternum, anterior trachea, and left pleura without gross invasion of adjacent structures. There are no enlarged mediastinal or hilar lymph nodes, and no pleural or pericardial effusion or nodularity. Laboratory studies reveal the presence of an antinicotinic acetylcholine receptor antibody with normal blood counts and chemistries. Her ocular symptoms improve with the administration of pyridostigmine. What is the most appropriate next step in the management of this patient?

A. Surgical resection
B. Neoadjuvant radiotherapy followed by surgical resection
C. Cisplatin-based chemotherapy
D. Definitive radiotherapy

Question 19.4. A 36-year-old woman presents with an anterior mediastinal mass that was identified incidentally on a chest radiograph done as part of an employment examination. She is asymptomatic and a lifelong nonsmoker, and has no significant medical history. Examination is unremarkable. CT scan shows a 3-cm, smooth, anterior mediastinal mass without local invasion. Resection of the mass reveals an encapsulated, lymphocyte-rich thymoma (World Health Organization [WHO] type B1) with no capsular invasion. She recovers from surgery without complications. What is the most appropriate next step in the management of this patient?

A. Clinical surveillance
B. Adjuvant radiotherapy alone
C. Adjuvant chemotherapy alone
D. Adjuvant chemotherapy plus radiotherapy

Question 19.5.   A 48-year-old man presents with progressive fatigue and dyspnea on exertion over the past 6 months. He is a former smoker, and his medical history is significant only for well-controlled hypertension. Examination reveals tachycardia with a regular rhythm, mild tachypnea at rest, and conjunctival and mucosal pallor without focal findings. Stool is guaiac negative. Laboratory studies show hemoglobin of 5.5 g/dL, hematocrit of 17%, white blood cell count of 6800/μL, platelet count of 343,000/μL, and normal electrolytes, renal function, and liver function test results. A chest radiograph reveals superior mediastinal widening. CT scan shows a large, irregular, anterior mediastinal mass. Bone marrow aspiration and biopsy show profound erythrocytic hypoplasia with no dysplasia and normal granulocytic and megakaryocytic maturation with no evidence of a clonal lymphoid proliferation. Serum LDH, α-fetoprotein, and β-hCG are normal. He is transfused with packed red blood cells, and his hemoglobin increases to 10.4 g/dL. Resection of the mass reveals a cortical thymoma (WHO type B2) with microscopic invasion of the capsule and negative surgical margins. He recovers without complications, and his hemoglobin is 11.5 g/dL 4 weeks after surgery. What is the most appropriate next step in the management of this patient?

A. Clinical surveillance
B. Adjuvant radiotherapy alone
C. Adjuvant chemotherapy alone
D. Adjuvant chemotherapy plus radiotherapy

Question 19.6.   A 62-year-old man presents with substernal chest pain. Cardiac evaluation is negative. CT angiogram shows no aortic dissection but does reveal an irregular, anterior mediastinal mass abutting the upper lobe of the left lung. Positron emission tomography (PET) scan shows a fluorodeoxyglucose (FDG)-avid anterior mediastinal mass without evidence of metastases. Resection of the mass with en bloc wedge resection of the left upper lobe shows high-grade thymic carcinoma (WHO type C) with invasion into the pericardium and left upper lobe. The surgical margins are positive on microscopic examination. He recovers from surgery without complications. What is the most appropriate next step in the management of this patient?

A. Clinical surveillance
B. Adjuvant radiotherapy alone
C. Adjuvant chemotherapy alone
D. Adjuvant chemotherapy plus radiotherapy

Question 19.7. A previously healthy 38-year-old man presents with facial and bilateral upper-extremity edema that has progressed over the past 2 weeks. Examination reveals moderate facial, cervical, and bilateral upper extremity edema with facial plethora and prominent anterior chest wall vasculature. He is tachycardic, but his heart sounds are regular and his lungs are clear. There is no lower-extremity edema. CT scan of the chest shows a large anterior mediastinal mass encasing the superior vena cava, displacing the aortic arch and trachea, and invading the pericardium and upper lobe of the left lung. The superior vena cava is compressed with numerous dilated, intrathoracic collateral vessels. An experienced thoracic surgeon deems that the lesion is primarily unresectable. Mediastinotomy with biopsy of the mass reveals well-differentiated thymic carcinoma (WHO type B3). PET scan shows a large FDG-avid mediastinal mass with no evidence of metastatic disease. What is the most appropriate management of this patient?

A. Palliative radiotherapy followed by chemotherapy
B. Definitive radiotherapy with concurrent chemotherapy
C. Neoadjuvant chemotherapy followed by surgical resection and post-operative radiotherapy
D. Palliative chemotherapy alone

Question 19.8. A 58-year-old woman presents with progressive dyspnea on exertion and diffuse right-sided chest pain over the past 2 months. Two years ago, she underwent resection of a stage III thymoma (WHO type B1) followed by adjuvant radiotherapy. Examination reveals decreased breath sounds and dullness to percussion over the lower half of the right lung field. Chest radiograph shows a moderate right pleural effusion and several pleural-based nodules. CT scan shows thickening of the anterior mediastinal soft tissues, a moderate, partially loculated right pleural effusion, and diffuse right pleural nodularity. A radiolabeled octreotide scan shows diffuse activity in the right pleura. She undergoes thoracocentesis, with removal of 1500 mL of fluid that contains malignant epithelial cells consistent with thymoma. She receives six cycles of cyclophosphamide, doxorubicin, and cisplatin (CAP) with good control of the pleural effusion and partial response of the pleural nodules, but she develops grade 3 peripheral neuropathy. Four months later, she has recurrent diffuse right chest pain and persistent neuropathy. CT scan shows a small, loculated right pleural effusion, increased diffuse right pleural thickening, and new enlargement of right hilar and pericardial lymph nodes. What is the most appropriate next step in the management of this patient?

A. Paclitaxel
B. Hemithorax radiotherapy
C. Extrapleural pneumonectomy
D. Prednisone plus octreotide

Question 19.9.   A 24-year-old man with multiple endocrine neoplasia type 1 has undergone two resections for pancreatic islet cell carcinoma metastatic to regional lymph nodes. He is asymptomatic. Examination shows well-healed abdominal scars. Surveillance CT scan identifies a new 3-cm, smooth, anterior mediastinal mass. Serum LDH, α-fetoprotein, and β-hCG are normal. Testicular ultrasonography is unremarkable. Which of the following is the most likely diagnosis?

A. Thymolipoma
B. Thymoma
C. Thymic carcinoid
D. Metastatic islet cell tumor

Question 19.10.   A 24-year-old man presents with anterior chest discomfort and cough of 3 weeks duration. Examination is unremarkable. Chest radiograph shows widening of the superior mediastinum. CT scan shows a 6-cm anterior mediastinal mass encasing the trachea and great vessels and three 1-cm pulmonary nodules. CT scan of the abdomen and pelvis and a testicular ultrasound examination are normal. Laboratory studies reveal a hemoglobin of 11.4 with normal white blood cell count and platelet count, LDH of 880 IU/L (normal, 120–240 IU/L), α-fetoprotein of 1800 ng/mL (normal, <8 ng/mL), and β-hCG of 1.2 mIU/mL (normal, <5 mIU/mL). What is the most likely diagnosis?

A. Hodgkin's lymphoma
B. Benign teratoma
C. Non-seminomatous germ cell tumor (NSGCT)
D. Seminoma

Question 19.11.   A 39-year-old woman presents with a cough and dyspnea that have progressed over the past 4 months. She is now dyspneic on walking less than 100 feet. Examination shows an anxious woman with a pulse rate of 110 beats/min, a respiratory rate of 24 breaths/min, and mild stridor. Lungs are otherwise clear to auscultation, and heart sounds are regular. Chest radiograph shows a large anterior mediastinal mass with narrowing of the mid-trachea. CT scan shows a 10-cm, highly heterogeneous anterior mediastinal mass with foci of dense calcification that compress the trachea and superior vena cava without obstruction. Laboratory studies reveal normal blood counts, chemistries, LDH, carcinoembryonic antigen (CEA), α-fetoprotein, and β-hCG. She undergoes complete resection of the mass, which is adherent to the trachea, superior vena cava, left pleura, and pericardium without gross invasion. Pathologic evaluation reveals a multicystic mass with foci of mature gland formation, respiratory epithelium, cartilage, and bone. There is no invasion into adjacent structures, and surgical margins are negative. What is the most appropriate management of this patient?

A. Clinical surveillance
B. Adjuvant radiotherapy
C. Cisplatin plus etoposide × four cycles
D. Doxorubicin plus ifosfamide × six cycles

Question 19.12.   A 23-year-old man presents with hoarseness, cough, and anterior chest pain. He has a 30 pack-year smoking history. Examination is normal. Chest radiograph shows a large left mediastinal mass and clear lung fields. CT scan of the chest shows only a 5-cm irregular left paratracheal mass. CT scan of the abdomen is normal. Serum CEA, β-hCG, and α-fetoprotein are normal. Bronchoscopy reveals extrinsic compression of the left mainstem bronchus without an endobronchial lesion. Left mediastinotomy reveals an anterior mediastinal mass that is biopsied and is suspicious for lymphoma on frozen-section histopathology. Final pathologic examination reveals a poorly differentiated malignant neoplasm that is immunohistochemically negative for leukocyte common antigen, vimentin, S100, TTF1, and chromogranin, but positive for low molecular weight cytokeratin. Genetic studies reveal no B- or T-cell rearrangements, and karyotypic analysis shows aneuploidy with an isochromosome 12p. Which of the following is the most appropriate therapy for this patient?

A.   Cisplatin plus etoposide
B.   Cisplatin, etoposide, and bleomycin
C.   Concurrent chemotherapy and radiation therapy
D.   Cyclophosphamide, doxorubicin, vincristine, and prednisone

Question 19.13.   A previously healthy 32-year-old man presents with fatigue and vague chest discomfort. A chest radiograph shows a widened mediastinum, and a CT scan confirms a large anterior mediastinal mass with focal areas of hemorrhage that fills the substernal space and invades into the upper lobe of the left lung. Laboratory studies show the following: LDH of 850 IU/L (normal, 120–240 IU/L), α-fetoprotein of 8700 ng/mL (normal, <8 ng/mL), and β-hCG of 220 mIU/mL (normal, <5 mIU/mL). Biopsy confirms embryonal carcinoma with elements of choriocarcinoma. After four cycles of cisplatin, etoposide, and bleomycin, a CT scan shows marked shrinkage of the mediastinal mass, now measuring 3 cm in maximal diameter. One month after completion of therapy, LDH is 150 IU/L, α-fetoprotein is 5.0 ng/mL, and β-hCG 2.4 is mIU/mL. Which of the following is the most appropriate management of this patient?

A.   Clinical surveillance
B.   Cisplatin, ifosfamide, and vinblastine (VIP)
C.   Two additional cycles of cisplatin, etoposide, and bleomycin
D.   Resection of the residual mediastinal mass

Question 19.14.   A 22-year-old man has a retrosternal mass identified on a chest radiograph done during his enlistment into military service. He is an asymptomatic nonsmoker with no significant medical history. CT scan shows a 2.5-cm smooth anterior mediastinal mass without local invasion. Serum LDH, β-hCG, and α-fetoprotein are normal. Testicular ultrasound is normal. He refuses primary surgical resection, and a percutaneous core biopsy shows pure seminoma. Which of the following is the most appropriate management of this patient?

A. Surgical resection
B. Radiotherapy
C. Cisplatin, etoposide, and bleomycin
D. Cisplatin plus etoposide followed by surgical resection

Question 19.15.   A 33-year-old man presents with chest tightness and shortness of breath. A chest radiograph shows a large mediastinal mass. CT scan shows a 9-cm lobulated anterior mediastinal mass invading the left lung and pericardium with a small pericardial effusion, a 3-cm right paratracheal lymph node, and a 5-cm subcarinal lymph node mass. Echocardiogram shows no tamponade. Serum LDH is 440 IU/L (normal, 120–240 IU/L), but α-fetoprotein and β-hCG are normal. Testicular ultrasound is normal. Bronchoscopic core biopsy of the subcarinal mass reveals seminoma. Which of the following is the most appropriate management of this patient?

A. Carboplatin plus etoposide
B. Radiotherapy
C. Surgical resection
D. Cisplatin, etoposide, and bleomycin

Question 19.16.   A previously healthy 52-year-old man presents with hoarseness and vague chest discomfort. A chest radiograph shows a widened mediastinum, and a CT scan confirms a large anterior mediastinal mass encasing the trachea and abutting the superior vena cava, left pleura, and superior pericardium. Serum α-fetoprotein is normal, but β-hCG is 10 mIU/mL (normal, <5 mIU/mL). Biopsy shows seminoma. He is treated with cisplatin, etoposide, and bleomycin. CT scan after treatment shows marked shrinkage of the mediastinal mass, now measuring 2 cm in maximal diameter. β-hCG is now 1.2 mIU/mL. Which of the following is the most appropriate management of this patient?

A. Clinical surveillance
B. Cisplatin, ifosfamide, and vinblastine (VIP)
C. Resection of the residual mediastinal mass
D. Involved-field radiotherapy

ANSWERS

Answer 19.1.   **The answer is D.**

This middle-aged woman has an anterior mediastinal mass that appears localized on radiologic imaging. Thymomas are the most common tumors arising in the anterior mediastinum. They occur in patients of all ages, and approximately one half of patients are symptomatic because of compression of mediastinal structures (e.g., pain, cough, superior vena cava syndrome) or associated paraneoplastic syndromes. Paraneoplastic syndromes can be identified in up to 70% of patients with thymoma but are uncommon in patients with thymic carcinoma. Myasthenia gravis is the most common paraneoplastic syndrome associated with thymoma, although a wide variety of other syndromes, primarily caused by autoimmune dysregulation, have been reported, including thyroiditis, polymyositis, pure red cell aplasia, hypogammaglobulinemia, scleroderma, and Addison's disease. Small cell lung cancer typically presents with a central lung mass and bulky mediastinal lymphadenopathy, and nearly all patients have a history of tobacco use. Pericardial cysts occur primarily in the middle mediastinum and, in adults, are usually asymptomatic. NSGCTs occur predominantly in young men, and 80% to 85% are associated with elevations of α-fetoprotein and/or β-hCG.

Answer 19.2.   **The answer is B.**

This child presents with radicular pain and a noninvasive-appearing posterior mediastinal mass arising from the paravertebral sulcus. Thoracic neurogenic tumors occur most commonly in the posterior mediastinum and account for 75% of tumors in this location. They are predominantly seen in children, in whom they are frequently malignant, and in young adults, in whom they are usually benign. In children, neurogenic tumors account for nearly half of all mediastinal neoplasms. Histologic subtypes of thoracic neurogenic tumors include neurofibroma, neurilemoma, neurosarcoma, ganglioneuroma, paraganglioma, and neuroblastoma. Because thoracic neurogenic tumors arise in the paravertebral sulcus, they frequently cause pain and a variety of neurologic symptoms, including spinal cord compression, paresthesia, Horner's syndrome, and muscular atrophy. Surgical resection is the primary treatment option for all thoracic neurogenic tumors if it can be accomplished with acceptable risk. Observation is an option for asymptomatic patients with benign tumors who are poor candidates for surgery. Thymomas are found predominantly in the anterior mediastinum, although ectopic thymic tissue can rarely result in tumors in other mediastinal compartments. Mediastinal germ cell tumors are uncommon in young children and nearly always arise in the anterior mediastinum. Lymphomas account for 26% of mediastinal tumors in adults, but only 9% in children, and are mainly noted in the anterior mediastinum.

Answer 19.3.   **The answer is A.**

This woman presents with typical symptoms, physical signs, and laboratory findings of myasthenia gravis (MG) associated with localized thymoma. MG is an autoimmune syndrome caused by antibodies to the postsynaptic nicotinic acetylcholine receptor that disrupt neuromuscular transmission. MG is the most common paraneoplastic syndrome associated with thymoma, occurring in 30% to 50% of patients, with women outnumbering men two to one. Diplopia is the most common initial symptom, but generalized weakness eventually develops in 80% of patients. Response to anticholinesterase-mimetic agents, such as pyridostigmine, is typical of MG and such treatment should be initiated before thymectomy to minimize postoperative complications. Surgical resection is the treatment of choice for all thymic neoplasms, and the completeness of resection remains the strongest prognostic factor. Five-year survival rates after resection of stage I, II, and III thymoma are 96%, 86%, and 69%, respectively. Preoperative biopsy, which violates the tumor capsule, is not necessary for patients with apparent thymic neoplasms that appear to be amenable to complete surgical resection. Multimodality therapy, consisting of neoadjuvant chemotherapy followed by surgery and postoperative radiotherapy, is preferred for patients with locally advanced tumors that are not amenable to primary complete resection. Definitive radiotherapy is used only for patients who are not candidates for resection. Although cisplatin-based chemotherapy can result in response rates of 30% to 50%, such treatment has no role in the management of patients with localized thymoma.

Answer 19.4.   **The answer is A.**

This woman has undergone complete resection of a noninvasive, low-grade thymoma. Several histologic classification schemes and staging systems have been developed for thymic neoplasms. The WHO histologic classification is most commonly used and includes both thymomas (types A, AB, B1, and B2) and thymic carcinomas (types B3 and C) with varying degrees of pathologic atypia and aggressiveness. The most commonly used staging system was derived by Masaoka: stage I, no microscopic capsular invasion (noninvasive); stage II, microscopic capsular invasion or gross invasion into perithymic fat; stage III, gross invasion into adjacent organs; stage IVa, pleural or pericardial dissemination; and stage IVb, lymphogenous or hematogenous metastases. Complete resection of Masaoka stage I low-grade thymoma is associated with 5- and 10-year survival rates of 90% to 100% and 70% to 80%, respectively. Neither adjuvant radiotherapy nor chemotherapy has been shown to benefit patients who have undergone complete resection of Masaoka stage I, or noninvasive, thymoma.

Answer 19.5.   **The answer is B.**

This middle-aged man presents with anemia and a mediastinal mass that is found to be a microscopically invasive, low-grade thymoma. The presence of capsular invasion is an adverse prognostic factor for patients with completely resected thymoma, leading to a classification of Masaoka stage II. Studies have suggested a survival advantage for adjuvant radiotherapy after complete resection in patients with invasion into the capsule (stage II) or adjacent organs (stage III). The role of adjuvant chemotherapy in such patients remains unclear. Pure red cell aplasia occurs in 5% of patients with thymoma and is believed to be caused by autoimmune dysregulation. Conversely, 30% to 50% of patients with pure red cell aplasia have an associated thymoma. Bone marrow examination shows marked reduction or absence of erythroid precursors. Approximately 30% of patients also have a reduction in megakaryocytes or leukocyte precursors. Thymectomy induces remission of pure red cell aplasia in only 40% of patients.

Answer 19.6.   **The answer is D.**

This man presents after incomplete surgical resection of a high-grade thymic carcinoma. Thymic carcinoma is a rare, aggressive malignancy that is frequently locally advanced or metastatic at diagnosis. The many histologic subtypes of thymic carcinoma generally fall into two clinically relevant categories: low grade or well differentiated (WHO type B3) and high grade (WHO type C). Low-grade thymic carcinomas can have a relatively indolent course leading to reported median survivals of 25 months to over 6 years. However, the median survival of patients with high-grade thymic carcinoma is only 11 to 15 months. Although the rarity of thymic carcinoma precludes evidence-based treatment guidelines, most patients undergo multimodality therapy because of the locally invasive nature of the disease. Adjuvant chemotherapy plus radiotherapy is recommended for patients with thymic carcinoma with either grossly (R2) or microscopically (R1) positive surgical margins. Clinical surveillance is recommended only for patients with no evidence of capsular invasion, and adjuvant radiotherapy alone is recommended for those with capsular invasion after complete surgical resection (R0). Recommendations are similar for patients with thymoma after R0 and R2 resections, except that adjuvant radiotherapy alone is usually used after R1 resection. Further surgical resection and adjuvant chemotherapy alone are not generally indicated for thymic tumors.

Answer 19.7.   **The answer is C.**

This young man presents with symptoms of superior vena cava syndrome caused by a locally advanced, primarily unresectable thymic carcinoma. Symptoms caused by compression or invasion of mediastinal structures, including anterior chest pain, cough, dyspnea, and superior vena cava syndrome, occur in up to 70% of patients with thymic carcinoma, whereas paraneoplastic syndromes are rare. Because completeness of resection is one of the most important predictors of outcome, multimodality therapy should be recommended for all patients with thymic neoplasms, both thymoma and thymic carcinoma, whose tumors are judged to be primarily unresectable because of the extent of local invasion. The most commonly studied approach includes neoadjuvant cisplatin-based chemotherapy followed by surgical resection and postoperative radiotherapy. Cumulative results reveal that neoadjuvant chemotherapy results in an objective response rate of 89% and a complete response rate of 31%. These studies included patients with both thymoma and thymic carcinoma. Long-term survival remains the goal of therapy for patients with locally advanced disease, with one trial noting a 7-year disease-free survival rate of 83% after trimodality therapy. Therefore, purely palliative approaches are only justifiable in patients whose performance status or comorbidities preclude potentially curative combined modality therapy. Although there are some data supporting the use of definitive chemotherapy plus radiotherapy without surgical resection, further studies are needed to define the utility of this approach.

Answer 19.8.   **The answer is D.**

This woman presents with recurrent stage IVb thymoma that has progressed shortly after initial response to neuropathy-inducing chemotherapy. Pleural "drop" metastases are the most common manifestation of advanced thymoma or thymic carcinoma. Palliative systemic therapy is the primary treatment for patients with metastatic thymoma. Cisplatin-based regimens, such as CAP or cisplatin plus etoposide, have been found to induce objective response in 50% to 60% of patients and complete response in 10% to 35% of patients. Even in the metastatic setting, thymoma tends to have a relatively indolent course with median survival times of 3 to 4.5 years. Several chemotherapy drugs have single-agent activity in patients with relapsed, metastatic thymoma, including ifosfamide, pemetrexed, and paclitaxel, although the latter should not be used in a patient with persistent peripheral neuropathy. In a cooperative group trial of patients with thymoma that demonstrated activity on radio-labeled-octreotide scan, treatment with octreotide with or without prednisone resulted in partial response rates of 32% and 12.5%, respectively. Surgical resection may be considered when there is evidence of limited pleural involvement, although the benefits of such an approach have not been well documented. Extrapleural pneumonectomy is not an appropriate option for patients with metastatic thymoma. Radiation therapy can be useful to palliate chest pain caused by pleural metastases that focally invade the chest wall but does not have a significant role for the management of diffuse pleural disease.

Answer 19.9.   **The answer is C.**

This young man with multiple endocrine neoplasia type I (MEN I) presented with a localized anterior mediastinal mass. Thymic carcinoid is a rare tumor that is associated with MEN I. Thymic carcinoids can produce adrenocorticotropic hormone (ACTH), leading to Cushing's syndrome, but rarely cause serotonin-induced carcinoid syndrome. The primary treatment is complete surgical resection, which results in a 5-year survival rate of 60%, although late recurrences and mortality are not uncommon. Adjuvant radiotherapy is reserved for patients with incomplete resections, and the role of chemotherapy is unclear. Thymolipomas are rare, benign tumors that occur mainly in young adults and consist of mature thymic and adipose tissue. Although they are noninvasive, thymolipomas can grow to a large size and cause symptoms resulting from compression of mediastinal structures. Complete resection is curative. Thymoma is not associated with any of the MEN syndromes. Malignant islet cell tumors tend to recur locally in the pancreatic bed or to metastasize to the peritoneum, regional lymph nodes, and liver.

Answer 19.10.   **The answer is C.**

This young man presents with an anterior mediastinal mass and an elevated α-fetoprotein (AFP) that is pathognomonic for a NSGCT. Germ cell tumors account for 10% to 12% of all mediastinal tumors in adults and 6% in children and usually arise in the anterior mediastinum. Approximately 10% of germ cell tumors originate in extragonadal sites, with 50% to 70% of these arising in the mediastinum. Serum tumor markers, namely, LDH, AFP, and β-hCG, are helpful in the diagnosis and management of germ cell tumors. Benign teratomas, the most common mediastinal germ cell tumors (60% to 70%), are not associated with significant tumor marker elevations. Pure seminoma can cause modest elevations of β-hCG but not AFP. AFP is produced by yolk sac elements, and in the setting of a mediastinal mass, an elevated serum AFP level is pathognomonic of NSGCT. Although lymphoma is commonly associated with elevations of LDH, AFP is not affected.

Answer 19.11.   **The answer is A.**

This woman has undergone complete resection of a tumor with radiologic and histologic characteristics of a benign, noninvasive teratoma. Benign teratoma is the most common mediastinal germ cell tumor. Unlike malignant germ cell tumors, benign teratomas, also known as dermoid cysts, occur with equal incidence in both men and women, primarily affecting patients between 20 and 40 years of age. Benign teratomas frequently present as large anterior mediastinal masses with normal serum tumor markers that cause symptoms resulting from compression of mediastinal structures. Although they may be adherent to adjacent structures, they are typically noninvasive. Histologically, both benign and malignant teratomas contain elements from all three germ cell layers: ectoderm (skin, hair, sweat glands, teeth); mesoderm (fat, muscle, bone, cartilage); and endoderm (bronchial or intestinal epithelium). Malignant teratomas, in which one or more of these elements have an invasive or metastatic phenotype, are aggressive tumors that usually have a poor response to therapy and are associated with an unfavorable prognosis. In contrast, surgical resection of benign teratoma results in excellent long-term survival rates with a low risk of recurrence. Neither adjuvant radiotherapy nor chemotherapy is indicated in the management of patients with benign teratoma.

Answer 19.12.   **The answer is B.**

This young man presents with a mediastinal poorly differentiated carcinoma of unknown primary site that is clinically and molecularly consistent with an extragonadal germ cell tumor. Poorly differentiated carcinoma arising in the midline structures of a young man is highly suggestive of an unrecognized extragonadal germ cell tumor, even in the face of nonelevated tumor markers. In this patient, immunohistochemical analysis is suggestive of carcinoma with positive cytokeratin and argues against lymphoma (common leukocyte antigen), neuroendocrine tumor (chromogranin), sarcoma (vimentin), lung cancer (TTF1), and melanoma (S100). Genetic analysis can frequently be useful in clarifying histogenesis in such situations. Isochromosome 12p (i[12p]) is pathognomonic of germ cell tumors and can be found in approximately 30% of patients in this setting. A long-term survival rate of 16% has been reported for patients with midline poorly differentiated carcinoma of unknown primary site treated with cisplatin-based chemotherapy appropriate for NSGCT. The presence of i(12p) has been favorably associated with response and survival. Because the International Germ Cell Cancer Collaborative Group considers mediastinal NSGCT a "poor-risk" tumor, appropriate treatment should consist of cisplatin, etoposide, and bleomycin for four cycles. Therapy aimed at good-risk NSGCT (answer A), stage III NSCLC (answer C), or lymphoma (answer D) would not be appropriate.

Answer 19.13.   **The answer is D.**

This young man had an excellent response to initial chemotherapy for mediastinal NSGCT with normalization of tumor markers and a small residual mediastinal mass. Mediastinal NSGSTs occur predominantly in young men and are associated with both Klinefelter's syndrome and acute megakaryocytic leukemia. They most commonly arise in the anterior compartment, and most patients are symptomatic at diagnosis. Elevations of β-hCG and α-fetoprotein are found in 30% to 50% and 60% to 80% of patients, respectively. NSGCTs frequently consist of a mixture of histologic subtypes, including choriocarcinoma, embryonal carcinoma, endodermal sinus (yolk sac) elements, and teratoma. Primary treatment of mediastinal NSGCTs is cisplatin, etoposide, and bleomycin, as per the guidelines for poor-risk nonseminomatous testicular cancer, which yields a complete response rate of 40% to 64% and a long-term survival rate of 45%. Surgical resection is recommended for patients with residual masses after completion of initial chemotherapy and normalization of tumor markers. If viable NSGCT elements are identified in the resected specimen, then two further cycles of cisplatin-based therapy are indicated. If the residual mass reveals only mature teratoma or necrosis, then clinical surveillance without further treatment is indicated. The role of surgical resection in patients with incomplete tumor marker responses has not been clearly defined, but such patients would typically proceed to salvage chemotherapy with a regimen such as VIP.

Answer 19.14.   **The answer is B.**

This young man presents with a localized mediastinal seminoma. Pure mediastinal seminoma is a rare disease, accounting for 35% of malignant mediastinal germ cell tumors and occurring mainly in men 20 to 40 years of age. Despite their slow growth rate, mediastinal seminomas tend to present as large tumors that cause symptoms resulting from compression of mediastinal structures. Serum β-hCG and LDH levels may be modestly elevated in patients with pure seminoma, but an elevated α-fetoprotein level would be indicative of a nonseminomatous germ cell component. Radiotherapy is the treatment of choice for localized mediastinal seminoma, yielding long-term survival rates of 60% to 80%. The total radiation dose should be in excess of 45 Gy, and the field should include the mediastinum and bilateral supraclavicular fossae. Although surgery followed by adjuvant therapy also yields high long-term survival rates, resection is not generally indicated in the management of mediastinal seminoma. Because of the exquisite sensitivity of seminoma to radiotherapy, the relatively low rates of recurrence after radiotherapy and the high cure rates associated with salvage chemotherapy, systemic treatment is not recommended for patients with localized disease.

Answer 19.15. **The answer is D.**

This man presents with locally advanced mediastinal seminoma that invades adjacent structures and involves regional lymph nodes. More than half of patients with mediastinal seminoma will have metastases at diagnosis, primarily to the intrathoracic lymph nodes, lung, or bone. Patients with locally advanced disease are usually treated with cisplatin-based chemotherapy with or without radiotherapy, whereas those with distant disease are treated with chemotherapy alone. Cisplatin-based treatment has been reported to result in an objective response rate that approaches 95% and a complete response rate of up to 85%, with a long-term disease-free survival rate of 80% to 85%. Carboplatin-based therapy is known to be inferior to cisplatin-based regimens. For patients with bulky, locally advanced mediastinal seminoma, the large radiation fields required to encompass all disease can result in excessive pulmonary or cardiac late toxicity. In addition, despite high rates of local control, 20% to 40% of patients with locally advanced disease who are treated with radiotherapy alone will develop distant metastases, leading to the recommendation for primary systemic chemotherapy in such patients. Surgery is not indicated in the primary treatment of mediastinal seminoma.

Answer 19.16. **The answer is A.**

This man has had an excellent response to initial chemotherapy for locally advanced mediastinal seminoma with normalization of β-HCG and a small residual mediastinal mass. The optimal management of patients with a residual mass on radiographic follow-up after treatment with initial chemotherapy or radiotherapy for seminoma remains controversial. Most studies have demonstrated that viable seminoma is rare in resected residual masses, and that 85% to 90% of such specimens consist entirely of scar tissue. Other studies have shown that up to 25% of residual masses more than 3 cm in size after initial chemotherapy contain viable seminoma. Nevertheless, resection of a residual mass is currently not recommended unless the mass enlarges during clinical surveillance. Similarly, the addition of radiotherapy after chemotherapy has not been shown to be of significant benefit. Salvage chemotherapy with a regimen such as VIP, with or without aggressive local therapy, is indicated for recurrent disease.

Cancer of the Gastrointestinal Tract

SECTION 1   Renuka V. Iyer

ESOPHAGUS AND STOMACH

Directions   Each of the numbered items below is followed by lettered answers. Select
the ONE lettered answer that is BEST in each case unless instructed
otherwise.

QUESTIONS

Question 20.1.1.   **Which of the following statements about the incidence of esophageal
cancer is TRUE?**

A. Esophageal cancer is relatively uncommon in the United States, and
the lifetime risk of being diagnosed with the disease is less than 1%.

B. Incidence rates among white men continue to increase and now
exceed 8 per 100,000 person-years, and reflect the marked increase
in the incidence of adenocarcinoma of the esophagus of more than
400% in the past 2 decades.

C. Although the incidence of adenocarcinoma in white women (2 per
100,000) is lower than that in white men, rates of adenocarcinoma
have increased in women by more than 300% during the past 20
years.

D. Only A and B.

E. All of the above.

Corresponding Chapter in *Cancer: Principles & Practice of Oncology,* Eighth Edition: 39, Section 2 (Cancer of the
Esophagus) and Section 3 (Cancer of the Stomach).

Question 20.1.2. **Which of the following statements about the risk factors for esophageal cancer are TRUE?**

A. Population-based studies demonstrate that tobacco and alcohol use are independent risk factors and that their effects are multiplicative, as evidenced by the association of the highest risk of developing esophageal cancer with heavy use of both agents.

B. For both squamous cell carcinoma and adenocarcinoma of the esophagus, case-control studies provide evidence of a protective effect of fruits and vegetables, especially those eaten raw.

C. Low socioeconomic status as defined by income, education, or occupation is associated with increased risk for esophageal squamous cell carcinoma and, to a lesser degree, adenocarcinoma.

D. Infection with *Helicobacter pylori,* particularly with cagA_ strains, is inversely associated with the risk of adenocarcinoma of the esophagus.

E. All of the above.

F. Only A and C.

Question 20.1.3. **A middle-aged white male patient recently read an article about Barrett's esophagus and visits his gastroenterologist requesting a screening upper endoscopy to rule out esophageal cancer. The patient is asymptomatic except for period of heartburn relieved with over-the-counter Prilosec for 3- to 4-week intervals after eating spicy foods. The patient has a screening endoscopy that reveals mild gastritis but no evidence of Barrett's. Which of the following statements best describes the follow-up recommendations for this patient?**

A. Practice guidelines published by the American College of Gastroenterology recommend surveillance endoscopy for patients with Barrett's esophagus, and the grade of dysplasia determines the endoscopy interval. Because he has no evidence of Barrett's, no further endoscopic surveillance is warranted.

B. The strategy of screening endoscopy for patients with long-standing symptomatic gastroesophageal reflux disease (GERD), especially those at high risk for Barrett's esophagus (middle-aged to elderly white men) and subsequent adenocarcinoma, is logical and has proven to be effective.

C. A randomized Veterans Affairs Cooperative Study of medical and surgical antireflux treatment in patients with severe GERD showed superior control of reflux symptoms in the surgical group, although no difference in the incidence of esophageal cancer; thus, he should be offered antireflux surgery.

Question 20.1.4.   **Which of the following statements about the role of epidermal growth factor receptor (EGFR) in premalignant and malignant conditions of the esophagus are TRUE?**

A.   EGFR is commonly overexpressed in early-stage esophageal cancer, and overexpression correlates with a poor prognosis.

B.   Increased expression of transforming growth factor (TGF)-β and EGF has been detected in Barrett's esophagus, esophageal adenocarcinoma (EAD), and esophageal squamous cell carcinoma (ESCC).

C.   EGFR overexpression may predict a poor response to chemoradiotherapy and is associated with decreased survival in patients with squamous cell carcinoma.

D.   EGFR overexpression may predict a better response to chemoradiotherapy and is associated with improved survival in patients with both squamous cell carcinoma.

E.   Only A, B, and C.

F.   Only A and B.

Question 20.1.5.   **A 22-year-old woman is diagnosed with metastatic gastric cancer, with diffuse involvement of the stomach and linitis plastica. Her father died of the same cancer at age 42 years. Her mother is concerned about familial gastric cancer and is asking for information about hereditary gastric cancer and appropriate screening for her other children. Which of the following would be the most appropriate recommendation to this family?**

A.   Hereditary gastric cancer is rare and unlikely. She may just have some environmental exposures or DNA mismatch repair gene mutations that cannot be screened for.

B.   She may very well have hereditary early-onset diffuse gastric cancer, but no surveillance or workup is recommended because this has yet to be confirmed in larger studies.

C.   E-cadherin mutation testing should be considered here, and, in fact, prophylactic gastrectomy should be considered strongly for her siblings if a germ line E-cadherin mutation is confirmed and mucosal abnormality can be documented by endoscopic examination of the stomach.

D.   E-cadherin mutation testing should be considered, and, in fact, prophylactic gastrectomy should be considered strongly for her siblings if a germ line E-cadherin mutation is confirmed even if no mucosal abnormalities are seen by endoscopic examination of the stomach.

Question 20.1.6.   **Which of the following statements is TRUE about molecular genetic alterations in gastric cancer?**

A.   Many sporadic diffuse gastric cancers display altered E-cadherin, a transmembrane, calcium-dependent adhesion molecule important in epithelial cell homophilic and heterophilic interactions.

B.   The p53 tumor suppressor gene is consistently altered in most gastric cancers.

C.   Microsatellite instability has been found in 13% to 44% of sporadic gastric carcinomas.

D.   All of the above.

Question 20.1.7.   **A 72-year-old man diagnosed with squamous cancer of the esophagus has questions regarding the benefit of chemoradiation + surgery for his locally advanced cancer. He would like to know about the natural history of his disease and the expected benefit of combined modality therapy. Which of the following statements best describes the likely outcome/prognosis of his cancer?**

A.   In patients with cancers of the upper and middle thirds of the esophagus, which are predominately squamous cell carcinomas, distant recurrence predominates over locoregional recurrence.

B.   Preoperative radiotherapy and chemoradiotherapy may reduce the rate of locoregional recurrence but have no obvious effect on the rate of distant metastases.

C.   Two recent prospective randomized trials evaluating chemoradiotherapy alone or chemoradiotherapy followed by surgery in squamous cancer indicate that improvement in local control with the addition of surgery also resulted in improved survival.

D.   Concurrent administration of chemotherapy and radiotherapy provides better local control than radiotherapy alone, and the administration of chemotherapy has been shown in follow-up studies to reduce systemic recurrence.

Question 20.1.8.   **Which of the following statements about the role of fluorodeoxyglucose positron emission tomography (FDG-PET) use in the diagnosis and management of esophageal cancers is TRUE?**

A.   In the detection of distant metastases, FDG-PET is superior to computed tomography (CT), with a sensitivity, specificity, and accuracy all in the range of 80% to 90%.

B.   PET in combination with CT (PET/CT fusion or hybrid FDG-PET/CT) further improves specificity and accuracy of noninvasive staging.

C.   FDG-PET seems to have value in evaluating response to chemotherapy and radiotherapy. A prospective validation study confirmed that a decrease in the standard uptake value of 35% or more predicts histologic response and is associated with improved survival and decreased recurrence.

D.   All of the above.

Question 20.1.9.   A 58-year-old Caucasian man with a long-standing history of alcohol abuse and 40 pack-year smoking history is evaluated by his primary care physician for symptoms of acid reflux. He is placed on a trial of proton pump inhibitor with partial relief of symptoms. He undergoes an upper endoscopy, and salmon pink color mucosa extending in a tongue-like fashion is identified at the gastroesophageal junction, extending 8 cm in length. Biopsy results reveal Barrett's esophagus with high-grade dysplasia and a 1.5-cm focus of submucosal adenocarcinoma. Staging PET/CT scan is negative for metastatic disease. The patient has neoadjuvant chemoradiation followed by esophagogastrectomy, and pathology is consistent with a residual 0.8-cm area of moderately differentiated adenocarcinoma extending into the muscularis, with no lymphovascular invasion or lymph node involvement with tumor. The patient is here for follow-up today 6 weeks postoperatively. He feels well and states he is thinking of returning to work. What are your recommendations?

A. Baseline postoperative restaging scan and annual radiographic surveillance, 3-month history, and physical examination
B. Adjuvant chemotherapy with cisplatin + 5-fluorouracil
C. Adjuvant chemoradiation therapy with cisplatin + 5FU
D. Follow-up in 4 months with complete blood count (CBC) and comprehensive metabolic panel (CMP)

Question 20.1.10.   In the case described in Question 9, what is the pathologic stage of the patient?

A. T1N0M0 stage I
B. T2N0M0 stage IIA
C. T3N0M0 stage IIB
D. T3N0M0 stage III

Question 20.1.11.   A 65-year-old African American man with a history of coronary artery disease and stroke has epigastric pain for 6 months. Upper endoscopy reveals a 3-cm fungating ulcer along the lesser curvature of the stomach. Biopsy is consistent with poorly differentiated adenocarcinoma. Physical examination results are nondiagnostic, and his Eastern Collaborative Oncology Group (ECOG) performance status is 1. Which of the following would not be appropriate preoperatively?

A. PET/CT
B. Radiation therapy consult
C. Epirubicin, cisplatin, and 5-fluorouracil chemotherapy for three cycles
D. Endoscopic ultrasound

Question 20.1.12. **In the United States, the use of preoperative chemoradiation for locally advanced esophageal cancer followed by esophagectomy is commonly used despite clear evidence that this approach offers a survival advantage over surgery alone. Which of the following statements about the benefits of neoadjuvant chemoradiation are TRUE?**

A. In approximately two thirds of patients, disease is downstaged.

B. A survival advantage exists for patients experiencing downstaging to pathologically confirmed complete response or minimal residual disease status.

C. Locoregional control is improved, whereas distant failure is frequent and is the major cause of death.

D. All of the above.

Question 20.1.13. **A 67-year-old man with dysphagia to solids and a 20-lb weight loss presents for evaluation and workup. Endoscopy reveals a 4-cm-long stricture from 28 to 32 cm, and biopsy confirms moderately differentiated squamous cell cancer, likely with regional nodal involvement noted on PET scan. The patient has long-standing diabetes mellitus, hypertension, and peripheral vascular disease and is not thought to be a good surgical candidate. The best treatment approach would be:**

A. Photodynamic therapy followed by salvage chemoradiation.

B. Chemoradiation with cisplatin, 5FU, and 64.8 Gy of radiation to tumor and involved nodal regions, including 5-cm margins above and below the tumor.

C. Chemoradiation with cisplatin, 5FU, and 50.4 Gy of radiation to tumor, including the nodes involved.

D. Radiation alone because he is unlikely to tolerate any kind of chemotherapy.

Question 20.1.14. **A 57-year-old Caucasian woman with long-standing reflux symptoms presented with hematemesis to a local emergency department. Endoscopy revealed a distal esophageal malignant ulcer with involvement of the gastroesophageal (GE) junction and 5 cm of the gastric cardia. Biopsy revealed intestinal metaplasia at the GE junction and confirmed a diagnosis of adenocarcinoma. CT shows thickened distal esophagus and proximal stomach, hiatal hernia, and enlarged celiac nodes. Which statement most accurately describes her cancer?**

A. She has a Siewert type I cancer: adenocarcinoma of the distal esophagus, which usually arises from an area with specialized intestinal metaplasia of the esophagus (i.e., Barrett's esophagus) and may infiltrate the esophagogastric junction from above.

B. She has a Siewert type II cancer: adenocarcinoma of the cardia, which arises from the epithelium of the cardia or from short segments with intestinal metaplasia at the esophagogastric junction.

C. She has a Siewert type III cancer: adenocarcinoma of the subcardial stomach, which may infiltrate the esophagogastric junction or distal esophagus from below.

Question 20.1.15.   **A 65-year-old woman underwent a D2 subtotal gastrectomy for a T3N1 moderately differentiated gastric cancer at a community hospital. On recovery from the operation, 9 weeks later, she was offered adjuvant fluoropyrimidine-based chemoradiation. Which of the following statements about adjuvant therapy for completely resected gastric cancer is TRUE?**

A. Comparable local control can be achieved with optimal surgery that includes D2 lymph node dissection, and if this can be confirmed by a second pathology review, she does not need additional therapy.

B. Adjuvant chemotherapy alone based on data from the MAGIC trial is indicated because she has had adequate surgery. Radiation will not add any further improvement in local control.

C. The recommendation is based on results of the Intergroup study where D2 dissections were performed in only 10% of patients; thus, this may not be the best approach for this patient.

D. Adjuvant 5FU-based chemoradiation with 45 Gy radiotherapy has been shown to have a major advantage in survival, disease-free survival, and local-regional control compared with surgery alone, with much of the advantage in terms of improved local and regional control.

Question 20.1.16.   **A 79-year-old African American man presents with advanced gastric cancer, peritoneal carcinomatosis, and malnutrition. Parenteral nutrition is initiated, and his performance status is slowly improving. He is now able to perform activities of daily living and has gained 8 lbs. His daughter would like to know what your recommendations are at this point. Your response would be:**

A. His survival with best supportive care alone is likely to be approximately 3 months. Now that he is strong enough to tolerate the side effects of chemotherapy, he could have a prolonged survival and better quality of life if he opts for chemotherapy.

B. His survival with best supportive care alone is likely to be 3 months; chemotherapy may improve his quality of life.

C. With chemotherapy, an improvement in survival is expected in patients with a performance status of 0 or 1, essentially only those who are fit and relatively asymptomatic from their cancer.

D. Intraperitoneal chemotherapy may be better in this case for better delivery of chemotherapy in the peritoneal cavity because it would avoid the toxicities of systemic therapy.

ANSWERS

Answer 20.1.1.   **The answer is E.**

Similar trends have been noted in western European countries. This trend of increased incidence of adenocarcinoma of the esophagus has paralleled the upward trend in rates of both GE reflux disease and obesity.

Answer 20.1.2.   **The answer is E.**

Approximately 65% and 57% of squamous cell carcinomas of the esophagus have been attributed to smoking tobacco for more than 6 months in white and African American men, respectively, in the United States. The risk of adenocarcinoma of the esophagus also increases twofold in smokers. Interestingly, the risk of squamous cancer of the esophagus decreases (up to 50%) with smoking cessation, although that is not the case with adenocarcinoma risk. This suggests that tobacco carcinogens may affect carcinogenesis early on in esophageal adenocarcinoma, and therefore the decline in prevalence of smoking in the United States has not had an impact on the risk for the disease. Raw fruits and vegetables contain several micronutrients and dietary components such as vitamins A, C, and E, selenium, carotenoids, and fiber that may prevent carcinogenesis. In the United States, it is estimated that 39% and 69% of squamous cell carcinomas of the esophagus in white men and African American men, respectively, are related to low annual income. Exposure of these patients to several occupational and industrial hazardous chemicals is implicated for this increase in risk. The mechanism of *Helicobacter pylori* infection causing cancer is unclear. *H. pylori* infection can result in chronic atrophic gastritis leading to decreased acid production, which negates the effects of chronic reflux, including the potential for development of Barrett's esophagus. Although infection by *H. pylori* cagA strains by itself may not increase the risk of squamous cell carcinoma, the concurrent presence of gastric atrophy and *H. pylori* infection has been reported to significantly increase the risk of squamous cell carcinoma.

Answer 20.1.3.   **The answer is A.**

The driving force behind this recommendation is the finding from non-controlled studies suggesting that adenocarcinomas identified by surveillance methods are detected at an earlier stage and associated with a more favorable outcome after esophagectomy. In addition, Barrett's esophagus can be identified in 80% to 100% of resected specimens from patients undergoing esophagectomy for esophageal carcinoma. However, the efficacy of surveillance endoscopy is unclear, and there are no convincing data demonstrating that surveillance prevents cancer or improves life expectancy. The utility of screening high-risk individuals has not been proven and is unlikely to have a significant impact on reducing death from cancer, because 40% of patients with adenocarcinoma of the esophagus have no history of reflux and less than 5% of patients undergoing resection for adenocarcinoma were documented to have Barrett's esophagus before seeking medical attention for their symptomatic cancer. Both medical and surgical antireflux therapies are effective at reducing or eliminating the symptoms of GE reflux, but no clear-cut evidence exists that either therapy reduces the risk of esophageal adenocarcinoma. A randomized Veterans Affairs Cooperative Study of medical and surgical antireflux treatment in patients with severe GE reflux disease demonstrated superior control of reflux symptoms in the surgical treatment group but no difference between medical and surgical therapy groups in the incidence of esophageal cancer. Overall survival was significantly decreased in the surgical treatment group as a result of an unexpected excess of deaths from heart disease; thus, surgery would not be an option in place of surveillance.

Answer 20.1.4.   **The answer is E.**

EGFR overexpression is typically the result of increased engagement with ligands and decreased turnover. However, deletion of the extracellular domain or mutation of a tyrosine residue in the cytoplasmic domain has yet to be described. Furthermore, EGFR overexpression was associated with recurrent disease and diminished overall survival in patients undergoing esophagectomy for ESCC. EGFR overexpression may predict a poor response to chemoradiotherapy and is associated with decreased survival in patients with squamous cell carcinoma. In contrast with EGFR, it is not clear whether erbB2 overexpression is consistently found in either ESCC or EAD.

Answer 20.1.5.   **The answer is D.**

Large families with an autosomal dominant, highly penetrant inherited predisposition for the development of gastric cancer are rare. However, early-onset diffuse gastric cancers have been described and linked to the E-cadherin/CDH1 locus on 16q and associated with mutations in this gene, which may be the case in this family. This seminal finding has been confirmed in other studies with gastric cancers at a relatively high (67% to 83%) penetrance rate. Thus, E-cadherin mutation testing should be considered in the appropriate clinical setting. In fact, prophylactic gastrectomy should be considered strongly in families with germ line E-cadherin mutation even without gross mucosal abnormalities by endoscopic examination of the stomach. Hereditary nonpolyposis colon cancer (HNPCC) involves germ-line mutations of DNA mismatch repair genes. Gastric adenocarcinoma may be observed in families with HNPCC.

Answer 20.1.6.   **The answer is D.**

A reasonably prevalent alteration is microsatellite instability, the result of changes in DNA mismatch repair genes (*PPO* Table 39.1.1). Microsatellite instability and associated alterations of the TGF-b II receptor, IG-FRII, BAX, E2F-4, hMSH3, and hMSH6 genes are found in a subset of gastric carcinomas. Microsatellite instability has been found in 13% to 44% of sporadic gastric carcinomas. A high degree of microsatellite instability occurs in gastric cancers of the intestinal type, reduced involvement of lymph nodes, enhanced lymphoid infiltration, and better prognosis. This is reminiscent of colon cancers associated with HNPCC. The p53 tumor suppressor gene is consistently altered in most gastric cancers. In a study of the promoter region of p16 in gastric cancers, a significant number (41%) exhibited CpG island methylation. Many cases with hypermethylation of promoter regions displayed the phenotype with a high degree of microsatellite instability and multiple sites of methylation, including the hMLH1 promoter region. Many sporadic diffuse gastric cancers display altered E-cadherin. E-cadherin may be downregulated in gastric carcinogenesis (especially diffuse gastric adenocarcinoma) by point mutation, allelic deletion, or promoter methylation. In addition, during epithelial-mesenchymal transition, E-cadherin transcription can be silenced by transcriptional factors such as Snail and Slug.

Answer 20.1.7.   **The answer is B.**

Median survival after esophagectomy for patients with localized disease is 15 to 18 months with a 5-year overall survival rate of 20% to 25%. Patterns of failure after esophagectomy suggest that both location of tumor and histologic type may influence the distribution of recurrence. In patients with cancers of the upper and middle thirds of the esophagus, which are predominately squamous cell carcinomas, locoregional recurrence predominates over distant recurrence. In patients with lesions of the lower third, where adenocarcinomas are more frequently located, distant recurrence is more common. Treatment failure patterns after definitive chemoradiotherapy without surgical resection reveal that concurrent administration of chemotherapy and radiotherapy provides better local control than radiotherapy alone, and that the administration of chemotherapy may reduce systemic recurrence; however, long-term follow-up of both randomized and nonrandomized patients treated with primary chemoradiotherapy failed to indicate a clear reduction in distant disease recurrence compared with radiation therapy alone. Although the addition of surgery further reduces local failure from 45% to 32%, it does not diminish systemic recurrence and, in fact, may enhance it by allowing patients to manifest distant disease because they do not succumb to locoregional failure. Two recent prospective randomized trials evaluating primary chemoradiotherapy alone or chemoradiotherapy followed by surgery in squamous cancer indicate that improvement in local control with the addition of surgery failed to improve survival. These patterns of relapse suggest that any further improvement in overall outcome for patients with esophageal cancer will be achieved through advances in systemic therapy.

Answer 20.1.8.   **The answer is D.**

The addition of CT to PET improves sensitivity and specificity, which translates into the detection of unsuspected metastatic disease (upstaging) in approximately 15% of patients and refutation of suspected disease (downstaging) in 10% of patients, which leads to alteration of the intended treatment plan in at least 20% of patients. Weber et al demonstrated that decreased FDG uptake significantly correlated with pathologically confirmed response in patients treated with induction chemotherapy before esophagectomy for esophageal adenocarcinoma.

Answer 20.1.9.   **The answer is A.**

The available data for postoperative adjuvant chemotherapy suggest a possible prolongation of survival for patients who have had a potentially curative (R0) resection and have lymph node-positive (N1) disease.

There are no data to indicate or suggest that administration of postoperative adjuvant chemotherapy will prolong survival for patients who have undergone a curative resection and have negative nodes (N0). Patients who have positive margins of resection should be considered for postoperative radiation. Those who have had R0 resections but have regional nodal metastases (stages IIB and III) should be enrolled in clinical trials evaluating adjuvant therapies.

Answer 20.1.10.   **The answer is B.**

Stage IIA.

Answer 20.1.11.   **The answer is B.**

The results of the MAGIC trial have shown that even regimens that are only moderately effective in palliating patients with advanced disease can have a small but real effect on survival when given in the perioperative setting. New effective cytotoxic agents and biologic agents are now being introduced in the treatment of patients with gastric and GE junction tumors. Studies involving perioperative chemotherapy using these agents are now in the advanced planning stage. The results of the MAGIC trial and the postoperative Intergroup 116 chemoradiation study support the use of systemic therapy as a portion of the treatment plan for patients with locally advanced GE junction and gastric cancers. The best strategy to pursue is to determine whether to give systemic therapy first followed by surgery or to proceed directly to operation followed by systemic treatment plus or minus radiation, which has not yet been compared in prospective trials.

Answer 20.1.12.   **The answer is D.**

Although two of the five randomized trials demonstrated a survival advantage for combined modality therapy, they are limited by small numbers of patients. The efficacy of preoperative combined modality treatment for patients with resectable esophageal cancer remains controversial. The accumulated experience from phase II and III trials support all of the statements listed here concerning chemoradiotherapy using cisplatin and infusional 5FU-based therapy followed by esophagectomy. Surgery seems to be an important component of treatment to eliminate persistent disease after chemoradiotherapy. Some 20% to 30% of this group will be long-term survivors. Rates of curative resection may be improved with preoperative chemoradiotherapy.

Answer 20.1.13.   **The answer is C.**

The INT 0123 trial was the follow-up to RTOG 85-01. In this trial, patients with either squamous cell carcinoma or adenocarcinoma who were selected for nonsurgical treatment were randomly assigned to receive a slightly modified RTOG 85-01 combined modality regimen with 50.4 Gy of radiation versus the same chemotherapy with 64.8 Gy of radiation. It was closed early after an interim analysis showed that the high-dose arm was unlikely to have a superior survival compared with the lower dose arm. In addition, 11 treatment-related deaths occurred in the high-dose arm compared with 2 deaths in the standard-dose arm, with 7 of the 11 deaths occurring in patients who had received 50.4 Gy or less.

Although the crude incidence of local failure or persistence of local disease (or both) was lower in the high-dose arm than in the standard-dose arm (50% vs. 55%), as was the incidence of distant failure (9% vs. 16%), these differences did not reach statistical significance. At 2 years, the cumulative incidence of local failure was 56% for the high-dose arm versus 52% for the standard-dose arm ($p = .71$). Although retrospective data from the M.D. Anderson Cancer Center suggests a positive correlation between radiation dose and locoregional control, based on results of the INT 0123 trial, the standard dose of external-beam radiation remains 50.4 Gy.

Answer 20.1.14. **The answer is B.**

The Siewert classification has important therapeutic implications. The lymphatic drainage routes differ for type 1 versus types II and III lesions. As shown on lymphographic studies, the lymphatic pathways from the lower esophagus pass both cephalad (into the mediastinum) and caudad (toward the celiac axis). In contrast, the lymphatic drainage from the cardia and subcardial regions is toward the celiac axis, splenic hilus, and para-aortic nodes. Thus, the Siewert classification provides a practical means for choosing among surgical options. For type I tumors, esophagectomy is required, whereas types II and III tumors can be treated by transabdominal extended gastrectomy (resection of the stomach and distal intra-abdominal esophagus).

Answer 20.1.15. **The answer is D.**

The major change in the past decade in the adjuvant radiation therapy of gastric cancer comes from the results of the Gastrointestinal Intergroup trial that tested the value of adjuvant postoperative radiation therapy and chemotherapy for patients with T2 to T4 and/or node-positive gastric cancer after surgery with no evidence of residual disease. A total of 550 patients were entered in the study, with patients generally having advanced stage disease; 85% of patients had node positive tumors and 69% of patients had T3 or T4 disease. Median overall survival in the Intergroup 116 study of observation versus postoperative chemoradiation therapy after potentially curative gastrectomy was 27 months in the surgery alone group and 36 months in the surgery plus chemoradiotherapy group. The hazard ratio for death in the surgery-alone group was 1.35 (95% confidence interval [CI], 1.09–1.66; $p = .005$). The Intergroup study has been criticized for not having good surgical quality control, with only a minimal number of nodes found in many surgical specimens and with D2 dissections having been performed in only 10% of patients. However, commentators often overlook the fact that the Intergroup protocol was a study of postoperative chemoradiation treatment for patients with completely resected high-risk gastric cancer; gastrectomy and lymph node dissection were not part of the protocol treatment because patients were evaluated for protocol eligibility only after successful recovery following gastrectomy. As such, the "surgical results" of the Intergroup trial are best viewed as a reflection of the standard practice of US surgeons and pathologists.

Answer 20.1.16.   **The answer is A.**

The results of the studies and supportive evidence from more recent trials indicate that fit patients with advanced incurable gastric cancer who can tolerate potential toxicities have a modest but real benefit in survival compared with best supportive care. The majority of studies that have evaluated intraperitoneal therapy for gastric cancer used mitomycin C, and most trials were performed in Asia. They have all examined intraperitoneal therapy in the adjuvant setting after surgery. A meta-analysis of these studies showed the majority involved less than 100 patients per arm. A total of 552 patients had a resection alone, and 609 patients were randomized to operation plus intraperitoneal treatment. The odds ratio (OR) was in favor of postoperative intraperitoneal therapy (OR 0.51; 95% CI, 0.4 to 0.65). However, the authors thought that only a few of the studies were high quality. They suggested that more rigorously designed trials with larger numbers of patients and greater power were necessary before definitive conclusions regarding the effectiveness of postoperative intraperitoneal treatment could be made. In summary, the use of intraperitoneal chemotherapy involving either technique is a reasonable experimental strategy, particularly until more effective systemic agents can be developed. The goal is improvement in overall survival, as well as prevention of abdominal carcinomatosis with its associated morbidities, such as recurrent bowel obstruction.

SECTION 2   Renuka V. Iyer

PANCREAS

Directions   Each of the numbered items below is followed by lettered answers. Select the ONE lettered answer that is BEST in each case unless instructed otherwise.

QUESTIONS

Question 20.2.1.   **Which of the following factors are not associated with an increased risk of pancreatic cancer?**

A.   Cigarette smoke
B.   Cirrhosis
C.   High-protein diet
D.   African American men

Question 20.2.2. **Which of the following statements regarding pancreatic cancer is NOT true?**

A. At diagnosis, 31% have evidence of distant metastases.
B. Pancreatic cancer tends to occur later in life.
C. Activation of the K-ras oncogene plus inactivation of tumor suppressor genes (p53, DPC4, p16, and BRCA2) are associated with the development of pancreatic cancer.
D. Pancreatic intraepithelial neoplasms (PanINs) are intraductal proliferative epithelial lesions that are precancerous.
E. Patients with advanced pancreatic cancer may have undetectable levels of CA 19-9 if they are Lewis antigen-a or -b negative.

Question 20.2.3. **A 56-year-old African American man with a medical history of hypertension and type II diabetes presented to his primary care physician with a 1-month history of gradually worsening painless jaundice and a 10-lb weight loss. Computed tomography (CT) scan of the abdomen and pelvis revealed a 3.3-cm pancreatic head mass adjacent to the superior mesenteric vein with no intervening fat plan and encasing both the superior mesenteric vein and artery. The common bile duct was dilated, with a diameter of 1.8 cm, and the pancreatic body and tail were atrophied with dilatation of the pancreatic duct. Portal lymphadenopathy measuring 2 cm was present. The patient underwent endoscopic retrograde cholangiopancreatography (ERCP), and a biliary stent was placed. Biopsy of the mass was consistent with moderately differentiated pancreatic adenocarcinoma. What is this patient's stage?**

A. Stage I
B. Stage II
C. Stage III
D. Stage IV

Question 20.2.4. **A 67-year-old woman presents to her local emergency department with a 2-month history of right upper quadrant pain, jaundice, and 20-lb weight loss. She has no fever and chills. Standard CT of the abdomen reveals a 2.5-cm, ill-defined soft tissue density within the head of the pancreas and mild celiac axis, porta hepatis, and porta caval adenopathy, with the largest being within the celiac axis region measuring 2.0 × 1.8 cm. Endoscopic retrograde cholangiopancreatography is done, and a biliary stent is placed. Biopsy of the mass reveals poorly differentiated adenocarcinoma. CA 19-9 is 798. Which of the following should be done next for staging?**

A. Multiphase multidetector helical computerized axial tomography
B. Magnetic resonance imaging
C. Ultrasonography
D. Staging laparoscopy
E. Endoscopic ultrasonography

Question 20.2.5.   A 71-year-old Hispanic woman undergoes Whipple resection for a T3, N1, M0 pancreatic adenocarcinoma. Postoperative recovery was uneventful, and she starts adjuvant therapy 7 weeks later with gemcitabine given intravenously weekly for 2 weeks, followed by a 1-week break. In a follow-up visit after her first cycle she reports a 5-lb weight loss, nausea, decreased appetite, occasional abdominal cramping, and diarrhea. What should be done next?

A. Increase pancreatic enzyme supplementation.
B. Admit the patient for small bowel obstruction.
C. Hold chemotherapy for 1 week and follow up on symptoms.
D. CT scan of the chest, abdomen, and pelvis to rule out metastatic disease.

Question 20.2.6.   Which of the following statements regarding adjuvant therapy is NOT true?

A. In patients with resected pancreatic head lesions, survival is superior with gemcitabine compared with infusional 5FU, when given after 5FU-based chemoradiation.
B. Gemcitabine when compared with observation is associated with prolonged disease-free survival and overall survival.
C. 5FU-based chemoradiation followed by chemotherapy with 5FU can also be considered for adjuvant therapy.
D. In the ESPAC-1 trial, patients who received chemotherapy did better than those who did not.

Question 20.2.7.   A 64-year-old Caucasian woman is diagnosed with locally advanced unresectable pancreatic cancer. She receives 2 months of gemcitabine, and restaging CT scan of the abdomen and pelvis shows a decrease in the size of the lesion and her CA19-9 decreases from 854 to 201. What should be done next?

A. Start 5FU-based chemoradiation.
B. Continue gemcitabine chemotherapy for another 2 months, and then reassess.
C. Start gemcitabine-based chemoradiation.
D. Add 5FU to her chemotherapy regimen.

Question 20.2.8.   A 52-year-old Asian woman is evaluated for chronic right upper quadrant abdominal pain. Workup leads to diagnosis of pancreatic adenocarcinoma with metastasis to the liver. She is extremely anxious and tearful and wants to do everything possible to prolong her life. Which of the following regimens has been shown to prolong overall survival compared with gemcitabine alone?

A. Gemcitabine and oxaliplatin
B. Gemcitabine and capecitabine
C. Gemcitabine and erlotinib
D. Gemcitabine and cisplatin and bevacizumab
E. Gemcitabine and cetuximab

ANSWERS

Answer 20.2.1. **The answer is C.**

Tobacco smoke exposure plays a significant role in the development of pancreatic adenocarcinoma. It has been estimated that tobacco smoking contributes to the development of 20% to 30% of pancreatic cancers. The strongest associations between cigarette smoking and pancreatic cancer have been observed when the smoking occurred within the previous 10 years. Smoking cessation can reduce this risk. Environmental tobacco smoke contains the same toxins, irritants, and carcinogens, such as carbon monoxide, nicotine, cyanide, ammonia, benzene, nitrosamines, vinyl chloride, arsenic, and hydrocarbons, as primary cigarette smoke. Host etiologic factors associated with an increased risk of pancreatic cancer include a history of diabetes mellitus (DM), chronic cirrhosis, pancreatitis, a high-fat/cholesterol diet, and prior cholecystectomy. Although not all studies have supported a relationship between DM and pancreatic cancer, a meta-analysis of 20 epidemiologic studies confirms that the pooled relative risk of pancreatic cancer in persons with DM for 5 years is double (relative risk, 2.0; 95% confidence interval [CI], 1.2 to 3.2) the risk of persons without DM. However, there is no association with a high protein diet. People of African American descent experience a higher rate of pancreatic cancer than those of European ancestry in the United States, with an annual incidence of 16.7 per 100,000 versus 10.9 per 100,000, respectively. Death from pancreatic cancer is similarly elevated, with an annual rate of 14.6 per 100,000 versus 10.6 per 100,000. The diagnosis is slightly but significantly earlier in African Americans compared with Caucasians, with a median age of diagnosis of 68 and 73 years, respectively. In developed countries, the incidence and mortality rates range from 7 to 9 per 100,000 for men and 4.5 to 6 per 100,000 for women.

Answer 20.2.2. **The answer is A.**

CA 19-9 is a clinically useful tumor marker. The epitope of this antibody is a sialylated lacto-Nfucopentaose II related to the Lewis-a blood group antigen. Limitations of CA 19-9 are that it is not specific for pancreatic cancer and has been found to be elevated in other tumor types, such as biliary tract, colon, and stomach cancers. Ten percent of patients are Lewis antigen-a or b negative and unable to synthesize this antigen, and therefore may have undetectable levels of CA 19-9, even in the setting of advanced pancreatic cancer. Cholestasis can falsely elevate serum CA 19-9 levels; therefore, in patients who present with obstructive jaundice, an elevated CA 19-9 is not specific for the presence of pancreatic malignancy. Despite these caveats, serum CA 19-9 levels seem to have prognostic utility, particularly when measured either preoperatively or postoperatively in patients with resectable pancreatic cancer. Pancreatic ductal adenocarcinoma arises from ductal epithelial cells. Neoplasia arising from these cells progresses from initial intraductal proliferative lesions (PanINs) to invasive carcinomas. The evidence that these lesions are precancerous includes the observation that after segmental resection of pancreata with PanINs in the resected tissue, pancreatic cancer can develop in the pancreatic remnant. The strongest evidence that PanINs are precancerous lesions is the stepwise progression of genetic mutational events that correlates with the stepwise progression of worsening PanINs culminating in adenocarcinoma. PanIN-1 lesions show a predominance of K-ras mutations and overexpression of HER-2/neu. In PanIN-2 lesions, p16 mutations are the typical mutational event, and in PanIN-3 lesions, p53, DPC4, and BRCA2 mutations predominate. The mutational pattern of PanIN-3 lesions is equivalent to mutations found in pancreatic adenocarcinoma. These events are the basis of a current progression model for pancreatic cancer in which point mutation of K-ras and overexpression of HER-2/neu are initiating early events, p16 inactivation is an intermediate event, and p53, DPCA, BRCA2 inactivation follow just before invasion outside of the duct. Approximately 90% of all cases have p16 mutations, 75% have p53 mutations, and 55% have DPC4 mutations. It is estimated that 10% to 20% of pancreatic cancers are hereditary or have a familial link. Of patients with available data in the United States who were diagnosed with pancreatic cancer from 1996 to 2002, 8% presented with local disease, 31% presented with regional disease, and 61% had distant metastases. Therefore, the majority of patients are metastatic at diagnosis. Five-year survival from all stages of disease is 5%. Pancreatic cancer tends to occur later in life. Only 10% of patients in Europe present before the age of 50 years, whereas those aged 50 to 54 years experience an incidence of 9.8 per 100,000, and those aged 70 to 74 years experience an incidence of 57 per 100,000. The median age of diagnosis with pancreatic cancer in the United States is 72 years.

Answer 20.2.3. **The answer is C.**

The patient has a stage III, T4N1M0 pancreatic cancer. As per the sixth edition of the American Joint Committee on Cancer staging system, this represents unresectable disease. The T-stage designation classifies T1 to T3 tumors as potentially resectable and T4 tumors as locally advanced (unresectable). Tumors with any involvement of the superior mesenteric or celiac arteries are classified as T4; however, tumors that involve the superior mesenteric, splenic, or portal veins are classified as T3 because these veins can be resected and reconstructed provided that they are patent.

Answer 20.2.4. **The answer is A.**

Laparoscopy and multiphase CT have evolved concurrently as methods to evaluate a pancreatic mass. Both have emerged as highly effective in evaluating the tumors, but CT as a noninvasive modality supplants the use of routine laparoscopy. Currently, routine use of laparoscopy is not warranted. The cornerstone of diagnostic evaluation of a pancreatic tumor is the multiphase CT scan, coordinating intravenous contrast administration with subsequent rapid thin-cut CT through the pancreas during arterial, portal venous, and parenchymal phases of enhancement. With this type of CT, extension of the tumor to the superior mesenteric artery, celiac axis, superior mesenteric vein/portal vein complex, and contiguous structures can be clearly determined, as well as an assessment of distant metastasis. Optimally, CT imaging should precede stent placement and biopsy because of the possibility of postprocedure inflammation from the biopsy and artifact from the stent that can confound interpretation of the images. Magnetic resonance imaging has not been widely used to assess pancreatic cancer. Endoscopic ultrasound (EUS) can image the primary cancer and be a means of obtaining a fine-needle aspiration (FNA) of pancreatic adenocarcinoma, but in general the procedure is noncontributory when CT scan characterizes the tumor. When a mass cannot be visualized on CT scan, sonography through the wall of the stomach or duodenum can image tumors in the body/tail and head of the pancreas, respectively. Although preoperative ultrasonography is useful in assessing tumor characteristics and resectability of pancreatic adenocarcinoma, it is particularly operator dependent. It has a high sensitivity and specificity (92.3% and 72.7%, respectively) in defining superior mesenteric vein and portal vein invasion, although lower than helical CT (98% and 79%, respectively).

Answer 20.2.5.   **The answer is A.**

Malabsorption is a frequent complication seen in patients after Whipple surgery because of pancreatic enzyme insufficiency. Most patients require adjustment of the pancreatic enzyme supplement for adequate control of this symptomatology. Although small bowel obstruction and metastatic disease can be seen, the patient's clinical picture does not go along with these diagnoses. The aim during adjuvant therapy is to administer the chemotherapy with minimal delays to obtain the full benefit from therapy.

Answer 20.2.6.   **The answer is B.**

The Radiation Therapy Oncology Group (RTOG) performed a prospective randomized trial (RTOG 9704) comparing gemcitabine with infusional 5FU as the systemic component of therapy with all patients also receiving 5FU-based chemoradiation. There was no survival difference between patients randomized to gemcitabine and those who received infusional 5FU. However, among the 380 patients with resected pancreatic head lesions, survival was superior for patients randomized to gemcitabine compared with those who received infusional 5FU (20.6 months vs. 15.9 months; hazard ratio [HR] for death 0.79; 95% CI, 0.63 to 0.99; p = .033). In CONKO-001, patients randomized to receive gemcitabine had a median disease-free survival of 13.9 months (95% CI, 11.4 to 15.3), whereas those patients who underwent surgery alone had a median disease-free survival of only 6.9 months (95% CI, 6.1 to 7.8; p = .001). However, there was no statistically significant difference in overall survival. 5FU-based chemoradiation followed by up to 2 years of weekly bolus 5FU was evaluated against observation alone in the GITSG trial. A preliminary analysis of survival was reported after only 43 patients had completed treatment and showed a striking survival advantage for patients receiving combined modality therapy compared with survival of patients who underwent surgery alone (median 21.0 months vs. 10.9 months, respectively; one-tailed $p = .03$). In ESPAC-1, patients receiving chemoradiation did worse (median survival of 15.9 months; HR for death 1.28; 95% CI, .99 to 1.66) than those not receiving chemoradiation (median survival of 17.9 months; $p = .05$). Conversely, patients who received chemotherapy had a median survival of 20.6 months (HR for death 0.71; 95% CI, 0.55 to 0.92) versus 15.5 months for those patients who did not receive chemotherapy, a statistically significant result ($p = .009$).

Answer 20.2.7. **The answer is B.**

The optimal treatment for locally advanced pancreatic cancer remains controversial. Locally advanced disease is generally incurable, and all therapies have significant limitations. Gemcitabine-based chemotherapy for 2 to 4 months followed by 5FU or capecitabine-based chemoradiation is the most appropriate choice for the majority of patients with locally advanced, unresectable disease. If patients are responding to chemotherapy (objective radiographic response or CA 19-9 level decline) after 2 months and tolerating therapy well, it is reasonable to continue for 2 more months. When there is radiographic local progression, a CA 19-9 level plateau or increase, local symptomatic progression, or chemotherapy is poorly tolerated, chemoradiation should be initiated. In patients in whom distant progression has become evident during chemotherapy, a 2-week course of 30 Gy of 5FU or capecitabine-based chemoradiation should be considered only in patients with symptomatic primary tumors. The patients who have not progressed after systemic therapy are most likely to benefit from chemoradiation, and typically a 5.5-week course (50.4 Gy) of radiation therapy is appropriate with concurrent chemotherapy.

Answer 20.2.8. **The answer is C.**

Thus far, only inhibition of epidermal growth factor receptor (EGFR) with erlotinib combined with gemcitabine has led to a small, but statistically significant improvement in survival compared with gemcitabine alone. In a study performed by the National Cancer Institute of Canada Clinical Trials Group, patients with advanced pancreatic cancer were randomized to receive gemcitabine alone at 1000 mg/m^2 weekly for 7 weeks, then 1 week off, followed by gemcitabine days 1, 8, 15, every 28 days, or the combination of gemcitabine with erlotinib at a dose of 100 to 150 mg orally daily. Overall survival was improved for patients randomized to receive gemcitabine and erlotinib compared with patients receiving gemcitabine alone (191 vs. 177 days, respectively; HR for death 0.82; $p = .02$).

Renuka V. Iyer

SECTION 3

HEPATOBILIARY

Directions

Each of the numbered items below is followed by lettered answers. Select the ONE lettered answer that is BEST in each case unless instructed otherwise.

QUESTIONS

Question 20.3.1.

A 52-year-old man is found to have abnormal liver function and an elevated serum alpha-fetoprotein (AFP). Workup reveals prior hepatitis B viral infection, but it was not previously known or treated. An ultrasound reveals a 4-cm lesion in the left hepatic lobe, and a computed tomography (CT) scan reveals no evidence of metastatic disease or vascular involvement. A needle biopsy reveals hepatocellular carcinoma. The patient undergoes successful partial hepatectomy, surgical margins are clear, and the patient recovers from surgery. Which of the following approaches should be followed?

A. Adjuvant chemotherapy with sorafenib
B. Combination chemotherapy that is doxorubicin based
C. Adjuvant radiation to surgical bed
D. None of the above

Question 20.3.2.

A 49-year-old man was recently diagnosed with hepatocellular cancer. This was confirmed by biopsy from a 3-cm growing liver mass, which was being followed by his primary care physician because of his history of chronic hepatitis C-related cirrhosis. The primary care physician contacts your office for guidelines for selection of patients appropriate for liver transplantation. Your response would be:

A. Patients with solitary tumors ≤5 cm
B. Patients with multifocal disease with ≤3 tumor nodules each ≤3 cm in size
C. Patients with Child's B or C cirrhosis
D. Patients who are not candidates for primary liver resection
E. Tumors with no evidence of macrovascular invasion
F. All of the above

Question 20.3.3. **Which of the following statements about staging systems for liver cancer is TRUE?**

    A. The Okuda system takes into account several clinical features that include tumor size (>50% of liver), ascites (positive or negative), hypoalbuminemia (<3 g/dL), and hyperbilirubinemia (>3 mg/dL).

    B. The Cancer of the Liver Italian Program (CLIP) system uses hepatic tumor morphology and extent of liver replacement, Child-Pugh score, portal vein thrombosis, and serum AFP levels.

    C. The Barcelona Clinic Liver Cancer (BCLC) scoring system combines assessment of tumor stage, liver function, and patient symptoms with a treatment algorithm and has been shown to correlate well with patient outcomes.

    D. All of the above.

Question 20.3.4. **Which of the following paraneoplastic syndromes have been associated with hepatocellular cancer?**

    A. Hypoglycemia (also caused by end-stage liver failure)

    B. Erythrocytosis

    C. Hypercalcemia

    D. Carcinoid syndrome

    E. Porphyria cutanea tarda

    F. All of the above

Question 20.3.5. **An increased risk of developing hepatocellular carcinoma is associated with all of the following, EXCEPT:**

    A. Wilson disease

    B. Hemochromatosis

    C. Alpha1-antitrypsin deficiency

    D. Primary biliary cirrhosis

Question 20.3.6. **Which of the following statements about screening and prevention is TRUE?**

    A. The advent of vaccination for hepatitis B has the potential to reduce hepatocellular carcinoma in endemic areas.

    B. A combination of AFP and ultrasound screening is used in high-risk populations.

    C. Aggressive screening programs for hepatocellular carcinoma have been shown to improve survival.

    D. None of the above.

    E. A and C.

    F. A and B.

Question 20.3.7. **Which of the following statements about the cause of cholangiocarcinoma is TRUE?**

    A. Primary sclerosing cholangitis (PSC) and choledochal cysts are the most common known predisposing factors found in the United States.

    B. Liver fluke infestation (estimated to afflict 17 million people worldwide, mostly in southeast Asia and China) is a parasite that can cause chronic inflammation of the bile duct, eventually leading to cholangiocarcinoma.

    C. Chronic portal bacteremia and portal phlebitis can lead to the development of intrahepatic pigmented stones. This is associated with an approximate 10% risk of cholangiocarcinoma.

    D. Exposure to Thorotrast (thorium dioxide), a radio contrast agent, used from 1930 to 1960, leads to cholangiocarcinoma after a latent period of 16 to 45 years.

    E. All of the above.

Question 20.3.8. **A 66-year-old man is noted to have painless jaundice on a routine follow-up at his primary care physician's office. Workup revealed biliary obstruction at the hilum. Endoscopic retrograde cholangiopancreatography (ERCP) was done that confirmed a high-grade stricture predominantly involving the left hepatic duct; however, brushings revealed atypical cells and no malignancy. He was seen at a tertiary care center and offered surgical management, an en bloc resection of the left hepatic lobe and extrahepatic bile duct, and a complete periportal lymphadenectomy. Which of the following statements about management/natural history of hilar cholangiocarcinoma are TRUE?**

    A. Surgical resection is associated with an operative mortality rate of 30%.

    B. Recurrences occur most commonly at the bed of resection, followed by retroperitoneal lymph nodes. Distant metastases occur in one third of cases.

    C. Less than 10% of patients have resectable cancer at the time of diagnosis.

    D. All of the above.

Question 20.3.9. **A 70-year-old man presents to an emergency department with a history of a 16-lb recent weight loss and persistent right upper quadrant pain. Computed tomography (CT) scan reveals a gall bladder stone and thickening of the anterior wall of the gall bladder. He undergoes a laparoscopic cholecystectomy. Pathology reveals a moderately differentiated 2-cm gall bladder adenocarcinoma invading the perimuscular connective tissue. Margins of resection are negative for tumor. What is the stage of this cancer?**

    A. Stage IA

    B. Stage IB

    C. Stage IIA

    D. Stage IIB

Question 20.3.10.   **The patient in Question 9 recovers after his surgery and receives a second opinion at a tertiary care center 5 weeks after his cholecystectomy. A follow-up CT scan 2 weeks after surgery shows mild periportal fullness. What would be the best approach at this time?**

    A. Perform en bloc resection of the gallbladder, resection of segments IVb and V of the liver, and regional lymph node dissection.

    B. No further therapy is warranted; surveillance with CT scans and laboratories done every 3 months.

    C. He requires a second laparotomy to assess the extent of remaining disease to guide further therapy.

    D. Perform ultrasound-guided biopsy of the periportal nodes; if positive, then fluoropyrimidine-based chemoradiation is indicated.

Question 20.3.11.   **Which of the following statements about adjuvant therapy for biliary cancers is TRUE?**

    A. Although there is no clear evidence from one prospective randomized trial, it appears patients treated in the adjuvant setting have a median survival of approximately 2 years.

    B. Adjuvant radiation is superior to chemotherapy alone.

    C. Adjuvant therapy can improve overall survival for patients with R0 resections.

    D. Fluoropyrimidine-based chemoradiation is standard, because it is superior to radiation alone.

ANSWERS

Answer 20.3.1.   **The answer is D.**

No adjuvant therapies have been shown to affect survival or delay progression thus far.

Answer 20.3.2.   **The answer is F.**

These are also referred to as the Milan criteria.

Answer 20.3.3.   **The answer is D.**

Multiple clinical staging systems for hepatic tumors have been described. The most widely used is the American Joint Committee on Cancer/Tumor-Node-Metastasis (AJCC/TNM). A staging system based entirely on clinical grounds that incorporates the contribution of the underlying liver disease was originally developed by Okuda et al. Adverse prognostic signs are as listed. Patients with Okuda stage III (advanced), namely, with three or more positive features, have a dire prognosis because they usually cannot be curatively resected and the condition of their liver typically precludes chemotherapy. The American Association for the Study of Liver Diseases (AASLD) has endorsed the use of the Barcelona Clinic (BCLC) system for staging of HCC. This has now been validated both internally and externally in several studies.

Answer 20.3.4.   **The answer is F.**

A variety of paraneoplastic syndromes have been described to occur in patients with hepatocellular cancer. Most of these are biochemical abnormalities without associated clinical consequences. The most important ones include hypoglycemia (also caused by end-stage liver failure), erythrocytosis, hypercalcemia, hypercholesterolemia, dysfibrinogenemia, carcinoid syndrome, increased thyroxin-binding globulin, sexual changes (gynecomastia, testicular atrophy, and precocious puberty), and porphyria cutanea tarda. Pathogenesis of hypoglycemia is unclear but may be related to production by the tumor of insulin-like growth factor I. Erythrocytosis occurs in 3% to 12% of patients. Hypercholesterolemia may occur in 10% to 40% of patients. This has been shown to be caused by an absence of normal feedback control in malignant hepatocytes and results from a deletion in beta-hydroxy-methylglutaryl coenzyme A reductase.

Answer 20.3.5.   **The answer is D.**

Primary biliary cirrhosis is associated with an increased risk of cholangiocarcinoma.

Answer 20.3.6.   **The answer is F.**

Although screening programs are in place in endemic areas of hepatocellular carcinoma (HCC) and in high-risk populations, it is unclear whether screening identifies patients at an earlier stage or improves patient survival.

Answer 20.3.7.   **The answer is E.**

In most patients, cholangiocarcinomas are sporadic and no precipitating factor can be identified. In a minority of patients, several risk factors can be identified. In early stages, PSC results in inflammation of the bile ducts. Subsequent chronic disease can lead to multifocal strictures of the biliary system. The risk of developing a biliary malignancy is approximately 160 times that of the general population, with approximately 10% to 36% of patients with PSC developing a hepatobiliary cancer. In patients with PSC, cholangiocarcinoma occurs at a young age, and approximately one third of cancers are diagnosed within 1 year of being diagnosed with PSC. These predisposing factors all cause chronic inflammation of the bile duct. Some 10% to 20% of patients with choledochal cysts will develop cholangiocarcinoma if left untreated or managed with surgical drainage alone. Early excision of the choledochal cyst may reduce the risk of cholangiocarcinoma. Chronic calculi of the bile duct (outside the gallbladder) rarely occur and may predispose one to cancer formation. Specific carcinogens, such as Thorotrast, that lead to cholangiocarcinoma have been reported; the evidence for other environmental carcinogens, such as cigarette smoke, is not as clear.

Answer 20.3.8.   **The answer is B.**

Approximately one third of patients presenting with the suspected diagnosis of cholangiocarcinoma will have resectable disease. Operative mortality averages approximately 8%, indicating the high-risk population that this tumor affects and the complexity of the procedure. Some 10% to 35% of patients survive 5 years after surgical resection. Recurrences occur most commonly at the bed of resection, followed by retroperitoneal lymph nodes. Distant metastases occur in one third of cases. The most common site is the lung or mediastinum, followed by liver and peritoneum. Comparisons of outcome over time suggest improved outcome in more recent series as a result of routine inclusion of liver resection. Prognostic factors for survival include negative microscopic margin status, lymph node metastases, tumor size, tumor grade, preoperative serum albumin, hepatic resection, and postoperative sepsis.

Answer 20.3.9.   **The answer is B.**

The patient's pathology reveals a T2 NX stage IB gall bladder cancer.

Answer 20.3.10.   **The answer is A.**

Numerous studies have demonstrated that simple cholecystectomy is curative for stage I disease (T1, N0). Recent studies have suggested that the prognosis is different for pT1a and pT1b tumors after simple cholecystectomy. Invasion of the muscular layer allows access to lymphatics and vessels, providing the rationale for extended cholecystectomy in this population. When an extended cholecystectomy is performed for T2 disease, the 5-year survival has been reported to be as high as 100%, but probably falls in the range of 70% to 90% (*PPO* Table 39.8.13). Simple cholecystectomy alone is associated with a 5-year survival rate of 20% to 40.5%. Lymph node metastases are seen in 46% of patients with T2 primary tumors, providing another reason in favor of radical repeat resection after simple cholecystectomy. In series of extended cholecystectomies, the operative morbidity ranges from 5% to 46%, and the mortality ranges from 0% to 21%. The risk of resection for each patient and each type of resection needs to be weighed against the chance of benefiting from the procedure on the basis of the tumor stage.

Answer 20.3.11.   **The answer is A.**

Balachandran et al. reported on 117 patients with gallbladder cancer, of whom 80 underwent simple cholecystectomy and 37 underwent extended resections. Seventy-three patients received adjuvant chemoradiotherapy and 44 patients did not. The median survival of all 117 patients was 16 months. On multivariate analysis, the T stage and use of adjuvant therapy were the only statistically significant independent predictors of survival. Median survival was 24 months and 11 months in patients with or without adjuvant chemoradiotherapy ($p = .001$), respectively, and this difference was most pronounced for patients with T3, node-positive disease, or after a simple cholecystectomy. Ben-David et al reported on 14 patients with gallbladder cancer treated at the University of Michigan with resection followed by radiotherapy or chemoradiotherapy. The median radiation dose was 54 Gy, and approximately half the patients received concurrent chemotherapy. The median survival was 23 months. Interestingly, there was no difference in survival between patients with R0 or R1 resection. No differences were observed in survival or pattern of failure between patients with gallbladder cancer and patients with bile duct cancer (distal or hilar). The high risk of systemic spread and locoregional failure associated with gallbladder cancer that extends beyond the mucosa has led most cancer centers in the United States to recommend consideration of adjuvant chemotherapy and radiotherapy. For external beam radiation therapy, the target volume should include the gallbladder fossa and adjacent liver, as well as the regional nodal areas.

SECTION 4   Benjamin R. Tan, Jr.

SMALL INTESTINE AND GASTROINTESTINAL STROMAL TUMORS

Directions   Each of the numbered items below is followed by lettered answers. Select the ONE lettered answer that is BEST in each case unless instructed otherwise.

QUESTIONS

Question 20.4.1.   **A 60-year-old previously healthy woman noted abdominal distension and discomfort for 6 months, associated with nausea and vomiting. A computed tomography (CT) scan confirms a 20 × 25-cm abdominal mass, and exploratory laparotomy demonstrated a pedunculated mass arising from the stomach. No other metastases were found. A partial gastrectomy was done, and pathology revealed a gastrointestinal stromal tumor (GIST) that strongly stains for CD117 and CD34. Fifteen mitoses were seen per high-power field (hpf). Which of the following is true regarding GISTs?**

A.   The most common mutation associated with GIST involves the inactivation of a tumor suppressor gene.

B.   Both tumor size and mitotic index predict response to imatinib therapy.

C.   Gastric GISTs are associated with relatively worse outcomes compared with small intestinal GISTs.

D.   Patients with metastatic GIST tumors harboring exon 9 mutations have a better prognosis and response to imatinib compared with those with exon 11 mutation.

E.   None of the above.

Question 20.4.2.   **After the patient in Question 1 has recovered from surgery, what would you recommend for this patient on the basis of current data?**

A.   Observation with serial scans
B.   Imatinib 400 mg per os (PO) daily for 1 to 2 years
C.   Imatinib 400 mg PO daily for 5 years
D.   Sunitinib 50 mg 4 weeks on/2 weeks off therapy for 5 years

Question 20.4.3.   **A 62-year-old patient with diabetes, hypertension, and chronic moderate renal insufficiency developed abdominal discomfort and early satiety. An esophagogastroduodenoscopy revealed a gastric mass measuring 6 cm, and biopsy confirmed GIST with three mitoses per hpf. A CT scan revealed at least three hepatic metastases and multiple omental lesions. His current creatinine clearance is 36 mL/min. You recommend:**

A.   No dose adjustment is necessary for moderate renal insufficiency, and start imatinib 400 mg PO daily.
B.   A 25% dose reduction and give 300 mg PO daily.
C.   A 50% dose reduction and give 200 mg PO daily.
D.   Give sunitinib because imatinib is contraindicated for patients with moderate renal insufficiency.

Question 20.4.4.   **A 52-year-old woman with metastatic gastric GIST had an initial complete response to daily imatinib 400 mg with resolution of her hepatic and peritoneal metastases after 6 months of therapy. Imatinib was continued for 18 months when her CT scan showed recurrent hepatic lesions. Imatinib was increased to 800 mg daily. However, subsequent scans revealed progressive disease. You recommend starting sunitinib for this patient. Which of the following statements is NOT true?**

A.   Secondary resistance to imatinib therapy may be associated with the development of secondary KIT or PDGFRA mutations.
B.   Sunitinib therapy for patients with imatinib-resistant GIST improved progression-free survival compared with placebo.
C.   Patients with GIST harboring exon 9 mutation have a higher response to sunitinib than those with exon 11 mutation.
D.   Patients with the wild-type GIST are resistant to both imatinib and sunitinib therapy.

Question 20.4.5. The patient in Question 4 started sunitinib 50 mg daily for 28 days followed by a 2-week break. After two cycles, repeat CT scans showed a decrease in her measurable lesions. In addition to hypopigmentation of her hair, she also noted progressive generalized fatigue. She denies any dyspnea on exertion, diarrhea, or pedal edema. Physical examination reveals an erythematous rash in her hands, clear lungs, no cardiac gallops or rubs, and no focal neurologic deficits. Pertinent laboratory tests are as follows:

White blood cell (WBC) 5.6 × 103 cells/μL
Hemoglobin 11.8 g/dL
Sodium 145 mmol/L
Potassium 4.5 mmol/L
Creatinine 0.8 mg/dL
Total bilirubin 0.5 mg/dL
Alkaline phosphatase 118 μ/L

What would you order next?

A. Magnesium level
B. Magnetic resonance imaging of the brain
C. Thyroid function tests
D. 25-Hydroxycholecalciferol level

Question 20.4.6. Familial and genetic syndromes associated with GIST include all of the following, EXCEPT:

A. Cowden's syndrome
B. Familial paraganglioma
C. Carney triad
D. Neurofibromatosis

Question 20.4.7. Conditions that predispose one to the development of small intestinal cancer are the following, EXCEPT:

A. Crohn's disease
B. Familial adenomatous polyposis
C. Celiac disease
D. Hereditary nonpolyposis colorectal cancer (HNPCC)
E. All of the above

Question 20.4.8. True statement(s) regarding the predominant small intestinal lymphomas arising in the setting of celiac disease is/are:

A. A clonal intestinal intraepithelial lymphocyte population expressing CD20 with clonal gene rearrangement is characteristic.
B. These are primarily located in the duodenum.
C. A gluten-free diet seems to increase the risk for the development of these lymphomas.
D. Generally, these lymphomas do not respond well to chemotherapy and are rapidly fatal.
E. A and D.

Question 20.4.9.   A 15-year-old woman presented to the emergency department with severe periumbilical abdominal pain for the past 10 hours associated with nausea and nonbilious vomiting. A CT scan showed small bowel intussusception. Exploration and resection of the intussuscepted small bowel was performed that revealed a 4 × 3-cm hemorrhagic polyp with multiple smaller polyps surrounding it. Pathology revealed multiple hamartomatous polyps with an arborized pattern of formation. She also was noted to have multiple pigmented lesions in her lips and buccal mucosa. TRUE statement(s) regarding this syndrome are:

A. This syndrome is associated with an increased risk for developing pancreatic cancer and sex-cord tumors.
B. It is an autosomal dominant disease.
C. Germline PTEN mutation is found in more than 60% of patients.
D. Only A and B are true.
E. Only B and C are true.

Question 20.4.10.   A 50-year-old man presented with severe anemia and melena requiring 6 units of packed red blood cell transfusion. Esophagogastroduodenoscopy and colonoscopy revealed no abnormalities. A CT scan of the abdomen and pelvis was also unrevealing. He also noted watery diarrhea and flushing. Which of the following tests would you perform next?

A. Simple small bowel follow-through with barium
B. Formal double-contrast enteroclysis study
C. Wireless capsule endoscopy
D. Double balloon enteroscopy
E. B, C, or D

Question 20.4.11.   The patient in Question 10 was found to have three ileal lesions. Exploratory laparotomy revealed a total of five 1 to 1.5-cm lesions in the ileum. A frozen biopsy of one of the lesions confirmed a well-differentiated neuroendocrine (carcinoid) tumor. Segmental resection of the small bowel with regional lymph node revealed two mesenteric lymph nodes involved with carcinoid. His diarrhea, flushing, and bleeding resolved after surgery. Other than obtaining baseline scans, chromogranin A level, 24-hour urine 5-HIAA, what would be the most optimal management?

A. Short-acting octreotide 150 μg three times per day.
B. Octreotide LAR 30 mg once per month.
C. Adjuvant chemotherapy with 5FU, streptozotocin, and doxorubicin.
D. No further therapy. The patient just needs follow-up with laboratory tests ± scans every 3 months.

Question 20.4.12.   In one of the largest reviews in literature examining the clinical outcomes of 1102 patients with jejunoileal carcinoids, the risk for locoregional or distant metastases from a carcinoid tumor measuring more than 1 cm is:

A. 83%
B. 73%
C. 31%
D. 15%
E. 0%

Question 20.4.13. The risk for progressive disease for a patient with small intestinal GIST measuring less than 2 cm with more than five mitoses/50 hpf is:

A. 0%
B. 4.3%
C. 24%
D. 50%
E. 85%

Question 20.4.14. A 20-year-old student presented to the emergency department with a 2-day history of right lower abdominal pain associated with fever. His abdomen was slightly distended with diffuse tenderness but without guarding or rebound tenderness. Rectal examination showed no masses and was negative for occult blood. Complete blood count (CBC) showed a slightly elevated WBC at 11,000. CT scan showed a mass in the terminal ileum with no evidence of free peritoneal air. Colonoscopy revealed a terminal ileum mass, the biopsy of which showed sheets of monotonous round nucleated cells with abundant basophilic cytoplasm with numerous macrophages. Ki-67 index is 100%. What is your diagnosis?

A. Mucosal-associated lymphoid tissue lymphoma
B. Burkitt's lymphoma
C. Peripheral T-cell lymphoma
D. Medullary carcinoma of the small intestine

ANSWERS

Answer 20.4.1. **The answer is E.**

In the majority of malignant GISTs, a gain-of-function mutation results in the constitutive activation of the KIT proto-oncogene. Approximately 80% of GISTs harbor mutations in the KIT receptor, whereas another 5% to 7% have activating PDGFRA mutations. The most common mutation is identified in the KIT juxtamembrane domain, exon 11. Other mutations in exon 9, 13, 17, and 18 have been described. In the Intergroup US-Finland study, higher response rates and better outcomes were observed among patients with GIST with the exon 11 mutation compared with those with exon 9 mutation. Objective responses to imatinib therapy among patients with GIST with exon 11 and exon 9 mutations are approximately 70% and 40%, respectively. Patients with wild-type GIST have a response rate of approximately 30%. Median time to progression also is longer for those with exon 11 compared with other genotypes. The higher prevalence of a specific exon 9 mutation among GISTs originating in the small intestine may explain in part the observation of worse prognosis of these tumors compared with gastric GISTs. Although tumor size and mitotic index carry prognostic significance for patients with GIST, both have not been associated with response to tyrosine kinase inhibition.

Answer 20.4.2.   **The answer is B.**

Current data on adjuvant therapy for patients with resected GIST are derived from the American College of Surgeons Oncology Group (ACO-SOG) studies, which demonstrated a 1-year relapse-free survival rate of 97% among patients who received imatinib at 400 mg PO daily for 1 year, compared with 83% for those who received placebo, with a hazard ratio of 0.325 (DeMatteo, J Clin Oncol 25:18S, abstract 10079). Although no survival benefit was demonstrated, those with tumors greater than 10 cm derived the most benefit from adjuvant imatinib. A Phase II study on adjuvant imatinib in resected high-risk GIST (tumor size ≥10 cm, tumor rupture, or ≤5 peritoneal metastases) demonstrated improved overall survival compared with historical controls (DeMatteo, Proc 2008 Gastrointestinal Cancers Symposium, abstract 8). Three-year recurrence-free survival and overall survival rates were 61% and 97%, respectively. Current studies are evaluating longer duration of adjuvant therapy, but there are no data on the benefit of adjuvant therapy beyond 1 to 2 years or on the use of sunitinib in the adjuvant setting.

Answer 20.4.3.   **The answer is A.**

No dose adjustment is necessary for patients with mild to moderate renal dysfunction receiving imatinib therapy based on the national Cancer Institute Organ Dysfunction Working Group Study published by Gibbons et al (Gibbons J, Egorin MJ, Ramanathan RK, et al. Phase I and pharmacokinetic study of imatinib mesylate in patients with advanced malignancies and varying degrees of renal dysfunction: a study by the National Cancer Institute Organ Dysfunction Working Group. J Clin Oncol 2008; 26:570–576). Although there was an increase in imatinib drug exposure in patients with mild to moderate renal dysfunction, this was not associated with any meaningful toxicities. Doses up to 600 to 800 mg daily were tolerable for those with moderate and mild renal dysfunction, respectively. In another study by Ramanathan et al (Gibbons J, Egorin MJ, Ramanathan RK, et al. Phase I and pharmacokinetic study of imatinib mesylate in patients with advanced malignancies and varying degrees of liver dysfunction: a study by the National Cancer Institute Organ Dysfunction Working Group. J Clin Oncol 2008;26:563–569), patients with mild hepatic dysfunction were able to tolerate imatinib doses up to 500 mg daily. No relationship was found between imatinib pharmacokinetics and severity of hepatic dysfunction. The authors recommended that for patients with moderate or severe hepatic dysfunction, patients can be dosed at 400 mg daily with close monitoring for toxicity or to start at 300 mg daily and rapidly escalate the dose to 400 mg daily if tolerated.

Answer 20.4.4.   **The answer is D.**

Primary resistance to imatinib, manifested by continued tumor growth within the first 6 months of imatinib therapy, occurs in a minority of GISTs. Secondary resistance generally occurs after a median of 24 months of continued tyrosine kinase inhibition. Acquired mutations in KIT or PDGFRA have been implicated in the development of drug resistance to imatinib. The emergence of KIT-independent genotypes may also result in imatinib resistance. Sunitinib was approved by the Food and Drug Administration for the treatment of GIST after disease progression or intolerance to imatinib. The pivotal Phase III study demonstrated a superior time to progression of 27.3 weeks for patients treated with sunitinib compared with 6.4 weeks for patients treated with placebo. Six-month survival rates also favor sunitinib at 79.4% compared with 56.9% for placebo. With the crossover design, the advantage for survival benefit on longer follow-up diminished. A subset analysis showed improvement in response rates and outcomes for patients with GIST harboring exon 9 mutation compared with those harboring exon 11 mutations. Responses were also observed among patients with wild-type genotype.

Answer 20.4.5.   **The answer is C.**

Biochemical and clinical hypothyroidism has been associated with sunitinib therapy. Rini et al reported an 85% rate of thyroid dysfunction associated with sunitinib use (Hypothyroidism in patients with metastatic renal cell carcinoma treated with sunitinib. J Natl Cancer Inst 2007;99: 81). Routine monitoring of thyroid function test is warranted, and thyroid hormone replacement therapy may alleviate symptoms. The precise mechanism for sunitinib-associated hypothyroidism is unclear. Destructive thyroiditis through follicular apoptosis has been postulated for sunitinib-associated thyroid dysfunction based on the observation of transient thyroid-stimulating hormone (TSH) suppression and subsequent absence of visualized thyroid tissue. Other causes of fatigue associated with sunitinib include adrenal insufficiency or congestive heart failure.

Answer 20.4.6.   **The answer is A.**

Carney triad, which encompasses multifocal GIST with pulmonary chondroma and extra-adrenal paraganglioma, familial paraganglioma, and neurofibromatosis type 1 are associated with GIST. These syndromes, along with pediatric GIST, can be characterized by the wild-type KIT gene. It is unclear whether GISTs associated with these syndromes have a similar response to imatinib therapy as sporadic GIST.

Answer 20.4.7.   **The answer is E.**

All of the conditions listed are associated with increased risk for the development of cancer in the small intestine. Other conditions include acquired immunodeficiency syndrome (AIDS), neurofibromatosis, Gardner's syndrome, Peutz-Jeghers, and a history of other primary tumors, such as uterine, ovarian, prostate, thyroid, skin, and soft tissue sarcomas.

Answer 20.4.8.   **The answer is D.**

The predominant lymphomas associated with celiac disease are referred to as enteropathy-associated T-cell lymphoma (EATL). Patients with refractory sprue may present with malabsorption syndromes, abdominal pain perforation, or obstruction. Although CD 20 + B-cell lymphomas are the most common non-Hodgkin's lymphoma occurring in the small intestine, lymphomas associated with celiac disease are often T cell. A clonal population of CD3+, CD8+ lymphocytes with T-cell gene rearrangement has been associated with the progression of refractory sprue and ulcerative jejunitis to malignant lymphoma. These generally occur in the jejunum, and a gluten-free diet may decrease the risk for malignancy. There is no evidence for a gluten-free diet increasing the risk for the development of these lymphomas. Generally, these are poorly responsive to therapy and can be rapidly fatal.

Answer 20.4.9. **The answer is D.**

Peutz-Jeghers disease is a rare autosomal dominant disease characterized by the presence of multiple gastrointestinal hematomas and a distinctive mucocutaneous pigmentation. Patients with this syndrome usually present in their second or third decade of life with abdominal pain, bleeding, anemia, small bowel obstruction, or intussusception. The cumulative risk for developing any type of cancer is more than 90%. Although patients are at high risk of developing enteric malignancies, such as small intestine, gastric, colon, and esophageal cancers, they are also at risk for other neoplasms, such as pancreatic cancer (132-fold) and breast, lung, and ovarian cancers. Benign lesions such as ovarian sex-cord tumors may also develop in women, and Sertoli-cell testicular tumors may develop in men. Germline mutations in the LKB1 tumor suppressor gene are common with Peutz-Jeghers, whereas germline mutations in PTEN are seen in a heterogenous hamartoma disorder that includes Cowden's syndrome. Cowden's syndrome is associated with an increased risk of breast, thyroid, and endometrial cancer. Other syndromes in this group include Proteus syndrome and Bannayan-Riley-Ruvalcaba syndrome (BRRS).

Answer 20.4.10. **The answer is E.**

Any of the answers would be an appropriate next test except for simple small bowel follow-through, which has a low sensitivity. A formal double-contrast enteroclysis will increase the sensitivity for detecting cancer in the small intestine. Emerging literature suggests that wireless capsule endoscopy is the standard of care for the diagnosis of small bowel malignancies. A more recent method, the contrast balloon enteroscopy, also yielded high detection rates but has not been formally compared with wireless capsule endoscopy.

Answer 20.4.11. **The answer is D.**

Although the patient is at high risk for developing recurrent or metastatic disease, there is currently no clear role for the use of adjuvant octreotide therapy or chemotherapy. Close follow-up is necessary, and if tumor markers are elevated, repeat CT or octreotide scans may be done to determine metastatic disease.

Answer 20.4.12. **The answer is B.**

According to one of the largest series on jejunoileal carcinoids by Soga et al, the risk for locoregional or distant metastasis from carcinoid tumors measuring more than 1 cm is 73%. The risks for tumors less than 6 mm and 6 to 10 mm are 15% and 31%, respectively.

Answer 20.4.13.   **The answer is D.**

GISTs arising from the small intestine appear to have a more malignant behavior at a smaller size compared with those found in the stomach or in the colon. For small tumors less than 2 cm, those with more than 5 mitoses per 50 hpf have a 0% risk of progression according to one study, whereas those with more than 5 mitoses per 50 hpf have a 50% risk for progression. GISTs larger than 10 cm with more than 10 mitoses per 50 hpf have a 90% risk of progression.

Answer 20.4.14.   **The answer is B.**

This patient has Burkitt's lymphoma arising from the terminal ileum presenting with appendicitis-like symptoms. This type of lymphoma accounts for less than 5% of all lymphomas in the small intestine. A "starry-eyed" pattern interspersed throughout monomorphic cells with abundant basophilic cytoplasm is characteristic and related to numerous macrophages with ingested apoptotic tumors within. A high proliferative index is also characteristic. Treatment consists primarily of aggressive chemotherapy.

SECTION 5   Benjamin R. Tan, Jr.

COLORECTAL AND ANAL CANCERS

Directions   Each of the numbered items below is followed by lettered answers. Select the ONE lettered answer that is BEST in each case unless instructed otherwise.

QUESTIONS

Question 20.5.1.   **A 30-year-old multigravid woman presents with a large abdominal mass associated with abdominal pain. She underwent a total proctocolectomy for colon cancer secondary to familial adenomatous polyposis (FAP) 4 years ago. She received adjuvant chemotherapy for node-positive disease. A recent esophagogastric endoscopy revealed only a tubulovillous adenoma in the duodenum. A computed tomography (CT) scan revealed a 10-cm mass filling the pelvis. Biopsy confirmed desmoid tumor. A TRUE statement regarding desmoids tumors is:**

A. Desmoid tumors represent the second most common cause of death for patients with FAP.

B. Desmoid tumors are uniformly aggressive and locally invasive.

C. Adjuvant radiation is recommended.

D. Adjuvant chemotherapy is recommended.

Question 20.5.2.   A 55-year-old woman underwent a right hemicolectomy for a cecal mass 15 years ago. Four years later, she was found to have a hepatic flexure adenocarcinoma and a total colectomy was performed. Four years ago, she presented with postmenopausal bleeding and was found to have endometrial adenocarcinoma. She also had multiple skin malignancies, including sebaceous adenomas and keratoacanthomas. One year ago, she underwent a Whipple procedure for a duodenal adenocarcinoma invading into the pancreas. She has three siblings and a paternal uncle with colorectal cancer all diagnosed in their late 30s. What is the most probable PRIMARY genetic explanation for her inherited colorectal cancer syndrome?

A.   Chromosomal instability characterized by the deletion or mutation of a tumor suppressor gene
B.   Chromosomal instability characterized by activation of an oncogene
C.   Microsatellite instability (MSI) caused by germline mutations in a DNA mismatch repair (MMR) gene
D.   MSI caused by epigenetic changes associated with hypermethylation in CpG islands

Question 20.5.3.   Other than genetic counseling, which test would you order to confirm the diagnosis?

A.   p53 mutation and loss of heterozygosity (LOH) of chromosome 18q
B.   APC mutation, including the I1307K allele
C.   MSI testing and methylation of CpG islands
D.   MSI test and MMR gene mutation including MLH1, MSH2, MSH6

Question 20.5.4.   The patient in Question 3 had a positive test result. What screening tests and surveillance program would you recommend to her three daughters aged 24, 22, and 20 years?

A.   Colonoscopy now and repeat every 1 to 2 years and transvaginal ultrasound for her daughters starting by age 30 to 35 years
B.   Colonoscopy for all and transvaginal ultrasound for her daughters starting at age 30 to 35 years
C.   Colonoscopy now and repeat every 1 to 2 years with transvaginal ultrasound at age 30 to 35 years only for her children confirmed to have the same genetic mutation as the patient; colonoscopy at age 40 to 50 years for those with no mutation
D.   Colonoscopy and transvaginal ultrasound at age 30 to 35 years only for those confirmed with the same mutation as the patient; colonoscopy by age 40 to 50 years for those with no mutation

Question 20.5.5.   Congenital hypertrophy of retinal pigment epithelium (CHRPE) is associated with which familial colorectal cancer syndrome?

A.   FAP
B.   Peutz-Jeghers syndrome
C.   Lynch syndrome variant, Muir Torre syndrome
D.   Bannayan-Riley-Ruvalcaba syndrome

Question 20.5.6. **A 65-year-old woman presented with intermittent constipation and diarrhea associated with abdominal cramping. A colonoscopy revealed a near-obstructing mass, and biopsy revealed a villoglandular polyp. She underwent an exploratory laparotomy and resection of a 5 × 5-cm circumferential necrotic and fungating mass. Pathology revealed a moderately differentiated adenocarcinoma invading into the pericolonic fat with 2 of 30 positive lymph nodes. Margins were negative. CT scan showed no evidence of metastatic disease. After recovery from her surgery, based on current evidence, you would recommend:**

    A. 5FU with leucovorin × 6 months
    B. Capecitabine × 6 months
    C. Irinotecan with 5FU (FOLFIRI) × 6 months
    D. Oxaliplatin with 5FU (FOLFOX) × 6 months
    E. Oxaliplatin with 5FU (FOLFOX) and bevacizumab × 6 months

Question 20.5.7. **One week after the first dose of chemotherapy, the patient in Question 6 developed a fever at 102°F associated with chills. She also developed diarrhea, mucositis, confusion, and ataxia. Repeat complete blood count (CBC) showed a white blood cell (WBC) count of 0.5×10^3 cells/μL with an absolute neutrophil count (ANC) of 100, hemoglobin of 11.7 g/dL, and platelet count of 42,000. Which one of the following pharmacogenetic conditions would best explain her clinical course?**

    A. The patient is homozygous for the thymidylate synthase (TYMS) *3/*3 polymorphism.
    B. The patient is homozygous for UGT1A1 *28 polymorphism.
    C. The patient is heterozygous for the IVS14 + 1 G>A DPYD*2A mutation.
    D. The patient is heterozygous for the ERCC2 Lys751Gln polymorphism.

Question 20.5.8. **A 62-year-old engineer was diagnosed with metastatic cecal adenocarcinoma with lung and liver metastases. He was initially treated with oxaliplatin plus infusional 5FU (FOLFOX6) and bevacizumab. After four cycles (2 months), his CT scan showed progressive disease. You discussed irinotecan 180 mg/m^2 every 2 weeks plus weekly cetuximab based on the results of the EPIC study. A test for UGT1A1 polymorphism was done, and results revealed him to be homozygous for UGT1A1 *28/*28. Which of the following statements is TRUE?**

    A. Patients homozygous for the UGT1A1 *28 polymorphism glucuronidate SN38 more efficiently than those with the wild-type *1 genotype.
    B. Patients homozygous for the UGT1A1 *28 polymorphism glucuronidate SN38 less efficiently than those with the wild-type *1 genotype.
    C. Patients homozygous for UGT1A1 *28 polymorphism are at greater risk for severe neutropenia with irinotecan compared with those with the wild-type *1 genotype.
    D. A and C are true.
    E. B and C are true.

Question 20.5.9.   **A 52-year-old teacher presents with a 2-month history of rectal bleeding. A rectal examination revealed a palpable mass 6 cm from the anal verge. Subsequent colonoscopy confirmed a friable, tethered mass biopsy that showed moderately differentiated adenocarcinoma. Transrectal ultrasound revealed a T3 N1 cancer. CT scans of the chest, abdomen, and pelvis revealed no metastatic sites. Which of the following treatment strategies would you recommend?**

   A.   Abdominoperineal resection (APR) with a total mesorectal excision (TME) followed by adjuvant chemoradiation
   B.   APR with TME followed by chemotherapy alone
   C.   Short-course 5-day neoadjuvant radiation (25 Gy) followed by APR with TME
   D.   Prolonged-course neoadjuvant 5FU-based chemoradiation followed by APR with TME and adjuvant chemotherapy

Question 20.5.10.   **Which of the following appropriately staged patients with rectal cancer would be the BEST candidate for transanal excision?**

   A.   A 48-year-old woman with a 2.5-cm T1 moderately differentiated rectal adenocarcinoma 4 cm from the anal verge
   B.   A 65-year-old man with a 4.5-cm T2 well-differentiated circumferential rectal mass 6 cm from the anal verge
   C.   A 30-year-old man with a 2-cm well-differentiated T1 mucinous adenocarcinoma 12 cm from the anal verge
   D.   A 52-year-old woman with a 3-cm well-differentiated T1N1 adenocarcinoma 5 cm from the anal verge
   E.   None of the above

Question 20.5.11.   **For the patient you have selected for transanal resection in Question 10, pathological review of the excised specimen showed no lymphovascular invasion and all margins were negative. Which of the following options would you recommend?**

   A.   No further therapy
   B.   Short-course (25 Gy/5 fractions) radiation
   C.   Intracavitary radiation
   D.   Adjuvant chemotherapy without radiation
   E.   Adjuvant chemotherapy with radiation

Question 20.5.12.   **The following are true statements regarding MYH-associated polyposis, EXCEPT:**

   A.   Inheritance is autosomal dominant.
   B.   Clinical features of MYH-related polyposis are similar to FAP.
   C.   The MYH-gene is a base-excision repair gene.
   D.   A deficiency in MYH leads to accumulation of somatic mutations in the APC gene.

Question 20.5.13. **A 49-year-old woman noted rectal bleeding for 2 months. She denied any pain, diarrhea, constipation, or weight loss. A colonoscopy was done that revealed a 2-cm low-lying mass 1 cm from the anal verge. A transrectal ultrasound revealed no lymph nodes. Biopsy confirmed basaloid squamous cell carcinoma. CT scans of the abdomen and pelvis did not reveal any metastatic disease. The BEST curative treatment option for this patient is:**

A. Abdominoperineal resection (APR)
B. Short-course (25 Gy/5 fractions) radiation followed by APR
C. Neoadjuvant chemoradiation with 5FU followed by APR
D. Chemoradiation alone with 5FU and mitomycin

Question 20.5.14. **A 58-year-old man presented with a 6-month history of anorexia, fatigue, and a vague right-sided abdominal discomfort. His physical examination was unremarkable except for mild pallor. Initial laboratory test revealed a hemoglobin level of 10.7 g/dL with a mean corpuscular volume (MCV) of 73. He also had mildly elevated alkaline phosphatase and hepatic transaminases. Colonoscopy revealed a nonobstructing transverse colon mass. Biopsy demonstrated moderately differentiated adenocarcinoma. CT scan revealed a 3-cm lesion in the left lobe of the liver and two other lesions measuring 1.5 to 2 cm in the right lobe of the liver. Positron emission tomography revealed uptake in the transverse colon and all three known hepatic lesions. Among the following options, what would be the best option for this patient based on current studies?**

A. Curative-intent resection of the transverse colon primary and all three hepatic lesions followed by active surveillance
B. Palliative-intent front-line chemotherapy with bevacizumab for metastatic colon cancer until progression, followed by palliative second-line chemotherapy
C. Curative-intent resection of the transverse colon primary and all three hepatic lesions with chemotherapy
D. Curative-intent resection of the transverse colon primary and all three hepatic lesions with radiotherapy

ANSWERS

Answer 20.5.1. **The answer is A.**

Desmoid disease is second only to colorectal cancer as a common cause of death among patients with FAP. There is heterogeneity in the clinical presentation of desmoid tumors from asymptomatic abdominal mass to bowel or ureteral obstruction. Sporadic desmoid tumors also occur. Retrospective studies have not confirmed the role of adjuvant radiation or chemotherapy for desmoid tumors. For unresectable tumors, chemotherapy, hormonal therapy, and targeted agents such as imatinib have been reported in literature as possible palliative options.

Answer 20.5.2.   **The answer is C.**

This patient meets the Amsterdam criteria for hereditary nonpolyposis colorectal cancer (HNPCC) with at least three affected relatives in at least two successive-generation relatives and one first-degree relative diagnosed with colorectal cancer before age 50 years. Unlike FAP, which is characterized by chromosomal instability caused by mutations in the APC tumor suppressor gene, HNPCC is characterized by MSI caused by mutations in the DNA MMR genes. HNPCC is the most common hereditary syndrome predisposing one to colorectal cancers. It accounts for approximately 2% to 3% of all colorectal cancer cases. The lifetime risk for developing colon cancer among patients with HNPCC approaches 80%. HNPCC is also associated with other malignancies, including endometrial, gastric, ampullary, biliary, and urinary tract cancers. This patient has Muir-Torre syndrome characterized by multiple colon cancers and multiple cutaneous neoplasia, including sebaceous adenomas.

Answer 20.5.3.   **The answer is D.**

HNPCC can be confirmed by the demonstration of the MSI-H phenotype and germline mutation in any of the DNA MMR genes, such as MLH1 on chromosome 3p, MSH2 on chromosome 2p, MSH6 on chromosome 2p, PMS1 on 2q, and PMS2 on 7q. Germline mutations involving MSH2 and MLH1 genes account for more than 60% of the known mutations present in patients with HNPCC. The National Comprehensive Cancer Network (NCCN) guidelines recommend the use of tumor screening with MSI and lack of expression of MMR protein expression by immunohistochemistry initially, followed by MMR mutation testing, although proceeding directly to MMR mutation testing is also acceptable. A negative MMR mutation test result does not rule out Lynch syndrome or HNPCC.

Answer 20.5.4.   **The answer is C.**

Once a germline MMR mutation is identified in a patient, genetic counseling and testing of at-risk family members are essential. The patient's three daughters, along with all her first-degree relatives, have a 50% probability of being a carrier of the mutant gene. In general, for family members who do not carry the known mutation, there is no need for intensive surveillance, and routine colorectal screening according to national guidelines is recommended. For family members who carry the germline MMR mutation, the National Comprehensive Cancer Network recommends colonoscopies every 1 to 2 years beginning at age 20 to 25 years or 5 to 10 years younger than the earliest age of diagnosis in the family, whichever comes first. For women with the MMR mutation, screening for endometrial cancer with transvaginal ultrasound with or without CA 125 for ovarian caner screening is recommended by age 30 to 35 years. Women who have completed childbearing could opt for prophylactic hysterectomy and bilateral salpingo-oophorectomy to reduce their risks for developing endometrial and ovarian cancers.

Answer 20.5.5. **The answer is A.**

Congenital hypertrophy of the retinal pigment epithelium (CHRPE) is one of the more common extracolonic manifestations associated with FAP. Other extracolonic manifestations include jaw cysts and osteomas. Other associated malignancies include hepatoblastoma, duodenal cancer, and brain tumors. CHRPE lesions are flat or slightly raised, oval, or round pigmented areas in the retinal pigment epithelium, which may be multifocal and bilateral when associated with intestinal polyposis.

Answer 20.5.6. **The answer is D.**

The standard adjuvant therapy for patients with stage III colon cancer is oxaliplatin with 5FU based on the MOSAIC and the NSABP-C07 studies. Recent updates of the MOSAIC study demonstrated a significant improvement in 6-year overall survival among patients with stage III colorectal cancer treated with FOLFOX compared with those treated with infusional 5FU/LV. Irinotecan-based regimens are not recommended for adjuvant therapy for patients with stage III according to the negative results of three large randomized studies. Current studies adding bevacizumab and cetuximab to oxaliplatin regimens are ongoing.

Answer 20.5.7. **The answer is C.**

More than 80% of the administered dose of 5FU is eliminated via the dihydropyrimidine dehydrogenase (DPD) enzyme. Patients with DPD deficiency are at high risk for 5FU toxicities, such as severe neutropenia, neutropenic fever, diarrhea, mucositis, cerebellar ataxia, neurotoxicity, and even death. The most common mutation associated with DPD deficiency is the IVS14 + 1 G > A, DPYD*2A mutation. Complete DPD deficiency has been reported in patients homozygous for this allele, whereas partial DPD deficiency occurs in patients heterozygous for this allele. More than 40 other mutations and polymorphism have been identified in the DPD gene, although the functional significance of these polymorphisms is not clear. Moreover, instances of low DPD activity have been reported in patients without any identified DPD mutation or polymorphism. The TSER *3/*3 genotype is associated with higher levels of thymidine synthase and lower tumor response to 5FU therapy. Although it is possible that this patient is homozygous for the UGT1A1*28 gene resulting in severe neutropenia and diarrhea, the constellation of the patient's symptoms, including cerebellar ataxia and mucositis, is more consistent with 5FU-related toxicities. Furthermore, irinotecan therapy would not have been given to this patient with stage III colon cancer.

Answer 20.5.8. **The answer is E.**

SN-38 is the active metabolite of irinotecan and is 100- to 1000-fold more potent than irinotecan as a topoisomerase I inhibitor. Glucuronidation is the principal elimination pathway for SN-38. UDP-glucuronosyltransferase 1 family polypeptide A1 mediates this glucuronidation of irinotecan encoded by the UGT1A1 gene. Patients who are homozygous for the UGT1A1*28 allele glucuronidate SN-38 less efficiently than patients who have one or two wild-type alleles; therefore, homozygous patients are exposed to higher plasma concentrations of SN-38 and are thus at a greater risk for severe neutropenia.

Answer 20.5.9. **The answer is D.**

The results of the German Rectal Cancer Study published by Sauer et al. confirmed the benefit of neoadjuvant prolonged course RT with 5FU-based chemotherapy for patients with T3 + / N0-2 rectal cancer. Although overall survival was similar for patients treated with neoadjuvant chemoradiotherapy compared with those treated with postoperative chemoradiotherapy, local recurrence rates and toxicities are more favorable with neoadjuvant chemoradiotherapy.

Answer 20.5.10. **The answer is A.**

Transanal excision should only be considered for select patients with early-stage rectal cancer with the following characteristics: small rectal cancers less than 3 cm; well to moderately differentiated T1 tumors within 8 cm from the anal verge and limited to less than 30% of the rectal circumference with no evidence of nodal metastases. Only patient A meets all of these criteria.

Answer 20.5.11. **The answer is A.**

After transanal resection of appropriately selected patients with early-stage rectal cancer, no further therapy is recommended.

Answer 20.5.12. **The answer is A.**

MYH-associated polyposis is an autosomal recessive disease affecting the MYH gene, a base excision repair gene. A deficiency in MYH leads to somatic, not germline, mutations in the APC gene. Thus, clinical features of patients with MYH-associated polyposis are similar to FAP.

Answer 20.5.13. **The answer is D.**

The standard therapy for early localized squamous carcinoma of the anus is chemoradiation with 5FU and mitomycin. This is associated with excellent cure rates. Salvage APR is reserved for recurrent anal cancer.

Answer 20.5.14. **The answer is C.**

This patient is potentially curable with an aggressive multidisciplinary approach. Resection of all tumor sites with close surveillance certainly is an option for this patient. However, the results of the recently published study, EORTC 40983, showed an improvement in progression-free survival for patients treated with perioperative chemotherapy with resection. Historically, cure rates of up to 35% have been observed even in patients with metastatic disease, as long as all tumor sites are resected. Thus, palliative chemotherapy would not be the best option for this patient. There is currently no role for radiotherapy for this patient.

Genitourinary Cancer

Directions   Each of the numbered items below is followed by lettered answers. Select the ONE lettered answer that is BEST in each case unless instructed otherwise.

QUESTIONS

Questions 21.1.–21.3.

A 56-year-old moderately obese woman with a medical history of chronic hypertension well controlled on a thiazide diuretic presents to the emergency department with a 1-day history of abdominal pain, diarrhea, nausea, and fever. General physical examination is significant only for some mild abdominal tenderness; negative stool guaiac; a white blood cell (WBC) count of 14.2/µL; hemoglobin of 14.5 g/dL; a normal platelet count; normal electrolytes, amylase, lipase, and transaminases; and a creatinine of 0.9 mg/dL. Workup includes an abdominal computed tomography (CT) scan, which is remarkable for a 1.5-cm enhancing left renal mass in the left lower pole that is interpreted by the radiologist as a "probable renal cell carcinoma" without evidence of other metastases. The patient's abdominal symptoms resolve without sequelae.

Question 21.1.   **All the following are reasonable, EXCEPT:**

A. Magnetic resonance imaging (MRI) with magnetic resonance (MR) angiography
B. Needle core biopsy
C. Open partial nephrectomy
D. Laparoscopic partial nephrectomy

Corresponding Chapter in *Cancer: Principles & Practice of Oncology*, Eighth Edition: 40 (Cancers of the Genitourinary System).

Question 21.2.   **The patient undergoes a laparoscopic partial nephrectomy. There are no postoperative complications, and she is back to work 3 weeks later. Postoperative creatinine is 1.3, and pathology reveals a 2.5-cm renal cell carcinoma, granular cell type, that is confined to the renal parenchyma. No lymph nodes were recovered. The next appropriate step is:**

    A. Open retroperitoneal lymph node dissection
    B. Adjuvant sunitinib
    C. Adjuvant local radiotherapy
    D. Submission of pathology specimen for second review

Question 21.3.   **Review of the pathologic specimen by an experienced genitourinary pathologist reveals clear cell carcinoma of the kidney, Fuhrman grade IV. The patient does well for 10 years, at which time she develops a pathologic intratrochanteric fracture of her left hip. CT scanning of the chest, abdomen, pelvis, and brain and bone scan reveal no other sites of disease. The MOST appropriate next step is:**

    A. Radiation alone
    B. High-dose interleukin (IL)-2 alone
    C. Orthopedic resection of the tumor with reconstruction followed by radiation
    D. Temsirolimus

Questions 21.4.–21.5.   **A 76-year-old man with chronic obstructive pulmonary disorder (COPD) and diabetes mellitus (DM) presents with back pain and confusion. Workup reveals extensive metastatic disease in the lungs, bones, and liver and a 6-cm tumor in the kidney. There is no evidence of cord compression. Laboratory studies reveal a calcium of 11.5 mg/dL and a creatinine of 2.0 mg/dL. After hydration and zoledronate, his calcium normalizes, hemoglobin is 9.5, creatinine decreases to 1.7, and Eastern Cooperative Oncology Group (ECOG) performance status is 2.**

Question 21.4.   **The poor-risk features present in this patient include all, EXCEPT:**

    A. His age of >75 years
    B. Hypercalcemia
    C. Performance status of 2
    D. Anemia

Question 21.5.   **The LEAST appropriate therapy in this case is:**

    A. Interferon-α
    B. Temsirolimus
    C. Sunitinib
    D. Sorafenib

Question 21.6. **A 25-year-old Caucasian man without a medical history presents with hematuria. Workup reveals bilateral renal cysts, at least one of them suspicious for malignancy. Family history is significant for a pheochromocytoma in his father and a pancreatic islet cell tumor and early death from kidney cancer in a paternal aunt. The MOST likely familial cancer syndrome is:**

A. Von Hippel-Lindau disease
B. Birt-Hogg-Dube syndrome
C. Hereditary papillary renal cancer
D. Hereditary leiomyomatosis and renal cancer

Question 21.7. **Which of the following statements about the VHL gene is INCORRECT?**

A. It is mutated or altered in greater than 60% of spontaneous clear cell carcinomas of the kidney.
B. It is critical for the normal oxygen sensing and response system in all cells.
C. It is part of a ubiquitin ligase complex.
D. Expression is regulated by vascular endothelial growth factor (VEGF).

Questions
21.8.–21.13. **A 63-year-old white male smoker presents to his physician with a 2-month history of urinary frequency, urgency, and dysuria without hesitancy or decreased stream. He denies hematuria, fever, chills, or abdominal pain. He has normal erections and is sexually active. His medical history is significant for hypertension, well-controlled on a beta-blocker and diuretic, hypercholesterolemia controlled on a 3-hydroxy-3-methylglutaryl coenzyme A (HMG-coA) reductase inhibitor, and diet-controlled type 2 diabetes. General physical examination is significant for scattered expiratory wheezes; cardiac and abdominal examination are normal. Rectal examination reveals a mildly enlarged prostate that is nontender.**

Question 21.8. **The appropriate initial workup should include which of the following?**

A. Urinalysis
B. Urine culture
C. Cystoscopy
D. All of the above

Question 21.9.   Urine dipstick reveals no protein or ketones, but there is 1+ blood. Microscopic analysis reveals 10 to 15 red blood cells (RBCs), 2 to 3 white blood cells (WBCs), 0 to 1 squamous epithelial cells, and no bacterial cells per high power field. Urine culture is negative. Prostate-specific antigen (PSA) is 2.5 ng/mL, complete blood count (CBC) is unremarkable, and general chemistries reveal normal electrolytes, normal liver function test results, and a creatinine of 1.2 mg/dL. Flexible cystoscopy in the urology office reveals a papillary tumor in the dome of the bladder that is approximately 3 cm, as well as diffuse erythema of the remainder of the bladder wall. In addition to scheduling a cystoscopic biopsy, the urologist should also schedule:

A.   Intravenous pyelogram (IVP)
B.   Contrast-enhanced CT scan of the abdomen and pelvis
C.   Abdominal ultrasound
D.   Fluorodeoxyglucose positron emission tomography (FDG-PET)

Question 21.10.   The patient is subsequently taken to the operating room, where an examination under general anesthesia reveals a mobile bladder. Resection of the papillary lesion reveals grade III urothelial papillary carcinoma, and multiple biopsies of the erythematous areas of the bladder all reveal diffuse carcinoma in situ. Muscle is present in the pathologic specimens, and there is no evidence for invasive tumor. The appropriate therapy is:

A.   Intravesical Bacillus Calmette–Guérin (BCG) vaccine
B.   Intravesical cyclophosphamide
C.   Radiation
D.   Cystectomy

Question 21.11.   The patient is treated with intravesical BCG weekly for 6 weeks, as well as with a follow-up maintenance program; however, 4 months after initiating the maintenance BCG program, the urologist notes multiple recurrent papillary lesions. Repeat biopsy reveals urothelial cancer invasive into muscle. CT scans of the chest, abdomen, and pelvis are unremarkable, creatinine remains normal at 1.2 mg/dL, and his performance status is excellent. Appropriate therapy at this point is:

A.   Reinduction with intravesical BCG
B.   Intravesical chemotherapy with mitomycin-C
C.   Partial cystectomy
D.   Cisplatin-based multiagent chemotherapy

Question 21.12. After consultation with an oncologist regarding the risks and benefits of neoadjuvant chemotherapy, the patient elects to proceed with a cystectomy and orthotopic neobladder. Pathologic specimen reveals a diffuse carcinoma in situ with an invasive tumor at the dome. The tumor invades into but not through the muscular layer, and evaluation of 15 lymph nodes shows no metastatic cancer. After additional discussion with the oncologist, the patient decides not to have adjuvant chemotherapy and opts only for routine follow-up. By 6 months, he feels well other than mild stress incontinence and impotence, but routine serum chemistries reveal a creatinine of 4.1 mg/dL. The MOST likely diagnosis is:

A. Acute glomerulonephritis
B. Calcium oxalate stone nephropathy
C. Obstructive nephropathy
D. Renal tubular acidosis

Question 21.13. The patient is found to have obstruction at the urethral anastomosis. This is surgically corrected, but the creatinine remains abnormal at 2.5 mg/dL. Six months later, a routine follow-up noncontrast-enhanced CT scan reveals two 3-cm lung nodules. Biopsy of one is consistent with metastatic urothelial cancer. Appropriate therapy at this time includes:

A. Surgical resection of all visible metastatic disease
B. Palliative care
C. Cisplatin-based multiagent chemotherapy
D. Interferon-based immunotherapy

Questions 21.14.–21.16. A 62-year-old woman is newly diagnosed with muscle-invasive bladder cancer. She quit smoking 10 years ago, had a non–ST-elevated myocardial infarction 4 years ago, underwent coronary artery bypass surgery and has had no residual cardiac symptoms, takes only a beta-blocker and a thiazide for hypertension, and has normal laboratory test results, including a creatinine of 0.9. Cystoscopic biopsy revealed a muscle invasive bladder cancer without associated carcinoma in situ (Tcis), and CT of the chest, abdomen, and pelvis is unremarkable.

Question 21.14. Which of the following statements about radical cystectomy is MOST correct?

A. An orthotopic neobladder is less effective in women than in men.
B. An abdominal wall diversion will require a urostomy bag.
C. An orthotopic neobladder will require the patient to be willing and able to perform self-catheterization.
D. Metabolic acidosis is not a significant problem with continent diversions.

Question 21.15.   **Which of the following statements about combined radiation and chemo-therapy is MOST correct?**

A.   Toxicity profile and tolerability of combined radiation and chemo-therapy are significantly better than that of radical cystectomy.
B.   Long-term cancer outcome is similar to cystectomy.
C.   It is preferred over cystectomy because of her cardiac history.
D.   It will obviate the need for cystectomy.

Question 21.16.   **Which of the following is CORRECT about neoadjuvant chemotherapy?**

A.   Three cycles of methotrexate, vinblastine, doxorubicin, and cisplatin (MVAC) before cystectomy is a standard of care.
B.   Gemcitabine/carboplatin should be considered to decrease the risk of renal failure with cystectomy.
C.   It increases the risk of surgical complications of cystectomy.
D.   It should always be used with an organ preservation approach but is optional if cystectomy is chosen.

Question 21.17.   **Which of the following statements about the molecular pathogenesis of urothelial cancer of the bladder is INCORRECT?**

A.   Chromosome 9 deletions are common and occur on both the short and long arms.
B.   p53 mutations are associated with carcinoma in situ and aggressive disease.
C.   pRb alterations are observed and correlate with poor prognosis.
D.   Activating FGFR3 mutations are most common in metastatic lesions.

Question 21.18.   **A 71-year-old man without significant medical history presents with hema-turia and flank pain. CT scan reveals a mass at the pelvic-ureteral junction with associated hydronephrosis, but no associated lymphadenopathy. Cystoscopy and ureteroscopy reveal an obstructing mass at the pelvic-ureteral junction, and cytology is diagnostic for a urothelial cancer. Which of the following is the MOST appropriate therapy?**

A.   Open nephroureterectomy and bladder cuff resection
B.   Open radical nephrectomy with retroperitoneal lymph node dissec-tion
C.   Laparoscopic radical nephrectomy without retroperitoneal lymph node dissection
D.   Definitive radiation and combined chemotherapy

Question 21.19. **A 51-year-old man with a strong family history of prostate cancer, a normal digital rectal examination, no significant comorbid medical problems, and a PSA of 2.9 seeks advice on prostate cancer prevention. He is sexually active in a monogamous relationship and denies any urinary or rectal symptoms. The following are all true, EXCEPT:**

A. Finasteride has been shown to decrease his risk of developing prostate cancer.

B. Taking supplemental vitamin E has been shown to decrease his risk of developing prostate cancer.

C. Taking finasteride will decrease the PSA.

D. 8q24 polymorphisms have been identified as risk alleles in patients such as this.

Questions 21.20.–21.24. **A 71-year-old white man with a history of hypertension, hyperlipidemia, coronary artery disease, and prior angioplasty with stent placement, but no prior myocardial infarction, is noted to have a increase in his PSA from 3.0 to 3.9 ng/mL and then to 4.6 ng/mL over 19 months. He is a semiretired accountant, swims actively three times per week, and helps care for his mildly demented 95-year-old father. General physical examination is unremarkable; a rectal examination reveals a mildly enlarged prostate gland without any palpable nodules.**

Question 21.20. **The MOST correct statement about this case is:**

A. Biopsy should be discussed because the PSA increase is greater than 0.75 ng/mL/y.

B. Biopsy should not be discussed because PSA is normal for his age.

C. Biopsy should not be discussed because his expected survival makes treatment not worthwhile, even if prostate cancer is discovered.

D. Biopsy should be discussed because the PSA is greater than 4 ng/mL.

E. The free-to-total PSA ratio will determine the need for biopsy.

Question 21.21. **Biopsy reveals Gleason 8 prostate cancer in six of six cores. CT scan of the abdomen and pelvis and bone scan are unremarkable. The MOST appropriate therapy is:**

A. Radical retropubic prostatectomy

B. Three-dimensional conformal radiotherapy with concomitant androgen ablation

C. Interstitial radiotherapy with 125I

D. All of the above

Question 21.22.   After discussion with a radiation oncologist and a urologist, the patient elects to undergo combined androgen ablation and external beam radiation therapy. The androgen ablation is administered before the radiation therapy and continued for 3 months thereafter. Radiotherapy is complicated only by a mild diarrhea that resolves once the radiation therapy is complete. The PSA nadirs at 1.2 ng/mL; however, 9 months after his last dose of the luteinizing hormone-releasing hormone (LH-RH) agonist, the PSA increases to 2.4 ng/mL and then to 3.6 ng/mL 1 month later. Testosterone level is normal at 350 ng/ml. The MOST appropriate next therapeutic and/or diagnostic maneuver is:

A. Perform MRI of the pelvis to assess for local recurrence.
B. Reinitiate androgen ablation.
C. Refer the patient to a urologist for salvage prostatectomy.
D. Initiate docetaxel-based chemotherapy.

Question 21.23.   The patient elects to undergo androgen ablation with an LH-RH agonist along with the antiandrogen bicalutamide. PSA declines to 0.8 ng/mL, but after 10 months, the PSA begins to slowly increase to a value of 3.7. He continues to feel well and has minimal urinary symptoms, no bone pain, and no weight loss. The MOST appropriate therapy at this point is:

A. Docetaxel-based chemotherapy
B. Discontinuing the antiandrogen bicalutamide
C. Hospice care
D. Radionuclide therapy with strontium-98 (Metastron)

Question 21.24.   The patient does not have a PSA response to antiandrogen withdrawal and in fact develops bone pain and documented bone metastases on bone scan. Appetite, weight, functional status, and organ function as assessed by routine chemistries remain normal. In addition to initiating docetaxel-based chemotherapy, other therapeutic maneuvers to be considered include:

A. Megestrol acetate
B. Estrogen therapy
C. Mitoxantrone chemotherapy
D. Bisphosphonates

Questions 21.25.–21.27.   A 51-year-old black male executive with no medical history undergoes a routine PSA screening evaluation and is found to have a PSA of 5.5 ng/mL. Biopsy reveals a Gleason 3 + 3 prostate cancer in two of six biopsy cores. After discussion with a radiation oncologist and urologist, he elects to receive treatment with a radical retropubic prostatectomy.

Question 21.25.   **Which of the following statements about the surgery is TRUE?**

A. Robotic laparoscopic prostatectomy is associated with a lower incidence of impotence than open retropubic prostatectomy.
B. The incidence of impotence under the assumption that a bilateral nerve sparing procedure can be performed is less than 10%.
C. Problems with incontinence persist in approximately 20% of patients.
D. Surgical experience has only a minimal impact on the positive margin rate.

Question 21.26.   **Surgical pathology confirms a Gleason score 6 tumor in both lobes of the prostate. There is a focal surgical positive margin. There is no evidence of seminal vesicle or lymph node invasion. His postoperative PSA is undetectable, and he has good continence. The MOST appropriate next step is:**

A. Adjuvant radiotherapy
B. Repeat surgical exploration with possible reexcision of the prostatic bed
C. Pelvic CT scan
C. Prostascint scan

Question 21.27.   **The patient maintains an undetectable PSA until 8 years later (at the age of 59 years), recurrent biochemical disease is noted. After appropriate discussion, androgen ablation with an LH-RH agonist alone is initiated, and the PSA once again becomes undetectable. The patient maintains an undetectable PSA while on androgen ablation for 3 years, when he develops sudden mid-back pain after lifting his grandson. There are no associated neurologic signs or symptoms. Bone scan shows marked uptake at the T8 vertebra, and PSA remains undetectable. The MOST appropriate therapeutic or diagnostic maneuver is:**

A. Immediate radiotherapy to T8
B. Therapy with ketoconazole, 400 mg three times daily with hydrocortisone replacement
C. Spinal MRI to rule out cord compression
D. Bone densitometry to assess for osteoporosis

Question 21.28.   **A 75-year-old man with diabetes, hypertension, and coronary artery disease who is receiving atorvastatin, glyburide, and an angiotensin-converting enzyme inhibitor is under surveillance after external beam radiotherapy for a Gleason 3 + 3 prostate cancer that was diagnosed and treated 10 years earlier when he was found to have a PSA of 4.3 on routine screening. His PSA level, which had been 0.2 ng/mL, has increased to 0.3, 0.35, and then 0.40 over the period of 18 months. The MOST appropriate therapy at this time is:**

A. Androgen ablation with an LHRH agonist
B. Continued active surveillance
C. High-intensity focused ultrasound to his prostate
D. High-dose (150 mg) bicalutamide

Question 21.29.   **A 65-year-old man has been receiving combined androgen ablation with leuprolide and bicalutamide for 4 years for biochemical recurrence after radical prostatectomy. His PSA has increased from an undetectable nadir to 1.1 ng/mL on serial measurement over the period of 6 months. The PSA continues to increase 2 months after discontinuation of bicalutamide to 1.5, with serum testosterone of 10 ng/mL. Bone scan and CT of the abdomen/pelvis do not reveal any metastatic disease, and he remains asymptomatic. Treatment options include all the following, EXCEPT:**

A.   Active surveillance
B.   Docetaxel-based chemotherapy
C.   Thalidomide
D.   High-dose ketoconazole

Question 21.30.   **All the following statements about prostate cancer epidemiology are correct, EXCEPT:**

A.   There is a marked difference in mortality from prostate cancer in different parts of the world.
B.   The difference in mortality between African Americans and Caucasian Americans can be completely explained by socioeconomic factors.
C.   Epidemiologic studies suggest a dietary or lifestyle component to prostate cancer development.
D.   There is molecular confirmation for genetic risk factors for prostate cancer.

Question 21.31.   **The following statements about prostate cancer biology are all correct, EXCEPT:**

A.   GSTπ loss is common in prostate intraepithelial neoplasia (PIN).
B.   TMPRSS2 translocations juxtapose an androgen responsive gene promoter with a transcription factor.
C.   PTEN loss is as common in PIN as in more advanced cancer.
D.   NKX3.1 has been postulated to be a gatekeeper tumor suppressor.

Question 21.32.   **Which of the following statements about the androgen receptor is MOST correct?**

A.   The majority of its activity in prostate cancer is due to its cytoplasmic effects.
B.   Upregulation of androgen receptor expression has been linked to prostate cancer development.
C.   Castration leads to complete inactivation of all androgen receptor-mediated pathways.
D.   Castrate-resistant prostate cancer is associated with upregulation of androgen receptor expression.

Question 21.33. **A 63-year-old uncircumcised man without any significant medical history presents to his physician with an inability to retract the foreskin. Examination reveals phimosis, with an underlying painless ulcerated mass of 1 × 2 cm. A 2.5-cm hard node is palpated in the left inguinal region. Biopsy of the penile lesion reveals squamous cell cancer. In addition to wide surgical resection of the primary lesion, other appropriate therapeutic and/or diagnostic maneuvers at this time include:**

A. Four-week course of a broad-spectrum antibiotic
B. Left inguinal lymph node dissection
C. Bilateral inguinal radiotherapy
D. Taxane-based chemotherapy

ANSWERS

Answer 21.1. **The answer is A.**

Although flank pain, hematuria, and a palpable abdominal mass have traditionally been considered the presenting symptoms for renal cancer, one of the most common manners in which this disease is currently diagnosed is during a CT scan performed for an unrelated reason. Contrast-enhanced CT scan has a high specificity for renal cancer, but the natural history of small incidental renal lesions is unknown and can be variable. Core needle biopsy can be performed safely, can provide definitive diagnostic information, and may provide information of possible prognostic importance, such as tumor histologic subtype and grade. Immediate partial nephrectomy, either by an open approach or depending on surgeon experience via a laparoscopic approach, is also reasonable. In this case, a partial nephrectomy would be preferred over a total nephrectomy to preserve renal function. MRI and MR angiography are useful for determining the extent of renal vein and inferior vena cava invasion, but this would be extremely unlikely with such a small tumor.

Answer 21.2. **The answer is D.**

Renal cell cancer is currently divided into clear cell and non-clear cell subtypes. The non-clear cell subtypes have been further divided into papillary, chromophobe, and collecting duct tumors. Several renal cancers cannot be accurately subtyped, often because of poor histologic differentiation such that the originating subtype cannot be easily recognized. Such tumors are often classified as "sarcomatoid." Granular cell carcinoma has been used in the past but is not currently an accepted pathologic classification. Thus, a second opinion and pathologic review should be requested. The risk of recurrence in this case is low, and adjuvant sunitinib has not been shown to decrease the risk of recurrence. Patients who do have recurrence after nephrectomy almost always recur systemically, and thus additional local radiotherapy is not indicated. Likewise, the role of extensive lymph node dissection is highly controversial and generally not recommended. In any case, formal retroperitoneal lymph node dissection as is carried out in testes cancer would certainly not be standard in patients with localized renal cell carcinoma.

Answer 21.3.   **The answer is C.**

Patients with renal cancer can develop recurrent disease more than 5 years after initial definitive therapy. Development of a single metastatic site is not unusual. Patients with a single site of metastatic disease and a long interval between initial diagnosis and recurrent metastatic disease typically have a good prognosis. Thus, aggressive surgical resection including orthopedic stabilization is indicated. Because orthopedic surgery such as this often leaves microscopic tumors behind in the surgical field, additional radiotherapy to the site is appropriate. Radiation alone is insufficient to completely eradicate metastatic renal cancer and does not repair the underlying structural bony abnormality. High-dose IL-2 is approved for metastatic renal cancer but is less effective than aggressive local surgery for complete eradication of disease when possible. Temsirolimus improves survival in patients with poor prognosis metastatic disease, which does not apply here. In addition, it is not curative.

Answer 21.4.   **The answer is A.**

Several prognostic factors have been identified that can help explain the highly heterogeneous natural history of metastatic renal cancer. Hypercalcemia, poor performance status, and anemia are significant prognostic factors in most studies. Age, in and of itself, is not a prognostic factor.

Answer 21.5.   **The answer is A.**

Of the choices, phase III data supportive of a survival benefit in a patient with poor prognosis such as this are available only for temsirolimus. The available data suggest that sunitinib or sorafenib could be considered. However, data suggest that interferon is not effective in patients with poor prognosis, and phase III data show that sunitinib is more effective than interferon for metastatic disease in patients with a good and intermediate prognosis.

Answer 21.6.   **The answer is A.**

Von Hippel-Lindau disease, caused by mutation of the VHL gene, is an autosomal-dominant cancer syndrome characterized by multiple renal cysts, early onset and multiple renal tumors, retinal angiomas and central nervous system hemangioblastomas, pheochromocytomas, and pancreatic islet cell tumors. The Birt-Hogg-Dube syndrome, caused by mutations of the BHD gene, is characterized by early onset chromophobe cancers, benign hair follicle tumors (fibrofolliculomas), and pulmonary cysts. Hereditary papillary renal cancer, caused by mutations of the MET gene, is characterized by multiple Type I papillary cancers. The hereditary leiomyomatosis and renal cancer syndrome, caused by mutation of the fumarate hydratase (FH) gene, is characterized by cutaneous and uterine leiomyomas and aggressive Type II papillary cancers.

Answer 21.7.   **The answer is D.**

VHL is part of the normal oxygen sensing and response system in all cells and is mutated or altered in greater than 60% of sporadic clear cell carcinomas of the kidney. Under normoxic conditions, VHL is part of a multiprotein complex that recognizes the hydroxylated HIF transcription factor, acts as a ubiquitin ligase, and thus targets it for proteasomal degradation. Under hypoxic conditions, HIF is not hydroxylated, not targeted to VHL and thus not degraded leading to upregulation of multiple genes critical for the hypoxic response including VEGF. The VHL gene is expressed constitutively.

Answer 21.8. **The answer is D.**

The differential diagnosis for dysuria, frequency, and urgency include cystitis, prostatitis, and obstructive uropathy, which is most commonly caused by benign prostatic hyperplasia in men. Notably, significant dysuria without hesitancy or decreased stream is unusual with obstruction caused by benign prostatic hyperplasia, and it is unusual to have a 2-month history of infectious cystitis without additional sequelae. It is also notable that prostate cancer, although occasionally presenting with local urinary obstructive symptoms, rarely presents with this constellation of findings unless there is obvious extensive local disease on rectal examination. This is because prostate cancer typically arises in the peripheral zone of the prostate, and thus obstructive symptoms are uncommon unless the tumor is more locally advanced. The appropriate workup thus includes urinalysis and urine culture to assess for infection and a flexible cystoscopy.

Answer 21.9. **The answer is B.**

The large tumor and erythema suggest that there might be associated muscle invasion and/or carcinoma in situ (Tcis). CT scanning is insensitive for local tumor staging but may detect lymphadenopathy or upper tract causes for hematuria with greater sensitivity than IVP or ultrasound. FDG-PET is less useful because of excretion of FDG in the urinary system, obscuring visualization of local lymph nodes.

Answer 21.10. **The answer is A.**

Indications for intravesical therapy are multiple recurrent Ta lesions, especially if they are high grade, or Tcis. It is critical that the pathologic specimen in patients diagnosed with superficial bladder cancer contains muscle to determine whether there is an invasive component. Most, but not all, studies have suggested that intravesical BCG is more effective than intravesical chemotherapy. Although other chemotherapeutic agents are being investigated, cyclophosphamide needs to be activated to 4-hydroxy-cyclosphosphamide in the liver to act as an alkylating agent, and thus bladder instillation of the parent compound is not expected to be effective. Radiation or cystectomy, although potentially useful for invasive carcinoma or refractory bladder cancer, is not appropriate as initial therapy in this patient.

Answer 21.11. **The answer is D.**

Patients with muscle-invasive bladder cancer require definitive local therapy. Additional intravesical therapy is inappropriate. Partial cystectomies are only rarely indicated and should be performed in only a very highly select group, which does not include patients with a history of Tcis or patients with multiple tumors. The standard definitive therapy for bladder cancer is cystectomy. Multiagent cisplatin-based neoadjuvant chemotherapy improves survival for patients with invasive urothelial bladder cancer and is considered a standard of care.

Answer 21.12.   **The answer is C.**

Complications of orthotopic neobladders include metabolic acidosis, renal calculi, and obstructive nephropathy. Of these, only obstruction commonly causes renal failure. Acute glomerulonephritis is not a recognized complication in the absence of other underlying medical history. Obstructive nephropathy can occur at the level of ureteral implantation or at the urethral sphincter anastomosis.

Answer 21.13.   **The answer is B.**

Metastatic urothelial cancer, even when only a limited number of metastatic deposits are visible on radiologic scanning, is almost always widely disseminated, and surgical resection alone has little role. Cisplatin-based multiagent chemotherapy is appropriate in patients with good performance status and normal organ function. MVAC has been shown to improve survival over other multiagent and single-agent chemotherapies, and gemcitabine/cisplatin has been shown to have outcomes similar to those of MVAC. However, less than 5% of patients have long-term survival with multiagent chemotherapy, and cisplatin is inappropriate for patients with abnormal renal function. Taxanes and carboplatin, which can be administered in patients with renal failure, do have anticancer activity in this disease and have the potential for being palliative. It is, however, unclear whether they provide any long-term benefit in patients such as this. Intravesical immunotherapy, although effective in superficial bladder cancer, is not effective in patients with systemic disease. Palliative care is thus the most appropriate option.

Answer 21.14.   **The answer is C.**

There are several options for urinary diversion after cystectomy, and no clear evidence has emerged that any is more or less desirable or effective based on patient gender. Diversion to the abdominal wall with a urostomy can be performed as a conduit, requiring a urine collection device, or as a continent diversion, requiring regular catheterization. Metabolic complications, including metabolic acidosis, can occur with both conduits and continent diversions. Complications of orthotopic continent diversions, or neobladders, include intermittent urethral obstruction and frequent requirement for intermittent or temporary self-catheterization.

Answer 21.15.   **The answer is B.**

Organ preservation with combined radiation and chemotherapy has been investigated in numerous trials, and long-term outcomes are similar to those observed in cystectomy series. The therapy is, however, an aggressive and potentially toxic approach in which approximately 30% of patients will require cystectomy for incomplete response. It is thus not more tolerable than cystectomy. The patient's cardiac history does not preclude major surgery, and in fact willingness to accept a cystectomy has been an inclusion criterion for most organ preservation trials.

Answer 21.16. **The answer is A.**

Randomized studies have demonstrated that cisplatin-based combination chemotherapy provides a survival advantage. The largest phase III studies used MVAC or a similar regimen in which the doxorubicin was eliminated (MVC). The strongest data supporting neoadjuvant chemotherapy are in the surgical setting, with no survival advantage demonstrated in modest-sized trials using combined chemotherapy and radiation for primary tumor treatment. The randomized data further demonstrate that there is no increase in surgical morbidity or complications after neoadjuvant chemotherapy. There are no data on the neoadjuvant use of carboplatin-based regimens, and data in the metastatic setting strongly suggest that carboplatin is an inferior agent in comparison with cisplatin for this disease.

Answer 21.17. **The answer is D.**

Chromosome 9 deletions are the most common alteration in urothelial carcinoma of the bladder, appear to be critical for the initiation of bladder cancer, and occur on both the long and short arms. Alterations of both p53 and pRb are most common in invasive disease and are markers of poor prognosis. Activating mutations of FGFR3 are common in papillary noninvasive cancers but are actually unusual in more invasive lesions.

Answer 21.18. **The answer is A.**

The standard definitive treatment for renal pelvis urothelial cancers is radical nephroureterectomy with resection of the bladder cuff at the ureteral insertion site. Radical nephrectomy without ureter resection is inappropriate because of the high incidence of undiagnosed or recurrent disease in the ureter. Definitive radiotherapy would also be inappropriate, because this would be expected to lead to kidney necrosis.

Answer 21.19. **The answer is B.**

The Prostate Cancer Prevention Trial randomized patients with normal rectal examination and PSA less than 3.0 ng/dL to finasteride or placebo, and required an end-of-treatment biopsy because of the decrease in PSA observed with 5-α reductase inhibitor therapy. It demonstrated an overall decrease in the incidence of prostate cancer but an increase in the number of high-risk prostate cancers. Single nucleotide polymorphisms (SNPs) on 8q24 have been identified as risk alleles for prostate cancer in multiple independent studies. Although dietary studies have suggested that vitamin E correlates with a decreased incidence of prostate cancer, early data from the phase III intervention study (SELECT) of selenium and vitamin E to prevent prostate cancer suggests that these supplements by themselves or in combination are not effective in preventing prostate cancer (JAMA 2009;301[1]:39–51).

Answer 21.20.   **The answer is A.**

The decision to screen for and diagnose prostate cancer always needs to be accompanied by a discussion between the physician and the patient regarding risks and benefits of screening. To this end, it should be recognized that the median survival of an average 70-year-old man without significant comorbidities is more than 10 years, and that such a patient could benefit from the treatment of localized disease. Nonetheless, there is a risk of treating disease that will never become clinically significant within the patient's lifetime. It also needs to be recalled that the sensitivity and specificity of all PSA-based screening methods are limited, and there are no absolute "normal" criteria. Therefore, no single test can determine the absolute need for a biopsy. Predictors of cancer on biopsy include PSA greater than 4.0 ng/mL, PSA greater than age-adjusted PSA norms (based on normal increasing PSA with age), free-to-total PSA ratio, and PSA velocity. Of these, and in this case, the rapid increase in the PSA is most predictive of malignancy, and this is also predictive of aggressive disease.

Answer 21.21.   **The answer is D.**

On the basis of the high Gleason score, the aforementioned rapid PSA doubling time, and the tumor in all cores, this patient is at a high risk for locally advanced disease and systemic recurrence. As such, staging CT scan and bone scan are reasonable, although not generally necessary in patients with lower-risk disease. Because of the presence of high-risk features and the general good health of the patient, watchful waiting is probably not an appropriate option in this case. Radiotherapy, with external beam radiotherapy or interstitial brachytherapy, or surgical prostatectomy are equally appropriate for patients with clinically localized disease. The choice is dependent on a discussion of expected risks and benefits.

Answer 21.22.   **The answer is B.**

Rapidly increasing PSA before diagnosis, high Gleason score, PSA nadir of greater than 1.0 after radiotherapy, short interval between definitive local therapy and biochemical recurrence, and rapid PSA increase once recurrence is identified are all associated with a poor prognosis. The probability of locally recurrent disease alone is extremely low, and there is not much value to pelvic MRI for assessing local recurrence. Despite the poor prognosis, the role of chemotherapy in patients whose testosterone axis is intact is controversial. Although timing of androgen ablation is not clearly defined, some retrospective data suggest that "early" ablation in high-risk patients such as this provides a long-term survival advantage over "later" ablation.

Answer 21.23.   **The answer is B.**

Approximately 10% to 15% of patients receiving treatment with an anti-androgen will experience an antiandrogen withdrawal response. Although the majority of these responses are of brief duration, it is obviously the easiest therapeutic maneuver. Docetaxel-based chemotherapy leads to improved survival in castrate-resistant prostate cancer, which is generally defined as a progressive disease after androgen ablation, an antiandrogen, and antiandrogen withdrawal. Radioactive nuclides are occasionally useful for the palliation of diffuse bone pain but have not been shown to have an impact on survival.

Answer 21.24.   **The answer is D.**

Docetaxel-based chemotherapy is appropriate, because it has been shown to improve survival of patients with hormone-refractory prostate cancer over that observed with mitoxantrone. Megestrol acetate has not been shown to have any impact in castrate-resistant prostate cancer. Randomized phase III data also suggest that the use of bisphosphonates in hormone-refractory prostate metastatic cancer decreases the incidence of bone complications and fractures, and the need for radiotherapy.

Answer 21.25.   **The answer is C.**

Although robotic laparoscopic prostatectomy has been touted as a less-invasive and potentially more effective approach, there is no reliable evidence that the risk of long-term complications, including impotence, is different than that observed in patients undergoing an open procedure with an experienced surgeon. In both groups, the incidence of impotence is at least 25%, even in young men with good erectile function before surgery. The risk of incontinence, when assessed by anonymized, validated quality of life instruments, is on the order of 20%. One of the most important variables for both pathologic outcome and complications is the surgeon's experience.

Answer 21.26.   **The answer is A.**

Adjuvant radiotherapy has been shown to decrease the risk of recurrence in patients with T3 disease. However, overall survival and clinical metastases-free survival have not been affected by this approach. Some have thus argued for close monitoring and salvage radiotherapy on biochemical recurrence in patients such as this. Imaging tests have not been shown to be helpful in identifying patients most likely to benefit from adjuvant therapy, and surgical reexploration is not indicated either.

Answer 21.27.   **The answer is D.**

Patients on long-term androgen ablation are at high risk for the development of osteoporosis and its complications, and an osteoporotic fracture must be considered in this patient before initiating any therapy for progressive metastatic disease. If progressive disease were to be diagnosed, ketoconazole is not an unreasonable second-line hormonal therapy, but the addition of an antiandrogen would likely be more appropriate. In the absence of neurologic signs or symptoms, an MRI is not necessary.

Answer 21.28.   **The answer is B.**

Patients with a slowly increasing PSA after definitive local therapy may have a very long natural history, with only a minority of patients having cancer-related mortality within 10 years. Androgen ablation, especially in elderly patients, is associated with osteoporosis, muscle loss, and changes in lipid metabolism that may have significant impact on cardio-vascular comorbidities. High-intensity focused ultrasound for treatment of possible localized recurrence is still investigational. Single-agent anti-androgen therapy is not approved and may lead to higher mortality in patients such as this.

Answer 21.29.   **The answer is C.**

This patient meets all the criteria for castrate-resistant prostate cancer, and the only therapy demonstrated to improve survival is docetaxel-based chemotherapy. Nevertheless, there remains controversy regarding the timing of such therapy in otherwise asymptomatic men. Active surveillance is thus reasonable. High-dose ketoconazole has been demonstrated to lead to PSA decreases in up to 30% of men in this situation in several studies. Although thalidomide has been investigated, it has minimal activity as a single agent and is not indicated.

Answer 21.30.   **The answer is B.**

Multiple studies confirm marked differences in prostate cancer incidence and mortality between various countries that are not explainable by any kind of ascertainment bias. Changes in incidence and mortality in populations migrating from a country with a low incidence to a country with a high incidence strongly suggest that there are significant dietary or lifestyle contributors to prostate cancer development. There is now also confirmation of a genetic risk component because genetic polymorphisms, including several on 8q24, have been found to be closely associated with prostate cancer. In fact, the large difference in prostate cancer mortality between African Americans and Caucasian Americans cannot be explained by socioeconomic factors alone.

Answer 21.31.   **The answer is C.**

NKX3.1 transcription factor inactivation can be detected in the earliest identifiable PIN lesions. In contrast, PTEN loss is far more common in advanced disease. GSTπ is also commonly seen at all disease stages, including PIN. Translocation of the androgen responsive gene promoter from TMPRSS2 to ETS family transcription factors is common in early tumors, but not in PIN.

Answer 21.32.   **The answer is D.**

Although the androgen receptor does have cytoplasmic effects, some of which may be important to prostate cancer oncogenesis, the majority of its effects occur in the nucleus where it modifies expression of genes with an androgen-responsive promoter. Upregulation of androgen receptor expression has been reported to be both necessary and sufficient for the castrate-resistant state, which is likely an adaptation to prolonged exposure to a low androgen environment. Such upregulation is not generally observed de novo and has not been linked to the development of prostate cancer. Castration dramatically lowers testosterone, but the levels of other androgenic steroids are sufficient to cause partial activation of androgen receptor-mediated pathways.

Answer 21.33. **The answer is A.**

Penile carcinoma is a rare malignancy that presents most commonly with phimosis in an uncircumcised patient. Metastatic spread of penile carcinoma is via superficial inguinal lymphatics, followed by deep inguinal lymphatics, and then to the pelvic lymphatics. Systemic metastatic disease almost never develops in the absence of pelvic lymphadenopathy. Therefore, surgery and occasionally radiotherapy form the cornerstone of treatment for lymph node-positive patients; however, half of the patients with clinically palpable nodes will have inflammatory lesions only. Thus, a course of antibiotics before any further therapy is indicated. If the nodes persist after a course of antibiotics, biopsy and surgical dissection are indicated. Management of patients with clinical N0 is more controversial, with some authors recommending immediate lymph node dissection and others recommending a watchful waiting approach. Pathologic risk factors as assessed in the primary lesion may assist in decision making. Lymphangiography before a course of antibiotics is generally not considered helpful.

Cancer of the Testis

Directions   Each of the numbered items below is followed by lettered answers. Select the ONE lettered answer that is BEST in each case unless instructed otherwise.

QUESTIONS

Question 22.1.   **Which germ cell tumor is associated with widespread hematogenous metastases and high levels of human chorionic gonadotropin (HCG)?**

A. Pure choriocarcinoma
B. Yolk sac tumor
C. Embryonal carcinoma
D. Seminoma

Question 22.2.   **Which factor is associated with increased risk of mediastinal germ cell tumors?**

A. Human immunodeficiency virus (HIV)
B. Klinefelter syndrome
C. Diethylstilbestrol exposure
D. None of the above

Question 22.3.   **What is the median time for progression from intratubular germ cell neoplasia to invasive disease?**

A. 1 year
B. 5 years
C. 10 years
D. 20 years

Question 22.4.   **Which immunohistochemical markers are commonly expressed in patients with seminoma?**

A. CD117
B. CD30
C. None of the above
D. All the above

Corresponding Chapter in *Cancer: Principles & Practice of Oncology*, Eighth Edition: 41 (Cancer of the Testis).

Question 22.5.   **All the following sentences are true regarding β-HCG, EXCEPT:**

A.   The probability of elevated serum levels in nonseminomas is directly related to the clinical stage.
B.   It is produced by syncytiotrophoblasts.
C.   The serum half-life is 5 days.
D.   The β subunit is identical to that of luteinizing hormone (LH) and follicle-stimulating hormone (FSH).

Question 22.6.   **Which of the following characterizes a pathological stage T2 testicular germ tumor?**

A.   Invasion of the tunica vaginalis
B.   Invasion of the tunica albuginea
C.   Invasion of the spermatic cord
D.   None of the above

Question 22.7.   **Which of the following is NOT recommended after orchiectomy for patients with stage I seminoma?**

A.   Radiation
B.   Retroperitoneal lymph node resection (RPLND)
C.   Observation
D.   None of the above

Question 22.8.   **Which of the following are TRUE regarding patients with stage I seminoma?**

A.   The relapse rate without radiation therapy is between 15% and 20%.
B.   The median time to relapse is 20 months.
C.   Approximately 10% of relapses occur 5 years after orchiectomy.
D.   All the above.

Question 22.9.   **Which of the following is recommended as the standard treatment after orchiectomy for patients with stage IB nonseminomatous germ cell tumors?**

A.   Observation
B.   Radiation
C.   RPLND
D.   All the above

Question 22.10.   **A 27-year-old man presented with a painless testicular mass. Computed tomography (CT) of the abdomen showed a 4-cm retroperitoneal lymph node. He underwent radical orchiectomy, and the pathology showed a pure seminoma invading the scrotum. Serum markers were within the normal range. What is this patient's stage?**

A.   IIA
B.   IIB
C.   IIC
D.   None of the above

Question 22.11.   **For the patient above, what is the recommended therapy of choice after orchiectomy?**

   A. Observation
   B. Two cycles of bleomycin, etoposide, and cisplatin (BEP)
   C. Two cycles of etoposide and cisplatin (EP)
   D. Radiation therapy

Question 22.12.   **What is the therapy of choice in a patient with a nonseminomatous germ cell tumor and normal serum markers who underwent orchiectomy and RPLND showing involvement of two lymph nodes measuring 1.5 cm and 0.8 cm?**

   A. Surveillance
   B. Radiation therapy
   C. Chemotherapy with BEP
   D. All the above

Question 22.13.   **What is the best treatment for a patient with seminoma, a single 6 × 5-cm retroperitoneal lymph node, normal serum markers, and no distant metastases?**

   A. Radiation therapy
   B. RPLND
   C. Three cycles of BEP
   D. Three cycles of EP

Question 22.14.   **Which of the following define a seminoma with poor prognosis?**

   A. Mediastinal primary site
   B. Brain metastases
   C. A and B
   D. None of the above

Question 22.15.   **Which of the following may be present in patients with good-risk seminoma?**

   A. Alpha-fetoprotein (AFP) of 20,000 ng/mL
   B. HCG of 35,000 mIU/mL
   C. Lung metastases
   D. All the above

Question 22.16.   **Which of the following patients have intermediate-risk germ cell tumor?**

   A. A 23-year-old man with testicular seminoma, lung metastases, and normal serum markers
   B. A 42-year-old man with nonseminoma arising in the mediastinum and lactate dehydrogenase (LDH) three times the upper normal limit
   C. A 32-year-old man with testicular nonseminoma, lung metastases, and LDH three times the upper normal limit
   D. A 22-year-old man with nonseminoma arising in the mediastinum and normal serum markers

Question 22.17.   **What is the expected 5-year survival for a patient with nonseminomatous germ cell tumor with lung metastases and AFP of 6000 ng/mL?**

A.   95%
B.   90%
C.   75%
D.   45%

Question 22.18.   **What is the standard chemotherapy regimen for patients with poor-risk germ cell tumors?**

A.   Three cycles of BEP
B.   Four cycles of EP
C.   Four cycles of BEP
D.   A or B

Question 22.19.   **Which of the following treatments have shown improved survival compared with BEP in patients with poor-risk germ cell tumors in a randomized phase III trial?**

A.   Four cycles of etoposide, ifosfamide, and cisplatin (VIP)
B.   Two cycles of BEP followed by high-dose chemotherapy and stem cell support
C.   A and B
D.   None of the above

Question 22.20.   **A 26-year-old man with intermediate-risk nonseminoma received induction chemotherapy with BEP. The previously elevated AFP returned to normal, but the repeated CT scan showed a 1.5-cm residual mass in the retroperitoneum. What is the best next step?**

A.   Observation
B.   Chemotherapy
C.   Surgery
D.   None of the above

Question 22.21.   **If the patient above undergoes surgery, what is the MOST likely pathological finding?**

A.   Necrosis
B.   Teratoma
C.   Viable tumor
D.   None of the above

Question 22.22.   **What is the best approach to a patient with seminoma who has normal serum markers and a residual mass after chemotherapy measuring 4 cm?**

A.   Observation
B.   Positron emission tomography (PET) scan
C.   RPLND
D.   Radiation therapy

Question 22.23.   **What is the best treatment for a patient with poor-risk germ cell tumor and compromised pulmonary function?**

A. Four cycles of EP
B. Four cycles of VIP
C. Three cycles of BEP
D. Four cycles of bleomycin, vincristine, and cisplatin (BOP)

Question 22.24.   **Which factor is a predictor for poor outcomes after salvage chemotherapy in germ cell tumors?**

A. Primary retroperitoneal site
B. Primary mediastinal site
C. Complete response to initial therapy
D. A and B

Question 22.25.   **Which chemotherapy agent used in the treatment of germ cell tumors has been associated with increased risk of Raynaud phenomenon?**

A. Cisplatin
B. Bleomycin
C. Etoposide
D. None of the above

ANSWERS

Answer 22.1.   **The answer is A.**

Metastases from testicular cancer usually follow the lymphatic drainage, reaching the retroperitoneal lymph nodes in a predictable way. This is the case for seminomas and almost all subtypes of nonseminomas. The main exception is pure choriocarcinoma, which is rare and associated with widespread hematogenous metastases. Choriocarcinomas are, by definition, composed of both cytotrophoblasts and syncytiotrophoblasts. Because HCG is produced by syncytiotrophoblasts, pure choriocarcinomas may be associated with high levels of this serum marker.

Answer 22.2.   **The answer is B.**

There is no established association between the use of diethylstilbestrol and the development of germ cell tumors. Although testicular cancer has been reported in patients with HIV, there is little evidence to support its increased incidence in this population. Klinefelter syndrome is diagnosed by a 47, XXY karyotype and is characterized by testicular atrophy, eunuchoid habitus, and gynecomastia. These patients are at increased risk for the development of mediastinal germ cell tumors.

Answer 22.3.   **The answer is B.**

Virtually all germ cell tumors develop from a preexistent carcinoma in situ or intratubular germ cell neoplasia (ITGCN). The median time to progression from ITGCN to invasive disease is approximately 5 years.

Answer 22.4. **The answer is A.**

CD30 is expressed in most embryonal carcinomas, but it is absent in seminomas. In contrast, virtually all seminomas express CD 117 (c-kit).

Answer 22.5. **The answer is C.**

There is a direct correlation between clinical stage and the probability of elevated β-HCG in nonseminomatous tumors, which ranges from 10% to 20% in patients with stage I to approximately 40% in those with stage III. Both the α and β subunits of HCG are produced by syncytiotrophoblasts, and the β subunit is identical to that of luteinizing hormone (LH), follicle-stimulating hormone (FSH), and thyroid-stimulating hormone (TSH). Unlike AFP, which has a serum half-life of 5 to 7 days, the half-life of β-HCG is only 18 to 36 hours.

Answer 22.6. **The answer is A.**

According to the sixth edition of the American Joint Committee on Cancer staging handbook, invasion of the tunica albuginea and spermatic cord characterize the pathological stages T1 and T3 respectively. Pathological stage T2 is defined by the involvement of the tunica vaginalis.

Answer 22.7. **The answer is B.**

After resection of the primary testicular cancer, the standard treatment for patients with stage I seminoma is radiation therapy. Because of the low risk of relapse and the high probability of cure with treatment of relapsed disease, observation after orchiectomy remains an alternative option. RPLND is usually not recommended in the management of patients with seminoma.

Answer 22.8. **The answer is D.**

After orchiectomy, the probability of relapse for patients with seminoma under surveillance is between 15% and 20%. The relapse, however, is typically 12 to 15 months longer than for nonseminomatous tumors, with the relapse rate after 2 and 5 years of approximately 30% and 5%, respectively.

Answer 22.9. **The answer is C.**

The relapse rate for unselected patients with nonseminomatous germ cell tumors undergoing observation is between 25% and 30%. This rate may be dependent on the pathological stage, ranging from 15% in patients with T1 (stage IA) to 50% in patients with stage T2 or higher (stage IB). Although surveillance may be considered an alternative therapy for patients with stage IA, the high relapse rate in stage IB makes this approach less desirable. Radiation therapy has a limited role in the management of stage I nonseminomatous germ cell tumors because of the higher rate of systemic relapse and the possibility of compromising the use of subsequent chemotherapy at relapse. RPLND is the standard treatment after orchiectomy in patients with nonseminomatous germ cell tumors. This procedure provides important staging information and is performed with curative intent.

Answer 22.10.   **The answer is B.**

Stage IIA is characterized by metastatic lymph nodes that are 2 cm or less (N1), whereas stage IIC is characterized by any involved lymph node that is more than 5 cm in greatest dimension. This patient has T4 (tumor invading the scrotum), N2 (lymph node measuring between 2 and 5 cm), M0 (no distant metastases), or stage IIB.

Answer 22.11.   **The answer is D.**

In patients with low tumor burden seminomas (stages IIA and IIB), radiation therapy is the treatment of choice. With this approach, relapses occur in less than 10% of patients and death from seminoma is uncommon because the majority of patients with relapse can be cured with chemotherapy. Observation is not a good option because of the high risk of relapse without treatment, and chemotherapy should be reserved for patients with relapsed disease. Two notable exceptions are patients with horseshoe kidney or inflammatory bowel disease. Radiation therapy may cause renal failure in the former and significant gastrointestinal toxicity in the latter. The alternative treatment for these patients is chemotherapy.

Answer 22.12.   **The answer is A.**

This patient has stage IIA disease treated with RPLND. Radiation therapy is not indicated because of the very low risk of infield recurrence. Because the overall risk of recurrence in patients with pathological stage IIA is between 10% and 20% after RPLND, the treatment of choice is surveillance. Chemotherapy is indicated in patients with poor compliance or in those with risk factors for increased probability of relapse, such as six or more lymph nodes involved, lymph nodes greater than 2 cm, or extranodal extension.

Answer 22.13.   **The answer is C.**

This patient has stage IIC disease. The risk of relapse in these patients is very high with radiation alone, and RPLND is usually not recommended in patients with seminoma. The standard treatment is chemotherapy with either three cycles of BEP or four cycles of EP. However, three cycles of EP is inferior to three cycles of BEP and should not be used.

Answer 22.14.   **The answer is D.**

Although either mediastinal primary site or brain metastases define poor-risk nonseminomas, the poor-risk category is not applicable for seminomas. Furthermore, whereas the presence of nonpulmonary visceral metastases, such as brain metastases, classifies seminomas as intermediate risk, primary mediastinal seminomas remain in the good-risk category.

Answer 22.15.   **The answer is D.**

The only criterion for the classification of seminomas as intermediate risk is the presence of nonpulmonary visceral metastases. Patients with pulmonary metastases remain good risk in nonseminomas as well, and the very high serum markers would define the high-risk category for nonseminomas.

Answer 22.16.   **The answer is C.**

The patient in option A has good-risk seminoma, and both options B and D constitute a high-risk nonseminoma because of the presence of primary mediastinal disease. The patient in option C has an intermediate risk because the LDH value is between 1.5 and 10 times the upper limit of normal.

Answer 22.17.   **The answer is C.**

This patient has intermediate risk nonseminoma because of the presence of AFP between 1000 and 10,000 ng/mL. The survival rate for patients with intermediate risk is approximately 75%. Survival rates between 90% and 95% are seen in patients with good risk, and only 45% of patients with poor risk are long-term survivors.

Answer 22.18.   **The answer is C.**

Options A and B are commonly used in patients with good-risk tumors with equivalent efficacy. In patients with high-risk disease, however, the standard approach consists of four cycles of BEP.

Answer 22.19.   **The answer is D.**

VIP has similar results compared with BEP and may be offered to patients with contraindications to BEP. In a large US trial comparing four cycles of BEP with two cycles of BEP followed by high-dose chemotherapy and stem cell support, the latter showed no significant survival benefit.

Answer 22.20.   **The answer is C.**

Observation is not a good option in this case, because further therapy may be curative depending on the histology of the residual mass. Chemotherapy would be indicated in the case of persistently elevated AFP because of the high risk of residual viable tumor. The best treatment option in patients with residual mass and normalization of tumor markers is surgical resection of all residual tumors.

Answer 22.21.   **The answer is A.**

The probability of residual teratoma is between 34% and 40%, whereas viable tumor may be present in 10% to 15% of cases. The most common finding, however, is necrosis and fibrosis, which are present in approximately 50% of the cases.

Answer 22.22.   **The answer is B.**

Observation is not a good option because of the high risk of residual tumor in patients with tumors greater than 3 cm. RPLND after chemotherapy is technically difficult because of desmoplastic reaction, obliteration of the tissue planes, and higher perioperative morbidity compared with nonseminomas. Because the probability of viable residual cancer in seminoma is significantly smaller in patients with tumors smaller than 3 cm, they can be treated with observation. In contrast, the recommended management for patients with tumors larger than 3 cm is further imaging with a PET scan. In this case, a negative PET scan is associated with a low probability of residual tumor, whereas a positive study may indicate the presence of residual seminoma and the need for additional therapy.

Answer 22.23.   **The answer is B.**

Although significant pulmonary toxicity from bleomycin is rare, it may be fatal. Because the predictive ability of pulmonary function tests such as vital capacity and diffusion capacity of carbon monoxide is not proven, this agent is typically avoided in patients with preexisting pulmonary compromise. Therefore, BEP and BOP should, if possible, not be used. Four cycles of EP are equivalent to three cycles of BEP in patients with good-risk germ cell tumors, but inferior to four cycles of BEP. The best option in this patient is four cycles of VIP.

Answer 22.24.   **The answer is B.**

Patients who fail to respond or relapse after first-line chemotherapy with BEP represent a heterogeneous population with a wide range of cure rates after salvage chemotherapy. The 3-year survival is approximately 35% in patients with primary tumors of the testicle or retroperitoneum and those who achieved a complete response to first-line chemotherapy. In contrast, the probability of cure from conventional therapy is less than 10% in patients with less than complete response to initial chemotherapy or relapsed mediastinal tumors.

Answer 22.25.   **The answer is B.**

Neither cisplatin nor etoposide is commonly associated with Raynaud phenomenon, which occurs in 6% to 24% of patients receiving weekly bleomycin. The incidence appears to be higher in bolus administration compared with continuous infusion.

Gynecologic Cancers

| SECTION 1 | David G. Mutch |

OVARIAN

Directions   Each of the numbered items below is followed by lettered answers. Select the ONE lettered answer that is BEST in each case unless instructed otherwise.

QUESTIONS

Question 23.1.1.   **A 35-year-old premenopausal woman of Ashkenazi Jewish ancestry presents to you because her 60-year-old paternal aunt was recently diagnosed with ovarian cancer, and she is concerned about her own risk for ovarian cancer. She has no siblings, and there is no other family history of cancer. She has two living children and is in good health, and her pelvic examination is unremarkable. You should advise her that:**

A. Ovarian cancer cannot be inherited through the paternal side, and she does not need any particular screening.

B. A single second-degree relative with cancer at age more than 50 years does not confer a significantly increased risk for her.

C. She should visit a genetic counselor.

D. Annual transvaginal ultrasound and CA-125 screening can reduce her risk of mortality.

E. She should have a prophylactic total abdominal hysterectomy/bilateral salpingo-oophorectomy (TAH/BSO) if/when she does not want to have any more children.

Corresponding Chapter in *Cancer: Principles & Practice of Oncology*, Eighth Edition: 42 (Gynecologic Cancers).

Question 23.1.2.   **A 35-year-old woman presents to you for recommendations regarding therapy of her newly diagnosed mucinous ovarian cancer. This was a 5-cm, grade 1, left-sided mass that was incidentally found at the time of surgery for endometriosis as part of an infertility workup. The ovary was removed, and the operative note states that there was no evidence of tumor on the external surface of the ovary or elsewhere in the abdomen, but full surgical staging was not performed. A postoperative computed tomography (CT) scan of the abdomen and pelvis is unremarkable, and CA-125 is within normal limits. Pelvic examination is unremarkable. The patient would like to have children but does not want to compromise her survival. You should advise her that:**

A.   She is unlikely to have any residual cancer or a recurrence, and further surgery or chemotherapy is not needed.

B.   She should have a positron emission tomography (PET) scan, and if there is no uptake, she does not need further surgery or chemotherapy.

C.   Because her CT scan and CA-125 are normal, she is unlikely to have any residual disease, and further surgery is not needed; however, because the mucinous subtype of ovarian cancer has a very poor prognosis, she will require three to six cycles of carboplatin/paclitaxel chemotherapy.

D.   She should have complete surgical staging, if possible, via laparoscopy, with the option of preserving her uterus and contralateral ovary if there is no further evidence of tumor; if no further tumor is found, she would have a greater than 90% chance of 5-year survival, and chemotherapy would not be required.

E.   She should have complete surgical staging, including TAH/BSO; if no further disease is found, she will need only three cycles of carboplatin/paclitaxel chemotherapy, but if there is disease outside the ovary, she will need six cycles.

Question 23.1.3.   **CA-125 is most useful in what aspect of ovarian cancer management?**

A.   Screening

B.   Diagnosis

C.   Monitoring treatment

D.   Equally useful in all of the above

Question 23.1.4.   **Which of the following increases the risk of a woman developing ovarian cancer?**

A.   Use of oral contraceptives for >5 consecutive years

B.   Nulliparity

C.   Breastfeeding

D.   Tubal ligation

Question 23.1.5.   **Which of the following is the most commonly mutated gene identified in patients with ovarian cancer to date?**

A. p53
B. Her2/neu
C. Vascular endothelial growth factor (VEGF)
D. K-ras

Question 23.1.6.   **A 50-year-old woman presents with a pelvic mass. She is found to have a tumor of low malignant potential. She undergoes a total abdominal hysterectomy bilateral salpingo-oophorectomy and staging. She has no gross disease but has positive washings on final pathology and one positive lymph node, making her disease stage IIIC. What is the most appropriate therapy postoperatively?**

A. Intraperitoneal cisplatin and intravenous (IV) taxane
B. IV platinum and a taxane
C. Hormonal therapy with tamoxifen or an aromatase inhibitor
D. No further therapy

Question 23.1.7.   **What percentage of the time will early-stage ovarian cancer have an elevated CA-125?**

A. 50%
B. 60%
C. 80%
D. 90%

Question 23.1.8.   **All of the following are founder mutations associated with individuals of Ashkenazi descent, EXCEPT:**

A. 185delAG
B. 5382insC
C. 617delT
D. 619delT

Question 23.1.9.   **A patient of Jewish heritage who has breast cancer, but no family history of breast or ovarian cancer, has what chance of having a BRCA1 or BRCA2 mutation?**

A. 5%
B. 10%
C. 40%
D. 90%

Question 23.1.10.   **Oral contraceptive use for ≥5 years is associated with what percentage decrease in the incidence of ovarian cancer?**

A. 5%
B. 10%
C. 20%
D. 50%
E. 80%

Question 23.1.11.   **A 25-year-old woman has a left ovary removed because of an ovarian mass. The final pathology shows that this is a moderately differentiated papillary serous cancer. There was no other evidence of disease in the abdominal cavity. What is the likelihood that this patient has a positive pelvic or para-aortic lymph node metastasis?**

    A. 5%
    B. 15%
    C. 30%
    D. 50%

Question 23.1.12.   **Patients with high-risk early ovarian cancer should generally be treated:**

    A. By observation
    B. With platinum-based chemotherapy
    C. With whole abdominal radiation therapy
    D. B or C

Question 23.1.13.   **A 55-year-old woman who has just achieved a complete clinical remission (normal CT scan, pelvic examination, and CA-125) after six cycles of chemotherapy for stage IIIC optimally debulked serous ovarian cancer presents to you for a second opinion regarding her prognosis and treatment options at this point. She is in excellent general health and tolerated chemotherapy well except for some numbness in her fingers and toes, which caused her treating oncologist to switch her treatment from paclitaxel/carboplatin to docetaxel/carboplatin after cycle three. You should advise her that:**

    A. The risk of eventual relapse for an optimally debulked patient with a complete clinical remission is approximately 30%; no therapy is proven to be of any further survival benefit at this point.
    B. She should have second-look surgery; if residual disease is found, she should have four to six cycles of intraperitoneal platinum-based therapy because this can improve survival in patients with platinum-sensitive, minimal residual disease.
    C. She should have a PET scan; if residual disease is found, she should have four to six cycles of a non–cross-resistant drug, such as topotecan.
    D. Her risk of eventual relapse is approximately 70%; she should be offered consolidation therapy with paclitaxel 175 mg/m^2 every 3 weeks for 12 months with the expectation of a 30% improvement in survival.
    E. Her risk of relapse is approximately 70%; no therapy is proven to be of any survival benefit at this point.

Question 23.1.14. **Which of the following statement(s) is/are TRUE about granulosa cell tumors of the ovary?**

A.   They usually occur in premenopausal women.
B.   They are usually stage III/IV.
C.   Survival of patients with stage I disease is generally good, but they may relapse late.
D.   Survival of patients with stage III/IV disease is poor, and they should consider chemotherapy.
E.   They may be associated with endometrial cancer.
F.   C, D, and E.

Question 23.1.15. **Which of the following statements is TRUE about germ cell tumors of the ovary?**

A.   They occur more often in younger women.
B.   They are usually stage III/IV.
C.   Appropriate therapy includes TAH/BSO/full surgical staging and chemotherapy regimens similar to those used in male testicular cancer.
D.   Survival of patients with stage III/IV disease is poor.
E.   The chemotherapy will usually result in infertility.

Question 23.1.16. **A 51-year-old woman presents to you for recommendations regarding the treatment of her recurrent ovarian cancer. She was optimally de-bulked for stage IIIC serous ovarian carcinoma and completed six cycles of carboplatin/paclitaxel 36 months ago with a clinical complete remission. She now has recurrent ascites, which is histologically positive for tumor compatible with her original primary. CT scan shows peritoneal carcinomatosis and a pelvic mass. You should advise her that:**

A.   Prognosis of recurrent ovarian cancer is poor; she may get short-term benefit from chemotherapy, but hospice is a reasonable option.
B.   Tamoxifen has a 40% chance of shrinking her disease.
C.   She has a very high likelihood of disease shrinkage and symptom palliation with further platinum-based chemotherapy.
D.   She has a chance of cure with autologous stem cell transplant.
E.   Liver metastases and liver failure will probably be her ultimate cause of death.

ANSWERS

Answer 23.1.1. **The answer is C.**

This woman should be referred for genetic counseling and possible genetic testing. Some 40% to 60% of patients of Jewish descent who have epithelial ovarian cancer carry one of three founder BRCA1 or BRCA2 mutations (irrespective of family history). These, like other BRCA mutations, are inherited in an autosomal dominant manner, through either the paternal or maternal side. If this woman carries a BRCA1 mutation, her lifetime risk of ovarian cancer is 20% to 60%, and her risk of breast cancer is even higher. Although transvaginal ultrasound and CA-125 screening are generally recommended for mutation carriers who have their ovaries in place, there is no good evidence that such screening will decrease mortality. Oral contraceptives have been suggested to decrease the risk of ovarian cancer by up to 50%. Removal of the ovaries likely confers the best method for reducing the risk of ovarian cancer; it remains controversial whether the uterus should be removed as well.

Answer 23.1.2. **The answer is D.**

Understaging is common, particularly when the preoperative diagnosis is that of a benign process. Earlier laparoscopic surgical staging series suggested that up to 30% to 40% of patients thought to have FIGO stage I or II disease actually had disease in the upper abdomen. The incidence of extraovarian spread will be lower with a grade 1 tumor. Nonetheless, complete surgical staging, if possible, is advised in this case, because the recommendation for a stage IA grade 1 mucinous tumor is no chemotherapy. Although some data have suggested that advanced-stage mucinous tumors may respond less well to chemotherapy than serous tumors, a low-grade early-stage mucinous tumor does not have a poor prognosis. However, chemotherapy would be recommended in the case of any extraovarian spread. In the hands of an experienced surgeon, laparoscopic staging, including omentectomy and para-aortic lymph node examination, is an option. Preservation of the uterus and contralateral ovary is reasonable if no further disease is found at the time of staging. CA-125 is frequently normal in women with mucinous ovarian tumors, even when of advanced stage. A PET scan will not detect microscopic disease, may not be positive in low-grade malignancies, and is not likely to be helpful.

Answer 23.1.3. **The answer is C.**

CA-125 is not useful for screening because early-stage ovarian cancer has an elevated CA-125 approximately 50% of the time. Furthermore, the positive predictive value of an elevated CA-125 is very low because many things cause an elevated CA-125 and the prevalence of the disease is quite low. It is not particularly useful in the diagnosis of ovarian cancer for the above reasons. It is useful in monitoring treatment.

Answer 23.1.4. **The answer is B.**

Anything that decreases ovulation decreases the risk of ovarian cancer. Thus, oral contraceptives, multiparity, and breastfeeding decrease the likelihood that an individual will develop ovarian cancer. Several population-based studies show that tubal ligation deceases the likelihood of developing ovarian cancer.

Answer 23.1.5. **The answer is A.**

p53 is mutated approximately 50% of the time in ovarian cancer. K-ras is rarely mutated. Her2/neu is overexpressed less than 8% of the time; thus, Herceptin is often not an effective treatment for patients with ovarian cancer. VEGF is often overexpressed, but less than 50% of the time.

Answer 23.1.6. **The answer is D.**

There are no data that suggest any adjuvant therapy will improve the survival in patients with tumors of low malignant potential.

Answer 23.1.7. **The answer is A.**

CA-125 is elevated only 50% of the time in early-stage ovarian cancers, and therefore is not a good marker for early-stage disease. This feature also makes it a poor marker for screening.

Answer 23.1.8. **The answer is D.**

The majority of inherited disease in the Jewish population is due to one of the three founder mutations in BRCA1 and BRCA2.

Answer 23.1.9. **The answer is C.**

Answer 23.1.10. **The answer is D.**

There are several published studies, at least two of which are referenced in the corresponding chapter (Chapter 42), that report this benefit.

Answer 23.1.11. **The answer is B.**

Answer 23.1.12. **The answer is B.**

There are several studies that address this issue. Most data suggest that platinum/taxane-based therapy is superior to others.

Answer 23.1.13. **The answer is E.**

Although the majority (almost 80%) of patients with advanced-stage (III–IV) ovarian cancer will achieve a clinically complete remission with taxane/platinum combination therapy, approximately 70% will ultimately relapse from a clinical complete remission. Even patients with a surgically confirmed complete remission (negative second look) have an eventual relapse rate of approximately 50%. Although patients with optimally debulked stage III disease are a relatively favorable subgroup, those optimally debulked patients who have a larger presurgical tumor burden (IIIC) fare worse that those with a lesser presurgical tumor burden (IIIA). One randomized trial has demonstrated that maintenance paclitaxel improved progression-free survival of women with a clinical complete response (66% with optimal stage III disease) from 21 to 28 months in a randomized trial, and this option should be discussed with this patient. However, no survival benefit was observed at the time the trial was ended and the randomization code was broken, and there is a significant incidence of neuropathy. No data exist on PET scans in this situation, and consolidation topotecan has shown no benefit in two randomized trials. Although intraperitoneal therapy is a theoretically attractive option, cisplatin, the most widely used drug, carries a significant risk of neurotoxicity, and there are no data showing any survival benefit to its use in the setting of minimal residual disease.

Answer 23.1.14.   **The answer is F.**

Sex cord–stromal tumors (of which granulosa cell tumors are the most common subtype) comprise only approximately 5% of all ovarian neoplasms. The peak incidence is in women aged more than 50 years, although a significant proportion occurs in premenopausal women. Granulosa cell tumors may secrete estrogen and be associated with endometrial hyperplasia and endometrial carcinoma. The majority are diagnosed in stage I, and these patients have 10-year survivals of 75% to 95%. However, late relapses may be observed. Patients with advanced-stage disease fare more poorly. Although the rarity of the tumor precludes randomized trial data, most such patients will be offered chemotherapy, traditionally with bleomycin, etoposide, cisplatin (BEP), or other regimens used in germ cell tumors.

Answer 23.1.15.   **The answer is A.**

Germ cell tumors almost always occur in young women, with a peak incidence in their early 20s. Some 60% to 70% are stage I at diagnosis. With the use of platinum-based chemotherapy regimens similar to those used for men with testicular cancer, even patients with an advanced stage have a good prognosis. Because most of these tumors occur in young women, often before they have had children, and because the type of chemotherapy used will not cause infertility in most young female patients, the surgical approach is critical; in many patients, the contralateral ovary and uterus can and should be spared.

Answer 23.1.16.   **The answer is C.**

Recurrent ovarian cancer is not generally curable with transplant or any other modality, but patients whose disease recurs with a disease-free interval of more than 1 year have more than a 50% chance of responding to platinum-based combination therapy and should usually be offered chemotherapy. Secondary debulking surgery may also be of benefit. Hormonal therapy in ovarian cancer generally produces response rates of only 10% to 15% and is usually reserved for patients who cannot tolerate other therapy. It has also been recommended as the initial salvage therapy in patients who have an increasing CA-125 as their only manifestation of recurrent disease.

SECTION 2   Matthew A. Powell

NONOVARIAN

Directions   Each of the numbered items below is followed by lettered answers. Select the ONE lettered answer that is BEST in each case unless instructed otherwise.

QUESTIONS

Question 23.2.1.   **Type I endometrial cancers have all of the following features, EXCEPT:**

A.   Commonly have mutations in PTEN
B.   Appear to arise via a progression pathway
C.   Commonly found to have mutations in p53
D.   Are usually related to estrogen exposure

Question 23.2.2.   **Microsatellite instability (MSI) in endometrial cancers have the following features, EXCEPT:**

A.   MSI phenotype is expressed in approximately 20% of type I endometrial cancers.
B.   The most common mechanism of MSI in endometrial cancer is through mutation in MSH2.
C.   MSI appears to be an early event in the development of endometrial cancer.
D.   The most common mechanism of MSI in endometrial cancer is through hypermethylation of the MLH1 promoter.

Question 23.2.3.   **PTEN mutations in endometrial cancer are characterized by all of the following, EXCEPT:**

A.   Are a late event in the development of endometrial cancer.
B.   Are the most common defect in type I endometrial cancer.
C.   Inactivation is caused by various mechanisms.
D.   Mutations have been demonstrated in many precancerous lesions, suggesting a "gatekeeper" role for the gene.

Question 23.2.4.   **B-catenin mutations in endometrial cancer are characterized by all of the following, EXCEPT:**

A.   Are an early event in the development of endometrial cancer.
B.   Are a feature of type I endometrial cancers.
C.   Gain of function mutations are common and result in transcriptional activation.
D.   Have not been demonstrated in precancerous lesions.

Question 23.2.5.   **Features of type II endometrial cancers include all of the following, EXCEPT:**

A.   Are more aggressive and characterized by p53 mutations.
B.   Arise in a background of complex hyperplasia.
C.   Her-2/neu amplification is a common feature.
D.   Do not appear to be associated with increased estrogen exposure.

Corresponding Chapter in *Cancer: Principles & Practice of Oncology*, Eighth Edition: 42, (Gynecologic Cancers).

Question 23.2.6.   **The majority of cervical, vaginal, and vulvar cancers appear to have a common cause and are usually caused by:**

    A.   Increased exposure to exogenous estrogen
    B.   Chronic bacterial and parasitic infections
    C.   Multiple prior herpes simple virus (HSV) infections
    D.   Human papilloma virus (HPV) infection with high-risk types

Question 23.2.7.   **In patients with gestational trophoblastic disease (GTD) with a complete mole, molecular features include all of the following, EXCEPT:**

    A.   Mutations in p53 have not been reported.
    B.   Most are diploid with duplication of a haploid paternal genome.
    C.   Predominance of maternal chromosomes is common.
    D.   Several genes, including CMYC, ERBB2, CFMS, and BCL2, have been implicated in the pathogenesis of complete moles.

Question 23.2.8.   **A 39-year-old married woman is seeing you in the office after recently having a cervical biopsy that demonstrated cervical cancer. She has no prior medical problems other than anemia and one prior uncomplicated child birth. You tell her all of the following epidemiologic factors are true, EXCEPT:**

    A.   During the past 80 years, death rates from cervical cancer have decreased primarily because of the adoption of routine screening programs with PAP smears.
    B.   Cervical cancer is the second leading cause of cancer deaths for women aged 20 to 39 years in the United States.
    C.   HSV is thought to be the causative agent for the majority of patients.
    D.   The incidence of cervical cancer is 30% and 100% higher in black and Hispanic women, respectively, compared with whites in the United States.

Question 23.2.9.   **She asks about prevention and treatment of HPV infections, and you advise her:**

    A.   The viral infections are rare, and promiscuity has caused her cancer.
    B.   Treatments for HPV infections with antiviral therapy are effective if taken within 4 days of exposure.
    C.   An HPV vaccine has recently been approved by the Food and Drug Administration (FDA) to help prevent infection from the most common HPV types.
    D.   An HPV vaccine has recently been FDA approved, and she should receive the vaccine now to help treat her cancer.

Question 23.2.10. **You counsel her about HPV and human immunodeficiency virus (HIV). After extensive discussion, you decide to proceed with testing for HIV with all of the following justifications, EXCEPT:**

A. HIV immunosuppression is correlated with an increased risk of cervical HPV infections.
B. Patients with HIV appear to have a faster rate of progression to high-grade dysplasia (cervical intraepithelial neoplasia [CIN]).
C. Antiretroviral therapy to manage HIV has demonstrated direct activity against HPV.
D. Cervical cancers in HIV-positive women may be more aggressive than in HIV-negative women.

Question 23.2.11. **She has done extensive reading about cervical cancer and asks you about factors that are associated with metastatic disease. You advise her the following are associated with extracervical disease, EXCEPT:**

A. Tumor size
B. Presence of microinvasion
C. Depth of invasion
D. Presence of lymph-vascular space invasion

Question 23.2.12. **If her initial biopsy returned with invasive squamous cell carcinoma with 2 mm of invasion and no lymphovascular space involvement (LVSI), you recommend that:**

A. She be referred back to her gynecologist for a simple hysterectomy.
B. She be referred to the radiation oncologist for consideration of radiation therapy with possible chemotherapy.
C. You begin therapy with cisplatin 40 mg/m^2 weekly for six cycles.
D. She undergo cervical conization.

Question 23.2.13. **The patient has a 3-cm visible tumor found on her cervix that is biopsied and is frankly invasive squamous cell carcinoma. She has several questions regarding staging of her cancer. You advise the following, EXCEPT:**

A. Staging for cervical cancer is clinical, involving pelvic examination.
B. If enlarged lymph nodes are seen on her computed tomography (CT) scan, her cancer would be staged appropriately as at least stage III.
C. If hydronephrosis is demonstrated on her CT scan, her cancer would be staged appropriately as at least stage III.
D. Positron emission tomography (PET) scanning appears to be the most sensitive noninvasive method of detecting nodal involvement.

Question 23.2.14.   **The patient's 3-cm visible tumor appears confined to the cervix and is staged appropriately as stage IB1. Which of the following therapies is most appropriate?**

    A.   Radiation and chemotherapy with weekly cisplatin dosed at 40 mg/m^2

    B.   Simple hysterectomy with removal of fallopian tubes and ovaries

    C.   Radiation therapy or radical hysterectomy with lymphadenectomy

    D.   Brachytherapy radiation with a dose of 75 Gy

Question 23.2.15.   **The patient's 5-cm tumor is found to include parametrial involvement with evidence of hydronephrosis on imaging. Her cancer is staged appropriately as stage IIIB. You elect to treat her with combined chemotherapy and radiation. You advise all of the following, EXCEPT:**

    A.   Several randomized trials involving patients with locally advanced cervical cancer have demonstrated a benefit to the addition of chemotherapy to standard radiation therapy.

    B.   Carboplatin appears to be the most appropriate agent to combine with radiation therapy for cervical cancer, and this should be followed by hysterectomy.

    C.   5FU with cisplatin is an acceptable regimen to combine with radiation therapy and has demonstrated improved survival.

    D.   Weekly cisplatin with radiation therapy appears as active as other regimen with manageable toxicity.

Question 23.2.16.   **After receiving definitive concurrent chemoradiotherapy for her stage IIIB cervical cancer, she develops a recurrence in the cervix, 18 months from the completion of therapy. Imaging studies suggest no extrapelvic disease. You recommend the following:**

    A.   Referral back to the radiation oncologist for consideration of further radiation

    B.   Chemotherapy with combined cisplatin and topotecan

    C.   Chemotherapy with combined cisplatin and paclitaxel

    D.   Referral for consideration of further surgery

Question 23.2.17.   **A 67-year-old woman presents for evaluation of a cancer found in the vagina. Before any examination or evaluation, you review with her that all of the following are true, EXCEPT:**

    A.   Prior in utero exposure to the synthetic estrogen diethylstilbestrol (DES) places a woman at an increased risk for development of vaginal clear cell adenocarcinoma.

    B.   Most cancers found in the vagina are actually metastases or direct extensions from other gynecologic tumors.

    C.   Vaginal squamous cell carcinoma is thought to be unrelated to the HPV.

    D.   Staging for primary vaginal cancers is similar to cervical cancer and is clinical.

Question 23.2.18. **This patient is found to have had a prior hysterectomy for mild dysplasia and benign indications. Her apparent primary vaginal cancer extends to the subvaginal tissues and is appropriately staged as a stage II cancer. You recommend:**

   A. Referral for total radical vaginectomy
   B. Chemotherapy with a cisplatin-based regimen
   C. Referral for radiation therapy
   D. Local excision followed by close observation

Question 23.2.19. **A 55-year-old patient with a history of abnormal PAP smears presents for evaluation of a 3-cm vulvar mass. It is located 1 cm lateral to the clitoris on the right and has an ulcerated appearance. She states she noticed it 2 years ago and has tried many different ointments to help control the itching and irritation. This was recently biopsied to reveal invasive squamous cell carcinoma. You review the epidemiology of invasive vulvar cancer with the patient and explain that all of the following are true, EXCEPT:**

   A. There appears to be two distinct types of invasive squamous vulvar cancer separated by the presence of HPV.
   B. HPV-associated vulvar cancer tends to occur in younger women (age <55 years) and be associated with prior cervical precancerous abnormalities.
   C. Melanoma of the vulva is also thought to be caused by exposure to HPV.
   D. These cancer tends to spread first to region lymph nodes in the groin before spread to the rest of the body.

Question 23.2.20. **You recommend this patient with a 3-cm vulvar cancer to undergo the following:**

   A. Neoadjuvant chemoradiation followed by local resection
   B. Concurrent chemoradiation
   C. Radical vulvectomy with bilateral inguinal (groin) lymphadenectomy
   D. Local resection followed by radiation and/or chemotherapy

Question 23.2.21. **Poor prognostic factors include all of the following, EXCEPT:**

   A. Presence of LVSI
   B. Tumor grade
   C. Depth of invasion and tumor thickness
   D. Number of positive lymph nodes

Question 23.2.22. **Her final pathology reveals a 3.3-cm invasive squamous cell carcinoma with two involved (positive) lymph nodes in the right inguinal/femoral lymph node dissection of 12 removed. The contralateral node dissection was negative. Margins around the primary tumor were negative and greater than 1 cm. Her appropriate FIGO and TNM stage are:**

A. IVA and T2N1M0
B. II and T2N2M0
C. III and T3N1M0
D. III and T2N1M0

Question 23.2.23. **The most appropriate therapy for this patient after she recovers from surgery is:**

A. Close observation
B. Chemotherapy with cisplatin plus 5FU
C. Referral for consideration of radiation therapy
D. Exploration with dissection of the pelvic lymph nodes

Question 23.2.24. **Unfortunately, despite the use of adjuvant therapy, this patient's cancer recurs locally on the vulva, and a 2-cm recurrence is documented. You advise the following:**

A. Repeat resection
B. Chemotherapy with bleomycin
C. Best supportive care
D. Chemotherapy with cisplatin plus 5FU

Question 23.2.25. **A 62-year-old woman has been diagnosed with a uterine corpus (body) cancer. You have not received her records for review, but she is seen in your office for consultation and asks many general questions. You tell her all of the following are true, EXCEPT:**

A. Approximately 90% of these cancers arise from the endometrial lining and are typically managed with hysterectomy and staging.
B. Most of these cancers are caused by exogenous estrogen use.
C. Uterine sarcomas are less common than endometrial cancers and represent approximately 10% of corpus cancers.
D. Endometrial cancer typically presents at an early stage with patients having abnormal uterine bleeding.

Question 23.2.26. **This patient's records arrive in the office, and the pathology verifies the diagnosis of a grade 2 endometrioid-type endometrial cancer from an office endometrial biopsy. She asks what has caused her cancer to develop. You tell her all of the following are considered to be independent risk factors for the development of endometrial cancer, EXCEPT:**

A. Obesity
B. Diabetes mellitus
C. Premature ovarian failure with early menopause
D. Presence of an estrogen-producing tumor

Question 23.2.27. **For this patient with an office biopsy demonstrating grade 2 endometri-oid endometrial cancer who is of apparent good heath with no other medical comorbidities, you recommend:**

A. Further evaluation with CT scan and PET scan to evaluate for meta-static disease

B. A formal dilation and curettage (D&C) to obtain a more accurate pathologic diagnosis

C. Hysterectomy with removal of the tubes and ovaries with considera-tion of pelvic and para-aortic lymphadenectomy

D. Referral for radiation therapy with possible chemoradiation

Question 23.2.28. **During the patient's initial visit, she reports her mother was diagnosed with endometrial cancer at age 42 years, her maternal aunt with colon cancer at age 51 years, and her sister with endometrial cancer at age 38 years. You are concerned her cancer may be hereditary. You advise that:**

A. She undergo colon assessment if she is not up to date with age-appropriate screening and consider counseling and possible testing for hereditary nonpolyposis colorectal cancer (Lynch II syndrome).

B. She undergo breast MRI and be tested for BRCA1 and BRCA2.

C. Colon and endometrial cancer are common, and no further evalua-tion is necessary at this time.

D. The maternal side of her family very likely has familial adenomatous polyposis and should be further evaluated.

Question 23.2.29. **The patient undergoes hysterectomy with full staging, including pelvic washing for cytology, removal of both tubes and ovaries; pelvic and para-aortic lymph nodes are removed. She is noted to have cancer involving three pelvic lymph nodes. Her stage is designated:**

A. IC

B. IIC

C. IIIC

D. IVA

Question 23.2.30. **For this patient with three positive pelvic lymph nodes and a grade 2 endometrioid endometrial cancer, you recognize adjuvant therapy is con-troversial but ultimately recommend:**

A. Hormone therapy with a progestational agent

B. Referral for pelvic radiation therapy

C. Chemotherapy with combined paclitaxel, cisplatin, and doxorubicin

D. Combination of radiation and chemotherapy

Question 23.2.31.   **The patient completes your recommended adjuvant therapy. Unfortunately, 18 months later she returns to your office with CT evidence of liver and lung recurrent cancer that is biopsy proven. All the following are correct regarding recurrent endometrial cancer, EXCEPT:**

A.   Recurrence typically occurs within 3 years of the original diagnosis.
B.   Approximately 50% of patients are symptomatic at time of recurrence.
C.   Serum CA-125 may be a useful surveillance marker for patients at high risk for recurrence.
D.   Isolated vaginal recurrence is rare in patients, and cure is only by ultra-radical surgery.

Question 23.2.32.   **The most active (improved disease-free and overall survival) chemotherapy regimen as determined in randomized clinical trials in women with advanced or recurrent endometrial cancer with measurable disease is:**

A.   Doxorubicin plus paclitaxel
B.   Cisplatin/doxorubicin
C.   Cisplatin/doxorubicin/paclitaxel
D.   Ifosfamide plus paclitaxel

Question 23.2.33.   **The following are true regarding uterine sarcomas, EXCEPT:**

A.   Represent approximately 10% of uterine corpus cancers.
B.   The malignant mixed mullerian tumor is also known as uterine carcinosarcoma.
C.   All different types of uterine sarcoma are treated similarly with resection followed by radiation therapy.
D.   Uterine leiomyosarcoma is more chemoresponsive than most other types of sarcomas.

Question 23.2.34.   **A 17-year-old female patient presents to your office with pelvic ultrasound suggesting intrauterine gestational trophoblastic neoplasia (GTN). The most common of the distinct clinicopathologic entities of GTN is:**

A.   Complete hydatidiform mole
B.   Partial hydatidiform mole
C.   Choriocarcinoma
D.   Placental site trophoblastic tumor

Question 23.2.35.   **This patient has a beta-human chorionic gonadotropin (hCG) of 122,300 and undergoes therapy with a suction D&C. Final pathology confirms the diagnosis of complete hydatidiform mole. The patient is followed with the following:**

A.   CT scan every 3 months
B.   Ultrasound of the pelvis every 3 months
C.   Pelvic examination with PAP smear every 6 weeks
D.   Beta-hCG weekly

Question 23.2.36. **This patient goes on to develop evidence of persistent gestational tropho-blastic neoplasia. You are concerned she may have "phantom" hCG. All of the following are correct regarding "phantom" hCG, EXCEPT:**

A. False-positive hCG test results are caused by the presence of heterophile antibodies.
B. False-positive hCG results have caused inappropriate therapies to be performed, including surgery and chemotherapy.
C. Phantom hCG is no longer a problem with modern testing equipment.
D. A urinary beta-hCG assay should be performed.

Question 23.2.37. **After a complete metastatic workup, the patient is determined to have low-risk disease. You recommend the following chemotherapy:**

A. Etoposide
B. Vincristine
C. Methotrexate
D. Cyclophosphamide

ANSWERS

Answer 23.2.1. **The answer is C.**

p53 mutations are typically a feature of type II endometrial cancers.

Answer 23.2.2. **The answer is B.**

The most common mechanism of MSI in endometrial cancer is through hypermethylation of the MLH1 promoter and NOT mutation in MSH2.

Answer 23.2.3. **The answer is A.**

Loss of PTEN expression through a variety of mechanisms appears to be an early event in the development of type I endometrial cancers and has been seen in many precursor lesions.

Answer 23.2.4. **The answer is D.**

B-catenin appears to be an early event in the development of endometrial cancer and has been seen in precancerous lesions.

Answer 23.2.5. **The answer is B.**

Type II endometrial cancers do not appear to arise in the typically estrogen-driven endometrial hyperplasias.

Answer 23.2.6. **The answer is D.**

Infection with high-risk HPV appears to be the common cause for these cancers.

Answer 23.2.7.   **The answer is C.**

Complete moles have a predominance of paternal chromosomes.

Answer 23.2.8.   **The answer is C.**

Cervical cancer is caused by exposure to high-risk strains of HPV. The presence of HPV DNA has been identified in more than 99% of cervical carcinomas. The epidemiologic information presented is correct. The increased incidence of cervical cancer in blacks and Hispanics in the United States is thought to be secondary to barriers in screening because of the lack of insurance, low income, and cultural differences.

Answer 23.2.9.   **The answer is C.**

HPV infections are not rare, and although promiscuity is more common for women with cervical cancer, it is certainly not required. There is no currently effective antiviral therapy that is active against HPV. Treatments of the precancerous and cancerous changes that develop from HPV are usually indicated, but the virus can still be often detected even after therapy. An HPV vaccine has recently been FDA approved as a preventative vaccine. It appears that primarily those patients who are naive to the virus benefit from vaccination. Young women between the ages of 9 and 26 years are currently approved for vaccination. Ideally, vaccination should occur before the onset of sexual activity.

Answer 23.2.10.   **The answer is C.**

All of the factors are correct except that current antiretroviral therapy has not demonstrated benefit against HPV.

Answer 23.2.11.   **The answer is B.**

The incidence of nodal (extracervical) involvement is directly correlated with tumor stage, size, histology, depth of invasion, and lymphovascular space invasion. For patients with stage I disease treated with radial hysterectomy, 15% to 20% and 1% to 5% of pelvic and para-aortic lymph nodes, respectively, will be involved. Cervical cancer usually follows an orderly pattern of spread from the cervix to the pelvic nodes, then to the common iliacs, and finally to the para-aortic lymph nodes before systemic spread. Distant metastatic sites can occur, and the most common are lung, extrapelvic lymph nodes, liver, and bone.

Answer 23.2.12.   **The answer is D.**

Microinvasive carcinoma of the cervix is often a source of confusion and mismanagement for patients with cervical cancer. Patient with stage IA1 cancers have been safely managed with conization only or simple hysterectomy. These patients typically are not treated with radiation and chemotherapy. The difficulty and confusion that arise result from practitioners attempting to make the diagnosis from small biopsies. To make the diagnosis, the patient should have less than 3 mm of invasion and no more than 7 mm of lateral spread, along with negative margins. LVSI remains controversial, but typically if present, patients should be treated as if they have frankly invasive disease. Thus, if superficial invasion is seen on a small biopsy and there is no visible tumor on the cervix, the patient should typically be evaluated with cervical conization before definitive therapy to properly stage the patient and allow for the most appropriate therapy.

Answer 23.2.13.   **The answer is B.**

Staging of cervical cancer is clinical, which is based on careful clinical examination and routine radiographic studies (e.g., chest radiograph, intravenous pyelogram, lower gastrointestinal) and procedures (cystoscopy, proctoscopy). Because cervical cancer is primarily a disease of the developing world, staging procedures have been kept simple to allow consistency staging throughout the world. Specific technology, such as CT and PET, is often used for treatment planning in the United States but should not be the basis for changing the stage.

Answer 23.2.14.   **The answer is C.**

For patients with small stage IB1 tumors, either radiation or radical hysterectomy with lymphadenectomy is appropriate. Factors such as patient preference, anesthetic, and surgical risks should be considered. Surgical treatment tends to be preferred for young women with small tumors because it permits preservation of the ovaries and likely better vaginal function. Radiation invariably leads to menopause with loss of ovarian hormone production and possible vaginal stenosis. Simple hysterectomy would be considered inadequate therapy for this size and stage of cancer. Chemoradiotherapy would typically be indicated for patients with more advanced cancers. Brachytherapy alone would also be inadequate because the patient is at risk for nodal involvement, and external beam therapy would also be indicated to treat the nodal area at risk.

Answer 23.2.15.   **The answer is B.**

Table 42.2.3 in *Cancer: Principles and Practice of Oncology* summarizes the randomized trials that have investigated the role of concurrent radiotherapy and chemotherapy for patients with locoregionally advanced cervical cancer. Although the 10 trials presented have a variety of regimens none included carboplatin, the use of hysterectomy after radiation and chemotherapy is no longer considered routine and should be abandoned except for rare circumstances. The use of chemotherapy when extended-field radiation (para-aortic) is used has not been well studied and appears to have greater toxicity. The use of neoadjuvant chemotherapy has been studied with a variety of regimens, and these have demonstrated little or no improvements in outcome. Concurrent treatment is thus preferred.

Answer 23.2.16.   **The answer is D.**

This patient has developed an apparently isolated central pelvic recurrence after combined chemoradiotherapy. Her only real curative option is surgical and will likely require pelvic exenteration. Patients typically receive the maximum tolerated dose of radiation during their primary therapy, and further meaningful doses of radiation are usually not possible. Chemotherapy is typically palliative in nature only. Recent randomized trials have suggested improved survival with combination chemotherapy over single-agent cisplatin, but this remains palliative.

Answer 23.2.17.   **The answer is C.**

All of the statements are correct except that vaginal cancers are thought to be related to HPV in at least 60% to 65% of cases. DES is a synthetic estrogen previously given to women during pregnancy primarily in women with a history of miscarriage or premature birth. First reported in 1971, an association between DES exposure in utero and clear cell vaginal cancer was made. Few cases of cancer in DES-exposed women have been reported in those aged more than 40 years, and these women continued to be followed closely. If a cancer in the vagina is in contact with the cervix or the vulva, then it is not classified as a vaginal cancer and the primary is consider either the cervix or the vulva, respectively. Staging for primary vaginal cancer is clinical, similar to cervical cancer.

Answer 23.2.18.   **The answer is C.**

Stage II vaginal cancer involves the subvaginal tissues and is typically not amendable to local resection without injury to the bladder or rectum. The most appropriate therapy is radiation, likely with both brachytherapy and external beam radiotherapy to treat the regional nodal areas. Chemotherapy is not indicated for primary therapy. Extrapolating from randomized studies in patients with cervical cancer, one could consider combination chemoradiotherapy for patients with vaginal cancer.

Answer 23.2.19.   **The answer is C.**

Vulvar melanoma is not thought to be related to HPV infection. There does appear to be two types of invasive squamous vulvar cancers. HPV-related cancers typically occur in younger women and can be multifocal and associated with vulvar-intraepithelial neoplasia (VIN). Non-HPV cancers occur in older women and are often associated with chronic vulvar inflammation or lichen sclerosis. The lymph nodes in the groin are usually the first site of spread of vulvar cancer.

Answer 23.2.20.   **The answer is C.**

Although all options are used to treat patients with invasive vulvar cancer, the apparent best option is typically radical vulvectomy with inguinal lymphadenectomy. Staging is then determined on the basis of the surgical findings, which also dictate adjuvant therapy. Typically, neoadjuvant and definitive chemoradiation are often necessary with very large cancers involving the urethra or anus and can help achieve organ preservation, but would not be typically used with a 3-cm tumor.

Answer 23.2.21. **The answer is B.**

Tumor grade has been inconsistent and is not typically been found to be an independent risk factor. LVSI is a very strong predictor of positive inguinal lymph nodes. Depth of invasion, tumor diameter, and tumor thickness are all directly related to lymph node involvement and the patient's ultimate survival.

Answer 23.2.22. **The answer is D.**

Staging for carcinomas of the vulva has been established by the International Federation of Obstetrician & Gynecologist (FIGO). In 1983, FIGO initially adopted a clinical TNM staging system. The reliability of clinical assessment of regional lymph node status was found to be poor. In 1988, FIGO adopted a surgical staging system, and this was updated in 1994 to include an additional substage for minimally invasive cancers (IA). Typically, both TNM and FIGO stages are provided.

Answer 23.2.23. **The answer is C.**

Radiation is indicated for patients with more than one positive lymph node and should be considered with any positive lymph nodes or if resection margins are positive and further resection is not possible. Chemotherapy has not been demonstrated to be of benefit in the adjuvant setting. A randomized trial evaluating the role of pelvic lymphadectomy for patients with positive groin lymph nodes was completed, suggesting there is no role for routine pelvic lymphadectomy for these patients. Pelvic radiation therapy should be delivered to patients with positive groin lymph nodes.

Answer 23.2.24. **The answer is A.**

Local recurrence of vulvar cancer is not uncommon. These patients can often be successfully managed with repeat resection. Large surgical defects from further resections in the vulva can be managed with the use of flaps and skin grafting. Chemotherapy is usually of limited efficacy and not needed if the lesion is resectable. Radical surgical resection, including pelvic exenterations, has been used successfully for large recurrent cancers.

Answer 23.2.25. **The answer is B.**

Exogenous estrogen use appears to cause a minority of endometrial cancers. In the past, when estrogens were given frequently to women without progestins to protect the endometrial lining, this was a more frequent cause of endometrial cancer. The majority (90%) of uterine corpus cancers arise from the endometrium with sarcomas representing less than 10% of cases. Abnormal uterine bleeding typically leads to early presentation and evaluation of patients with endometrial cancer.

Answer 23.2.26. **The answer is C.**

Risk factors for the development of endometrial cancer are typically related to chronic estrogenic stimulation. Estrogen therapy, obesity, early age of menarche, late age of menopause, anovulation, and estrogen-producing tumors have all been associated with the development of endometrial cancers. Interestingly, diabetes mellitus imparts a increased relative risk of 3, even when controlling for other known factors.

Answer 23.2.27.   **The answer is C.**

Hysterectomy, whether performed through a large open incision, laparoscopically, or vaginally, is indicated. Ovarian preservation has been performed in rare circumstances but is typically discouraged. Preoperative imaging, beyond a chest radiograph for patients with disease apparently confined to the uterus on clinical examination, is rarely helpful. Thus, CT, MRI, and PET scan are not typically recommended as a preoperative evaluation for these patients. The office endometrial biopsy is sufficiently accurate in this setting, and a D&C would not offer any further benefit to the preoperative evaluation. Radiation can be used as primary therapy for the treatment of endometrial cancer but is typically reserved for patients with severe medical comorbidities in whom surgery is thought to be too high risk. These patients will still typically require general anesthesia to allow for brachytherapy implantation into the uterine fundus.

Answer 23.2.28.   **The answer is A.**

The family history presented is worrisome for Lynch II syndrome. Approximately 5% of endometrial cancers are hereditary, with the majority being Lynch II (hereditary nonpolyposis colorectal cancer syndrome). Lynch syndrome is caused by a defect in mismatch repair genes. Women who carry one of these abnormal genes have a 22% to 60% chance of developing endometrial cancer, which is similar to their risk of developing colorectal cancer. Patients with the diagnosis of endometrial cancer with a strong family history should be counseled and offered genetic testing. Families with BRCA1 or BRCA2 mutations confer an increased risk in breast and ovarian cancer. There is no convincing evidence that these patients are at an increased risk for the development of endometrial cancer. Endometrial cancer is not related to familial adenomatous polyposis (FAP) syndrome.

Answer 23.2.29.   **The answer is C.**

Staging of endometrial cancer is typically surgical. Both a clinical and surgical staging system exist. A minority of patients with major medical comorbidities would typically not undergo surgical management and require staging via the older clinical staging system. Since 1988, the surgical staging system has been used as directed by FIGO. This patient is correctly staged as IIIC.

Answer 23.2.30.   **The answer is D.**

Adjuvant therapy for patients with stage IIIC disease remains controversial. GOG-122 compared whole abdomen/pelvic radiation therapy with chemotherapy (cisplatin plus doxorubicin × eight cycles) and demonstrated a progression-free and overall survival benefit to chemotherapy. GOG-184 evaluated "volume-directed" radiation therapy that included pelvic and para-aortic lymph nodes when indicated, followed by chemotherapy. Patients were randomized to two differing chemotherapy arms (cisplatin plus doxorubicin vs. cisplatin, doxorubicin, and paclitaxel). There was no significant benefit to the addition of paclitaxel for these patients. Methods to reduce toxicity of radiation therapy including intensity-modulated radiotherapy (IMRT) are being investigated. Lower toxicity with potentially sparing the pelvic bone marrow should allow for combination of radiation and chemotherapy to maximize efficacy.

Answer 23.2.31.   **The answer is D.**

Recurrent endometrial cancer occurs most often in patients with high-risk histologic subtypes (serous, clear cell, or carcinoma) or initial advanced stage. Patients are typically followed after adjuvant therapy and evaluated for recurrence with pelvic examination and serum CA-125. One third of recurrences in patients with early-stage disease have recurrence with disease apparently confined to the pelvis. Isolated vaginal and pelvic recurrences are important to identify because these patients have a favorable cure rate with therapy. Patients with systemic disease would rarely be cured, and treatment is palliative.

Answer 23.2.32.   **The answer is C.**

The Gynecologic Oncology Group (GOG) has conducted several randomized trials in patients with advanced or recurrent endometrial cancer. GOG-177 demonstrated the combination of cisplatin, doxorubicin, and paclitaxel to have an improved progression-free and overall survival benefit that was statistically significant. This regimen had a response rate of 57% compared with 34% in the cohort treated with cisplatin and doxorubicin alone. Ifosfamide plus paclitaxel is a regimen that has been developed and demonstrated superiority in uterine carcinosarcomas.

Answer 23.2.33.   **The answer is C.**

There are many different types of uterine sarcomas, including endometrial stromal sarcoma, leiomyosarcoma, malignant mixed mullerian tumor, and adenosarcoma. They each have differing presentations and prognosis. Typically all are treated surgically when possible. Adjuvant therapy is controversial, but there does not appear to be a survival benefit to adjuvant radiation therapy for most uterine sarcomas. Uterine leiomyosarcoma has been shown to have a reasonable response to chemotherapy. The combination of gemcitabine and docetaxel in a group of previously treated patients demonstrated a response rate of 53%.

Answer 23.2.34.   **The answer is A.**

Gestational trophoblastic neoplasia (GTN) includes rare gynecologic tumors that represent less than 1% of gynecologic malignancies. These tumors are potentially life threatening but usually should be highly curable when treated appropriately. The most common pathologic entity in GTN is complete hydatidiform mole.

Answer 23.2.35. **The answer is D.**

Beta-hCG is an extremely sensitive and specific marker used in the management of these patients. Patients are typically followed post-evacuation with weekly beta-hCG determinations. The diagnosis of persistent gestational trophoblastic neoplasia is based on the following: a plateau in the level for at least 3 weeks, a 10% or greater increase in the level for three or more values during a 2-week time period, persistence of beta-hCG levels greater than 6 months after evacuation, or histologic evidence of choriocarcinoma.

Answer 23.2.36. **The answer is C.**

Phantom hCG has only recently been recognized. Heterophile antibodies interfere with some immunoassays used to determine hCG levels. This has led to dramatic overtreatment and loss of fertility (hysterectomy) for some patients. If phantom hCG is suspected, urine hCG should be obtained. The heterophile antibodies are not present in the urine, and this test should be negative.

Answer 23.2.37. **The answer is C.**

Treatment for gestational trophoblastic neoplasia is based on risk assessment either by the WHO or FIGO guidelines. Low-risk disease is typically treated with methotrexate or actinomycin-D. Treatment is continued until the hCG levels are normal for 3 consecutive weeks. The patient is then followed monthly for 12 months. Hysterectomy can be offered for patients who have completed child bearing.

Cancer of the Breast

Directions Each of the numbered items below is followed by lettered answers. Select the ONE lettered answer that is BEST in each case unless instructed otherwise.

QUESTIONS

Question 24.1. **Most of the known genes involved in inherited breast cancer are involved in:**

A. Signal transduction
B. DNA repair
C. DNA methylation
D. Cell–cell and cell–matrix interactions

Question 24.2. **Which of the following about BRCA1 is FALSE?**

A. It is located on chromosome 17 (position q12–21).
B. It contributes to multiple functions, including cell-cycle checkpoint control.
C. It shares functional, but not sequence, similarity with BRCA2.
D. It is not a classic tumor suppressor gene because both alleles must be lost or mutated to confer an increased risk of cancer.

Question 24.3. **Compared with sporadic breast cancers, BRCA1-associated breast cancers have a distinct phenotype characterized by:**

A. Intermediate tumor grade
B. Overexpression of TP53
C. Overexpression of C-MYC and cyclin E
D. Estrogen receptor (ER) positive, progesterone receptor (PR) negative by immunohistochemical (IHC) staining

Corresponding Chapter in *Cancer: Principles & Practice of Oncology*, Eighth Edition: 43 (Cancer of the Breast).

Question 24.4.   **Which of the following statements about trastuzumab is FALSE?**

A. It activates natural killer cells and triggers antibody-dependent cytotoxicity.
B. It disrupts heterodimer formation between HER2 and epidermal growth factor receptor (EGFR).
C. It does not alter the expression of Her-2/neu receptors.
D. It decreases tumor microvessel density.

Question 24.5.   **ER-α has both genomic and nongenomic effects. In contrast with the genomic effects, nongenomic effects:**

A. Occur 24 hours after stimulation by estrogen
B. Result in phosphorylation of EGFR and IGF-1R
C. Rarely result in tamoxifen resistance
D. Require binding of ER-α to an estrogen response element (ERE) in regulatory regions of DNA

Question 24.6.   **You are seeing a non-Ashkenazi Jewish woman for a high-risk screening evaluation. Which of the following factors in her family history would be suggestive of a BRCA1 or BRCA2 mutation?**

A. Mother with breast cancer at age 65 years and paternal aunt with breast cancer at age 45 years
B. Maternal cousin (daughter of mother's brother) with initial breast cancer at age 36 years and a second contralateral breast cancer at age 57 years
C. Mother with breast cancer at age 65 years, paternal aunt with breast cancer at age 67 years, and sister with breast cancer at age 47 years
D. Mother with breast cancer at age 52 years and maternal great grandmother with ovarian cancer at age 78 years

Question 24.7.   **Factors that increase the risk of developing breast cancer include all of the following, EXCEPT:**

A. Early menarche or late menopause
B. Age >30 years at time of first pregnancy
C. Nulliparity
D. First or second trimester abortion

Question 24.8.   **Based on the Women's Health Initiative (WHI) Study, the use of postmenopausal combined estrogen and progestin therapy:**

A. Increased the frequency of abnormal mammograms after 1 year
B. Doubled the risk of developing breast cancer after 4 years
C. Doubled the risk of developing breast cancer after 2 years
D. Did not alter the likelihood of having nodal involvement at diagnosis

Question 24.9.   **Which of the following is associated with the highest risk of breast cancer?**

A. Postmenopausal obesity
B. Dense breasts on mammogram
C. Postmenopausal estrogen plus progestin therapy
D. Nulliparity

Question 24.10.   **Current evidence does NOT support the addition of screening breast magnetic resonance imaging (MRI) for which of the following patients?**

A. A 25-year-old woman with a deleterious mutation in BRCA2
B. A 66-year-old woman who underwent lumpectomy and radiation for a high-grade ductal cancer in situ (DCIS) 2 years ago
C. A 32-year-old woman whose sister tested positive for a deleterious mutation in BRCA1 (she has declined testing)
D. A 35-year-old woman who underwent mantle radiation for Hodgkin's disease at age 16 years

Question 24.11.   **The Gail model includes all of the following risk factors, EXCEPT:**

A. First-degree relatives with breast cancer
B. Previous breast biopsies
C. Age at menarche
D. Age at menopause

Question 24.12.   **You are advising a 42-year-old premenopausal woman with a history of atypical hyperplasia on prevention strategies. Which of the following is CORRECT?**

A. Tamoxifen reduces her risk by ~50%.
B. Oophorectomy reduces her risk by ~50% to 65%.
C. Bilateral mastectomy completely eliminates her risk of breast cancer.
D. Raloxifene would provide similar benefit as tamoxifen.

Question 24.13.   **A 58-year-old woman presents to your office with a new palpable breast mass; a biopsy has been recommended based on the results of mammogram and ultrasound. In discussing the options, you explain that:**

A. A biopsy can be deferred if a breast MRI does not show significant enhancement.
B. The false-negative rate of core biopsy is 5% to 10%.
C. Diagnosis by core biopsy decreases the number of surgical procedures required, even in women ultimately found to have cancer.
D. A fine-needle biopsy can distinguish DCIS from invasive cancer.

Question 24.14.   You are asked to advise a woman who underwent core-needle biopsy for evaluation of suspicious microcalcifications detected on screening mammogram. A surgical biopsy should be recommended in all of the following, EXCEPT:

A. Ductal hyperplasia without atypia, calcifications are seen associated with the hyperplasia
B. Radial scar
C. Lobular carcinoma in situ
D. Sclerosing adenosis, no calcifications are identified in the specimen

Question 24.15.   All of the following statements about DCIS are true, EXCEPT:

A. DCIS accounts for 15% to 30% of mammographically detected cancers.
B. DCIS is most common in premenopausal women.
C. Younger women have a higher rate of local recurrence after breast-conserving therapy.
D. Preoperative MRI does not improve surgical planning.

Question 24.16.   The use of radiation therapy (RT) after lumpectomy in patients with DCIS:

A. Improves overall survival
B. Reduces the risk of recurrent DCIS, but not invasive disease, in the treated breast
C. Does not decrease local recurrence when tamoxifen therapy is administered
D. None of the above

Question 24.17.   Which of the following are pathologic subtypes of breast cancer associated with a more favorable prognosis?

A. Metaplastic
B. Scirrhous
C. Tubular
D. Medullary

Question 24.18.   Which of the following findings indicates the presence of stage IV disease?

A. Inflammatory changes in the breast
B. Involvement of the ipsilateral supraclavicular node
C. Extension into the pectoralis muscle
D. None of the above

Question 24.19. **For which of the following patients is a full staging evaluation NOT mandatory?**

A. A patient with a 4-cm tumor with two positive axillary lymph nodes
B. A patient with peau d-orange and palpable axillary lymph nodes
C. A patient with a 4-cm tumor with six involved nodes with extracapsular extension
D. A patient with a 6-cm tumor with clinically apparent internal mammary lymph nodes

Question 24.20. **Which of the following patients is at greatest risk of local recurrence after breast-conserving therapy?**

A. A 65-year-old with a 2-cm grade 1, ER+ tumor, closest margin 3 mm, treated with whole breast radiation therapy (WBRT) (no boost), and an aromatase inhibitor (AI)
B. A 25-year-old with a 2-cm grade 3, ER− tumor, closest margin <1 mm, treated with WBRT (with boost) and no systemic therapy
C. A 35-year-old with a 2-cm grade 2 ER− tumor, closest margin 6 mm, treated with WBRT (with boost) and adjuvant chemotherapy
D. A 65-year-old with a 4-cm grade 1, ER+ tumor, closest margin 4 mm, treated with WBRT (with boost) and an AI

Question 24.21. **Which of the following is an absolute contraindication to breast-conserving surgery (BCS)?**

A. Pregnancy
B. Diffuse malignant-appearing microcalcifications
C. Active rheumatoid arthritis
D. Primary tumor size of 4.8 cm

Question 24.22. **Compared with the use of adjuvant therapy, the use of neoadjuvant therapy:**

A. Increases the potential for BCS
B. Does not provide an opportunity to test the chemosensitivity of the tumor
C. Increases overall survival
D. Decreases the risk of local recurrence

Question 24.23.   **Which of the following statements regarding autologous tissue breast reconstruction is FALSE?**

A. Autologous reconstruction may be performed in patients who will require postmastectomy RT without an excessively high risk of flap loss.
B. Immediate autologous reconstruction does not delay the administration of systemic chemotherapy and may be performed in patients with stage II or III disease.
C. Skin-sparing mastectomy should be avoided because there is a 2% to 4% increase in the risk of local recurrence.
D. Patients undergoing autologous tissue reconstruction may still require a complementary prosthetic implant to achieve a satisfactory cosmetic result.

Question 24.24.   **Which of the following factors is associated with failure to identify the sentinel node?**

A. Tumor located in the lower inner quadrant
B. Increased body mass index
C. Excisional biopsy before sentinel node biopsy (SNB)
D. Invasive lobular carcinoma

Question 24.25.   **Which statement regarding SNB is TRUE?**

A. SNB can be safely performed during pregnancy.
B. SNB is less accurate in patients with multicentric tumors.
C. The incidence of lymphedema is <2% at 12 months.
D. The false-negative rate in multicenter trials is ~10%.

Question 24.26.   **Identify the CORRECT statement:**

A. Radiation after BCS reduces the risk of local recurrence but does not improve overall survival.
B. Radiation after BCS improves breast cancer-specific survival but does not improve overall survival.
C. Radiation improves overall survival when administered after BCS but does not improve overall survival in patients who underwent mastectomy.
D. Improved local control at 5 years results in a proportional improvement in overall survival at 15 years.

Question 24.27.   **Which of the following is both a prognostic and predictive factor?**

A. Axillary node involvement
B. Estrogen receptor
C. Patient age
D. Lymphovascular invasion

Question 24.28.   **The gains associated with adjuvant tamoxifen:**

    A. Are independent of patient age
    B. Are less in patients who also receive adjuvant chemotherapy
    C. Are dependent on patient menopausal status
    D. Decline 10 years after diagnosis

Question 24.29.   **The use of aromatase inhibitors in the adjuvant treatment of postmenopausal women:**

    A. Improves overall survival when used as initial therapy, but not when used after 2 to 5 years of tamoxifen
    B. Increases the risk of fracture for 10 years
    C. Effectively lowers estrogen levels by 90%
    D. Provides increased benefit when administered for 10 years

Question 24.30.   **You are following a 32-year-old with stage II (ER+ /PR+ /HER2−) breast cancer. She completed adjuvant chemotherapy 22 months ago. She continued to menstruate during her chemotherapy and is now receiving tamoxifen. She reports that 3 months ago her primary care physician (PCP) started paroxetine for worsening depressive symptoms. You should:**

    A. Continue tamoxifen and paroxetine.
    B. Discontinue tamoxifen and begin additional hormonal therapy with an AI.
    C. Discuss alternate antidepressant therapy with her PCP.
    D. Continue tamoxifen and paroxetine but add a luteinizing hormone-releasing hormone (LHRH) agonist.

Question 24.31.   **You are seeing a 42-year-old premenopausal patient with newly diagnosed stage I, ER+ /HER2− breast cancer. Her surgeon had requested an OncotypeDX recurrence score assay, which returned with a score of 36. On the basis of her recurrence score, the absolute improvement in her risk of recurrence with the addition of adding cyclophosphamide (CMF) to tamoxifen is predicted to be:**

    A. <5%
    B. 14%
    C. 22%
    D. 30%

Question 24.32.   **You are seeing a 58-year-old woman with stage I breast cancer. She has been taking tamoxifen for 30 months and you have advised switching her hormonal therapy to exemestane on the basis of the IES trial results. In discussing the potential benefits of this strategy compared with continuing tamoxifen for the planned 5 years, you tell her that exemestane:**

    A. Improved disease-free survival by ~25%
    B. Improved overall survival in patients with ER+ disease
    C. Reduced contralateral breast cancers by ~40%
    D. All of the above

Question 24.33. You are seeing a 52-year-old woman with newly diagnosed stage III breast cancer (5.5 cm tumor, 6 + LN, grade 3, ER − /PR − /HER2 + by FISH with ratio 8.7). She asks about the benefits of trastuzumab. On the basis of the updated analysis of the Intergroup adjuvant trials (N9831 and B31), you tell her that the addition of trastuzumab to adjuvant AC>T chemotherapy:

A. Improves relative disease-free survival by 35%
B. Improves relative overall survival by 40%
C. Reduces the probability of distant recurrence by 50%
D. Results in death from congestive heart failure in 5%

Question 24.34. On the basis of the overview analysis, the relative benefits of adjuvant chemotherapy are:

A. Independent of ER status
B. Independent of administration of hormone therapy
C. Greater with anthracycline compared with CMF-type regimens
D. All of the above

Question 24.35. Identify the correct statement regarding the use of taxanes in the adjuvant setting:

A. Concurrent administration with anthracyclines provides superior efficacy compared with sequential regimens.
B. Sequential anthracycline > taxane therapy is superior to anthracycline therapy alone.
C. Docetaxel administered every 3 weeks has greater efficacy than paclitaxel administered weekly.
D. Incorporation of taxanes into adjuvant therapy increases the risk of cardiotoxicity.

Question 24.36. The addition of bevacizumab to paclitaxel as initial chemotherapy for metastatic breast cancer increases all of the following, EXCEPT:

A. Disease-free survival
B. Overall survival
C. Response rate
D. Hypertension

Question 24.37. The addition of lapatinib to capecitabine in patients with advanced HER2 + breast cancer increases all of the following, EXCEPT:

A. Time to progression
B. Rash
C. Diarrhea
D. Overall survival

Question 24.38. **A 67-year-old woman has been taking anastrazole as adjuvant therapy for stage I breast cancer for 4 years. She was recently found to have bone metastases. After RT to a painful lesion at T8, she is asymptomatic. You recommend:**

A. Fulvestrant.
B. Exemestane.
C. Either will be equally effective.
D. Neither will be effective.

Question 24.39. **In a recently reported Phase III trial, the addition of ixapebilone to capecitabine**

A. Increased progression-free survival (PFS) from 4.2 to 5.8 months
B. Increased objective response rate (ORR) based on investigator, but not independent review facility, assessment
C. Increased neutropenia, but not neutropenic fevers
D. All of the above

Question 24.40. **A urologist tells you his mother has just been diagnosed with Paget's disease based on a punch biopsy of an area of crusting on her nipple. You tell him:**

A. It is associated with in situ or invasive breast cancer in only 50% of cases.
B. Approximately half of Paget's disease cases are hormone-receptor positive.
C. It tends to be associated with underlying low-grade disease.
D. Underlying breast cancers are almost always located within 2 cm of the nipple.

Question 24.41. **Which of the following regarding treatment of breast cancer in the pregnant patient is FALSE?**

A. Breast irradiation is contraindicated in the pregnant patient.
B. Mastectomy has no place in the treatment of pregnant patients who have tumors amenable to breast conservation.
C. Adjuvant chemotherapy should be avoided in the first trimester, because almost all chemotherapeutic agents cross the placenta and are associated with a 15% to 20% risk of fetal malformation.
D. Chemotherapy can generally be administered safely during the second and third trimesters of pregnancy; the risk of fetal malformation is 1% to 3% during this time, similar to the risk of fetal malformation in healthy women.

Question 24.42. **Which of the following regarding locally advanced breast cancer is TRUE?**

    A. Chemotherapy given in the adjuvant setting obviates the need for postmastectomy radiation.

    B. Hormonal therapy does not improve outcome.

    C. There is no difference in outcomes regardless of whether chemotherapy is given in the neoadjuvant or the adjuvant setting.

    D. Surgery should be done first to debulk disease and achieve local control.

Question 24.43. **Which of the following does NOT accurately characterize inflammatory breast cancer (IBC)?**

    A. Almost all women with IBC have lymph node involvement.

    B. The 10-year survival rate exceeds 30%.

    C. IBC is staged as T4d, overall stage IIIC.

    D. Dermal lymphatic invasion must be seen on biopsy to confirm IBC.

Question 24.44. **With regard to the clinical and pathologic characteristics of male breast cancer, which of the following is FALSE?**

    A. Male breast cancer is found, more often than female breast cancer, to be estrogen-receptor positive, and the older a man is with breast cancer, the more likely the cancer is estrogen-receptor positive.

    B. Both lobular carcinoma in situ and invasive lobular carcinoma have been reported in male patients.

    C. The most common presenting symptom is a painless, firm subareolar mass, seen in more than 75% of patients.

    D. In addition to a palpable mass, common physical examination findings include changes in the areola with nipple retraction, inversion or fixation, or eczematous skin changes.

Question 24.45. **Concerning the staging and treatment of male breast cancer, which of the following is FALSE?**

    A. The same TNM staging system is used to stage male breast cancer.

    B. Stage and axillary node status are the more important prognostic indicators in male breast cancer.

    C. In cases of DCIS in men, simple mastectomy with axillary node dissection is the treatment of choice.

    D. For localized disease, a simple mastectomy, or modified radical mastectomy, with local radiation treatment is an effective therapy; there are no data to suggest that more extensive surgical resection improves survival.

Question 24.46. **With regard to surveillance for patients with early-stage breast cancer, all of the following are true, EXCEPT:**

A. Screening mammography and breast ultrasound are the only imaging studies recommended for routine surveillance.
B. There is no role for intense surveillance, because early detection of relapse has not been shown to improve overall survival or other meaningful clinical end points.
C. Survival data from surveillance strategies to detect early recurrence of disease may be affected by lead-time bias.
D. Survival data from surveillance strategies to detect early recurrence of disease may be affected by length bias.

ANSWERS

Answer 24.1. **The answer is B.**

Most of the known genes implicated in inherited breast cancer are tumor suppressor genes that have functions involved in DNA repair and replication of genome fidelity. (See text: Molecular Biology of Breast Cancer.) Recent genome-wide screening has also identified common low penetrance single nucleotide polymorphisms (SNPs) in genes that control cell-cycle progression, steroid hormone metabolism, and cell signaling pathways that are associated with an increased risk.

Answer 24.2. **The answer is D.**

BRCA1 is a classic tumor suppressor gene. One inherited defective copy is sufficient for cancer predisposition, but the loss of the second wild-type allele is required for tumorigenesis. (See text: Molecular Biology of Breast Cancer.)

Answer 24.3. **The answer is C.**

BRCA1-associated breast cancers are typically high grade and aggressive, with gene expression profiles similar to the basaloid or triple negative groups. They overexpress C-MYC and cyclin E, and have loss of TP53 and downregulation of p27. (See text: Molecular Biology of Breast Cancer.)

Answer 24.4. **The answer is C.**

Trastuzumab results in downregulation of the HER2 receptor. (See text: Molecular Biology of Breast Cancer.)

Answer 24.5. **The answer is B.**

Nongenomic effects of ER-α occur within seconds to minutes and result from activation of membrane-bound or cytosolic ERs. These nonnuclear ERs rapidly activate other kinases including EGFR and IGF-1R, resulting in both acquired and de novo tamoxifen resistance. (See text: Molecular Biology of Breast Cancer.)

Answer 24.6.   **The answer is C.**

The family history in this scenario includes breast cancer in two first-degree relatives, one diagnosed by the age of 50 years. (See *PPO* Table 43.2.1 for other considerations.)

Answer 24.7.   **The answer is D.**

Hormonal factors that increase total estrogen exposure increase the risk of developing breast cancer. Abortion, whether spontaneous or induced, does not increase breast cancer risk. (See text: 43.2 Hormonal Factors.)

Answer 24.8.   **The answer is A.**

In the WHI study, combined estrogen and progestin increased the risk of developing breast cancer with a hazard ratio of 1.24. The increase in breast cancer was detected at 2 years, but an excess of abnormal mammograms was apparent at 1 year. Hormone replacement therapy (HRT) users were more likely to have nodal involvement or distant metastases at diagnosis. (See text: 43.2 Hormonal Factors.)

Answer 24.9.   **The answer is B.**

Hormonal risk factors typically have relative risks of less than 2. Mammographic breast density is an underappreciated risk factor with a relative risk of 2 to 4. Factors associated with a relative risk more than 4 include atypical hyperplasia, LCIS, BRCA1, or BRCA2 mutation and radiation exposure before age 40 years. (See *PPO* Table 43.2.2.)

Answer 24.10.   **The answer is B.**

American Society of Clinical Oncology (ASCO) guidelines for MR screening were revised in 2007. Current evidence supports screening MR in patients with a known BRCA mutation, untested first-degree relatives of BRCA mutation carriers, or patients with an estimated 20% to 25% lifetime risk of breast cancer (e.g., someone who received mantle radiation at age 16 years). There is currently insufficient evidence to recommend for or against MR screening for patients with a personal history of breast cancer. (See *PPO* Table 43.2.3.)

Answer 24.11.   **The answer is D.**

The Gail model estimates a woman's risk of developing breast cancer on the basis of age at menarche, age at first live birth, number of previous breast biopsies and presence of atypia, and the number of first-degree female relatives with breast cancer. It may underestimate the risk in women with a strong family history, because it does not include second-degree relatives, men with breast cancer, or relatives with ovarian cancer. (See text: Management of the High-Risk Patient.)

Answer 24.12.   **The answer is B.**

In the P1 trial, tamoxifen reduced the risk of breast cancer by 84% in patients with atypical hyperplasia. Although raloxifene provided similar benefits with a more favorable safety profile than tamoxifen in the STAR trial, this trial only included postmenopausal women. Oophorectomy before menopause decreases the risk of breast cancer by 50% to 65% depending on age at the time of surgery. Although bilateral mastectomy decreases the risk by more than 90%, the risk is not completely eliminated. (See text: Management of the High-Risk Patient.)

Answer 24.13.   **The answer is C.**

If cytopathologist expertise is available, FNA can reliably diagnosis cancer but cannot distinguish DCIS from invasive disease. The false-negative rate is 5% to 10% for FNA but less than 4% for core biopsy. In a prospective study of 1550 patients undergoing biopsy for mammographic abnormalities, core biopsy reduced the number of surgical procedures. (See text: Diagnosis and Biopsy.)

Answer 24.14.   **The answer is A.**

Ductal hyperplasia without atypia (a.k.a. usual type hyperplasia) is not an indication for surgical biopsy. (See *PPO* Table 43.2.8 for other indications.)

Answer 24.15.   **The answer is B.**

DCIS is most common among women ages 49 to 69 years. Several studies have reported an increased risk of local recurrence in younger women. Initial studies suggested that MRI can both over- and underestimate the extent of DCIS and does not improve surgical planning. (See text: Ductal Carcinoma In Situ.)

Answer 24.16.   **The answer is D.**

The use of RT after BCS for DCIS reduces both invasive and noninvasive recurrences but does not alter overall survival. (See text: Ductal Carcinoma In Situ.)

Answer 24.17.   **The answer is C.**

Subtypes with a more favorable prognosis include breast cancers with tubular, mucinous, papillary, or cribriform features. (See text: Pathology of Breast Cancer.)

Answer 24.18.   **The answer is D.**

Stage IV disease is defined as the presence of distant metastatic involvement. None of the examples given are considered distant sites by the current American Joint Committee on Cancer Staging Criteria. (See *PPO* Table 43.2.10.)

Answer 24.19.   **The answer is A.**

The first patient has T2N1 disease (stage IIB). Staging data for more than 400 patients have been reviewed to ascertain which patients are more likely to have metastatic disease, and therefore, for whom a complete staging workup is more likely to yield useful information (Ravaioli A, Tassinari G, Pasini G, et al. Staging of breast cancer: what standards should be used in research and clinical practice? Ann Oncol 1998;9: 1173–1177). Three different risk groups were defined. Groups I (T1N0-1) and II (T2N0-1) were found to be at relatively low risk for having metastatic disease; the detection rate for metastatic disease was less than 3%. Group III (T4N1, or patients with N2 disease) had substantially higher risk. The yield for an evaluation for metastatic disease was closer to 15%. As such, staging is asymptomatic patients presenting with stage I or II disease is not recommended.

Answer 24.20.   **The answer is B.**

This patient has multiple risk factors for local recurrence, including young age (<35 to 40 years), close (though not frankly involved) margins, high-grade histology, and lack of use of systemic therapy. (See text: Risk Factors for Local Recurrence.)

Answer 24.21.   **The answer is B.**

Although pregnancy is an absolute contraindication to breast radiation, it is possible to perform BCS in the third trimester and RT after delivery. Although patients with active scleroderma or systemic lupus are at higher risk for complications of RT, rheumatoid arthritis is not a contraindication. There is no absolute upper size limit for BCS, but the impact of removing a larger tumor on cosmesis must be considered. (See text: Contraindication to Breast-Conserving Surgery.)

Answer 24.22.   **The answer is A.**

Although administering chemotherapy in the neoadjuvant setting does not confer a survival benefit, it may allow breast conservation in patients who would have otherwise required mastectomy. However, there is a slightly higher risk of local recurrence in patients who require neoadjuvant chemotherapy to undergo BCS compared with patients who are initial candidates for BCS. (See text: Preoperative Systemic Therapy.)

Answer 24.23.   **The answer is C.**

Skin-sparing mastectomy does not alter the risk of local recurrence. Contrary to initial concerns, immediate reconstruction does not alter the risk of local recurrence, limit ability to detect local recurrence, or delay initiation of systemic therapy. Although fat necrosis, fibrosis, and volume loss are common with RT after autologous reconstruction, complete flap loss is rare. (See text: Mastectomy.)

Answer 24.24.   **The answer is B.**

In the ACOSOG Z10 trial, increasing age, body mass index, and surgical sites with fewer than 50 patients enrolled were associated with a decrease in sentinel node identification rate. (See text: Management of the Axilla.)

Answer 24.25.   **The answer is D.**

Pregnancy and lactation are contraindications to SNB. Although T3 and multicentric tumors were initially thought to be contraindications, recent data suggest that SNB is accurate in these situations. Although lymphedema is less common after SNB than with traditional axillary dissection, lymphedema was reported in approximately 5% of patients at 12 months in the ALMANAC trial. (See text: Management of the Axilla.)

Answer 24.26.   **The answer is D.**

On the basis of the most recent Early Breast Cancer Trialists' Collaborative Group findings, improved local control at 5 years results in a proportional improvement overall survival at 15 years. This was true whether improved local control was obtained by more extensive surgery or the addition of radiation. (See text: Local-Regional Therapy and Survival.)

Answer 24.27.   **The answer is B.**

A prognostic factor is defined as a measurement taken at diagnosis that is associated with outcome. A predictive factor is a measurement that predicts response or lack of response to a specific therapy. Estrogen receptor is both prognostic and predictive of benefit from hormonal therapies. The other factors are prognostic but not predictive. (See text: Prognostic and Predictive Factors.)

Answer 24.28.   **The answer is A.**

Adjuvant tamoxifen results in an improvement in overall survival for at least 15 years. The benefits are independent of age, menopausal status, and the use of chemotherapy. (See text: Adjuvant Endocrine Therapy.)

Answer 24.29.   **The answer is C.**

AIs lower estrogen levels by 90% in postmenopausal women. To date, no study has shown a survival advantage, and the optimal duration of therapy is unknown. AIs increase the risk of fracture during therapy, but that risk appears to revert to baseline levels once therapy has been discontinued. (See text: Adjuvant Endocrine Therapy.)

Answer 24.30.   **The answer is C.**

Tamoxifen must be converted to its active metabolite endoxifen via CYP2D6-mediated hydroxylation. Both CYP2D6 genotype and coadministration of potent CYP2D6 inhibitors such as paroxetine decrease the plasma concentration of endoxifen. Retrospective analyses suggest that in postmenopausal women receiving tamoxifen for early breast cancer, impaired CYP2D6 metabolism, whether by genetic variation and enzyme inhibition, is associated with a higher risk of recurrence. (See text: Adjuvant Endocrine Therapy. See also Stearns V, Johnson MD, Rae JM, et al. Active tamoxifen metabolite plasma concentrations after coadministration of tamoxifen and the selective serotonin reuptake inhibitor paroxetine. J Natl Cancer Inst 2003;95:1758–1764; Jin Y, Desta Z, Stearns V, et al. CYP2D6 genotype, antidepressant use, and tamoxifen metabolism during adjuvant breast cancer treatment. J Natl Cancer Inst 2005;97: 30–39.)

Answer 24.31.   **The answer is C.**

The OncotypeDX assay classifies patients by expression of 16 cancer-related genes (normalized to the expression of five reference genes) into low-, intermediate-, and high-risk groups. In NSABP B-20, the addition of chemotherapy to tamoxifen did not improve distant recurrence-free survival (DRFS) at 10 years in patients with a low or intermediate recurrence score (RS). However, in patients with a high RS, the DRFS at 10 years improved from 60% to 82% with the addition of CMF. (See text: Molecular and Genomic Factors.)

Answer 24.32.   **The answer is D.**

Disease-free survival (DFS) was improved by 24%, and time to contralateral breast cancer was reduced by 43%. Although overall survival was not improved in the entire study population ($p = .08$), analysis of patients with known ER+ disease did find a significant improvement in survival. (See text: Adjuvant Endocrine Therapy. See also Coombes RC, Hall E, Gibson LJ, et al. A randomized trial of exemestane after two to three years of tamoxifen therapy in postmenopausal women with primary breast cancer. N Engl J Med 2004;350:1081–1092; Coombes R, Paridaens R, Jassem J, et al. First mature survival analysis of Intergroup Estemestane Study: A randomized trial in disease-free patients with early breast cancer randomized to continue tamoxifen or switch to exemestane following an initial 2–3 years of adjuvant tamoxifen. Proc Am Soc Clin Oncol 2006; 24:9s.)

Answer 24.33.   **The answer is C.**

Despite the crossover effects after the trial was unblinded, the most recent update of the combined analysis continued to show a similar impact on DFS (~50%), distant DFS (~50%), and overall survival (OS) (~30%). Among 875 patients randomized to trastuzumab and chemotherapy, there were 22 cases of congestive heart failure but no cardiac deaths. In the control arm there was only one case of CHF, and one cardiac death was reported. (See text: Adjuvant Trastuzumab. See also Romond EH, Perez EA, Bryant J, et al. Trastuzumab plus adjuvant chemotherapy for operable HER2-positive breast cancer. N Engl J Med 2005; 353:1673–1684.)

Answer 24.34.   **The answer is D.**

The relative benefits of chemotherapy are independent of age, ER status, and use of hormonal therapy, although the absolute benefits will differ according to baseline risk. (See text: Adjuvant Chemotherapy.)

Answer 24.35.   **The answer is B.**

Approximately 12 studies have evaluated the incorporation of the tax-anes, either sequentially or concurrently, into anthracycline-based adju-vant therapy. Although most studies report an improved outcome, no clearly superior regimen has emerged. In the E1199 trial, no difference was identified with docetaxel or paclitaxel administered weekly or every 3 weeks. (See text: Adjuvant Chemotherapy.)

Answer 24.36.   **The answer is B.**

The addition of bevacizumab to paclitaxel significantly prolonged PFS (11.8 vs. 5.9 months; hazard ratio [HR] = 0.60, $p < .001$) and increased objective response rate (36.9% vs. 21.2%; $p < .001$), but median overall survival was similar in both groups (26.7 vs. 25.2 months; HR = 0.88, $p = .16$). Grade 3/4 hypertension (15% vs. 0%; $p = .001$) and cerebro-vascular ischemia (2% vs. 0%; $p = .009$) were both more frequent in patients receiving paclitaxel + bevacizumab. (See text: Antiangiogenesis Therapy for Advanced Breast Cancer. See also Miller K, Wang M, Gralow J, et al. Paclitaxel plus bevacizumab versus paclitaxel alone for metastatic breast cancer. N Engl J Med 2007;357:2666–2676.)

Answer 24.37.   **The answer is D.**

The addition of lapatinib to capecitabine in patients with advanced HER2+ breast cancer increased time to progression (TTP) (HR 0.49; $p < .001$). The most common toxicities were diarrhea, hand-foot syn-drome, nausea, fatigue, vomiting, and rash. Diarrhea and rash were sig-nificantly more frequent in patients receiving combined therapy. Al-though OS data are not yet mature, to date there is no improvement in OS. (See text: Anti-HER2 Therapy for Metastatic Breast Cancer. See also Geyer CE, Forster J, Lindquist D, et al. Lapatinib plus capecitabine for HER2-positive advanced breast cancer. N Engl J Med 2006;355:2733.)

Answer 24.38.   **The answer is C.**

The EFECT trial compared fulvestrant and exemestane in postmenopau-sal women progressing on a nonsteroidal AI. Response rate, clinical bene-fit, and time to progression were identical, suggesting either fulvestrant or exemestane would be reasonable options. However, the EFECT trial used a loading dose of fulvestrant (500 mg on day 0, 250 mg on days 14 and 28, and then monthly) to achieve steady-state potentially therapeutic levels within the first month. (See text: Endocrine Therapy for Metastatic Breast Cancer. See also Gradishar W, Chia S, Piccart-Gebhart M, et al. Fulvestrant versus exemestane following prior non-steroidal aromatase inhibitor therapy: first results from EFECT, a randomized phase II trial in postmenopausal women with advanced breast cancer. Breast Cancer Res and Treat 2006;100:S8–S9.)

Answer 24.39.   **The answer is A.**

Ixabepilone increased ORR by both the investigator (23% vs. 42%) and independent radiologic review (IRR) (14% vs. 35%). Ixabepilone causes significantly more neutropenia (11% vs. 68%) than capecitabine alone. Neutropenic fevers were uncommon but were increased with ixabepilone (<1% vs. 4%, $p <.001$). (See Thomas ES, Gomez HL, Li RK, et al. Ixabepilone plus capecitabine for metastatic breast cancer progressing after anthracycline and taxane treatment. J Clin Oncol 2007;25: 5210–5217.)

Answer 24.40.   **The answer is B.**

An underlying malignancy is found in approximately 97% of patients with Paget's disease, frequently with high-grade histology. It is not uncommon for an underlying tumor to be several centimeters away from the nipple. Half of cases are hormone-receptor negative, consistent with the higher rate of underlying high-grade tumors. (See text: Paget's Disease. See also Chaudary Ma, Millis RR, Lane EB, et al. Paget's disease of the nipple: a ten year review including clinical, pathological, and immunohistochemical findings. Breast Cancer Res 1986;8:139–146; Marshall JK, Giffith KA, Haffty BG, et al. Conservative management of Paget disease of the breast with radiotherapy; 10- and 15-year results. Cancer 2003; 97:2142–2149.)

Answer 24.41.   **The answer is B.**

Because breast irradiation is contraindicated in the pregnant patient, mastectomy may prove to be a more appropriate management approach even in patients with tumors amenable to breast conservation, particularly in women early in pregnancy. (See text: Breast Cancer and Pregnancy.)

Answer 24.42.   **The answer is C.**

Neoadjuvant chemotherapy plays a multifaceted role in the treatment of locally advanced breast cancer. It may downsize a tumor, making it more amenable to breast-conserving treatment or helping to achieve a more acceptable cosmetic result. It may downstage the patient's disease by decreasing the number of positive axillary lymph nodes, thereby improving survival. Giving neoadjuvant chemotherapy allows the oncologist to gauge the chemosensitivity of the tumor. Regardless of whether chemotherapy is given in the neoadjuvant or adjuvant setting, postsurgical radiation is still required, and the outcome is the same. Hormonal therapy improves outcome and should be given after any additional adjuvant treatment. (See text: Locally Advanced and Inflammatory Cancer.)

Answer 24.43.   **The answer is D.**

IBC is a clinical diagnosis. Dermal lymphatic invasion on full-thickness skin biopsy is often seen but is not required for diagnosis. Most women will have lymph node involvement. In the absence of distant metastases, IBC is staged as T4d, stage IIIC disease (See text: Locally Advanced and Inflammatory Cancer.)

Answer 24.44.   **The answer is A.**

Approximately 80% of cases of male breast cancer are estrogen-receptor positive, presumably because men are effectively postmenopausal. There does not appear to be a difference in the chances a tumor will be estrogen-receptor positive depending on the age of a male patient with breast cancer. (See text: Male Breast Cancer.)

Answer 24.45.   **The answer is C.**

As in women, DCIS is primarily a local disease with excellent prognosis, and axillary node dissection is not necessary. (See text: Male Breast Cancer.)

Answer 24.46.   **The answer is A.**

It is not clear that early detection of distant metastatic disease improves clinically important outcomes. As such, screening mammography is the only imaging study recommended for routine surveillance in asymptomatic patients. A woman should have a mammogram of her conserved breast annually, beginning no more than 6 months after completion of radiotherapy. (See *PPO* Table 43.2.21.)

Rami Y. Haddad
Mouhammed Amir Habra

Cancer of the Endocrine System

| Directions | Each of the numbered items below is followed by lettered answers. Select the ONE lettered answer that is BEST in each case unless instructed otherwise. |

QUESTIONS

Question 25.1. A 37-year-old woman presents with a right anterior neck mass. She denies dysphagia or hoarseness. There is no history of radiation exposure or family history of cancer, and no palpable nodes are detected on physical examination. Neck ultrasound reveals a 2.5-cm right thyroid solid nodule without enlarged cervical lymph nodes. Fine-needle aspiration (FNA) suggests the diagnosis of papillary thyroid carcinoma. You recommend which one of the following as the initial management plan?

   A.   Total thyroidectomy
   B.   Right thyroid lobectomy
   C.   Total thyroidectomy with modified right neck dissection
   D.   Total thyroidectomy with bilateral neck dissection

Question 25.2. A 39-year-old woman underwent right thyroid lobectomy and isthmusectomy after the incidental discovery of a 0.8-cm right thyroid nodule with indeterminate FNA. On preoperative neck ultrasound, the left thyroid lobe appeared normal and there was no evidence of abnormal lymph nodes. Pathological examination revealed a 0.75-cm intrathyroidal papillary carcinoma. The most appropriate management now is:

   A.   Thyroid hormone replacement if needed without further resection.
   B.   Radioactive iodine scan followed by radioactive iodine ablation if there is neck uptake.
   C.   Surgical resection of remaining thyroid tissue followed by radioactive iodine ablation.
   D.   Radioactive iodine ablation followed by thyroid hormone suppression.

Corresponding Chapter in *Cancer: Principles & Practice of Oncology*, Eighth Edition: 44 (Cancer of the Endocrine System).

Question 25.3.   A 42-year-old woman underwent FNA of a 3-cm left thyroid mass. No palpable nodes were detected on physical examination or imaging. FNA was suspicious of thyroid malignancy. What is the most appropriate next step?

A. Total thyroidectomy.
B. Left lobectomy but with fresh-frozen section to plan immediate further resection.
C. Left complete lobectomy and isthmusectomy, to be followed by total thyroidectomy later if malignancy is confirmed.
D. Plan to repeat FNA for further tissue evaluation.

Question 25.4.   A 41-year-old woman, who was treated 4 years ago for papillary thyroid carcinoma with total thyroidectomy and bilateral neck dissection followed by radioactive iodine ablation, is found on follow-up to have an elevated thyroglobulin (TG) level (16 ng/mL) with negative TG antibodies. Diagnostic whole-body iodine scan is negative, and thyroid-stimulating hormone (TSH) is suppressed. What is the most appropriate next step?

A. Chest radiograph
B. Positron emission tomography (PET) scan
C. Surveillance
D. Neck imaging

Question 25.5.   A 24-year-old woman underwent FNA of a left thyroid nodule, which showed cells suspicious of neuroendocrine origin. She has been experiencing intermittent diarrhea for the past 4 months. Family history includes kidney stones in several members. The rest of the history and physical examination results are normal. What is the most appropriate next step?

A. Obtain metanephrines and catecholamines/serum calcium/serum calcitonin/carcinoembryonic antigen (CEA)/RET proto-oncogene.
B. Obtain serum calcitonin/thyroglobulin/calcium/RET proto-oncogene, and then perform a total thyroidectomy.
C. Measure metanephrines and catecholamines/serum calcium/calcitonin/CEA.
D. Perform a total thyroidectomy now, and then obtain postoperative evaluation.

Question 25.6.   A 54-year-old man underwent total thyroidectomy for suspected papillary thyroid carcinoma on FNA. Pathological examination confirmed a 3-cm papillary carcinoma in the right lobe, without extracapsular extension; all nodes examined were free of cancer. You recommend which one of the following?

A. Radiation therapy
B. Radioactive iodine ablation
C. Chemotherapy
D. Concurrent chemotherapy and radiotherapy
E. Observation only

Question 25.7.   A 64-year-old man was found to have an abnormal PET scan on follow-up. He was diagnosed with papillary thyroid carcinoma 10 ago. He was treated with total thyroidectomy and radioactive iodine ablation; follow-up iodine scans have always been normal. He presents now with dysphagia. TG level is found to be 80 ng/mL with negative anti-TG antibodies and suppressed TSH. Computed tomography (CT) chest scan reveals a 3-cm mass in the upper chest causing mild esophageal compression corresponding to PET findings. You recommend which one of the following as the best initial approach?

A. Esophageal stent placement
B. External beam radiotherapy
C. Cytotoxic chemotherapy
D. Radioactive iodine ablation
E. Surgical resection to achieve local control, possibly followed by external beam radiation therapy

Question 25.8.   A 34-year-old woman who was treated with external beam radiation for Hodgkin's lymphoma when she was 14 years old was recently diagnosed with papillary thyroid carcinoma. Which genetic defect is expected to be found in this case?

A. BRAF mutation
B. APC gene mutation
C. RET proto-oncogene mutation
D. RET/PTC rearrangement

Question 25.9.   Which of the following factors is (are) considered poor prognostic features of papillary thyroid carcinoma?

A. Age; men >40 years
B. Tumor size >5 cm
C. Extracapsular invasion
D. All of the above

Question 25.10.   A 35-year-old woman is found to have bilateral lung nodules on chest CT scan. Six years ago she underwent total thyroidectomy for a 3-cm papillary thyroid carcinoma, followed by radioiodine ablation. She was lost to follow-up until she recently presented with a cough. Serum TG level is found to be 192 ng/mL. Chest CT with intravenous contrast shows small bilateral lung nodules. Biopsy obtained by thoracoscopy shows papillary histology. A whole-body radioiodine scan reveals no iodine-avid lesions. TSH is suppressed. A well-healed scar is seen on the neck, with no palpable nodes detected, and the rest of the examination shows normal results. Which is the most appropriate next step?

A. Chemotherapy
B. Repeat iodine scan in 6 to 8 weeks
C. Surgical resection of the lung nodules
D. External beam radiation

Question 25.11.   **Which of the following is TRUE regarding medullary thyroid carcinoma (MTC)?**

A. Genetic testing is not indicated in the absence of family history of MTC.

B. Plasma metanephrines should be obtained within a few weeks after thyroidectomy.

C. It is associated with radiation exposure.

D. It arises from the parafollicular C cells in the thyroid gland.

Question 25.12.   **A 67-year-old man presents with a rapidly growing mass on the anterior part of the neck that is associated with progressive hoarseness. He also reports a 12-lb weight loss. The remainder of his history is significant for hypertension. Physical examination reveals mild respiratory distress, a 6-cm mass on the anterior part of the neck, and adequate air entry. Core needle biopsy confirms anaplastic thyroid carcinoma. CT scan shows a thyroid mass with local invasion and multiple bilateral lung nodules. Laboratory test results are normal. What is the most appropriate management now?**

A. Surgical debulking followed by adjuvant radioiodine

B. Radioactive iodine alone

C. Concurrent chemoradiation

D. Doxorubicin-based chemotherapy

Question 25.13.   **Which one of the following should be considered in the staging of medullary thyroid carcinoma?**

A. Complete contrast-enhanced CT scan

B. Serum CEA and calcitonin

C. Bone survey

D. Octreoscan

E. All of the above

Question 25.14.   **All of the following are true regarding Hurthle cell carcinoma, EXCEPT:**

A. It is a papillary carcinoma variant.

B. It is also known as Oxyphil cell carcinoma.

C. It has a worse prognosis than papillary or follicular carcinoma.

D. It is less iodine-avid than papillary or follicular carcinoma.

Question 25.15.   **Which of the following is TRUE about anaplastic thyroid carcinoma?**

A. 6% of all thyroid cancers

B. Always stage IV

C. Slow growing and can be curable

D. Treated mainly with radioactive iodine

Question 25.16.   **The most commonly used chemotherapeutic agent(s) in metastatic thyroid carcinoma is (are):**

     A.   Methotrexate (MTX)
     B.   Cisplatin
     C.   5-fluorouracil (5FU)
     D.   Doxorubicin (Adriamycin)

Question 25.17.   **Parathyroid carcinoma is suspected in a 48-year-old man. He presented with symptoms of hypercalcemia and was treated with standard approach. Parathyroid hormone (PTH) level is markedly elevated; calcium level is 16 mg/dL on presentation. PTH sestamibi scan showed an intense uptake in the left superior parathyroid gland. CT of the neck showed a 3-cm mass corresponding to the PTH scan findings. What is the most appropriate management?**

     A.   Total or subtotal parathyroidectomy
     B.   Single gland resection followed by external beam irradiation to the neck
     C.   External beam irradiation alone
     D.   Radioactive iodine ablation

Question 25.18.   **Which of the following can be used to treat malignant hypercalcemia related to metastatic parathyroid carcinoma?**

     A.   Cinacalcet (Sensipar)
     B.   Mithramycin
     C.   Intravenous (IV) hydration
     D.   IV bisphosphonates
     E.   All of the above

Question 25.19.   **Which of the following genetic defects is most likely associated with parathyroid carcinoma?**

     A.   Mutations of the HRPT2 gene (1q25-31)
     B.   Allelic loss in several chromosomes
     C.   RET proto-oncogene mutation
     D.   All of the above

Question 25.20.   **Which of the following is a TRUE statement regarding parathyroid carcinoma?**

     A.   If a neck mass is palpated, parathyroid carcinoma should be suspected.
     B.   Reported overall 5-year survival rate is approximately 30%.
     C.   TNM staging corresponds to prognosis.

Question 25.21. A 36-year-old man presents to his primary physician reporting reduced libido for the past 9 months. He also reports periodic epigastric pain associated with occasional heartburn. His medical history includes two episodes of kidney stones in the past 10 years. Family history includes kidney stone formation in his father. Physical examination results are unremarkable. Laboratory evaluation showed prolactin level of 180 ng/mL, testosterone level of 90 ng/dL, serum calcium of 10.9, and PTH level of 110 pg/mL. Magnetic resonance imaging (MRI) of the brain revealed a 1.5-cm mass in the sella without evidence of damage of the surrounding structures. CT scan of the abdomen did not reveal any abnormality. What is the appropriate management of this patient?

A. Subtotal parathyroidectomy

B. Dopamine agonists (bromocriptine) with subtotal parathyroidectomy

C. Transsphenoidal pituitary resection with subtotal parathyroidectomy

Question 25.22. All of the following are considered to be part of MEN1, EXCEPT:

A. Pituitary adenoma

B. Carcinoids

C. Medullary thyroid carcinoma

D. Benign adrenal tumors

Question 25.23. The following are considered to be part of MEN2A syndrome, EXCEPT:

A. Medullary thyroid carcinoma

B. Pheochromocytoma

C. Parathyroid adenoma

D. Diffuse neuronal hypertrophy

Question 25.24. What is the best approach to individuals with kindreds with MEN2A who are interested in screening and prevention?

A. Screen for RET mutation

B. Periodic imaging

C. Periodic laboratory tests

D. Clinical surveillance

Question 25.25. What is the genetic defect that is likely to be associated with MEN1?

A. RET proto-oncogene

B. MENIN gene

C. APC gene

D. HRPT2 gene

Question 25.26. **RET proto-oncogene mutation is associated with which of the following condition(s)?**

A. MEN2
B. Hirschsprung disease
C. MTC
D. A and B

Question 25.27. **A 48-year-old woman presents with amenorrhea for the past 5 months. She also reports appearance of facial hair, development of new acne lesions on the face, and recent unexplained weight gain. Medical history is unremarkable. On physical examination, blood pressure (BP) is 130/82 mm Hg, weight is 195 lbs, thick facial hair and multiple acne-like lesions on the face are noted, and the remainder of the examination is normal. CT scan of the abdomen reveals a 6-cm mass in the left adrenal gland without other identified lesions. What is the most appropriate plan of management?**

A. Percutaneous image-guided needle biopsy
B. Metabolic workup followed by surgical resection
C. Observation and reassurance that symptoms are related to menopause
D. Metabolic workup followed by mitotane

Question 25.28. **Recurrent metastatic pheochromocytoma can be treated by all of the following, EXCEPT:**

A. Systemic chemotherapy combination chemotherapy cyclophosphamide, vincristine, and doxorubicin (CVD)
B. High-dose meta-iodo-benzyl-guanidine (MIBG) therapy
C. External beam radiation
D. Mitotane

Question 25.29. **All of the following are true regarding carcinoid tumors, EXCEPT:**

A. The most common site is the small bowel, followed by the rectum.
B. Diarrhea, flushing, and bronchospasm are classic features.
C. Complete surgical resection of all neoplastic tissue is the preferred therapy.
D. Diarrhea can be controlled with long-acting octreotide.
E. External beam radiation is ineffective in treating this disease.

Question 25.30. **Adrenocortical carcinoma is favored over adenoma by which of the following CT scan features?**

A. Size >6 cm
B. Density of <10 Hounsfield units on nonenhanced CT
C. Washout of >50% at 15 minutes after contrast
D. Homogenous appearance

Question 25.31. **All of the following are true about pheochromocytoma, EXCEPT:**

A. It arises from the adrenal medulla in 50% of the cases.
B. Most tumors of adrenal origin are not malignant.
C. Extra-adrenal tumors have increased risk of malignancy.
D. It may be associated with mutated RET proto-oncogene.

Question 25.32. **All of the following statements are true regarding mitotane, EXCEPT:**

A. It treats metastatic adrenocortical carcinoma.
B. It has significant gastrointestinal and neurological side effects.
C. It can improve hormonal production.
D. Mitotane levels should be monitored.
E. Overall survival benefit has been confirmed.

Question 25.33. **All of the following statements are true regarding insulinoma, EXCEPT:**

A. Whipple's triad consists of symptoms of hypoglycemia when blood glucose decreases and relief of symptoms with correction of glucose levels.
B. It is frequently malignant.
C. Surgery is indicated in most cases.
D. MEN1 should be suspected.

Question 25.34. **Excessive secretion of all the following will lead to diarrhea, EXCEPT:**

A. Gastrin
B. Serum vasoactive intestinal peptide (VIP)
C. 5-hydroxy indole acetic acid (5-HIAA)
D. Insulin

Question 25.35. **All of the following are true regarding pancreatic endocrine tumors, EXCEPT:**

A. Classified as APUDomas.
B. Gastrinoma is the least malignant.
C. Malignancy is established by the presence of metastasis.
D. Glucagonoma arises from alpha cells.
E. Insulinoma arises from beta cells.

ANSWERS

Answer 25.1. **The answer is A.**

Total thyroidectomy alone and without neck dissection is the appropriate initial management in this patient with well-differentiated papillary thyroid carcinoma, especially in the absence of palpable lymph nodes or abnormal lymph nodes on ultrasound.

Answer 25.2. **The answer is A.**

The patient has microscopic papillary thyroid carcinoma, typically defined as a solitary tumor, less than 1.0 to 1.5 cm, with the absence of lymph node involvement. There is no need for further surgical resection beyond lobectomy and intraoperative examination of the contralateral lobe in this case. Thyroid hormone replacement might be needed post-operatively.

Answer 25.3.   **The answer is C.**

The appropriate management is complete lobectomy and isthmusec-tomy, to be followed by total thyroidectomy later if malignancy is con-firmed. This is especially true in cases of suspected follicular carcinoma, because FNA does not distinguish benign from malignant follicular pa-thology. Intraoperative frozen section would not be of great help in this regard. The finding of vascular or capsular invasion on final pathological examination will help to determine the diagnosis.

Answer 25.4.   **The answer is B.**

Patients with thyroid carcinoma are typically followed up with TG levels and iodine scan. TG levels are very sensitive, particularly when TSH is suppressed. In the face of negative iodine scan, and particularly when TG level is greater than 10, distant metastatic disease is suspected. PET scan is most helpful in these cases where thyroid cancer dedifferentiates and loses iodine uptake.

Answer 25.5.   **The answer is A.**

Medullary thyroid carcinoma (MTC) is a neuroendocrine tumor. The hallmark is elevated serum calcitonin, which is produced by the parafol-licular cells (thyroid C cells). CEA is another tumor marker of this dis-ease, but less specific, because it can be elevated in other malignancies. MTC can be part of MEN2A, which includes pheochromocytoma, and it must be ruled out before any surgery. Germline mutation causes famil-ial non-MEN MTC, MEN2A, and MEN2B. RET proto-oncogene has be-come a standard test in the evaluation of newly diagnosed MTC.

Answer 25.6.   **The answer is B.**

Radioactive iodine ablation is indicated in patients with high-risk features despite complete excision. Male patients aged more than 40 years are considered to be in this category. Other high-risk features include female patients aged more than 50 years, incomplete excision, capsular invasion, and tumor size more than 5 cm.

Answer 25.7.   **The answer is E.**

This is an example of dedifferentiated papillary thyroid carcinoma, where the cancer no longer shows uptake of iodine but can be detected on PET scan. Another caveat in this case is the recognition of recom-mended long-term follow-up, perhaps indefinitely. In thyroid carcinoma, TG level is very sensitive, particularly when TSH is suppressed, and this is also true in dedifferentiated thyroid carcinoma. Chemotherapy has been disappointing in this disease. Surgical resection, and perhaps external beam radiation, is his best option to achieve local control and relief of symptoms.

Answer 25.8.   **The answer is D.**

RET/PTC rearrangements are found in about 20% of papillary thyroid carcinoma in general, and in 60% to 80% of those occurring after irradiation. BRAF mutation can be found in patients with papillary thyroid carcinoma, but it is not associated with radiation exposure. APC gene mutation is found in patients with familial adenomatous polyposis, and some of these patients might develop differentiated thyroid carcinoma. RET proto-oncogene mutations are associated with MEN2.

Answer 25.9.   **The answer is D.**

All of the listed features indicate poor prognosis. Additional poor prognostic features include women aged more than 50 years and the presence of distant metastasis. These features can be remembered by the acronym AMES (age, metastasis, extracapsular invasion, size).

Answer 25.10.   **The answer is B.**

This case highlights the importance of the fact that intravenous contrast with diagnostic CT scan interferes with the thyroid cancer uptake of iodine during radioactive iodine scan. This test should be done at least 6 to 8 weeks after iodine-contrast CT scan to allow the excretion of the circulating iodine pool; 24-hour urinary iodine can be measured before repeat iodine scanning in these cases.

Answer 25.11.   **The answer is D.**

MTC arises from the parafollicular C cells in the thyroid gland and is not associated with radiation exposure. RET proto-oncogene testing is indicated even in the absence of family history. Pheochromocytoma must be ruled out before any surgical resection by measuring metanephrine levels.

Answer 25.12.   **The answer is C.**

Anaplastic thyroid carcinoma remains an incurable cancer. It grows rapidly, and 20% to 50% of cases are associated with distant metastasis. Median survival is between 3 and 4 months. Surgery is typically reserved for local disease control, particularly in the absence of distant disease. Radioactive iodine is ineffective in the treatment of anaplastic thyroid cancer, and chemotherapy alone has modest effects on local response. This patient is best served with concurrent chemoradiation.

Answer 25.13.   **The answer is E.**

MTCs tend to metastasize early to cervical and mediastinal lymph nodes and later to the liver, bones, and lungs. CEA and calcitonin are useful tumor markers reflecting the disease burden. MTC is of neuroendocrine origin and expresses a high level of somatostatin receptors; thus, it binds to pharmacological-radiolabeled somatostatin analogs. Octreoscan can be used in selected cases with elevated calcitonin. Only limited evidence showed that PET scan can also be helpful in the imaging of MTC.

Answer 25.14.   **The answer is A.**

Hurthle cell carcinoma, or Oxyphil cell carcinoma, is a variant of follicular cell carcinoma. It has the same malignant features, is known to have poorer outcomes, and is less apt to concentrate radioactive iodine.

Answer 25.15.   **The answer is B.**

Anaplastic thyroid carcinoma represents 1% to 3% of all thyroid cancers and is typically fast growing. It is treated mainly with chemoradiation and perhaps debulking surgery in selected cases, but is considered incurable. It is always considered stage IV because of its extremely poor prognosis, with a median survival of only 3 to 4 months.

Answer 25.16.   **The answer is D.**

Doxorubicin is the most commonly used single chemotherapeutic agent in metastatic thyroid carcinoma, with a modest partial response rate reported to be approximately 30%. Taxanes are another group of agents that has also been used in the treatment of metastatic thyroid carcinoma.

Answer 25.17.   **The answer is B.**

Parathyroid carcinoma is a rare cancer. Surgery is the standard treatment approach. Adjuvant external beam irradiation has been shown to reduce the rate of recurrence. Resection of other uninvolved parathyroid glands is not indicated, because parathyroid carcinoma typically originates from one parathyroid gland. Radioactive iodine, as well as chemotherapy, is not generally effective in the treatment of parathyroid carcinoma. Bone pain, pathologic fracture, or other evidence of bone disease occurs in approximately 90% of patients, and renal stones occur in 50% to 80% of patients.

Answer 25.18.   **The answer is E.**

All of the mentioned options can be used in this case, but perhaps not all are needed at the same time. IV hydration and IV bisphosphonate represent the most widely used methods to treat malignant hypercalcemia. Mithramycin has been used in the past to treat metastatic parathyroid carcinoma. Cinacalcet (Sensipar) directly lowers PTH levels by increasing the sensitivity of calcium-sensing receptors on chief cells of the parathyroid gland to extracellular calcium. It also results in concomitant serum calcium decrease. Calcitonin can also be used to treat hypercalcemia and has an analgesic effect in cases of pathological fracture.

Answer 25.19.   **The answer is A.**

Several genetic defects have been reported to be associated with parathyroid cancer. Mutations of the HRPT2 gene (1q25-31) have been described in this disease, most commonly in association with the hyperparathyroidism jaw tumor syndrome. However, many sporadic parathyroid carcinomas exhibit defects in this gene. This gene codes for a tumor suppressor protein called "parafibromin," whose function is not yet known. Allelic loss in several chromosomes has been noted, but other than HRPT2, no gene has definitively been associated with parathyroid carcinoma. RET proto-oncogene mutation is not associated with parathyroid carcinoma.

Answer 25.20.   **The answer is A.**

Parathyroid cancer is rare enough that no staging system has been established. A palpable mass is virtually never present with benign parathyroid adenomas or hyperplasia. The reported overall 5-year survival rate is approximately 50% to 75%.

Answer 25.21.   **The answer is B.**

This patient has MEN1 syndrome, because his presentation includes pituitary adenoma and hyperparathyroidism. Prolactin-producing pituitary adenomas are treated initially with dopamine agonists; transsphenoidal resection is reserved as a second-line treatment. Subtotal parathyroidectomy (or total parathyroidectomy with autotransplantation of a parathyroid tissue in the arm) is the standard approach in treating hyperparathyroidism in MEN1 syndrome. Further evaluation is warranted to exclude pancreatic neuroendocrine tumors possibly producing gastrin, especially in the presence of gastrointestinal symptoms.

Answer 25.22.   **The answer is C.**

Hyperparathyroidism is the most common manifestation in this disorder. The other endocrine disorders include pituitary adenomas, pancreatic neuroendocrine tumors (PNETs), carcinoid tumors, and occasionally adrenocortical adenomas. Other manifestations include lipomas, collagenomas, and angiofibromas.

Answer 25.23.   **The answer is D.**

Virtually 100% of patients with MEN2A have C-cell hyperplasia or MTC; 50% have pheochromocytoma, and 20% to 30% have hyperparathyroidism. Diffuse neuronal hypertrophy is part of MEN2B.

Answer 25.24.   **The answer is A.**

The gene MEN2A is the RET proto-oncogene, located at the centromeric region of chromosome 10 (10q11-2). Data are accumulating regarding genotype-phenotype correlations and mutations in various RET codons. A negative family history is not reliable, because of the variable age of clinical presentation that can affect the identification of clinical cases. Thus, family members should be screened.

Answer 25.25.   **The answer is B.**

The MENIN gene was recently identified, and it is localized on the long arm of chromosome 11.

Answer 25.26.   **The answer is D.**

The RET proto-oncogene mutation is associated with MEN2 and Hirschsprung disease.

Answer 25.27.   **The answer is B.**

The development of amenorrhea, acne, hirsutism, and rapidly progressive Cushing's syndrome in a woman is a typical presentation of adrenal carcinoma. Complete metabolic workup is indicated before any intervention. Approximately 50% of adrenocortical neoplasms have features of hormonal hypersecretion. Surgical resection represents the standard treatment in localized tumors. Mitotane is given in metastatic disease and as adjuvent therapy. Hormonal hypersecretion can be medically controlled: Effective agents include ketoconazole, aminoglutethimide, and metyrapone.

Answer 25.28.   **The answer is D.**

The CVD regimen has been the most used chemotherapy regimen in patients with metastatic pheochromocytoma. External beam radiation can palliate metastatic bone lesions. I131 MIBG leads to a response rate of approximately 40%. Mitotane is used to treat metastatic adrenocortical carcinoma and not pheochromocytoma.

Answer 25.29.   **The answer is E.**

Carcinoid tumors are responsive to higher doses of external beam radiation, with a response rate of 40% to 50%.

Answer 25.30.   **The answer is A.**

Size more than 6 cm should raise the possibility of adrenocortical carcinoma. The other features are suggestive of benign adrenal adenoma.

Answer 25.31.   **The answer is A.**

Pheochromocytoma arises from the adrenal medulla in 90% of cases, where most are not malignant. Extra-adrenal lesions have increased risk of malignancy. The diagnosis is based on measuring catecholamines and metabolites in the serum and/or urine. Mutated RET proto-oncogene has been associated with bilateral pheochromocytomas, but it has not been associated with extra-adrenal pheochromocytoma.

Answer 25.32.   **The answer is E.**

Only limited evidence from retrospective reviews suggested improved disease-free survival with adjuvant mitotane therapy. Mitotane is associated with a wide range of side effects, especially gastrointestinal and neurological symptoms. Mitotane levels must be followed closely to guide therapy.

Answer 25.33. **The answer is B.**

Insulinomas are usually benign, with only 5% to 10% of cases being malignant. Documentation of metastasis is the only definitive way to diagnose malignant disease.

Answer 25.34. **The answer is D.**

Secretory diarrhea is commonly associated with all the listed hormones except insulin.

Answer 25.35. **The answer is B.**

The percentage of tumors of the endocrine pancreas that are malignant ranges from 10% for insulinoma, to 50% for glucagonoma, and to at least 65% for gastrinoma.

Sarcomas

Directions   Each of the numbered items below is followed by lettered answers. Select the ONE lettered answer that is BEST in each case unless instructed otherwise.

QUESTIONS

Question 26.1.   **Which of the following are NOT predisposing factors to the development of soft tissue sarcoma?**

A.   Prior radiation exposure
B.   Chronic lymphedema
C.   Neurofibromatosis type I
D.   Multiple endocrine neoplasia (MEN) type I

Question 26.2.   **Which of the following is NOT true about radiation-induced sarcomas?**

A.   Cancer history usually includes breast cancer, lymphoma, and cervical cancer.
B.   These sarcomas have a favorable prognosis.
C.   Osteogenic sarcoma, malignant fibrous histiocytoma, angiosarcoma, and lymphangiosarcoma are the usual histologic subtypes.
D.   They usually occur 10 to 30 years after radiation exposure.

Question 26.3.   **Which clonal cytogenetic abnormality is associated with the correct sarcoma subtype?**

A.   Ewing's sarcoma and t (11; 22) (q24; q12)
B.   Synovial sarcoma and t (12; 16) (q13; p11)
C.   Myxoid liposarcoma and t (x; 18) (p11; q11)
D.   Alveolar rhabdomyosarcoma and t (17; 22) (q22; q13)

Corresponding Chapter in *Cancer: Principles & Practice of Oncology,* Eighth Edition: 65 (Rehabilitation of the Cancer Patient).

Question 26.4.   **Which of the following statements about soft tissue sarcomas is NOT true?**

A.   Histologic subtype is an important determinant of prognosis, natural history, and therapy.

B.   Nodal metastases are common.

C.   Histologic tumor grade is the most important prognostic factor.

D.   Immunohistochemical status frequently yields evidence used to define the histologic subtype.

Question 26.5.   **Which of the following is TRUE about the clinical presentation of soft tissue sarcoma?**

A.   Most patients present with a painful mass.

B.   Fine-needle aspirate is recommended for the primary diagnosis.

C.   For extremity tumors, most metastases go to the lung.

D.   Positron emission tomography (PET) scans are the best radiologic method to determine the extent of the disease.

Question 26.6.   **Which of the following is NOT true regarding the staging of soft tissue sarcomas?**

A.   Stage II includes small (<5 cm) high-grade tumors without metastases.

B.   Stage IV includes distant but not nodal metastases.

C.   All low-grade tumors are classified as stage I if not metastatic.

D.   Histologic grade, size, depth, and presence or absence of nodal and distant metastases are variables used to determine tumor stage.

Question 26.7.   **A 52-year-old man underwent resection of a 3-cm mass from the lateral left thigh. Pathology revealed a high-grade leiomyosarcoma, and the lateral surgical margin was positive. The most appropriate next step in the treatment of this patient's cancer would be:**

A.   Radiation

B.   Adjuvant chemotherapy

C.   Reresection

D.   Observation

Question 26.8.   **A 68-year-old woman presented with a purplish nodular lesion in the occipital scalp. Resection revealed an angiosarcoma measuring 3 cm. Surgical margins were negative. What is the most appropriate next step in the treatment of this patient's cancer?**

A.   Radiologic imaging to look for nodal metastases and referral for adjuvant radiation

B.   Monitoring

C.   Adjuvant chemotherapy with an anthracycline

D.   Adjuvant chemotherapy with paclitaxel

Question 26.9.   A 65-year-old woman presented with abdominal pain and iron-deficiency anemia. Workup revealed a gastric mass and multiple large intra-abdominal masses and liver hypodensities. Biopsy of the gastric mass revealed a spindle cell neoplasm thought to be a leiomyosarcoma. After three cycles of doxorubicin and ifosfamide, imaging showed disease progression. The appropriate next step in the management of this patient's cancer would be:

A. Docetaxel and gemcitabine
B. Dacarbazine
C. Request the pathologist to perform a CD117 (C-Kit) stain
D. Palliative radiation

Question 26.10.   A 55-year-old man presented with a 10-cm mass in the medial left thigh. Biopsy revealed a high-grade liposarcoma. Imaging revealed no evidence of distant metastases. The most appropriate treatment for this patient's cancer would be:

A. Definitive radiation
B. Definitive radiation and concurrent doxorubicin
C. Limb-sparing resection followed by adjuvant radiation
D. Preoperative chemotherapy followed by resection

Question 26.11.   A 52-year-old man with metastatic unresectable gastrointestinal stromal tumor (GIST) was treated with imatinib (400 mg/d). Imaging showed initial disease response; however, the disease progressed after 28 months on therapy. The most appropriate treatment would be:

A. Erlotinib
B. Sunitinib
C. Doxorubicin
D. Imatinib 600 or 800 mg/d

Question 26.12.   The following factors are independent predictors of poorer disease-specific survival in patients with nonmetastatic soft tissue sarcoma, EXCEPT:

A. Large tumor size (>10 cm)
B. High-grade histology
C. Extremity site
D. Older age (>60 years)

Question 26.13.   A 48-year-old woman underwent complete resection of a 9-cm high-grade leiomyosarcoma arising in the lower extremity. Postoperative adjuvant radiation was administered. Two years later, a chest computed tomography (CT) scan revealed a new single 3-cm, round, noncalcified pulmonary nodule. What is the most appropriate next treatment?

A. Complete resection of the lung nodule
B. Radiation
C. Ifosfamide and doxorubicin
D. Docetaxel and gemcitabine

Question 26.14. Which of the following are FALSE about patients with metastatic or locally recurrent soft tissue sarcoma?

A. Median survival is 12 months, although 20% to 25% of patients are alive 2 years after diagnosis.
B. Complete resection of oligometastases to the lung can result in 5-year survivorship in 20% to 30% of patients.
C. Reresection is the preferred treatment for a locally recurrent sarcoma.
D. Combination chemotherapy improves overall survival compared with single-agent chemotherapy.

Question 26.15. Which of the following is TRUE about chemotherapy treatment of metastatic soft tissue sarcoma?

A. Escalating doses of doxorubicin or ifosfamide does not improve tumor response rates over standard doses of these agents.
B. Leiomyosarcoma is uniquely sensitive to ifosfamide, whereas synovial cell sarcoma is not.
C. Paclitaxel shows broad-spectrum activity.
D. Dacarbazine has modest activity.

Question 26.16. A 30-year-old man presents with a permeative bone tumor in the distal femur. Open biopsy reveals a malignant fibrous histiocytoma (MFH). Radiologic imaging does not find distant metastases. What is the most appropriate treatment?

A. Limb-sparing resection with wide margins
B. Definitive radiation
C. Chemotherapy
D. Preoperative chemotherapy, limb-sparing resection, and adjuvant chemotherapy

Question 26.17. Which of the following is NOT true regarding osteosarcoma?

A. Approximately 20% of patients with localized high-grade disease treated with resection alone remain disease free 5 years later.
B. Approximately 60% to 80% of patients with localized high-grade disease treated with resection and chemotherapy remain disease free 5 years later.
C. Parosteal (low-grade cortical) osteosarcoma is best treated with resection and chemotherapy.
D. Periosteal osteosarcoma is best treated with resection and chemotherapy.

Question 26.18. Which of the following is NOT true regarding chondrosarcomas?

A. Most are low-grade tumors.
B. Most are treated with resection.
C. Children have a poorer prognosis than adults.
D. Adjuvant chemotherapy has no role in the management of nonmetastatic disease.

Question 26.19.   **A 22-year-old woman presents with a giant cell tumor (GCT) of the distal femur. Appropriate treatment would be:**

A.   Curettage and debridement
B.   Amputation
C.   Radiation
D.   Preoperative chemotherapy, resection, and adjuvant chemotherapy

Question 26.20.   **A 16-year-old female patient presents with a painful rapidly growing scapular mass. Core needle biopsy reveals a Ewing's sarcoma. Staging evaluation shows no evidence of metastatic disease. The most appropriate therapy is:**

A.   Resection
B.   Preoperative chemotherapy (with vincristine, doxorubicin, and cyclophosphamide alternating with ifosfamide and etoposide), resection, and adjuvant chemotherapy
C.   Resection and radiation
D.   Preoperative chemotherapy (with vincristine, doxorubicin and cyclophosphamide), resection, and adjuvant chemotherapy

ANSWERS

Answer 26.1.   **The answer is D.**

Prior radiation exposure increases the risk for development of malignant fibrous histiocytoma, angiosarcoma, lymphangiosarcoma, and osteogenic sarcoma. Chronic lymphedema increases the risk for development of lymphangiosarcoma, most often occurring in women with a history of breast cancer treated with mastectomy and radiation. Neurofibromatosis type I increases the risk for the development of malignant peripheral nerve sheath tumors. MEN type I is not associated with increased risk for sarcomas.

Answer 26.2.   **The answer is B.**

Radiation-induced sarcomas usually occur 10 to 30 years after exposure to radiation. The most common cancers for which radiation was administered include breast and cervical cancer, and lymphoma. Most radiation-induced sarcomas are osteogenic sarcoma or MFH, and the prognosis is poor.

Answer 26.3.   **The answer is A.**

Ewing's sarcoma is associated with five known cytogenetic abnormalities, including t (11; 22) (q24; q12). Synovial sarcoma is associated with t (x; 18) (p11; q11), whereas myxoid liposarcoma is associated with t (12; 16) (q13; p11). Alveolar rhabdomyosarcoma is associated with t (2; 13) (q35; q14).

Answer 26.4. **The answer is B.**

Nodal metastases are uncommon in soft tissue sarcoma, except with epithelioid and synovial cell sarcoma, angiosarcoma, and rhabdomyosarcoma. The natural history and prognosis of sarcomas are dependent on the histologic subtype and tumor grade. High-grade tumors have a poorer prognosis than low-grade tumors. Immunohistochemistry frequently is used by the pathologist to provide supportive evidence of the histologic subtype of the sarcoma.

Answer 26.5. **The answer is C.**

Most patients with soft tissue sarcoma present with a painless mass. A core needle, incisional, or excisional biopsy is more likely to accurately define the histologic subtype of sarcoma, compared with fine-needle aspirate. Most metastases from an extremity sarcoma go to the lung, in contrast with retroperitoneal sarcomas, which usually go to the liver. The role of PET scans in staging of sarcoma is controversial. For example, fluorodeoxyglucose (FDG)-PET scans may not show known sites of disease (defined by CT or magnetic resonance imaging [MRI]) in the case of low-grade sarcomas, but may be more useful in high-grade sarcomas. CT and MRI scans remain the standard for radiologic imaging of sarcomas.

Answer 26.6. **The answer is B.**

Stage IV disease includes the presence of nodal or distant metastases. The prognosis of patients with small (<5 cm) high-grade soft tissue sarcomas without metastases is similar to that of other patients with stage II disease. Stage I disease includes only low-grade tumors. Staging of soft tissue sarcoma requires knowledge of histologic grade, size, depth, and presence of metastatic disease.

Answer 26.7. **The answer is C.**

Positive surgical margin predicts a higher risk of local recurrence. Re-resection in an attempt to achieve negative surgical margins would be the next most appropriate step in the management of this patient. If negative surgical margins are achieved after re-resection, adjuvant radiation would not be required. Adjuvant chemotherapy would have no clear benefit in this case.

Answer 26.8. **The answer is A.**

Soft tissue sarcoma of the head and neck is associated with a poor prognosis. Angiosarcoma has a higher risk of nodal metastases and local recurrence after resection alone. Adjuvant radiation reduces the risk of local and regional disease recurrence. Although angiosarcomas tend to be sensitive to anthracyclines and taxanes, there would be no known benefit of adjuvant chemotherapy in this case.

Answer 26.9.   **The answer is C.**

Intra-abdominal leiomyosarcomas and GISTs have similar characteristics by light microscopy; however, GISTs stain positive for the CD117 (C-Kit) protein, whereas leiomyosarcomas usually do not. Leiomyosarcomas frequently respond to chemotherapy, whereas GISTs do not. However, GISTs are uniquely responsive to C-Kit inhibitors. In this case, a C-Kit immunostain should be requested to determine whether the sarcoma is a GIST and not a leiomyosarcoma. Because this patient has metastatic disease, systemic therapy would be favored over palliative radiation.

Answer 26.10.   **The answer is C.**

Resection of the primary tumor with intent to achieve negative surgical margins followed by adjuvant radiation would be the most appropriate treatment of a large high-grade extremity liposarcoma. Definitive radiation with or without concurrent chemotherapy would be less effective treatment. Preoperative chemotherapy may be used when the tumor is marginally resectable, but its role in this situation is controversial.

Answer 26.11.   **The answer is D.**

Studies have demonstrated that approximately one third of patients with GIST resistant to imatinib 400 mg/d will benefit with increasing the dose of imatinib to 600 or 800 mg/d. Should that step fail, sunitinib would be the next most appropriate therapy. GIST is generally resistant to chemotherapy drugs, such as doxorubicin. Epidermal growth factor receptor (EGFR) inhibitors, such as erlotinib, would not be expected to benefit patients with GIST.

Answer 26.12.   **The answer is C.**

Independent predictors of prognosis of patients with nonmetastatic soft tissue sarcoma include age, histologic subtype, histologic grade, tumor site, and tumor size. Factors predictive of better disease-specific survival include younger age, selected histologic subtypes (fibrosarcoma), low histologic grade, smaller (<5 cm) tumor size, and extremity location. Nomograms are available that accurately predict the prognosis of patients with nonmetastatic soft tissue sarcoma treated with surgery with or without adjuvant radiation.

Answer 26.13.   **The answer is A.**

In this patient, the most likely cause of the new lung nodule is metastases of the leiomyosarcoma. Retrospective series have observed that 20% to 30% of such patients who undergo complete resection of the lung metastases were alive 5 years later. Factors that predict for a lower success rate with resection in such patients include more than four lung nodules, bilateral lung nodules, and disease-free interval of less than 12 months. Chemotherapy and radiation provide only palliative intent in this case.

Answer 26.14.   **The answer is D.**

For locally recurrent sarcoma without distant metastases, reresection is the preferred treatment. For patients with metastatic sarcoma, median survival is 1 year; however, a subset of these patients live for more than 2 years. It is important to consider complete resection of oligometastases to the lung because approximately 25% of those patients will be alive 5 years later. Nearly all randomized trials have shown no overall survival benefit with combination (vs. single agent) chemotherapy, although tumor response rates were consistently higher. A single, recent randomized trial demonstrated a modest survival benefit with the addition of docetaxel to gemcitabine in patients with metastatic sarcoma.

Answer 26.15.   **The answer is D.**

Several studies have shown higher tumor response rates (but not improved survival) with larger doses of doxorubicin and ifosfamide; however, this does result in greater toxicity. Ifosfamide is an active agent in synovial cell sarcoma but has little activity in leiomyosarcoma. Paclitaxel appears to only be effective in the treatment of angiosarcoma and Kaposi's sarcoma. Perhaps the first drug identified to be active in adult soft tissue sarcoma, dacarbazine resulted in tumor response rates of 10% to 30%.

Answer 26.16.   **The answer is D.**

In contrast with MFH of soft tissue, which is primarily treated with resection, MFH of bone is treated like high-grade osteosarcoma with preoperative chemotherapy, limb-sparing resection, and adjuvant chemotherapy. Outcomes of patients with MFH of bone and with osteosarcoma are similar when treated this way. Limb-sparing resection alone or definitive radiation would offer lower chances of success. Chemotherapy alone would provide palliation, but the chance of cure is unclear.

Answer 26.17.   **The answer is C.**

Parosteal osteosarcoma is usually a low-grade tumor that involves the bone cortex and is associated with a better prognosis than classic osteosarcoma. Resection is the preferred treatment, and there is no clear role for chemotherapy. In contrast, periosteal osteosarcoma is an aggressive, high-grade cortical sarcoma that is best treated like classic osteosarcoma with resection and chemotherapy. For classic high-grade osteosarcoma, resection alone is curative in 20%, but the addition of chemotherapy to resection improves cure rates to 60% to 80%.

Answer 26.18.   **The answer is D.**

The preferred therapy for chondrosarcoma is resection. Although chondrosarcomas as a group are known to be resistant to chemotherapy, mesenchymal chondrosarcoma has a high metastatic potential and appears to benefit from adjuvant chemotherapy. Most chondrosarcomas are low grade and usually occur in patients aged more than 40 years. Children have a worse prognosis than adults.

Answer 26.19.   **The answer is A.**

GCT of bone is a tumor with a high risk for local recurrence but a low risk for distal metastases. Appropriate treatment is resection, preferably by curettage and debridement. Amputation is reserved for massive local recurrences. Radiation is reserved for lesions of the spine that can lead to cord compression. There is no benefit of preoperative or adjuvant chemotherapy for GCT of bone.

Answer 26.20.   **The answer is B.**

A randomized trial of patients with Ewing's sarcoma treated with either vincristine, doxorubicin, and cyclophosphamide (VAC) alone or alternating with ifosfamide and etoposide (IE) given as preoperative and adjuvant chemotherapy clearly showed an overall survival and progression-free survival advantage with the alternating regimen of VAC and IE versus VAC alone in patients with nonmetastatic (but not in patients with metastatic) disease. Resection alone or with radiation would be significantly less effective than when used in combination with chemotherapy.

Benign and Malignant Mesothelioma

Directions   Each of the numbered items below is followed by lettered answers. Select the ONE lettered answer that is BEST in each case unless instructed otherwise.

QUESTIONS

Question 27.1.   **Regarding chromosomal alternations in patients with malignant mesothelioma, which is the most common?**

A.   Deletion in the short arm of chromosome 1
B.   Deletion in the short arm of chromosome 3
C.   Deletion in the long arm of chromosome 6
D.   Loss of a copy of chromosome 22

Question 27.2.   **All of the following are forms of malignant mesothelioma, EXCEPT:**

A.   Epithelial type
B.   Sarcomatoid type
C.   Multicystic type
D.   Biphasic type

Question 27.3.   **Malignant mesothelioma will stain positive for the following markers, EXCEPT:**

A.   Pankeratin
B.   TTF-1
C.   Calretinin
D.   WT1

Corresponding Chapter in *Cancer: Principles & Practice of Oncology,* Eighth Edition: 46 (Benign and Malignant Mesothelioma).

Question 27.4. **Solitary fibrous tumors of the pleura are characterized by all of the findings, EXCEPT:**

A. Well-circumscribed lobulated heterogenous tumor by radiologic films.
B. Immunohistochemically negative for cytokeratins.
C. Surgical resection is the treatment of choice in first-line and recurrent treatment.
D. Five-year survival rates are less than 20%.

Question 27.5. **Patients affected by mesothelioma tend to have a clinical presentation of:**

A. Female gender
B. Age less than 50 years
C. History of work in shipbuilding, construction, insulation, and oil and chemical industries
D. History of work in clerical positions

Question 27.6. **In patients with mesothelioma, poor prognostic indicators include the following, EXCEPT:**

A. Female gender
B. Poor performance status
C. Nonepithelioid histology
D. Elevated lactate dehydrogenase

Question 27.7. **Supportive care in the treatment of mesothelioma include the following modalities:**

A. Control of pleural effusion via thoracentesis, pleurodesis, shunting, and Pleurx catheter
B. Narcotics for pain control
C. Local radiotherapy for chest wall pain or nodules
D. All of the above

Question 27.8. **Surgical management of mesothelioma include all of the following options, EXCEPT:**

A. Thoracoscopy
B. Pleurectomy/decortication
C. Extrapleural pneumonectomy
D. All of the above

Question 27.9. **Regarding the use of radiotherapy in mesothelioma, which of the following is TRUE?**

A. Single modality radiotherapy is used as definitive treatment.
B. Useful as a postadjuvant treatment after extrapleural pneumonectomy.
C. Definitive chemoradiotherapy is curative.
D. Radiotherapy is not useful in palliation of chest wall pain.

Question 27.10. **Current chemotherapeutic options in the treatment of mesothelioma include:**

A. Platinum agent (cisplatin, carboplatin)
B. Gemcitabine
C. Pemetrexed
D. All of the above

Question 27.11. **Regarding malignant peritoneal mesothelioma, which is NOT true?**

A. Systemic chemotherapy is the mainstay of treatment.
B. Patients present with ascites, pain, and weight loss.
C. This must be differentiated from papillary tumors of the peritoneum.
D. Multimodality treatment with intraperitoneal chemotherapy and surgical debulking is the treatment of choice.

ANSWERS

Answer 27.1. **The answer is D.**

Commonly seen chromosomal abnormalities in malignant mesothelioma include deletions in the short (p) arm of chromosomes 1, 3, and 9, as well as the long (q) of chromosome 6. However, loss of a copy of chromosome 22 is the most common chromosomal alternation.

Answer 27.2. **The answer is C.**

There are many types of mesothelioma. Some of the benign types include multicystic mesothelioma, adenomatoid mesothelioma, well-differentiated papillary mesothelioma, and localized mesothelioma/localized fibrous tumor of the pleura. Some of the malignant types include epithelial type, fibrous/sarcomatoid type, and mixed/biphasic type.

Answer 27.3. **The answer is B.**

Malignant mesothelioma tends to stain positive for pankeratin, keratin 5/6, calretinin, and WT-1. They tend to be negative for the epithelial markers carcinoembryonic antigen (CEA), CD15, Ber-EP4, Moc-31, TTF-1, and B72.3. Sarcomatoid mesothelioma may be difficult to elucidate because only a fraction are positive for calretinin and WT1.

Answer 27.4. **The answer is D.**

Solitary fibrous tumors of the pleura (FTP) are generally benign, with a 10% occurrence of a malignant variant. They tend to be immunohistochemically negative when stained for cytokeratins. They can cause symptoms (dyspnea, lower-extremity edema, osteoarthropathy) in up to 60% of patients. These lesions are well-circumscribed lobulated heterogenous-appearing tumors that arise from a pedicle to the visceral pleura. Surgical resection is the treatment of choice, with 5-year survival rates of 97%. For recurrences, reexcision is the treatment of choice, if possible.

Answer 27.5.   **The answer is C.**

Because of the long latency period between exposure to asbestos (generally from occupations such as shipbuilding, construction, insulation, and oil and chemical manufacturing), patients tend to be older than 50 years of age. The male to female ratio is approximately 3 to 5:1, likely because of the gender differences in occupational exposure.

Answer 27.6.   **The answer is A.**

Poor prognostic indicators in mesothelioma include poor performance status, nonepithelioid histology, male gender, low hemoglobin, high platelet count, high white blood cell count, and high lactate dehydrogenase (LDH). The clinical prognostic scoring systems from the European Organization for Research and Treatment of Cancer (EORTC) and Cancer and Leukemia Group B (CALGB) are the best known.

Answer 27.7.   **The answer is D.**

Pleural effusions can be controlled through the use of repeated thoracenteses, talc pleurodesis, pleuroperitoneal shunting, or placement of a Pleurx catheter. Narcotics can be used to control the chest pain associated with mesothelioma. Local radiotherapy can be used to control chest wall pain and nodules.

Answer 27.8.   **The answer is D.**

There is a lack of randomized controlled trials looking at the role of surgery in mesothelioma. Both the role of surgery and the type of surgery in mesothelioma remain controversial. Management is dependent on the presentation of the patient and the experience of the treating center.

Answer 27.9.   **The answer is B.**

Radiotherapy, as a single modality or in combination with chemotherapy, has little role in definitive treatment. However, radiotherapy is useful in reduction of pain when doses greater than 4500 cGy were used. High-dose thoracic radiotherapy after an extrapleural pneumonectomy was found to have improved survival compared with historical data.

Answer 27.10.   **The answer is D.**

The combination of cisplatin and pemetrexed is associated with improved survival, response rates, quality of life, and time to disease progression compared with cisplatin alone. Other doublet regimens containing a combination of a platinum agent and either gemcitabine or pemetrexed have also shown activity in mesothelioma.

Answer 27.11.   **The answer is A.**

Patients with malignant peritoneal mesothelioma tend to present with increased abdominal girth from ascites, pain, and weight loss. They can also present with a hernia or pelvic mass along with fever, leukocytosis, and thrombocytosis. Papillary tumors of the peritoneum have a different natural history and must be differentiated from malignant peritoneal mesothelioma. Chemotherapy alone has poor results, so the treatment of choice is multimodality treatment with either induction therapy followed by surgery or surgical debulking followed by intraperitoneal chemotherapy.

Cancer of the Skin and Melanoma

Directions   Each of the numbered items below is followed by lettered answers. Select the ONE lettered answer that is BEST in each case unless instructed otherwise.

QUESTIONS

Question 28.1.   **Which of the following statements is TRUE? According to the National Cancer Database:**

A.   Ninety-one percent of melanomas are cutaneous in origin.
B.   Five percent of melanomas are ocular in origin.
C.   One percent of melanomas are mucosal in origin.
D.   Two percent of melanomas are of unknown primary.
E.   All of the above.

Question 28.2.   **Recent epidemiologic data suggest that the incidence and mortality of melanoma is increasing in which of the following populations:**

A.   Young adults
B.   Women aged 50 to 64 years
C.   Infants
D.   Men aged 65 to 74 years

Question 28.3.   **Which of the following statements regarding the anatomic distribution of melanoma is FALSE?**

A.   Cutaneous melanoma can occur at any body site.
B.   Acral and mucosal melanoma occur at a much higher frequency in non-Caucasians compared with Caucasian populations.
C.   Ocular melanoma is more common in Caucasians.
D.   The most common sites for cutaneous melanoma in women are the back and head and neck area.

Corresponding Chapters in *Cancer: Principles & Practice of Oncology*, Eighth Edition: 47 (Cancer of the Skin) and 48 (Melanoma).

Question 28.4.   **Risk factors for cutaneous melanoma include all of the following, EXCEPT:**

    A. Prior scalp radiation
    B. Inherited mutation of p16(CDKN2A)
    C. Higher socioeconomic status
    D. Pregnancy

Question 28.5.   **A healthy 42-year-old woman was recently found to have a 2.4-mm Breslow thickness nonulcerated primary cutaneous superficial spreading melanoma. The pigmented lesion was excised from her left lower extremity by her local dermatologist. The physician calls you for advice regarding further evaluation. Your recommendation is which of the following:**

    A. Referral to a medical oncologist for a clinical trial
    B. Body positron emission tomography/computed tomography (PET/ CT) scan for initial staging
    C. Referral to a surgeon for wide local excision and sentinel lymph node mapping
    D. Annual follow-up for skin checks

Question 28.6.   **A 56-year-old man was recently diagnosed with a stage IIa primary cutaneous melanoma (T2b N0 Mx). What is the most appropriate recommendation for clinical follow-up?**

    A. Annual visit with a dermatologist
    B. Office visits with a dermatologist every 3 months for 3 years, every 6 months for 2 years, and then annually for life
    C. Office visits with a dermatologist every 3 months for 3 years, every 6 months for 2 years, and then annually for life plus body PET-CT imaging every 6 months for life
    D. Office visits with a dermatologist every 3 months for life

Question 28.7.   **Indications for radiation therapy in the treatment of melanoma include which of the following:**

    A. Symptomatic brain metastases
    B. Symptomatic unresectable nodal metastases
    C. Symptomatic bone metastases
    D. All of the above

Question 28.8.   **The MOST common first metastatic site for ocular melanoma is:**

    A. Brain
    B. Lung
    C. Liver
    D. Skin

Question 28.9.   **The MOST appropriate staging evaluation for a newly diagnosed patient with stage IV (metastatic) melanoma includes:**

    A. Whole-body PET-CT scan
    B. Body (chest/abdomen/pelvis) CT scan with contrast
    C. Brain magnetic resonance imaging (MRI) scan with gadolinium and body (chest/abdomen/pelvis) CT scan with contrast
    D. None of the above

Question 28.10.   **Which of the following statements regarding adjuvant therapy is TRUE?**

    A. Isolated limb perfusion has been shown to increase the overall survival for patients with surgically resected stage III melanoma in randomized clinical trials.
    B. High-dose interferon has been shown to increase the relapse-free survival for patients with surgically resected stage III melanoma.
    C. Radiation therapy has been shown to increase the overall survival for patients with surgically resected stage III melanoma.
    D. High-dose chemotherapy with hematopoietic stem cell transplantation can increase the overall survival for patients with stage III surgically resected melanoma.

Question 28.11.   **Surgical resection for metastatic melanoma may be appropriate in which of these instances?**

    A. Symptomatic brain metastases
    B. Bowel obstruction caused by small bowel metastases
    C. Symptomatic adrenal metastases
    D. All of the above

Question 28.12.   **Dacarbazine is considered the standard of care as systemic treatment for metastatic melanoma. Which of the following statements is TRUE regarding dacarbazine?**

    A. Dacarbazine has a significantly higher response rate compared with temozolomide.
    B. Peripheral neuropathy is the most common major toxicity.
    C. Dacarbazine is associated with improved overall survival compared with observation or placebo.
    D. Dacarbazine-based combination chemotherapy results in a higher response rate compared with single-agent dacarbazine but is not shown to improve overall survival.

Question 28.13.   **Recent advances in the treatment of intracranial melanoma metastases suggest that which of the following statements is TRUE?**

A.   Addition of concurrent low-dose temozolomide (75 mg/m^2) by mouth daily during radiation therapy provides superior disease control and improved response rate.
B.   The median overall survival of patients with surgically resected solitary intracranial metastases is approximately 9 months.
C.   Stereotactic radiosurgery followed by whole-brain radiation therapy confers an overall survival benefit compared with whole-brain radiation therapy alone.
D.   All of the above.

Question 28.14.   **A 65-year-old man with metastatic Merkel cell carcinoma is referred to you for evaluation. CT imaging reveals bilateral pulmonary metastases. What is the MOST appropriate initial therapy?**

A.   High-dose interleukin-2
B.   Platinum-based chemotherapy
C.   Imatinib
D.   Referral to a surgical oncologist

Question 28.15.   **Treatment for actinic keratoses includes:**

A.   Cryosurgery
B.   Photodynamic therapy
C.   Imiquimod
D.   All of the above

Question 28.16.   **The MOST common skin malignancy affecting the eyelid is:**

A.   Basal cell carcinoma
B.   Melanoma
C.   Squamous cell carcinoma
D.   None of the above

ANSWERS

Answer 28.1.   **The answer is E.**

Skin is the most common site for melanoma.

Answer 28.2.   **The answer is D.**

SEER statistics continue to show increasing rates for older men. The median age at diagnosis is 59 years. The age-adjusted incidence is 19.4 per 100,000 men and women per year. The most recent age-adjusted incidence rate for men (aged 65 to 74 years) is 91 (per 100,000) and has increased steadily since 1975. In comparison, the rate for women (aged 65 to 74 years) is 37 (per 100,000).

Answer 28.3.   **The answer is D.**

The most common site of primary cutaneous melanoma in women is the lower extremities. In men, the most common sites are the head and neck area and the back.

Answer 28.4.   **The answer is D.**

Prior scalp radiation (during childhood), familial p16 mutation, and higher socioeconomic status have all been shown to be risk factors for cutaneous melanoma. In contrast, pregnancy is not considered to be a risk factor for the development of primary or recurrent melanoma.

Answer 28.5.   **The answer is C.**

The management of primary cutaneous melanoma is straightforward. It is essential that primary care providers have a firm understanding of the guidelines to expedite referral to the appropriate surgical specialist. Excisional biopsy is the preferred method for diagnosis of most pigmented lesions and permits the accurate assessment of primary depth (Breslow's thickness). Intraoperative lymphatic mapping with sentinel node biopsy remains the standard approach at major centers. Sentinel node mapping is performed for primary lesions 1 mm or more in depth and selected thin (<1 mm) lesions with features of regression or ulceration, high mitotic rate, and positive deep margin.

Body fluorodeoxyglucose (FDG) PET-CT imaging as an initial staging procedure is not recommended unless clinically indicated on the basis of history and physical examination. Clinical research provides strong evidence that the sensitivity of standard FDG PET imaging is inadequate to detect micrometastasis in draining nodal basins. Finally, there is no standard adjuvant therapy currently recommended for patients with stage IIA (T3a N0 Mx) cutaneous melanoma. Oncology referral should be made after the pathologic staging is completed.

Answer 28.6.   **The answer is B.**

The current National Comprehensive Cancer Network (NCCN) guidelines call for physical examination focused on skin and regional lymph nodes plus any new areas of clinical concern based on patient history. Routine imaging is limited to annual chest radiography in asymptomatic patients. Routine surveillance PET-CT scans every 6 months are not indicated in stage I/II melanoma. However, if clinically indicated (i.e., new symptoms), appropriate imaging is warranted for patients with a history of stage I-II-IIIA melanoma. For patients at higher risk for recurrence (stage IIIB to IIIC and surgically resected stage IV), periodic surveillance imaging is warranted.

Answer 28.7.   **The answer is D.**

Palliative radiation therapy is indicated for these three indications. In addition, patients with symptomatic cutaneous or subcutaneous metastases can often be palliated by radiation therapy.

Answer 28.8. **The answer is C.**

Liver metastases are common in recurrent ocular melanoma. More than 90% of patients with metastatic ocular melanoma have liver metastases, often as the initial and sole site of distant disease. Brain metastasis from ocular melanoma is less frequent (>5%) compared with cutaneous melanoma and typically occurs late in the disease course. The median survival for patients with metastatic ocular melanoma is 7 months.

Answer 28.9. **The answer is C.**

MRI with gadolinium is the most sensitive imaging modality for the brain offered at most institutions, and for this reason, MRI is suggested as part of the initial staging evaluation. Whole-body FDG PET-CT imaging is a sensitive modality for the initial evaluation but is suboptimal for the detection of small intracranial metastases. Most disease specialists recommend brain MRI together with CT of the chest/abdomen/pelvis as routine imaging. For patients with suspected gastrointestinal metastasis, FDG PET-CT imaging is considered particularly useful.

Answer 28.10. **The answer is B.**

Various clinical trials provide convincing evidence for the relapse-free survival benefit of adjuvant interferon. There are no data to suggest that limb perfusion, radiation therapy, or high-dose chemotherapy can improve survival in patients with surgically resected melanoma.

Answer 28.11. **The answer is D.**

The three clinical situations listed are all accepted indications for surgical resection in selected patients with metastatic melanoma.

Answer 28.12. **The answer is D.**

No treatment has been shown to prolong survival for patients with metastatic melanoma according to a controlled randomized clinical trial. Although dacarbazine-based combination chemotherapy promotes higher response rates as recorded in many randomized clinical trials, there is no survival benefit; thus, most disease experts consider single-agent dacarbazine as the standard of care. When evaluated in a randomized clinical trial, temozolomide is comparable to dacarbazine in response rate. Temozolomide has the advantage of better central nervous system penetration and thus is often recommended for patients with intracranial disease. The most common major toxicities of dacarbazine are myelosuppression and nausea.

Answer 28.13. **The answer is B.**

Data from the Sidney Melanoma Unit in Australia suggest that the median survival is 8.9 months for patients with surgically resected intracranial melanoma metastasis (Fife KM, Colman MH, Stevens GN, et al. Determinants of outcome in melanoma patients with cerebral metastases. J Clin Oncol 2004;22:1293–1300). Many patients in this retrospective series received postoperative whole-brain radiation therapy. The addition of concurrent temozolomide to whole-brain radiation has been studied but has never been shown to provide benefit by any outcome measure.

Answer 28.14.   **The answer is B.**

Although response rates are relatively high (>50%) with platinum-based chemotherapy, it is unclear if chemotherapy prolongs survival. In addition to platinum and etoposide, topotecan and doxorubicin are considered active agents in Merkel cell carcinoma. Interleukin-2 and imatinib have not been extensively studied for this disease. Surgical resection would appear to be an option for selected patients with a single distant site in instances that could be rendered disease free; however, most patients with bilateral pulmonary metastases are not generally considered for surgery.

Answer 28.15.   **The answer is D.**

All are accepted treatments for actinic keratoses.

Answer 28.16.   **The answer is A.**

Mohs micrographic surgery is the preferred approach for eyelid skin cancers. Referral to an oculoplastic surgeon is often necessary for optimal management.

Janakiraman Subramanian

Neoplasms of the Central Nervous System

Directions   Each of the numbered items below is followed by lettered answers. Select the ONE lettered answer that is BEST in each case unless instructed otherwise.

QUESTIONS

Question 29.1.   **Linkage studies have identified genes associated with neurofibromatosis type 2 (NF2), Turcot syndrome, and Li Fraumeni syndrome in which of the following chromosomes?**

A. 10q, 22q, and17q
B. 5q, 17p, and 22q
C. 5q, 10q, and 17p
D. 5q, 10q, and 17q

Question 29.2.   **Of the following, the MOST common primary brain tumor in adults in the United States is:**

A. Glioblastoma
B. Meningioma
C. Astrocytoma
D. Oligodendroglioma

Question 29.3.   **The gene that is frequently altered and plays a key role in the development of diffuse fibrillary astrocytoma is:**

A. p53
B. K-ras
C. MDM2
D. MDM4

Corresponding Chapter in *Cancer: Principles & Practice of Oncology*, Eighth Edition: 49 (Neoplasms of the Central Nervous System).

Question 29.4.   The chromosomal alteration that is most frequently associated with World Health Organization (WHO) grade 3 anaplastic astrocytoma is:

A. Loss of 9p
B. Loss of 10q
C. Gain in 12q
D. Loss of 19q

Question 29.5.   Primary (de novo) glioblastoma multiforme (GBM) is commonly associated with all of the following, EXCEPT:

A. PTEN inactivation
B. p53 mutation
C. CDKN2A deletion
D. Median age <60 years

Question 29.6.   Patients with secondary GBM are characterized by all of the following, EXCEPT:

A. Age >50 years
B. p53 mutation
C. Loss of chromosome 19
D. Gain in chromosome 4

Question 29.7.   Upregulation of the transcript for YKL-40 in GBM is associated with:

A. Loss of chromosome 9
B. Loss of chromosome 10
C. Gain in 12q
D. Loss of chromosome 19

Question 29.8.   Loss of heterozygosity of chromosomes 1p and 19q are common in:

A. GBM
B. Ependymoma
C. Oligodendroglioma
D. Meningioma

Question 29.9.   The central nervous system (CNS) tumor that is commonly associated with NF2 mutations is:

A. GBM
B. Spinal ependymoma
C. Cerebral ependymoma
D. Oligodendroglioma

Question 29.10.   **Patients with GBM have a higher likelihood of responding to therapy with epidermal growth factor receptor tyrosine kinase (EGFR TK) inhibitors if which of the following biomarkers is present?**

    A. Methyl guanine methyl transferase (MGMT) gene cytosine methylation

    B. Activated EGFRvIII

    C. Retained PTEN function

    D. B and C

Question 29.11.   **The primary CNS neoplasm that is associated with Epstein-Barr virus (EBV) is:**

    A. Primary CNS lymphoma

    B. Ependymoma

    C. Oligodendroglioma

    D. GBM

Question 29.12.   **Which of the following tumors exhibits contrast enhancement on magnetic resonance imaging (MRI) scan?**

    A. Pilocytic astrocytoma

    B. Grade 2 oligodendroglioma

    C. Grade 2 astrocytoma

    D. None of the above

Question 29.13.   **All of the following are associated with poor prognosis in patients with low-grade gliomas, EXCEPT:**

    A. Age $\geq$40 years

    B. Tumor diameter $\geq$6 cm

    C. Tumor crossing midline

    D. Oligodendroglioma

Question 29.14.   **A 45-year-old man presents with generalized seizures, and magnetic resonance imaging (MRI) of the brain reveals a nonenhancing mass measuring 7 cm. Biopsy is done, and the tumor histology is reported as grade 2 astrocytoma. The patient undergoes surgery, and a near total resection is achieved. Further treatment should include:**

    A. Watchful waiting

    B. Chemotherapy

    C. Radiotherapy, 50.4 Gy in 1.8 Gy fractions

    D. Radiotherapy with chemotherapy (procarbazine, CCNU, and vincristine)

Question 29.15.   **A 29-year-old woman presents with seizures that are readily controlled with antiepileptic medications. MRI of the brain reveals a nonenhancing lesion measuring 3 cm in diameter. She undergoes a biopsy that reveals a grade 2 oligodendroglioma. Treatment should include:**

A. Watchful waiting
B. Chemotherapy
C. Radiotherapy, 50.4 Gy in 1.8 Gy fractions
D. Radiotherapy with procarbazine, CCNU, and vincristine (PCV) chemotherapy

Question 29.16.   **A 55-year-old man presents with headache and mental status changes. MRI scan of the brain reveals a 5-cm contrast-enhancing mass with surrounding edema. He undergoes stereotactic biopsy revealing GBM. The patient undergoes resection of the tumor, and further treatment should include:**

A. Focal external beam irradiation with 45 Gy in 30 fractions plus concurrent temozolomide
B. Focal external beam irradiation with 60 Gy plus a 10 Gy boost plus concurrent temozolomide
C. Focal external beam irradiation with 60 Gy in 30 fractions plus concurrent temozolomide
D. Hyperfractionated dose of 72 Gy in 1.2 Gy fractions plus concurrent temozolomide

Question 29.17.   **A 62-year-old man presents with nausea, vomiting, and severe headache. MRI scan of the brain reveals a 5-cm mass in the posterior fossa. The patient undergoes surgical resection of the mass, and pathology is reported as ependymoma. Further treatment should include:**

A. Radiation therapy
B. Concurrent chemoradiation with temozolomide
C. Check MGMT methylation status
D. Chemotherapy alone with cisplatin plus etoposide

Question 29.18.   **A 53-year-old woman presents with mental status changes; brain MRI identifies a left frontal tumor with dural marginal thickening. She undergoes a resection of the tumor and the involved dural attachments. The histopathology is meningioma. Further treatment should include:**

A. Watchful waiting
B. Adjuvant radiation therapy
C. Chemotherapy
D. Radiosurgery

Question 29.19.   **All of the following are embryonal tumors, EXCEPT:**

A. Medulloepithelioma
B. Ependymoblastoma
C. Atypical rhabdoid tumor
D. Cerebellar liponeurocytoma

Question 29.20.   **All of the following hormones are commonly oversecreted in patients with pituitary adenoma, EXCEPT:**

A. Prolactin
B. Thyroid-stimulating hormone (TSH)
C. Growth hormone
D. Adrenocorticotropic hormone (ACTH)

Question 29.21.   **Which of the following is LEAST commonly associated with craniopharyngioma?**

A. Sexual dysfunction
B. Visual dysfunction
C. Hypothyroidism
D. Diabetes insipidus

ANSWERS

Answer 29.1.   **The answer is B.**

Linkage studies have revealed the NF1 gene to reside in chromosome 17q and the NF2 gene to reside in chromosome 22q. For Turcot's syndrome, the APC gene has been identified in chromosome 5q. For Li-Fraumeni syndrome, the cancer disposition has been shown to be associated with chromosomes 17p and 22q.

Answer 29.2.   **The answer is B.**

According to data from the Central Brain Tumor Registry of the United States (1998 to 2002), the proportionate distribution of incidence is 30.1% for meningioma, 20.3% for glioblastoma, 9.8% for astrocytoma, and 2.3% for ependymoma.

Answer 29.3.   **The answer is A.**

Alterations of p53 gene are found in 30% of all three grades of astrocytoma. Other reported gene alterations include the amplification of MDM2 or MDM4 gene. Chromosome 9p deletions resulting in loss of the p14 product of the CDKN2A gene have also been reported.

Answer 29.4.   **The answer is A.**

Chromosome 9p loss occurs in approximately 50% of grade 3 astrocytomas. These alterations target the CDKN2A locus that encodes the p16 and ARF proteins. Chromosome 10 loss is a frequent finding in GBM. Amplification of the CDK4 gene, located in chromosome 12q13–14, is found in 15% of malignant gliomas. Chromosome 19q loss has been observed in up to 40% of anaplastic astrocytomas and GBM.

Answer 29.5.   **The answer is D.**

Primary (de novo) GBM is associated with age greater than 62 years, amplified EGFR, wild-type p53, PTEN inactivation, CDKN2A deletion, and decreased survival.

Answer 29.6.   **The answer is A.**

Patients with secondary GBM have a median age of <40 years. Loss of chromosome 19, p53 mutation, and gain in chromosome 4 (in the K3-2 subgroup) are all commonly observed in these tumors.

Answer 29.7.   **The answer is B.**

Upregulation of the YKL-40 transcript is common in GBM with loss of chromosome 10. The molecular significance of this finding is unclear; however, upregulation of the YKL-40 transcript in GBM is associated with poor survival.

Answer 29.8.   **The answer is C.**

Allelic loss of chromosome 1p and 19q occurs in 40% to 80% of grade 2 and 3 oligodendrogliomas. The loss of tumor suppressor genes from these chromosomes is believed to play an important role in the early stage of oligodendroglial tumorigenesis.

Answer 29.9.   **The answer is B.**

Chromosome 22q loss is common in ependymomas; in spinal ependymomas, this loss is associated with mutations of the NF2 gene. In cerebral ependymomas, loss of chromosome 22q is not associated with NF2 mutations.

Answer 29.10.   **The answer is D.**

In a randomized phase III trial, patients with GBM who were positive for MGMT gene methylation and treated with combined temozolomide and radiation had significantly improved survival when compared with patients who were either negative for MGMT gene methylation or received radiation only. In another study, patients with GBM had improved survival when treated with EGFR TK inhibitors when the tumors expressed the common form of mutated EGFR (activated EGFRvIII) and retained PTEN function compared with patients not expressing both of these biomarkers.

Answer 29.11.   **The answer is A.**

There has been no reported association between primary CNS neoplasms and viral infections in humans, except for primary CNS lymphoma, which is strongly associated with EBV. The majority of primary CNS lymphomas are large B-cell histology, and EBV DNA is detectable in most of these tumors. In addition, the incidence of primary CNS lymphoma is higher in patients with human immunodeficiency virus (HIV) infection.

Answer 29.12.   **The answer is A.**

Contrast-enhanced MRI images help differentiate between different types of CNS tumors. MRI also helps to differentiate between high- and low-grade tumors. Low-grade CNS tumors generally do not enhance, except for pilocytic astrocytoma and pleomorphic xanthoastrocytoma.

Answer 29.13.   **The answer is D.**

Multivariate analysis from two large European phase III trials have reported age ≥40 years, tumor diameter ≥6 cm, tumor crossing the midline, astrocytoma histology, and neurologic deficits to be associated with adverse prognosis.

Answer 29.14.   **The answer is C.**

Radiotherapy is not routinely recommended in patients undergoing resection for low-grade gliomas. In the European Organization for Research and Treatment of Cancer (EORTC) 22845 trial, patients receiving immediate postoperative radiotherapy had a progression-free survival (PFS) advantage compared with those receiving radiation therapy on tumor progression (5.3 vs. 3.4 years, *p* <.0001). There was no significant difference in overall survival (7.4 years vs. 7.2 years). In another study, age ≥40 years, tumor diameter ≥6 cm, astrocytoma histology, and incomplete resection were identified as adverse prognostic factors, with the presence of three or more of these factors conferring poor prognosis. In such patients, immediate postoperative radiotherapy is recommended. Currently, there is no evidence to recommend chemotherapy in adult patients diagnosed with astrocytoma.

Answer 29.15.   **The answer is A.**

Watchful waiting until progression is recommended in patients with small, low-grade oligodendroglioma without poorly controlled seizures. Surgical resection is recommended in patients with large tumors or significant neurologic deficits. In addition, postoperative radiation therapy is recommended in incompletely resected tumors and anaplastic oligodendrogliomas. The RTOG 9402 and EORTC 26951 trials demonstrated superior PFS in patients with anaplastic oligodendrogliomas and oligoastrocytomas with adjuvant PCV chemotherapy with radiation compared with radiation therapy alone. Furthermore, PFS was significantly better in patients whose tumors had chromosomes 1p/19q loss. However, there was no overall survival advantage, and further evidence is required to define the role of chemotherapy in patients with 1p/19q loss and the use of single-agent temozolomide in these patients.

Answer 29.16.   **The answer is C.**

For patients with GBM, standard radiation therapy is 60 Gy in 30 or 33 fractions. The Medical Research Council study reported a survival advantage in patients receiving a 60 Gy dose versus a 45 Gy dose (12 vs. 9 months, *p* = .007). In an RTOG/ECOG study, patients receiving 60

Gy followed by a 10 Gy boost did not have a survival advantage over patients receiving the standard 60 Gy dose. Hyperfractionated and accelerated regimens have likewise not shown survival advantage. In the phase I/II RTOG 8302 study, hyperfractionated doses with 64.8 Gy, 72 Gy, 76.8 Gy, and 81.6 Gy in 1.2 Gy twice daily fractions did not show a survival benefit between the different treatment arms. This study included treatment arms with accelerated hyperfractionated regimens of 48 Gy and 54.4 Gy in 1.6 Gy twice daily fractions, which also did not lead to survival benefit. Adjuvant temozolomide with radiation was shown to improve overall survival compared with radiation alone in a randomized, phase III trial for patients with GBM (14.6 vs. 12.1 months).

Answer 29.17.   **The answer is A.**

Surgical resection is the primary treatment for patients with ependymoma. There are no definitive recommendations for the addition of radiotherapy to the treatment. However, tumors in the posterior fossa cannot always be fully resected, and patients undergoing resection alone have a very high incidence of local recurrence. Therefore, adjuvant focal radiotherapy to the site of the tumor may be added in the treatment of patients with ependymoma. In one study, patients receiving focal radiotherapy of more than 45 Gy to the tumor bed had 5- and 10-year survival rates of 67% and 57%, respectively. The addition of focal radiotherapy has been shown to improve 10-year survival from 67% in patients treated with gross total resection (GTR) alone to 83% in patients treated with GTR and radiotherapy. MGMT gene methylation is associated with better survival in patients with GBM. In ependymomas, there has been no reported association between MGMT gene methylation and survival. There is no evidence to date supporting the use of chemotherapy for treating ependymoma.

Answer 29.18.   **The answer is A.**

Surgical resection is the mainstay for the treatment of meningioma, and it is classified into Simpson grades based on the extent of surgery. Grade 1 is GTR of the tumor, with removal of the dural attachments and hyperostotic bone. The relapse rate after this procedure is 9%. Grade 2 does not include removal of hyperostotic bone (relapse rate 19%). Grade 3 is GTR of the tumor alone (relapse rate 29%). Grade 4 is partial resection (relapse rate 44%). Grade 5 refers to biopsy alone without resection. Adjuvant radiotherapy is not recommended for patients with low-grade meningioma who undergo Simpson grade 1 to 2, and sometimes grade 3, resection. The patient in this case has undergone grade 2 resection for a low-grade meningioma and therefore does not require further radiotherapy. For patients with resected anaplastic and malignant meningioma, adjuvant radiotherapy is recommended. Radiosurgery can be used in patients with unresectable disease, but there is no evidence to support the use of chemotherapy in patients with meningioma. Tamoxifen, mifepristone, and hydroxyurea have not been shown to be effective in this disease.

Answer 29.19.   **The answer is D.**

Cerebellar liponeurocytoma is a posterior fossa tumor commonly diagnosed in patients aged more than 50 years. All the other choices are embryonal tumors and typically occur in infants and young children.

Answer 29.20.   **The answer is B.**

Oversecretion of TSH in patients with pituitary adenomas is uncommon. In a retrospective study with 800 patients undergoing surgical resection for pituitary adenomas, 79% were associated with oversecretion of pituitary hormones. Of these, 52% secreted prolactin, 27% secreted growth hormone, 20% secreted ACTH, and 0.3% secreted TSH.

Answer 29.21.   **The answer is D.**

Some degree of sexual dysfunction occurs in approximately 90% of all adult patients presenting with craniopharyngioma. Visual dysfunction occurs in 40% to 70% of these patients. Hypothyroidism occurs in 40% of patients, and diabetes insipidus occurs in 10% to 20% of patients. However, the incidence of diabetes insipidus after surgical resection increases substantially; in one study, it increased from 16.1% in the preoperative setting to 59.4% after surgery.

Cancers of Childhood

Directions   Each of the numbered items below is followed by lettered answers. Select the ONE lettered answer that is BEST in each case unless instructed otherwise.

QUESTIONS

Question 30.1.   **Pediatric malignancies exhibit all the following characteristics, EXCEPT:**

A. Aggressive, rapid growth
B. Short latency period
C. Associated with exposure to carcinogens
D. Familial association in 10% to 15% of cases

Question 30.2.   **Genetic abnormalities predispose to malignant disorders in children because of:**

A. Abnormal mechanisms of genomic DNA repair
B. Constitutional activation of molecular pathways of deregulated cellular growth and proliferation
C. Increased function of oncogenes or inactivation of tumor suppressor genes
D. All of the above

Question 30.3.   **Which of these cancer predisposition syndromes do not have associated physical stigmata?**

A. Beckwith-Wiedemann syndrome
B. Fanconi anemia
C. Li-Fraumeni syndrome
D. Von Hippel-Lindau disease

Corresponding Chapter in *Cancer: Principles & Practice of Oncology,* Eighth Edition: 32 (Cancers of Childhood).

Question 30.4. All cancer predisposition syndromes listed below have a dominant mode of inheritance, EXCEPT:

A. Neurofibromatosis type I
B. Xeroderma pigmentosum
C. Peutz-Jeghers syndrome
D. Multiple endocrine neoplasia (MEN) 2

Question 30.5. The correct order of associated cytogenetic abnormalities that correlate respectively with Ewing's sarcoma, rhabdomyosarcoma (RMS), rhabdoid tumor, synovial sarcoma, and retinoblastoma is:

A. t(11;22), t(2;13), delq22.11, t(X;11), and del13q14
B. del13q14, t(2;13), delq22.11, t(X;11), and t(11;22)
C. t(2;13), delq22.11, del13q14, t(X;11), and t(11;22)
D. t(11;22), delq22.11, t(X;11), t(2;13), and del13q14

Question 30.6. Retinoblastoma is a heritable tumor that is often bilateral. All the following statements regarding retinoblastoma are true, EXCEPT:

A. Loss of heterozygosity of the wild-type allele at the Rb1 locus results in the disease.
B. Rb1 loss abrogates control of cell-cycle regulation from the G1 to S phase.
C. Both Rb1 and EWS genes are implicated in the development of retinoblastoma.
D. In a developing retina, inactivation of Rb1 is necessary and sufficient for tumor formation.

Question 30.7. Which of the following pediatric conditions is NOT associated with known genetic events that predispose to tumor development in children?

A. Retinoblastoma
B. Neuroblastoma
C. Ewing's sarcoma
D. Hodgkin's lymphoma

Question 30.8. Children with WAGR, Denys-Drash, and Beckwith-Wiedemann syndromes are all predisposed to develop the same tumor. Pick the CORRECT answer:

A. Retinoblastoma
B. Neuroblastoma
C. Neurofibromatosis
D. Wilms' tumor

Question 30.9. Which of the following tumors is uncommon in the pediatric age group?

A. RMS
B. Neuroblastoma
C. Wilms' tumor
D. Colon carcinoma

Question 30.10.   **WAGR, a syndrome complex with deletions at chromosome 11q13, the locus of the WT1 gene, predisposes to Wilms' tumor and involves the following structures (choose one answer):**

A. Iris, genitourinary (GU) system, IQ
B. Ovaries, gut, and central nervous system (CNS)
C. CNS, heart, and kidneys
D. None of the above

Question 30.11.   **Strong correlations are present between all of the following, EXCEPT:**

A. Wilms' tumor, intersex disorders, and progressive renal failure
B. Macroglossia, hyperinsulinemia, and Wilms' tumor
C. Neurofibromas, café au lait spots, and optic glioma
D. Mental retardation, spinal abnormalities, and neuroblastoma

Question 30.12.   **The NF1 gene on chromosome 17 has which of the following functions:**

A. Encoding a ubiquitously expressed protein neurofibromin
B. Facilitating the hydrolysis of GTP to GDP by ras oncoprotein
C. Sending inhibitory signals to cell division
D. All of the above

Question 30.13.   **Each of the following is associated with poor prognosis neuroblastoma, EXCEPT:**

A. N-myc amplification
B. trkA gene activation
C. LOH at 1p36 and 11q23
D. Telomerase expression and increased telomere length

Question 30.14.   **The fusion transcript associated with t(11;22), EWS-ETS, or EWS-FLI-1, and loss of p53 and/or p16 signaling are associated with all the following tumors, EXCEPT:**

A. Osteosarcoma
B. Ewing's sarcoma
C. Askin's tumor
D. Peripheral primitive neuroectodermal tumor (pPNET)

Question 30.15.   **Which of the following statements regarding the molecular basis for the development of embryonal RMS is FALSE?**

A. They are characterized by loss of heterozygosity (LOH) at the 11p15 locus.
B. Insulin-like growth factor (IGF)-2 gene activity is increased twofold.
C. IGF-2 tumor suppressor gene activity is lost with the LOH.
D. There is loss of paternal imprinting of IGF-2.

Question 30.16. **Alveolar RMS has all the following molecular characteristics, EXCEPT:**

A. t(2;13) or t(1;13) translocation (PAX-3-FKHR or PAX-7-FKHR fusion)
B. Increased expression of myoblast growth factor (MGF)
C. Increased c-met expression
D. Increased hepatocyte growth factor (HGF) expression

Question 30.17. **The Li-Fraumeni syndrome is characterized by the following:**

A. Germline mutations in the tumor suppressor gene p53
B. Expression of a stabilized mutant protein in affected cells
C. Mutation or deletion of the second wild-type p53 allele in tumors
D. All of the above

Question 30.18. **Therapeutic interventions targeted at known molecular abnormalities and pathways are being tested using the following intervention strategies:**

A. Agents blocking growth hormone IGF-1 pathways
B. Agents targeting mutant transcription factors
C. All agents listed
D. Agents targeting tyrosine kinase enzymes that transduce growth factor signals

Question 30.19. **A 2-year-old girl is brought to the doctor after her mother feels a hard lump near the umbilicus that is not painful. On physical examination, she is noted to be a large child with hemihypertrophy. A large (6 × 6-cm) hard mass is palpable in the left flank. The remainder of his examination is normal. Laboratory evaluation of blood counts, urinalysis, serum electrolytes, and liver and renal function test results are normal. An ultrasound confirms the presence of a mass involving the superior pole of the left kidney. Which of the following anatomic areas are unlikely to be involved by this tumor?**

A. Lung
B. Muscle
C. Lymph nodes
D. Renal vein

Question 30.20. **Which of the tests listed below is necessary to correctly stage this tumor?**

A. Head computed tomography (CT)
B. Bone scan
C. Plain chest radiograph
D. Skeletal survey

Question 30.21.   **The patient is taken to surgery. Which of the following is the ideal surgical approach for accurate diagnosis and staging?**

A.   Start preoperative chemotherapy followed by resection at a later date because of the size of mass.
B.   Biopsy the mass and sample draining lymph nodes.
C.   Resect the mass and renal vein if involved.
D.   Resect the mass with renal vein if involved, explore the opposite kidney, and sample drain lymph nodes.

Question 30.22.   **After surgical resection and staging, the tumor is confirmed to be consistent with stage III favorable histology Wilms' tumor. Treatment should include which of the following:**

A.   Surgical resection only
B.   Surgery and radiation therapy to kidney
C.   Radiation and chemotherapy
D.   Surgery, radiation, and chemotherapy

Question 30.23.   **Factors associated with good prognosis during the evaluation of Wilms' tumor include which of the following:**

A.   Tumor size <550 g
B.   Favorable histology with only focal anaplasia
C.   Isolated single pulmonary metastatic nodule
D.   Limited extension into renal vein

Question 30.24.   **A 2-year-old child is brought to the emergency department with low-grade fever, pallor, lethargy, extensive bruising, and "raccoon" eyes (periorbital hematomas). On examination, it is noted that the child appears ill and has a left-sided abdominal mass that is firm and nontender. He also has involuntary rapid eye movements, noticed over 2 to 3 weeks. A biopsy of the mass confirms the presence of a neuroblastoma. All of the following procedures are helpful for further staging and workup, EXCEPT:**

A.   CT scan of the chest and abdomen, bone scan, skeletal survey
B.   Splenectomy, liver biopsy, and exploratory laparotomy
C.   Biopsy of local lymph nodes, bone marrow aspiration/biopsy
D.   Radiolabeled (123)I-metaiodobenzylguanidine (MIBG) scan and determination of urine catecholamines

Question 30.25.   **Staging workup reveals stage IV neuroblastoma involving the periorbital area, multiple bones, and bone marrow. Treatment modalities include all of the following, EXCEPT:**

A.   Combination chemotherapy: carboplatinum, cyclophosphamide, doxorubicin, and etoposide
B.   High-dose chemotherapy and autologous stem cell rescue
C.   Allogeneic stem cell transplant
D.   Radiotherapy and biologic response modifiers, such as 13-cis retinoic acid

Question 30.26. **Therapy planning for infants with a small adrenal mass and bone marrow involvement and non-myc amplification includes:**

A. Resection of the mass and short-course chemotherapy
B. Resection of the mass, radiation if residual disease, and short-course chemotherapy
C. Monitoring for spontaneous regression
D. 13-cis retinoic acid therapy only

Question 30.27. **Which of the following statements about the genetics of retinoblastoma transmission is NOT true?**

A. It is transmitted as a highly penetrant autosomal dominant trait and is the most common pediatric ocular tumor.
B. The majority of retinoblastomas are hereditary, bilateral, and caused by germline mutations of 13q14; only 10% to 15% are sporadic and unilateral.
C. All sporadic bilateral retinoblastomas also have a germline mutation transmitted in an identical manner as familial retinoblastoma.
D. The parents and siblings of all patients with retinoblastoma should have a thorough ophthalmoscopic evaluation whether or not there is family history of the disease.

Questions 30.28.–30.31. **An 11-month-old boy who has just learned to walk is noticed to consistently bump into objects in his path. There is no history of major medical illness in this healthy child. The parents report a "white-looking" eye on the right side that was not observed during a regular pediatric checkup at 6 months of age. There is no family history of ophthalmic disease or tumors. On examination, he has a white pupillary reflex on the right side. In addition, mild proptosis and a sixth nerve palsy are noticed in the right eye. The remainder of the physical examination is normal. A biopsy confirms the presence of retinoblastoma.**

Question 30.28. **All patients with retinoblastoma should undergo the following staging studies, EXCEPT:**

A. CT of the orbit
B. Magnetic resonance imaging (MRI) of the orbit and head to include the optic nerve
C. Meticulous inspection under general anesthesia of both eyes
D. Lumbar puncture and cerebrospinal fluid (CSF) cytology

Question 30.29. **Further staging studies reveal complete visual loss in the affected eye and tumor involving the right orbit and optic nerve. The left eye is normal. CSF, bone, and bone marrow studies are normal. Therapy should include:**

A. Cryotherapy or hyperthermia
B. Plaque radiotherapy and chemotherapy
C. Enucleation with a sufficient length of the affected optic nerve
D. Enucleation with a sufficient length of the affected optic nerve and local radiation

Question 30.30.   **Enucleation instead of vision-sparing interventions is indicated for all of the following, EXCEPT:**

A.   Bilateral neuroblastoma with multiple lesions in both eyes
B.   Unilateral retinoblastoma that completely fills the globe
C.   Painful glaucoma and loss of vision in one eye
D.   Bilateral retinoblastoma with no useful vision in either eye

Question 30.31.   **The potential side effects of therapy for this patient include all of the following, EXCEPT:**

A.   Second cancers
B.   Orbital hypoplasia
C.   Cataract formation in the contralateral eye
D.   Recurrent disease

Question 30.32.   **The most common site(s) of origin of RMS is/are:**

A.   Head and neck
B.   Extremities and trunk
C.   Abdomen and GU tract
D.   Spinal canal

Question 30.33.   **Survival is excellent (>70%) with current therapy in all of the following groups of patients, EXCEPT:**

A.   Embryonal extremity Group III tumors
B.   Group III orbital tumors
C.   Embryonal Group III nonorbital tumors
D.   Embryonal tumors in children between 1 and 10 years of age

Question 30.34.   **Staging studies for RMS should include all the following, EXCEPT:**

A.   CT or MRI of the primary site
B.   MIBG scan
C.   Bone scan and bilateral bone marrow sampling
D.   Lymph node sampling

Question 30.35.   **A 6-year-old boy presents with a soft tissue mass involving the right cheek, noticed by his mother to cause facial asymmetry and proptosis, worsening over 3 to 4 weeks. He has no other systemic symptoms. Physical examination reveals a large, hard, right, lower orbital mass. An upper cervical lymph node is also palpable on the right side of his neck, measuring 2 cm in diameter. CT scan of the face and neck confirm the presence of a large tumor involving the right orbit and maxillary sinus. An incisional biopsy confirms the presence of embryonal RMS, and the lymph node is positive for tumor. Which of the following would NOT be appropriate therapy for this child?**

A.   Gross total resection of tumor with facial reconstruction at initial diagnosis
B.   Chemotherapy: vincristine, dactinomycin, and cyclophosphamide
C.   Radiation therapy to the site of tumor and lymph node metastasis
D.   Second-look surgery to assess chemotherapy responsiveness to chemotherapy

Question 30.36. **All of the following statements about treatment of RMS are true, EXCEPT:**

A. Treatment for parameningeal RMS with intracranial extension should include radiation.
B. Local radiation should be used for all patients with microscopic or gross residual RMS.
C. Hyperfractionated radiotherapy is better than conventional fractionated radiation for control of local, regional, or metastatic RMS.
D. Surgical intervention in RMS should aim for complete tumor resection with negative margins whenever possible.

Question 30.37. **Small round blue cell tumors of childhood include all of the following, EXCEPT:**

A. Ewing's sarcoma
B. Neuroblastoma
C. RMS
D. Wilms' tumor

Question 30.38. **The most frequent site of metastasis in Ewing's sarcoma is:**

A. Liver
B. Lung
C. Spleen
D. Lymph nodes

Question 30.39. **The most important feature that distinguishes osteosarcoma from Ewing's sarcoma, chondrosarcoma, and fibrosarcoma is:**

A. Metaphyseal rather than diaphyseal origin
B. The production of osteoid
C. A "sunburst" pattern on radiologic examination
D. Specificity of chromosomal translocations by karyotyping

Question 30.40. **All of the following treatment modalities are useful in osteosarcoma, EXCEPT:**

A. Isolated surgery in low-grade tumors
B. Chemotherapy regimen that includes cisplatin, doxorubicin, and methotrexate
C. Ifosfamide combined with biologic response modifier liposomal muramyl tripeptide phosphatidylethanolamine (MTP-PE)
D. Radiation therapy

Question 30.41. **All of the following are good prognostic factors in the outcome of Ewing's sarcoma, EXCEPT:**

A. Localized tumor less than 8 cm in diameter and volume less than 100 mL
B. Primary pelvic tumors
C. Low serum lactate dehydrogenase level
D. Type 1 EWS-FLI1 fusion transcripts

Question 30.42.   **All of the following treatment approaches have decreased recurrence rates in Ewing's sarcoma, EXCEPT:**

A. The addition of ifosfamide and etoposide in nonmetastatic patients
B. The addition of irradiation to both the primary tumor and whole lung and/or bone in the case of metastatic disease
C. Preoperative chemotherapy followed by surgical resection
D. Myeloablative chemotherapy and stem cell rescue

Questions 30.43.–30.45.   **A 12-month-old boy who had hemihypertrophy at birth presents with abdominal distension and a right-sided abdominal mass. The mass is confirmed to be arising from the right lobe of the liver by ultrasound of the abdomen. No calcification is identified. The serum alpha-fetoprotein (AFP) level is increased markedly.**

Question 30.43.   **The most likely histologic diagnosis of this mass is:**

A. Hepatoblastoma
B. Neuroblastoma
C. Hepatocellular carcinoma
D. Choriocarcinoma

Question 30.44.   **Family history in this patient can include all of the following, EXCEPT:**

A. Beckwith-Wiedemann syndrome
B. Adenomatous polyposis coli
C. Extreme low birth weight
D. Hepatitis B infection

Question 30.45.   **Staging workup for this patient should include the following, EXCEPT:**

A. Liver and renal function tests
B. Chest radiograph or chest CT
C. MRI of the head
D. CT and/or MRI with magnetic resonance (MR) angiography of the abdomen

Question 30.46.   **The most important treatment for hepatoblastoma is:**

A. Adjuvant chemotherapy
B. Concomitant radiation
C. Cryoablation or radiofrequency ablation of tumor
D. Complete resection of tumor and liver transplantation, if necessary

Question 30.47.   **Which of the following statements is NOT true?**

A. Gonadal tumors are commonly germ cell tumors in adults.
B. Extragonadal germ cell tumors are more frequent in adults than in children.
C. The sacrococcygeal region is the most common site for extragonadal germ cell tumors in children.
D. Extragonadal germ cell tumors may involve the pineal gland, mediastinum, vagina, or retroperitoneum.

Question 30.48.　　**Which of the following is NOT a variety of germ cell tumor?**

　　　A.　Teratoma or teratocarcinoma
　　　B.　Seminomas or dysgerminomas
　　　C.　Embryonal carcinoma
　　　D.　Cholangiocarcinoma

Question 30.49.　　**Which of the following statements about germ cell tumors is NOT true?**

　　　A.　Staging should include CT or MRI scans of the mass and the lymph node region involved, the chest for metastatic disease, a bone scan, and tumor markers.
　　　B.　A transscrotal biopsy of a testicular mass should be performed to confirm the diagnosis of a germ cell tumor.
　　　C.　Cisplatinum-based chemotherapy (cisplatin, vinblastine, and bleomycin [PVB] or cisplatin, etoposide, and bleomycin [PEB]) has resulted in excellent survival, even in advanced-stage disease in children but does not need to be considered in completely resected pediatric germ cell tumors, especially if tumor markers such as AFP return to normal.
　　　D.　Radiation therapy is indicated as second-line therapy for patients who have relapsed after surgery and chemotherapy.

Question 30.50.　　**Which of the following pediatric germ cell tumors would be characterized as low risk?**

　　　A.　A localized completely resected testicular tumor by high inguinal orchiectomy
　　　B.　An ovarian tumor that is completely resected and with only microscopic residual disease
　　　C.　An extragonadal germ cell tumor that has metastasized only to locally draining lymph nodes
　　　D.　An extragonadal germ cell tumor that is fully resected with only microscopic residual disease

ANSWERS

Answer 30.1.　　**The answer is C.**

Pediatric malignancies generally cannot be traced to long-term exposure to known carcinogens because they occur in the young, without time for prolonged exposure and transition to a malignant change.

Answer 30.2.　　**The answer is D.**

The mechanisms listed above are some of the known pathways of carcinogenesis in the pediatric age group and predispose to specific groups of malignant disorders.

Answer 30.3.   **The answer is C.**

Many hereditary premalignant disorders, such as Li-Fraumeni, hereditary retinoblastoma, and familial adenomatous polyposis, are devoid of physical stigmata making them difficult to diagnose without a detailed family history.

Answer 30.4.   **The answer is B.**

Xeroderma pigmentosum predisposes to melanoma and leukemia and is caused by multiple gene mutations.

Answer 30.5.   **The answer is A.**

Each of the tumors listed have specific cytogenetic markers associated with them that promote tumor development and aid in diagnosis and evaluation.

Answer 30.6.   **The answer is C.**

EWS is not implicated in retinoblastoma formation but is involved in the development of Ewing's sarcoma. Amplification of MDMX results in retinoblastoma progression.

Answer 30.7.   **The answer is D.**

Retinoblastoma is associated with deletions or mutations of Rb1. In neuroblastoma, there are deletions or mutations in the short arm of chromosome 1, and rarely chromosomes 10, 14, 17, and 19; neuroblastoma is also associated with amplification of the N-myc oncogene. Ewing's sarcoma is characterized by a reciprocal t(11;22) translocation, fusing a transcription factor FLI-1 with oncogene EWS.

Answer 30.8.   **The answer is D.**

The WAGR syndrome has a constitutional deletion of chromosome 11q13. Patients with DDS have germline mutations in WT1. The BWS gene maps to 11p15.

Answer 30.9.   **The answer is D.**

Multiple genetic events are necessary for the development of colon cancer resulting in tumor formation predominantly in adults. All others are common pediatric malignancies.

Answer 30.10.   **The answer is A.**

Three hereditary syndromes genetically predispose to Wilms' tumor. WAGR manifests with aniridia, GU abnormalities, and mental retardation. Denys-Drash syndrome manifests with intersex disorders and progressive renal failure. Beckwith-Wiedemann syndrome, the most common, is a hereditary overgrowth syndrome characterized by macroglossia, visceromegaly, and hyperinsulinemia.

Answer 30.11.   **The answer is D.**

Wilms' tumor and neurofibromatosis are often associated with syndromic manifestations that are easy to recognize. No association is described between neurologic abnormalities and neuroblastoma.

Answer 30.12.   **The answer is D.**

Loss of neurofibromin activity (on both alleles) because of mutations in NF1 results in elevated levels of GTP-bound ras oncoprotein that transduces signals for cell division. This is one of the mechanisms of tumor development in neurofibromatosis type 1. The NF2 gene located on chromosome 22 has been implicated in tumor genesis when nonfunctional in neurofibromatosis type 2 by interfering with the function of the protein it encodes, called "merlin."

Answer 30.13.   **The answer is B.**

Nerve growth factor (NGF) receptor trkA gene amplification shows ganglionic differentiation and has a favorable prognosis. All other markers, including trkB receptor expression, herald poor prognosis neuroblastoma.

Answer 30.14.   **The answer is A.**

EWS-ETS fusion transcripts or related variants can be found in >90% of peripheral PNET group of tumors by reverse transcriptase polymerase chain reaction (RT-PCR) or fluorescence in situ hybridization.

Answer 30.15.   **The answer is C.**

Paternal gene duplication or loss of imprinting (LOI) of the normally transcriptionally silent maternal allele results in overexpression of IGF-2 in embryonal RMS.

Answer 30.16.   **The answer is B.**

Except for MGF, all other statements regarding alveolar RMS are true. Additional mutations on p53 are also described. Interestingly, the mouse model with overexpression of PAX-3-FKHR develops no tumors, but mice expressing an HGF transgene develop embryonal RMS.

Answer 30.17.   **The answer is D.**

Some 60% to 80% of Li-Fraumeni families have detectable germline mutations in p53. The others may be associated with modifier genes, promoter defects, or involvement of other as yet known candidate genes involved in the p53 tumor suppressor pathway. hCHK2, a checkpoint kinase, is a potential candidate.

Answer 30.18.   **The answer is C.**

Identification of various altered molecular signaling pathways (e.g., growth factor, tumor suppressor, tyrosine kinase) has shown that novel and more effective treatment approaches may lie within reach when these pathways are targeted against tumors.

Answer 30.19.   **The answer is B.**

The presentation is classic for Wilms' tumor. This often silent tumor can metastasize or invade all the structures listed and can perforate through the capsule if very large. It is, however, unlikely to invade muscle tissue. The common pathologic variety is termed "favorable histology Wilms' tumor."

Answer 30.20.   **The answer is C.**

Pulmonary metastasis is the most common site of distant dissemination. The need for a chest CT in addition to a chest radiograph is controversial because small nodules identified by CT scans are often negative on biopsy. Pulmonary nodules should be biopsied to prove tumor dissemination. Brain and bone imaging are only necessary if the diagnosis includes rare renal tumors, such as clear cell sarcoma or rhabdoid tumor.

Answer 30.21.   **The answer is D.**

The National Wilms Tumor Study Group (NWTSG) supports tumor resection. There is a 19.8% operative complication rate that includes intestinal obstruction and hemorrhage. Although the SIOP has promoted the use of preoperative chemotherapy before biopsy, there is a 7.6% to 9.9% rate of benign or other malignant disorders involving the kidney in children. The risk of rupture of the tumor during surgery is 14% and may be associated with an increased risk of local recurrence. Preoperative chemotherapy after a biopsy is recommended for solitary kidneys, bilateral renal tumors, tumor in a horseshoe kidney, or patients who are anesthesia risks because of extensive lung involvement. Exploring the opposite kidney is also recommended by the NWTSG because there is a small chance that involvement of the opposite kidney may be missed by all other imaging studies.

Answer 30.22.   **The answer is D.**

Surgical resection of the tumor is combined with lymph node sampling and examination of the contralateral kidney (bilateral tumor is present in 5% of patients) to complete staging. Stage III disease involves the presence of residual nonhematogenous tumor confined to the abdomen. The chemotherapy combination used through serial NWTSG trials is vincristine and dactinomycin for patients with a low stage (I and II) and doxorubicin with or without cyclophosphamide for patients with a higher stage and those with unfavorable histology, such as anaplastic Wilms' tumor or clear cell sarcoma.

Answer 30.23.   **The answer is A.**

Some of these prognostic factors no longer pertain because of the development of effective therapy via the NWSTG (trials 1 to 5) and other international trials. Histology and lymph node involvement remain the most important prognostic factors. Survival for most children with favorable histology Wilms' tumor now approaches 90%. The presence of extension or metastatic spread results in intensification of therapy.

Answer 30.24.   **The answer is B.**

Neuroblastoma, a tumor of the sympathetic nervous system, disseminates frequently to the bone, bone marrow, and lymph nodes. Clinical symptoms depend on the location of the tumor and may include Horner syndrome and spinal cord compression. Hematogenous dissemination is evident in 62% of patients at diagnosis. Undifferentiated tumor (Shimada histology), low DNA ploidy, N-myc amplification, and disseminated disease are associated with poor prognosis. Other poor prognostic markers include low Trk A and high Trk B expression, chromosome 1p deletion, and chromosome 17q gains. In a unique small group of infants, small primary tumors with metastatic disease restricted to the liver, skin, and bone marrow without bone involvement (stage IV S) have favorable prognosis. Tumors in infants often have the capacity to regress spontaneously. For the new International Neuroblastoma Staging System (INSS), see *PPO* Table 50.2.2 on page 2047.

Answer 30.25.   **The answer is C.**

Intense chemotherapy alone achieves a remission rate of 22% ± 4% in disseminated neuroblastoma and can be improved to 34% ± 4% with autologous bone marrow transplant. The addition of 13-cis retinoic acid improves the 3-year relapse free survival rate to 46% ± 6% in these patients. Those with residual disease or positive lymph nodes have better control with local radiation therapy (24 to 30 Gy) to involved areas. Low-risk patients (stage I, stage II with N-myc amplification <10 or >10 with favorable Shimada histology, stage IVS, and hyperdiploidy) often require no treatment. Allogeneic transplants have not demonstrated a definite benefit to date.

Answer 30.26.   **The answer is C.**

Neuroblastoma as described in the question is a special entity. It has a high rate of spontaneous remission and excellent survival. Intermediate-risk neuroblastomas, a rare subgroup (10% to 15%) generally in older children, are generally large and localized. Surgery and moderately intense chemotherapy results in 4-year event-free survival (EFS) rates of 54% to 100%.

Answer 30.27.   **The answer is B.**

The majority of retinoblastomas are sporadic and unilateral (70% to 75%). The median age at diagnosis is 1 to 2 years. Between 10% and 15% of patients with unilateral retinoblastoma have germline mutations of chromosome 13q14. Between 25% and 30% of children with sporadic retinoblastoma have bilateral disease and carry germline mutations of 13q14. The median age at diagnosis is less than 12 months.

Answer 30.28.   **The answer is D.**

The risk of dissemination of retinoblastoma is determined by the extent of ocular tumor and is increased by involvement of the choroid, optic nerve, anterior chamber, ciliary body, and orbit. Lumbar puncture, bone marrow, and bone scan should only be performed in patients with extraocular involvement or in the presence of symptoms and signs of involvement of distant sites.

Answer 30.29.   **The answer is D.**

Cryotherapy, hyperthermia, and photocoagulation can be used instead of enucleation for unilateral or bilateral localized disease that does not involve the globe or the anterior chamber to preserve vision. Enucleation, where indicated, should include a 10- to 15-mm length of optic nerve to obtain a tumor-free margin. External beam radiation including the entire orbit and optic nerve up to the optic chiasm (44 to 50 Gy) is indicated for orbital involvement. For intraocular or recurrent disease, chemotherapy agents (vincristine, etoposide, cyclophosphamide, doxorubicin, cis-platinum, and cyclosporin A as an multidrug resistance [MDR]-reversing agent) are used in combination with other modalities to preserve vision or avoid enucleation, or as salvage. They are most useful on group I to IV tumors. However, chemotherapy alone rarely achieves durable control.

Answer 30.30.   **The answer is A.**

There is excellent response to vision-sparing interventions in retinoblastoma. These include photocoagulation, cryotherapy, hyperthermia, plaque radiotherapy, and so forth. Enucleation should only be undertaken if there is severe inflammation, no salvageable vision, or extraocular extension at risk for metastatic disease. For staging and classification of retinoblastoma see *PPO* Tables 50.2.6 and 50.2.7 on page 2055.

Answer 30.31.   **The answer is D.**

Radiation therapy increases the risk of second malignancies, especially bone tumors in the area of radiation, predisposes to cataracts, and interferes with normal development of the orbit.

Answer 30.32.   **The answer is A.**

In the head and neck area, orbital tumors are the most common, accounting for 13% of all RMS diagnosed. The second common site includes the abdomen and GU tract and tends to affect younger children, sometimes in infancy. Tumors at both these sites tend to be embryonal in histology. Genital tumors (cervical, vaginal) are likely to be of botryoid histology with excellent prognosis (6%). Trunk and extremity tumors are likely to be diagnosed in the second decade of life. These tumors are more likely to have an alveolar histology. Twenty-five percent of all newly diagnosed cases are metastatic at initial presentation. Embryonal histology RMS has a better prognosis than alveolar histology tumors.

Answer 30.33. **The answer is A.**

Recent analyses of prognostic factors in patients with nonmetastatic disease have identified distinct risk groups for failure-free survival. For staging and grouping classifications see *PPO* Tables 50.2.10 and 50.2.11. Stage I group I/IIa or III orbit (90% survival), stage II group I and II embryonal tumors, and stage III group I and II embryonal tumors have greater than 85% survival. Survival is poor (<50%) despite all treatment modalities in patients with embryonal extremity or alveolar tumors (see *PPO* Table 50.2.12 on page 2070), and children with metastatic disease. Younger children aged less than 10 years fare better.

Answer 30.34. **The answer is B.**

MIBG scans are indicated for neuroblastoma and not RMS. The other scans and bone marrow samples are necessary in view of dissemination patterns of RMS that include both hematogenous spread and lymphatic spread to the draining lymph nodes. Treatment decisions are based on TNM staging (see *PPO* Table 50.2.10 on page 2069), and clinical group is based on extent of resection (see *PPO* Table 50.2.11 on page 2070). Prognosis depends on stage, age, clinical group, histology, and primary site. Orbital, vaginal, and paratesticular tumors have the best prognosis, whereas extremity and parameningeal tumors are unfavorable. Tumors that are more than 5 cm and that present in children less than 10 years of age have a worse prognosis.

Answer 30.35. **The answer is A.**

Orbital tumors are usually of embryonal histology and have excellent response to radiation and chemotherapy. Surgical resection is only indicated for recurrent disease. The dose of radiation is 45 to 55 Gy over 5 to 6 weeks. Children with group II or III RMS of the orbit have a 5-year progression-free survival rate of 90%. Parameningeal disease (usually group III) has a 5-year progression free survival rate of 78% without CNS involvement and 70% with CNS involvement. Extensive surgeries are not necessary to sites that produce significant surgical morbidity.

Answer 30.36. **The answer is C.**

Radiation therapy for RMS is indicated only for gross or microscopic residual disease or regional and metastatic extension. The dose for microscopic residual disease is 41 to 50 Gy. Tested in IRS IV, hyperfractionated radiation had no added benefit over conventional fractionated radiation. Surgical resection should be attempted in the place of an incisional biopsy upfront only if the tumor is completely resectable. No radiation is necessary in the event of complete resection of the tumor without microscopic residual or regional extension.

Answer 30.37. **The answer is D.**

All the other tumors have similar light microscopy features that group them into this category.

Answer 30.38.   **The answer is B.**

The lung, bones, and bone marrow are the most common sites of hematogenous spread of Ewing's sarcoma. Lesions that originate in long bones characteristically involve the diaphysis. Parallel lamellated periosteal new bone formation frequently presents with an "onion skin" appearance. Radionuclide scans determine the presence of bone metastases. CT or MRI scans detect the presence of associated soft tissue masses and lung lesions.

Answer 30.39.   **The answer is B.**

The main feature that distinguishes osteosarcoma from other tumors that arise from primitive mesenchymal cells is the production of osteoid and thus is the *sine qua non* for this tumor.

Answer 30.40.   **The answer is D.**

Osteosarcomas are not very sensitive to radiation therapy. All other treatment modalities are used. Adjuvant chemotherapy has increased osteosarcoma survival rates to more than 60%. Juxtacortical osteosarcomas (parosteal and periosteal) that do not invade the medullary cavity may be treated with surgical resection alone.

Answer 30.41.   **The answer is B.**

Pelvic tumors, even when nonmetastatic, herald a poor prognosis perhaps because of poor resectability at this location. Patients with type 1 fusion transcripts of EWS-FLI1 have a 5-year EFS of 70% in contrast with 20% for all other types of fusion transcripts. Low lactate dehydrogenase levels and good response to therapy are other predictors of a better prognosis in Ewing's sarcoma.

Answer 30.42.   **The answer is D.**

Although it is still being explored, previous studies have shown no benefit to adding myeloablative chemotherapy and stem cell rescue to standard chemo/radiotherapy and surgery in patients with high-risk disease.

Answer 30.43.   **The answer is A.**

Hepatoblastoma is the most common primary hepatic tumor in the young with a median age at presentation of 1 year. In contrast, the median age at which hepatocellular carcinoma (HCC) presents is 12 years. Both demonstrate a male predominance. Patients with hepatoblastoma frequently have additional abnormalities, such as hemihypertrophy, congenital absence of the kidney or adrenal gland, and umbilical hernia. AFP levels are increased in 90% of patients with hepatoblastoma and in 78% of adult patients with HCC. HCC is associated with hepatitis B, biliary atresia, galactosemia, Fanconi anemia, and a1-antitrypsin deficiency. Malignant tumors of the liver are rarely calcified.

Answer 30.44. **The answer is D.**

Familial adenomatous polyposis coli has been identified in mothers and maternal relatives of several patients with hepatoblastoma. The risk of hepatoblastoma arising in children from kindreds with the APC gene on the long arm of chromosome 5 is 1000 to 2000 times higher than in sporadic cases. In Japanese children, hepatoblastoma accounted for 58% of cancer diagnoses in children with extremely low birth weight (<1000 g). HCC is strongly associated with hepatitis B infection, acquired by vertical transmission from infected mothers or contaminated blood products. HCC is also associated with other disorders, such as tyrosinemia, galactosemia, biliary atresia, giant cell hepatitis of infancy, and Fanconi anemia.

Answer 30.45. **The answer is C.**

Intracranial metastasis is not a common feature of malignant hepatic tumors. The grouping system used in therapeutic studies segregates patients according to resectability and lymph node or hematogenous metastases. Laboratory tests are not useful for a differential diagnosis of malignant hepatic tumors in children. Pulmonary metastases are identified on a plain chest radiograph in approximately 10% of patients with hepatic tumors. The PRETEXT staging system by the European liver study group divides the liver into four sectors and characterizes tumors by the sectors involved; it was devised to facilitate the assessment of neoadjuvant chemotherapy in rendering tumors resectable and appears to have prognostic value.

Answer 30.46. **The answer is D.**

Resection is the primary treatment for hepatoblastoma and HCC. Long-term survival is rare in the absence of successful resection. Hepatoblastoma is generally unifocal, and approximately one half of all hepatoblastomas are resectable at initial presentation. HCC has an invasive pattern of spread across anatomic planes and is unresponsive to current forms of chemotherapy. Complete resection of HCC is frequently difficult because of multifocality and invasiveness. Only 30% of HCC tumors can be fully resected at diagnosis.

Answer 30.47. **The answer is B.**

Only 5% to 10% of germ cell tumors are extragonadal in adults, whereas 60% are extragonadal in children. Forty percent of all childhood germ cell tumors involve the sacrococcygeal region. Germ cell tumors are relatively rare in children and account for 3% of pediatric malignancies.

Answer 30.48. **The answer is D.**

All the others are varieties of germ cell tumors, each with characteristic histologic features. High AFP levels are common in pediatric patients with testicular, ovarian, presacral, and vaginal primary yolk sac tumors. AFP is a glycoprotein produced in the liver, gastrointestinal tract, and yolk sac of the human fetus. It has a long half-life of 7 days. Human chorionic gonadotropin (hCG) is a glycoprotein secreted by the placenta. Patients with non–yolk sac tumors, such as embryonal carcinoma, choriocarcinoma, and malignant germ cell tumors of the ovary, have elevated hCG levels. hCG has a short half-life of 24 to 36 hours.

Answer 30.49. **The answer is B.**

Transscrotal biopsy contaminates the scrotum and the lymphatic drainage to the inguinal lymph nodes and prevents high ligation of the spermatic cord. All scrotal masses should be explored through an inguinal incision. If the tumor is malignant, high ligation of the spermatic cord should be performed at the internal ring. With adjuvant chemotherapy consisting of PVB or PEB, 5-year survival rates for germ cell tumors are more than 80%, even for advanced stage disease. Radiation is reserved only for recurrent or refractory disease.

Answer 30.50. **The answer is A.**

A localized testicular tumor that is resected in the right fashion by high orchiectomy qualifies for close observation only. All others use adjuvant chemotherapy.

Lymphomas

Directions   Each of the numbered items below is followed by lettered answers. Select the ONE lettered answer that is BEST in each case unless instructed otherwise.

QUESTIONS

Question 31.1.   **Which is NOT true of leukemias and lymphomas of childhood?**

A. Demonstrate better outcomes than adults with leukemia and lymphomas.

B. Cure rates range from 60% to 90%, and more than two thirds of children are treated in clinical trials.

C. Young adults (<30 years) display similar clinical and molecular features as seen in children.

D. Young adults are not eligible for enrollment in pediatric clinical trials.

Question 31.2.   **Which of the following statements is NOT true regarding leukemias in childhood?**

A. The ratio of acute myeloid leukemia (AML) to acute lymphoblastic leukemia (ALL) cases in children is 1 to 4. Black and Hispanic children develop higher risk forms of ALL than white children.

B. Age 1 to 9 years, trisomy 4 and 10, high hyperdiploidy (>50 chromosomes), and absence of central nervous system (CNS) lymphoblasts (CNS-1) are good prognostic features in ALL.

C. Electromagnetic field exposure is not associated with increased incidence of leukemia.

D. Juvenile myelomonocytic leukemia (JMML) is more common than chronic myeloid leukemia (CML) in children.

Corresponding Chapter in *Cancer: Principles & Practice of Oncology*, Eighth Edition: 51 (Lymphomas).

399

Question 31.3.   **All of the following statements about childhood leukemias are true, EXCEPT:**

A. Bloom's, ataxia telangiectasia, Schwachman-Diamond, Sotos, Noonan's syndromes, and neurofibromatosis are associated with increased incidence of leukemia.
B. ALL relapses involve testicular and CNS extramedullary sites, requiring localized therapy and a second full course of systemic therapy.
C. Down's syndrome (trisomy 21) is associated with ALL in the neonatal period.
D. ALL treatment protocols contain an intensive induction/consolidation phase within 6 to 12 months followed by prolonged maintenance/continuation phases lasting 2 to 3 years.

Question 31.4.   **All of the following inherited syndromes are associated with a higher risk of childhood lymphomas, EXCEPT:**

A. Wiskott-Aldrich
B. X-linked lymphoproliferative syndrome
C. Ataxia telangiectasia
D. Human immunodeficiency virus (HIV)-acquired immunodeficiency syndrome

Question 31.5.   **The following are true regarding childhood Burkitt's lymphomas, EXCEPT:**

A. Burkitt's and atypical Burkitt's lymphoma are uncommon.
B. Rasburicase reduces hyperuricemia in tumor lysis.
C. The majority display t(8;14) (q24;q32) translocation.
D. The c-myc oncogene is overexpressed, leading to increased B-cell proliferation and transcriptional activation.

Question 31.6.   **The following are true regarding childhood Hodgkin's lymphoma (HL), EXCEPT:**

A. Occurs mostly in children aged more than 10 years, mostly localized.
B. Mediastinal involvement is common in nodular sclerosing HL.
C. Epstein-Barr virus (EBV) is detected in 40% of pediatric HL cases.
D. Nodular lymphocyte-predominant Hodgkin's lymphoma (NLPHL) occurs in 15% of cases and is usually disseminated.

Question 31.7.   **Regarding the epidemiology of lymphoma, all of the following are true, EXCEPT:**

A. Non-Hodgkin's lymphoma (NHL) and HL are the most commonly occurring hematologic malignancies in the United States and the fifth leading cause of cancer death in the United States.
B. Nasal T-cell lymphomas are more common in China.
C. The largest increases have occurred in low-grade lymphomas.
D. Higher rates of gastric lymphoma have been reported in Northern Italy.

Question 31.8.　**The following statements about bacterial infectious agents linked to lymphoma genesis are all true, EXCEPT:**

A.　*Helicobacter pylori* is linked to gastric mucosa-associated lymphoid tissue (MALT) lymphomas.

B.　*Chlamydia psittaci* is associated with periorbital marginal zone lymphomas in the United States.

C.　*Borrelia burgdorferi* is detected in skin lesions in primary cutaneous B-cell lymphoma.

D.　*Campylobacter jejuni* has been linked to immunoproliferative small intestinal disorder (alpha-chain disease).

Question 31.9.　**Which viral infectious agent is NOT linked to lymphoma?**

A.　Human herpesvirus-8 is associated with primary effusion lymphoma.

B.　Hepatitis C is associated with monocytoid B-cell lymphomas, lymphoplasmacytoid lymphomas, and chronic lymphocytic leukemia (CLL)/small lymphocytic leukemia (SLL), primarily in Northern Italy.

C.　Human T-cell leukemia virus 1 is always found in adult T-cell leukemia/lymphoma.

D.　Coxsackie B virus is linked to enteropathy-type intestinal T-cell lymphoma.

Question 31.10.　**All of the following statements about lymphocyte differentiation are true, EXCEPT:**

A.　Follicular lymphomas are derived from germinal center B cells in which centrocytes fail to undergo apoptosis because of the translocation t(14;18) (q32;q21), which prevents the switching off of bcl-2.

B.　Burkitt's lymphoma corresponds to the early surface immunoglobulin (Ig)M positive (sIgM +) B blast found in the early germinal center reaction; they express sIg, CD10, and CD20, and are negative for CD23, CD5, and cyclin D1.

C.　Antigen-specific effector T cells, either CD4 or CD8 type or memory T cells, evolve from antigen-stimulated T-cell reactions. CD4 T-helper cells (Th1 and Th2) produce cytokines that affect B-cell function and modulate antigen-presenting cells (APCs) and the immune response.

D.　Th1 T cells produce interleukin (IL)-4, 5, 6, and 10, which help B cells produce antibodies.

Question 31.11.　**Genetic abnormalities in CLL/SLL can influence prognosis and include all of the following, EXCEPT:**

A.　t(11;18)(q21;q21) and/or i(7q)(q10)

B.　11q23 deletion involving the ATM gene, which is also seen in T-cell prolymphocytic leukemia (T-PLL)

C.　17p13 deletion involving the p53 tumor suppressor gene

D.　Trisomy 12 and/or 13q14 deletion (the latter also seen in myeloma)

Question 31.12.   **All of the following are true about CLL/SLL, EXCEPT:**

A. Deletion 17p13 predicts poor survival and fludarabine resistance.
B. CD38 expression and ZAP-70 are associated with poor prognosis.
C. Unmutated Ig V region is associated with good prognosis.
D. Autoimmune hemolytic anemia and immune thrombocytopenia require therapy with glucocorticoids, intravenous gammaglobulin, and/or rituximab.

Question 31.13.   **Initial therapy of CLL/SLL may include all, EXCEPT:**

A. Bendamustine
B. Fludarabine, cyclophosphamide, and rituximab (antibody to CD20)
C. Alemtuzumab (Campath-1H) (antibody to CD52)
D. Reduced-intensity allogeneic stem cell transplantation or autologous stem cell transplantation

Question 31.14.   **All of the following apply to lymphoplasmacytic lymphomas, EXCEPT:**

A. It is a neoplasm of small B lymphocytes, plasmacytoid lymphocytes, and plasma cells lacking CD5, CD10, and CD23, with strong expression of sIg and CD20, differentiating it from CLL/SLL.
B. Translocation of t(9;14)(p13;q32) and rearrangement of the PAX-5 gene.
C. Thalidomide (an immunomodulatory agent derivative) and bortezomib (a proteosome inhibitor) are not active in these lymphomas.
D. Monoclonal serum IgM paraproteinemia, with or without hyperviscosity, characterizes Waldenstrom's macroglobulinemia. Clinical presentation commonly involves the marrow, nodes, and spleen, but rarely involves pulmonary, small bowel, and renal sites (the latter seen with mixed cryoglobulinemia and hepatitis C virus [HCV]).

Question 31.15.   **All of the following apply to International Prognostic Index (IPI) for diffuse large B-cell lymphoma (DLCBL) and the Follicular Prognostic Index (FL-IPI) for follicular lymphoma, EXCEPT:**

A. The IPI in DLCBL includes age >60 years, abnormal serum lactic dehydrogenase (LDH), progression-free survival (PFS) ≥2, >2 nodal sites, and advanced-stage disease.
B. IPI in DLCBL was developed after the introduction of rituximab and cytoxan, hydroxydoxorubicin, oncovin, prednisone (CHOP) chemoimmunotherapy.
C. The FL-IPI includes >4 nodal sites, age >60 years, Ann Arbor staging, LDH > normal, and hemoglobin <12 g/dL.
D. Five-year overall survival (OS) rates were 90% for low-risk patients (FL-IPI 0-1) and 50% for poor-risk patients with FL-IPI >3.

Question 31.16. **Higher risk of CNS relapse may occur in all of the following large cell lymphoma presentations, EXCEPT:**

A. Paranasal sinus involvement; epidural involvement
B. Bone marrow involvement and high IPI score
C. Testicular involvement
D. Tonsillar involvement

Question 31.17. **Regarding the staging workup of NHL and HL, all are true, EXCEPT:**

A. The fluorodeoxyglucose (FDG) positron emission tomography (PET) scan is highly reliable in finding disease activity in intermediate/high-grade lymphoma and HL.
B. The FDG-PET scan is less reliable in detecting extranodal marginal zone lymphoma.
C. The FDG-PET scan has replaced gallium scans in staging lymphoma.
D. The FDG-PET scan is not useful in the evaluation of splenic involvement.

Question 31.18. **Regarding splenic marginal zone lymphoma (SMZL), all are true, EXCEPT:**

A. Patients can have circulating ''villous'' lymphocytes; most tumors are CD5 negative and express CD19, CD20, CD22, and bcl-2.
B. Hemoglobin <12 g/dL, LDH > normal, and albumin <3.5 g/dL are risk factors predicting a shorter survival of 50%.
C. Disease is confined only to the spleen.
D. Observation, splenectomy, and chemotherapy with alkylating agents and purine analogs similar to follicular lymphoma are used in these patients.

Question 31.19. **Regarding follicular lymphoma, all are true, EXCEPT:**

A. Radiotherapy (RT) is the standard of care in early-stage disease (CS I and II).
B. Radioimmunotherapy, novel monoclonal antibodies, proteosome inhibitors, and tumor vaccines have all been associated with responses.
C. Autologous stem cell transplantation is curative for patients with advanced-stage disease.
D. Translocations involving BCL6 are seen in DLCBL transformation.

Question 31.20. **All of the following apply to mantle cell lymphoma (MCL), EXCEPT:**

A. t(11;14)(q13;q32) is seen in mantle cell lymphoma, along with cyclin D1 overexpression.
B. Bortezomib and temsirolimus have not shown activity in MCL.
C. MCL accounts for 7% of adult NHL in the United States and Europe, and most patients present in stage IV disease (70%).
D. Hyper-CVAD + rituximab and/or clinical trials incorporating autologous or allogeneic stem cell transplantation with or without bortezomib maintenance should be considered in MCL in younger patients.

Question 31.21. **All of the following are true about MCL, EXCEPT:**

    A. Tumor cells strongly express sIgM and IgD (often of lambda light chain type) and B-cell–associated antigens, and arise from antigen-naïve B cells of the inner mantle zone.

    B. Some 70% of patients have stage IV at diagnosis: Lymph node, bone marrow, spleen, Waldeyer's ring, and gastrointestinal involvement (lymphomatous polyposis) are common.

    C. Median OS is 3 years, with no plateau in the curve in historical series.

    D. R-CHOP has improved survival compared with CHOP in de novo MCL.

Question 31.22. **All of the following are true of diffuse large B-cell lymphoma (DLBCL), EXCEPT:**

    A. It is the most common lymphoma (31% in REAL series); patients often have rapidly enlarging nodal masses and B symptoms. Up to 40% of DLBCLs are extranodal, and marrow involvement is seen in 16%.

    B. At least two subtypes have been defined by gene expression profiling (GEP), germinal center B cell (GCB), and activated B cell (ABC). GCB survival is better than ABC survival and has the t(11;14)(q32; q21) translocation, supporting the hypothesis that this DLBCL sub-type is of follicular cell origin.

    C. GCB and ABC DLBCL subtypes cannot be differentiated by immu-nochemistry.

    D. Known subtypes of DLBCL include T-cell–rich B histiocyte cell var-iant, plasmablastic type seen in HIV-positive patients, and a rare ALK-positive variant.

Question 31.23. **Regarding diffuse DLBCL, which of the following statements is NOT correct?**

    A. Abbreviated CHOP chemotherapy plus involved field RT is excellent therapy for patients with low-risk, nonbulky, early-stage DLBCL.

    B. Standard initial treatment for advanced-stage DLBCL is CHOP plus rituximab; ongoing clinical trials are focusing on the role of upfront autologous stem cell transplantation in patients with high IPI.

    C. In a subset analysis of the GELA R-CHOP trial, rituximab appeared to confer greater benefit in patients with DLBCL who do not express bcl2 on immunocytochemistry.

    D. Autologous stem cell transplantation is the treatment of choice for patients with relapsed DLBCL that is shown to be chemosensitive.

Question 31.24.　A 61-year-old physician is seen by her gastroenterologist because of persistent upper abdominal pain that is not relieved with antacids. The physical examination is unremarkable. The complete blood cell count (CBC) shows the following: hemoglobin of 10 g/dL, mean corpuscular volume of 82 (fl), white blood cell count (WBC) of 5000/μL, and platelet count of 500,000/μL. Upper gastrointestinal (GI) endoscopy reveals several superficial raised lesions in the gastric antrum. Biopsy of the lesions show features consistent with low-grade MALT lymphoma. *H. pylori* is present in the biopsy specimen. A computed tomography (CT) scan of the chest, abdomen, and pelvis does not show lymphadenopathy or hepatosplenomegaly. Bone marrow examination reveals no evidence of lymphoma. You recommend:

A.　Antibiotic therapy
B.　Chemotherapy with CHOP
C.　Rituximab at 375 mg/m^2 intravenously (IV) weekly for four doses.
D.　RT and/or surgical consult for gastrectomy

Question 31.25.　A 25-year-old college student has had a sore throat for 4 weeks associated with pain on swallowing. A 4-cm mass in the right tonsil is found showing diffuse large B-cell lymphoma by biopsy. Further staging reveals no other adenopathy or hepatosplenomegaly. CT scan of the neck, chest, and abdomen reveals no further abnormality. The patient is classified as Eastern Collaborative Oncology Group (ECOG) performance status (PS) 0. A bone marrow biopsy does not reveal evidence of lymphoma involvement. The CBC and LDH are normal. You recommend:

A.　CHOP every 3 weeks for eight cycles
B.　CHOP and rituximab every 3 weeks for eight cycles
C.　CHOP for three cycles followed by RT
D.　CHOP and rituximab for three cycles followed by RT

Question 31.26.　A 42-year-old woman presents with enlarged cervical lymph nodes 16 months after initial therapy with R-CHOP chemoimmunotherapy for diffuse large B-cell lymphoma, stage IVB. She now has no "B" symptoms and her physical examination results are unremarkable except for multiple enlarged left cervical lymph nodes, the largest being 2.5 × 4 cm. CBC shows a hemoglobin level of 11 g/dL, WBC of 4300/μL with absolute neutrophil count (ANC) of 3000/mm^3, and platelet count of 300,000/μL. LDH is normal. The patient is classified as ECOG PS 0. A biopsy of a left cervical lymph node reveals diffuse large B-cell lymphoma. PET-CT scan of the chest, abdomen, and pelvis shows no detectable disease elsewhere. A bone marrow biopsy does not reveal evidence of lymphoma. What would you recommend?

A.　CHOP and rituximab for three cycles followed by RT
B.　Radioimmunotherapy (Bexxar or Zevalin)
C.　Two cycles of rituximab-ifosfamide, cisplatin, and etoposide (R-ICE) chemotherapy followed by autologous peripheral blood stem cell transplantation with BEAM
D.　Fludarabine, busulfan, and thymoglobulin reduced-intensity allogeneic stem cell transplantation

Question 31.27. **Primary mediastinal (thymic) large B-cell lymphomas (PMBCLs) are characterized by all of the following, EXCEPT:**

A. Involve the thymus. Tumor cells correspond to B cells in the thymic medulla and are Ig negative but express B-cell–associated antigens CD19, CD20, CD22, CD79a, and CD45. Most cases are BCL6 positive and Ig heavy, and light-chain genes are rearranged, whereas BCL2 and BCL6 are germline.

B. Express FIG1 and amplified REL oncogene on chromosome 9p and overexpress the MAL gene at chromosome 2p13-15.

C. Gene expression profiling (GEP) of PMBCL is similar to DLCBL with overexpression of the MAL and FIG1 genes.

D. OS at 5 years in patients aged less than 65 years treated with MACOP-B/VACOP-B, R-CHOP, and CHOP is 87%, 81%, and 71%, respectively (Vancouver series). Addition of RT did not improve survival in this series.

Question 31.28. **Which statement is FALSE about natural killer (NK)/T-cell neoplasms?**

A. Extranodal NK/T-cell lymphoma is EBV+, is common in Asia and Peru, and can affect children and adults. Hemophagocytic syndrome may occur.

B. Extranodal sites involve the nose, palate, upper airway, gastrointestinal tract, and skin.

C. Atypical cells are CD2+, CD56+, surface CD3−, cytoplasmic CD3+, and many are CD4− CD8− and express cytoplasmic granule proteins (granzyme B and TIA-1).

D. Relapse after RT alone is rare. Patients with disseminated disease are cured by CHOP therapy.

Question 31.29. **Which statement is FALSE about T-cell neoplasms?**

A. Enteropathy-type T-cell lymphoma occurs in adults with gluten-sensitive enteropathy (antigliadin antibodies). Outcomes in patients with advanced celiac disease are very poor.

B. Anaplastic large T/null cell lymphoma expresses ALK-1, CD30, and usually CD25; therapy with DLCBL active regimen without rituxan is used; the outcome of ALK− patients is worse (31% to 37%) than that of ALK+ patients (71% to 95%). Responses have been seen with CD30-directed monoclonal antibodies.

C. Subcutaneous panniculitis T-cell lymphoma is a cytotoxic T-cell neoplasm that infiltrates subcutaneous tissues. Hemophagocytic syndrome is common with fever and serositis, myalgias, and joint pains. Disease prognosis is very good with chemotherapy.

D. Hepatosplenic T-cell lymphoma is rare, and diagnosis is often difficult. Patients present with organomegaly and sinusoidal infiltrates in the liver, spleen, or marrow. It is CD2+CD3+CD5−, CD4−CD8−CD16+CD56+/−. TCRg and TCRd genes are rearranged; isochromosome 7 is common and trisomy 8 may be seen.

Question 31.30. **Which statement about CTCL is FALSE?**

A. The skin is the most common extranodal site of lymphomas.

B. The World Health Organization European Organization for Research and Treatment of Cancer (WHO-EORTC) classification identifies three groups as CTCL: cutaneous T/NK cell lymphoma (mycosis fungoides [MF]) and its Sézary subtype, now viewed as a distinct entity; the cutaneous B-cell lymphomas; and the precursor hematologic neoplasms.

C. B-cell CTCL includes marginal zone (mucosa-associated lymphoid tissue) lymphoma, primary cutaneous follicular cell lymphoma, diffuse cutaneous B-cell lymphoma, intravascular large B-cell lymphoma, lymphomatoid granulomatosis, and cutaneous involvement of MCL, CLL, and Burkitt's lymphoma.

D. Precursor hematologic neoplasms include the blastic NK/cell dermal neoplasms, precursor lymphoblastic leukemia/lymphomas, and myeloid leukemia.

Question 31.31. **All is true about Sézary syndrome (SS), EXCEPT:**

A. Sézary cells are peripheral blood atypical lymphocytes with hyperconvoluted nuclei. SS is defined as diffuse erythroderma with circulating neoplastic SS cells at >1000 cells/mm^3.

B. IL-11 is an autocrine and paracrine growth factor for Sézary cells.

C. Loss of antigens CD2, CD7, and CD4 is seen in MF/SS.

D. CTCL express cutaneous T-cell antigen (CLA) that binds E selectin on activated endothelial venules and facilitates homing to the skin via CCL17/CCR4 chemokine receptor interactions.

Question 31.32. **All are true about MF, EXCEPT:**

A. Outcome of MF/SS is not correlated with clinical stage.

B. Features include patches, plaques, erythroderma, and cutaneous tumors or ulcers. T-cell receptor rearrangement is used in the differential diagnosis (psoriasis, eczema, large plaque parapsoriasis, and drug eruptions).

C. Therapy for localized disease includes topical carmustine or mechlorethamine, bexarotene, ultraviolet B, plus near ultraviolet light (PUVA) $\pm$ interferon alpha and electron beam radiation.

D. Systemic therapy may include chemotherapy (EPOCH, pentostatin, fludarabine + interferon alpha, gemcitabine, and doxorubicin), extracorporeal photochemotherapy, denileukin diftitox $\pm$ bexarotene, histone acetylase inhibition (vorinostat), and the monoclonal antibodies alemtuzumab and zanolimumab.

Question 31.33. **Which statement is FALSE regarding primary CNS lymphoma (PCNSL)?**

A. PCNSL was once a rare tumor accounting for 0.5% to 1.25% of intracranial neoplasms, usually associated with congenital, acquired, or iatrogenic immunodeficiency states.

B. PCNSL has increased threefold from 1985 to 1997 in immunocompetent individuals. This increase was part of an overall increase in all extranodal NHLs.

C. Frontal lobe presentation is the least frequent in brain PCNSL.

D. Brain lesions are multifocal in 40% of normal patients and 100% of patients with acquired immunodeficiency syndrome (AIDS). The frequency of AIDS PCNSL has dramatically decreased since the institution of highly active antiretroviral therapy (HAART).

Question 31.34. **Which statement is FALSE regarding PCNSL?**

A. The eye distinct from the orbit is a direct extension of the brain, and approximately 20% of patients with PCNSL have ocular involvement at presentation.

B. Ocular lymphoma involves the vitreous, retina, or choroid, but optic nerve infiltration does not occur.

C. Primary leptomeningeal lymphoma in the absence of a brain mass is rare, approximately 7% of PCNSL. Symptoms of progressive leg weakness, urinary incontinence or retention, cranial neuropathies, and confusion may be present for months before diagnosis; delayed therapy is common because of difficulty of diagnosis.

D. MRI should be the standard imaging technique for patients with PCNSL. Prominent contrast enhancement is characteristic in 90% of patients.

Question 31.35. **Management and therapy of PCNSL include all, EXCEPT:**

A. Corticosteroids should be avoided before diagnostic biopsy, and resection should be avoided.

B. Polymerase chain reaction for EBV on cerebrospinal fluid in AIDS-associated PCNSL.

C. RT must be whole brain (3600 to 4500 cGy) and may be deferred in patients >60 years of age. Primary treatment of ocular disease is 3500 to 4500 cGy RT to both eyes.

D. Chemotherapy should be considered at diagnosis for every patient, must penetrate the blood–brain barrier (high-dose methotrexate and leucovorin rescue), must be lipophilic (procarbazine), and should be administered after RT.

Question 31.36. **ALL are true of HL, EXCEPT:**

    A. The malignant cells known as Hodgkin cells or Reed-Sternberg (HRS) cells represent 0.15% to 1% of the entire cell population in classic Hodgkin's lymphoma (cHL).

    B. In lymphocyte-predominant Hodgkin's lymphoma (LPHL), HRS cells express B-cell antigens like CD19 and CD20.

    C. In cHL, these HRS cells express the activation marker CD30, and in many cases are CD15 positive and lack major B and T-cell lineage antigens.

    D. HRS cells express IL-13 but lack IL-5.

Question 31.37. **All of the following statements are true, EXCEPT:**

    A. The activator protein (AP)-1 and the nuclear factor-kappa B (NF-kB) transcription factors are constitutively active in cHL.

    B. NF-kB is the central mediator of survival and proliferation of HRS cells in cHL.

    C. Mutations of the NF-kB inhibitory gene IkBa are not important transforming events in cHL in the absence of EBV or other viruses.

    D. Activation of the signal transducer and activator of transcription family (STAT3, STAT6, and STAT5a) have been found in cHL. STAT3 activation was constitutive and did not depend on IL-6, whereas STAT6 depended on IL-13 signaling.

Question 31.38. **All statements are true about the immunology of HL, EXCEPT:**

    A. Eosinophils stimulated by IL-5 and attracted by eotaxin inhibit the Th2 response.

    B. T cells within the HL lymphoma are CD4+, TCRab+, express the CD38, CD69, and CD71 activation markers, but lack CD26 and the IL-2 receptor CD25.

    C. Secretion of IL-10 and TGF-βb by HRS cells and the inability of T cells to secrete IL-2 suppress an effective immune response.

    D. HRS cells are not able to mount an effective immune response.

Question 31.39. **NLPHL differs in several ways from the subtypes of cHL, nodular sclerosing, mixed cellularity, and lymphocyte depleted. All of the following statements about NLPHL are true, EXCEPT:**

    A. Approximately 80% of patients with NLPHL have stage I or II disease at the time of diagnosis.

    B. In contrast with cHL, the atypical cells in NLPHL are CD45+, express B-cell antigens (CD19, CD20, CD22, CD79a, and PAX5), the transcription factors Oct2 and BOB.1, and the germinal center-associated proteins Bcl6 and EMA, but lack CD15 and CD30.

    C. NLPHL does not transform to diffuse large B-cell lymphoma (DLCBL).

    D. NLPHL accounts for 5% of the cases of HL. More than 90% of patients have a clinical remission and are alive at 10 years.

Question 31.40.   **The term "lymphocyte rich classic Hodgkin's lymphoma" (LRCHL) has been proposed in the Revised European–American Lymphoma (REAL) classification for cases of HL with RS cells that appear classic by morphology and immunophenotype and have a background infiltrate consisting predominantly of lymphocytes, with rare or no eosinophils. True statements about LRCHL include all of the following, EXCEPT:**

A.   LRCHL can closely resemble NLPHL morphologically, and immunophenotyping may be required to differentiate the two entities. Cases of LRCHL have the same immunophenotype of cHL with expression of CD15 and CD30 by the HRS cells. CD20 is coexpressed in 3% to 5% of cases.

B.   Follicular meshworks of follicular dendritic cells (FDCs) are seen with antibodies to CD21 or CD35, and RS cells are found within the mantle and interfollicular regions.

C.   Patients with LRCHL usually lack bulky disease or B symptoms and tend to present with early-stage disease. The clinical features at presentation seem to be intermediate between those of NLPHL and cHL.

D.   OS of LRCHL is slightly better than that of NLPHL in the German Hodgkin Study Group studies.

Question 31.41.   **All are true about the association of cHL with other lymphomas, EXCEPT:**

A.   cHL can be associated with high-grade DLCBL, Burkitt's, or Burkitt's-like lymphoma.

B.   Cases of cHL associated with follicular lymphoma or DLCBL may precede, follow, or occur simultaneously with the lymphoma.

C.   B-cell CLL does not transform into HL.

D.   Mediastinal grey zone lymphoma has features of both cHL and DLCBL at diagnosis.

Question 31.42.   **Staging procedures for HL have become simpler and less invasive with the advent of new staging modalities and the use of combined modality treatment. Which of the following statements is TRUE?**

A.   Patients with large mediastinal adenopathy, mediastinal mass >50% of the thoracic diameter at T5-6, or a ratio >50% of the transverse diameter of the mediastinal mass over the diameter of the diaphragmatic thorax have increased risk of relapse (nodal or extranodal sites) after RT alone.

B.   For a patient with early-stage HL treated initially with chemotherapy, if a PET scan is subsequently negative, there is good evidence that the patient does not need adjuvant-involved field RT after chemotherapy.

C.   Staging laparotomy has been replaced by FDG-PET scanning but should be used in rare circumstances in early-stage HL, in which the use of limited RT alone depends on pathologic staging.

D.   Evidence of contiguous spread of HL is most convincing in patients with LP disease.

Question 31.43. **A 25-year-old man with stage IIA nodular sclerosing HL was treated with total nodal RT 3 years ago. The patient now presents with a new enlarged lymph node in the groin. A biopsy of the node confirms a diagnosis of recurrent HL, nodular sclerosing type. The patient has no "B" symptoms. A restaging workup includes a CT scan of the chest, abdomen, and pelvis, and PET scanning. Recurrent disease is found in nodes above and below the diaphragm. A bone marrow biopsy is negative for HL. The patient is classified with clinical stage IIIA. Which of the following statements is TRUE?**

A. Because the patient has recurrent disease after initial curative therapy, he should be treated with allogeneic or autologous high-dose chemotherapy and stem cell transplant (ASCT).

B. Patients with early-stage HL who relapse after RT fare worse than patients who relapse after initial conventional chemotherapy, suggesting that RT affects drug resistance and can compromise chemotherapy outcome.

C. Treatment with Adriamycin, bleomycin, vinblastine, dacarbazine (ABVD) chemotherapy results in superior disease-free survival compared with nitrogen mustard, oncovin, procarbazine, prednisone (MOPP) regimen in patients with recurrent HL after RT.

D. Advanced relapsing patients with "B" symptoms after prior RT have a low 10-year survival when treated with conventional salvage chemotherapy (<10%) and should be considered for ASCT as initial therapy rather than conventional chemotherapy.

Question 31.44. **The following statements about standard treatment strategy in HL are true, EXCEPT:**

A. Early stages, favorable patients: radiation alone (extended field).

B. Early stages, unfavorable patients: moderate amount of chemotherapy (typically four cycles) plus radiation.

C. In patients who receive pelvic irradiation for subdiaphragmatic HL, men have a high risk of loss of fertility. The risk of loss of fertility in women is minimal, particularly in women aged less than 25 years at the time of treatment.

D. Advanced stages: extensive chemotherapy (typically eight cycles) with or without consolidation RT (usually local).

Question 31.45.   **All of the following statements about HL during pregnancy are true, EXCEPT:**

    A. CT scanning is to be avoided because it exposes the fetus to ionizing radiation. Magnetic resonance imaging (MRI) may be used for staging because it is nonteratogenic.

    B. Chemotherapy drugs that act as antimetabolites, such as methotrexate, have a high risk of causing teratogenesis. The long-term survival of women with HL who were pregnant at the time of initial presentation is worse than that of nonpregnant women with similar stages of disease.

    C. In the second or third trimester of pregnancy, if there is rapid progression of supradiaphragmatic lymphadenopathy, RT alone can be used. If involved field or mantle radiation is used with abdominal shielding, the risk of adverse sequelae for the fetus is low.

    D. If HL is diagnosed in the first trimester of pregnancy, therapeutic options in early pregnancy are limited and include supradiaphragmatic irradiation or pregnancy termination. If the woman wants to continue the pregnancy, treatment should be deferred until at least the second trimester, if possible.

Question 31.46.   **Patients with HL develop treatment-related complications after curative therapy for HL. All of the following statements such as secondary malignancies are true, EXCEPT:**

    A. Secondary AML appears to be higher in patients treated with ABVD regimen, compared with patients treated with MOPP.

    B. Treatment-related AML has a latency period of 3 to 5 years, and most cases occur within 10 years of the initial treatment.

    C. Most cases of NHL occurring after HL have intermediate or high-grade histology.

    D. Solid tumors tend to occur in the second decade after therapy and include lung cancer in smokers and breast cancer in women.

Question 31.47.   **All of the following statements about long-term complications in patients with HL are true, EXCEPT:**

    A. Myocardial damage from radiation and anthracycline exposure can be serious.

    B. Lung fibrosis is not seen after exposure to RT plus bleomycin or BCNU-based high-dose therapy (i.e., BEAM or BEC)/autologous SCT.

    C. Hypothyroidism after mantle RT can be detected by finding an elevated thyroid-stimulating hormone (TSH) level.

    D. The risk of postsplenectomy sepsis can be minimized by immunization with pneumococcal vaccine; vaccines have also been developed against Neisseria and Haemophilus, which are also associated with postsplenectomy sepsis.

Question 31.48. **The German Hodgkin Study Group (GHSG) recently conducted a series of clinical trials to look at the role of dose intensification in advanced HL. The BEACOPP regimen (bleomycin, etoposide, doxorubicin, cyclophosphamide, vincristine, procarbazine, and prednisone) was used as a standard combination for dose escalation. The GHSG designed a three-arm study comparing COPP/ABVD, standard BEACOPP, and escalated BEACOPP in patients with advanced HL. Approximately two thirds of the patients also received consolidation RT. In 1996, at an interim analysis, the COPP/ABVD arm was closed to accrual because it was inferior to the BEACOPP arm. All of the following statements about the GHSG trial are true, EXCEPT:**

A. At a median of 5 years, the freedom from treatment failure rate was 69% for COPP/ABVD, 76% for standard BEACOPP, and 87% for the escalated BEACOPP.

B. There were nine cases of AML/MDS in the escalated BEACOPP arm, whereas there were two cases in the standard BEACOPP arm; also, the total rate of second neoplasms was highest in the escalated BEACOPP arm.

C. Escalated BEACOPP was associated with greater hematologic toxicity, requiring more red cell and platelet transfusions, but there were no differences in hematologic toxicity between the standard BEACOPP arm and the COPP/ABVD arm.

D. Rates of early progression were significantly lower with the escalated BEACOPP compared with standard BEACOPP and COPP/ABVD.

Question 31.49. **Several trials have looked at the use of less-toxic chemotherapy combined with RT. These combinations would allow a reduction in the amount and toxicity of chemotherapy and the use of smaller radiation volumes. All of the following statements are true, EXCEPT:**

A. A less-toxic regimen, vinblastine, bleomycin, and methotrexate (VBM) was developed at Stanford. A trial treating patients with PS IA to IIIA compared subtotal nodal/total nodal irradiation with involved field irradiation followed by VBM. There was no significant difference in OS.

B. The British National Lymphoma Investigation (BNLI) trial found that the combination of VBM with involved field irradiation produced unacceptable pulmonary and hematologic toxicity.

C. In a later Stanford trial, patients with CS IA-IIIA HL received subtotal nodal and splenic irradiation or two cycles of VBM, followed by regional mantle irradiation and then four more cycles of VBM with dose-reduced bleomycin. There was no difference in PFS or OS.

D. The German Hodgkin Lymphoma Study Group (GHSG) HD7 (1994 to 1998) trial randomized 643 CS IA-IIB patients to either subtotal nodal and splenic irradiation alone or to two courses of ABVD and the same RT. No difference was seen in the freedom from treatment failure between the two groups.

Question 31.50.   **All of the following statements about new treatment modalities in HL are true, EXCEPT:**

A. Vinorelbine, idarubicin, and gemcitabine have been found to have activity in HL.

B. Native monoclonal antibodies have been tested in HL: CD20-based antibodies are not active in LPHL.

C. Anti-CD30 antibodies and bispecific anti-CD30 antibodies (CD16/CD30; CD30/CD64) are currently under development.

D. In EBV-positive HL, mostly LMP2a-specific autologous cytotoxic CD8 T cells have been generated in vitro and shown to be active in vivo.

ANSWERS

Answer 31.1.   **The answer is D.**

Patients aged less than 30 years are eligible for treatment in pediatric clinical trials. Many findings and methods first shown to be useful in pediatric oncology (including the clinical trial mechanism itself) have been successfully applied to adult oncology.

Answer 31.2.   **The answer is D.**

ALL is the most common malignancy arising from precursor T or B-lymphoid cells. JMML accounts for less than 1% of childhood leukemia cases, whereas CML occurs in approximately 3% to 4% and AML occurs in 15% to 20% of childhood leukemia cases. JMML is a myeloproliferative disorder characterized by extreme monocytosis and hepatosplenomegaly, thrombocytopenia and increased fetal hemoglobin, dysplastic hypercellular marrow, and often monosomy 7 by cytogenetics. Mutations of PTN11 and RAS pathway genes have been noted in JMML.

Answer 31.3.   **The answer is C.**

Patients with trisomy 21, Down syndrome have a higher risk for ALL up to age 13 years, but not in the neonatal period. Extra copies of chromosome 21 are a common finding but carry no prognostic meaning. In neonates, a transient myeloproliferative disease is seen that resolves spontaneously. AML M7 develops in patients with Down syndrome aged less than 2 years and is associated with GATA-1 mutations.

Answer 31.4.   **The answer is D.**

HIV infection is an acquired infection and is associated with increased secondary lymphomas possibly related to EBV infection and a low CD4 count. Common variable immunodeficiency is also a risk factor, but its cause is not known and may be a function of environmental exposure and genetic predisposition.

Answer 31.5. **The answer is A.**

Burkitt's and atypical Burkitt's lymphoma are common histologies seen in 40% to 50% of pediatric NHL cases. Endemic Burkitt's lymphoma in Africa is more common (100 cases per million children), presents in the head and neck, involves the jaw, and is associated with EBV in 95% of cases. Sporadic Burkitt's lymphoma is seen in the United States, presents with an abdominal mass in one to two cases per million children, and only 15% are EBV associated.

Answer 31.6. **The answer is D.**

NLPHL affects 10% to 15% of pediatric patients, is usually clinically localized (low stage), and is more common among male and younger patients. It needs to be distinguished from progressive transformation of germinal centers (PTGC), a reactive process associated with follicular hyperplasia. Nodular sclerosing HL is the most frequent histology seen in >50% of cases (40% in younger patients and 70% in adolescents).

Answer 31.7. **The answer is C.**

The largest NHL increase is in patients with aggressive histologies. In primary central nervous system lymphoma, diffuse large B-cell NHL occurs increasingly in patients with AIDS. Adult T-cell leukemia/lymphoma (ATL) is common in Southern Japan and the Caribbean, whereas certain small intestinal lymphomas are commonly seen in the Middle East.

Answer 31.8. **The answer is B.**

Chlamydia psittaci is found in periorbital marginal zone lymphomas in Italy, not in the United States, and unlike *H. pylori* does not show strain specificity.

Answer 31.9. **The answer is D.**

Coxsackie virus infection is not linked to enteropathy type lymphoma but has been implicated in insulin-dependent diabetes mellitus via molecular mimicry. EBV infection can be associated with HHV-8 in primary effusion lymphomas, early posttransplant lymphoproliferative disease (PTLD), and HL. SV40 DNA has been detected in 40% of tumor specimens examined in lymphoma, and further studies are ongoing to evaluate this in specific lymphoma subtypes.

Answer 31.10. **The answer is D.**

Th1 T cells produce IL-2 and interferon gamma, which activate macrophages and cytotoxic T cells, whereas Th2 T cells produce IL-4, 5, 6, and 10, which help B cells produce antibodies.

Answer 31.11. **The answer is A.**

The t(11;18)(q21;q21) translocation seen in MALT lymphomas produces the antiapoptotic API2-MLT fusion protein, which is activated as a consequence of the fusion. Isochromosome 7q deletion is characteristic of hepatosplenic T-cell lymphoma and not CLL.

Answer 31.12.   **The answer is C.**

Unmutated Ig V region is associated with aggressive disease and correlates with ZAP-70 expression (a tyrosine kinase protein normally expressed in T and NK cells) and CD38 antigen expression. (Rassenti LZ, Jain S, Keating MJ, et al. Relative value of ZAP-70, CD38, and immunoglobulin mutation status in predicting aggressive disease in chronic lymphocytic leukemia. Blood 2008;112:1923–1930.)

Answer 31.13.   **The answer is D.**

Allogeneic or autologous stem cell transplantation is not performed as part of front-line therapy in CLL/SLL. Reduced-intensity allogeneic stem cell transplantation offers a chance of long-term cure in high-risk patients with advanced CLL. Bendamustine is a combination alkylator and purine nucleoside analog that has been compared with oral chlorambucil in front-line CLL and has been shown to have activity in relapsed refractory CLL/SLL culminating in full Food and Drug Administration (FDA) approval for both indications. (Keating, MJ, Bach C, Yasothan U, et al. Bendamustine. Nat Rev Drug Discov 2008;7:473–474.)

Answer 31.14.   **The answer is C.**

IMIDs such as thalidomide and lenalinomide, as well as bortezomib, have demonstrated activity in lymphoplasmacytic lymphomas. Like most CD20 positive B-cell lymphomas, the combined use of chemotherapy and immunotherapy with rituxan has improved the disease-free interval and led to greater complete remissions.

Answer 31.15.   **The answer is B.**

The IPI was introduced before the application of chemoimmunotherapy in DLCBL. A retrospective analysis in British Columbia of patients with DLCBL treated with R-CHOP showed that the IPI remained predictive but identified only two risk groups and no longer identified a risk group with <50% chance of survival.

Answer 31.16.   **The answer is D.**

Patients with paranasal sinus, testicular involvement, epidural lymphoma, and bone marrow involvement with large cells are especially prone to meningeal spread and should have a diagnostic lumbar puncture unless their therapy includes agents that penetrate the cerebrospinal fluid, such as high-dose methotrexate and leucovorin rescue. In addition, a lumbar puncture is favored for highly aggressive large cell lymphoma in immunocompromised patients with HIV infections.

Answer 31.17.   **The answer is D.**

The majority of studies evaluating FDG-PET in intermediate/high-grade NHL and HL have shown high standardized uptake value in areas of active disease. FDG-PET is highly reliable in detecting splenic involvement and has rendered laparotomy obsolete in the staging workup of these patients. Many studies have shown the lack of reliability in detecting marginal zone lymphoma, particularly the extranodal marginal type. The available data strongly demonstrate increased sensitivity of FDG-PET compared with the gallium scan in the staging of NHL and has supplanted that test in the workup of patients with lymphoma.

Answer 31.18. **The answer is C.**

SMZL accounts for up to 25% of low-grade B-cell neoplasms in splenectomy samples and 1% to 2% of chronic lymphoid leukemia. The lack of CD103 and CD25 differentiates it from hairy cell leukemia. SMZL is not only found in the spleen but involves the bone marrow, peripheral blood, and unusual sites, such as the central nervous system (leukemic meningitis).

Answer 31.19. **The answer is C.**

Follicular lymphoma arises from the germinal center B cells (centrocytes and centroblasts). Tumors are CD10 +, CD20 +, CD5 −. Most cases are bcl-2 +, and some neoplastic cells have nuclear bcl-6. Rituxan immunotherapy has improved all chemotherapy modalities in this disease, and radioimmunotherapy with I131 Tositumomab (Bexxar) or Ytrium90 ibritumomab tiuxetan (Zevalin) has produced objective responses and is currently under evaluation when combined with chemotherapy (CHOP) and/or autologous stem cell transplantation. Myelodysplastic syndrome has been reported after radioimmunotherapy and high-dose therapy and autologous stem cell transplantation. The latter is not curative in follicular lymphoma, but the addition of rituxan purging has improved disease-free survival and delayed onset of relapses. Rituxan maintenance therapy has been used in various stages of the disease, but its ultimate benefit may reside in patients who are receiving chemotherapy for relapsing disease. Reduced-intensity allogeneic stem cell transplantation has been successfully applied to patients with advanced relapsed follicular lymphoma.

Answer 31.20. **The answer is B.**

Bortezomib and the mTOR inhibitor temsirolimus have demonstrated activity in MCL and are under evaluation in clinical trials. Bortezomib maintenance after autologous stem cell transplantation is being evaluated in clinical trials.

Answer 31.21. **The answer is D.**

No differences were observed in PFS (in months) or OS (in years) in a German trial randomizing patients with de novo MCL to R-CHOP versus CHOP. R-CHOP had superior overall response rates and complete remission rates underscoring the importance of rituxan immunotherapy in that setting. Relapses occur from residual MCL cells that have disseminated to remote sites. Recently, rituxan maintenance has been reported to improve progression-free and overall survival rates after combined (R-Fcm) in patients with relapsed follicular and mantle cell lymphoma.

Answer 31.22.   **The answer is C.**

A panel of three immunohistochemical stains (CD10, BCL6, and MUM1) has been validated for distinction of the CGB and ABC subtypes of DLCBL. Localized stage I and II extranodal disease is seen in 30% of cases. Host response, B-cell receptor/proliferation, and oxidative-phosphorylation have been found by GEP to be associated with favorable outcome.

Answer 31.23.   **The answer is C.**

The benefit of rituximab was greater in patients with lymphoma that overexpressed bcl-2 on immunochemistry.

Answer 31.24.   **The answer is A.**

The standard treatment of low-grade MALT lymphoma of the stomach associated with *H. pylori* is antibiotic therapy and follow-up with endoscopy 3 to 6 months later. *H. pylori* eradication can result in lymphoma regression in more than 50% of patients with low-grade MALT lymphoma of the stomach. Patients who have complete response should be followed without further treatment. Patients who have a partial response and remain *H. pylori* positive should receive a second course of antibiotics before proceeding to more definitive treatment. Patients who are negative for *H. pylori* are unlikely to respond to antibiotics and should be considered for RT or chemotherapy.

Answer 31.25.   **The answer is D.**

The Southwest Oncology Group Trial in a recent pilot study has shown that R-CHOP × 3 plus RT led to outstanding results. The mabThera International Trial (Min T) used six cycles of CHOP-like chemotherapy in young patients with favorable risk factors (75%) with early-stage disease. In that study the rituximab-containing arm had outstanding results without added RT. Ongoing clinical trials are comparing radioimmunotherapy with and without radiation and increasingly relying on FDG-PET imaging to define optimal amount of therapy.

Answer 31.26.   **The answer is C.**

Abbreviated chemotherapy followed by RT has been shown to be superior to a full course of chemotherapy in patients with untreated limited-stage DLBCL, but this has not been shown to be beneficial in patients relapsing after chemotherapy. The role of R-CHOP (a regimen that was previously used) in the treatment of relapsed aggressive lymphoma is less optimal and may expose the patient to increased cardiac toxicity. On the basis of the Parma trial, this patient would benefit from cytoreductive chemotherapy followed by autologous stem cell transplantation if her lymphoma is still chemosensitive. The addition of granulocyte-macrophage colony-stimulating factor (GM-CSF)/granulocyte colony-stimulating factor (G-CSF) to augment antibody-mediated cellular cytotoxicity may be used to purge residual circulating DLCBL cells before peripheral blood stem cell collection. Radioimmunotherapy is active in large-cell lymphoma, but its role as a single agent in this disease has not been studied prospectively. Reduced-intensity allogeneic stem cell transplantation may be used in patients with less optimal responses or in whom autologous stem cell collection is not possible.

Answer 31.27. **The answer is C.**

The GEP in PMBCL shows a distinct signature from nodal DLCBL, whereas MAL and FIG1 genes were observed; similarities to HL were apparent with loss of B-cell receptor signaling genes and activation of the JAK-2 and NF-kb pathways. Ongoing studies are evaluating bortezomib in combination with R-CHOP therapy in PMBCL.

Answer 31.28. **The answer is D.**

Patients with localized NK/T-cell lymphoma in the nasal pharynx can be cured with a combination of chemotherapy and local RT. With RT alone, treatment failure is frequent. Genetic abnormality includes del(6)(q21;q25); T-receptor genes are germline. Patients with disseminated NK/T-cell lymphoma have an extremely poor outlook and should be enrolled in clinical trials. Early application of high-dose chemotherapy and autologous stem cell transplantation may be curative in some patients after relapse from standard therapy.

Answer 31.29. **The answer is C.**

Subcutaneous panniculitis T-cell lymphoma is associated with atypical lymphoid cells and often with necrosis and karyorrhexis. Responses to RT and chemotherapy are transient, and the long-term outlook is very poor. Early consideration of aggressive approaches, such as autologous or allogeneic stem cell transplantation, is recommended.

Answer 31.30. **The answer is A.**

CTCLs are a heterogeneous group of both T and B lymphocytes that localize to the skin, which is the second most common site of extranodal lymphoma estimated at 1:100,000.

Answer 31.31. **The answer is B.**

Sézary cells are clonal CD4 + CD45RO + T cells; some CTCL variants are CD8 + . Antigen loss is characteristic of the disease (loss of CD7, CD5, or CD2 and dim CD3) and display a Th2 phenotype secreting IL-4, 5, 6, 10, and 13. The pruritus characteristic of this disease is related to IL-5 and other chemokines. IL-7, not IL-11, is an autocrine and paracrine growth factor for these cells. Clinical features of SS include extensive skin involvement with erythroderma that may progress to lichenification, palmoplantar hyperkeratosis, and diffuse exfoliation.

Answer 31.32. **The answer is A.**

Overall outcome in MF is correlated with clinical stage (skin involvement and visceral stage). Staging for MF is based on estimating the degree of skin involvement and the amount of infiltration of lymph nodes and viscera. T1 and T2 are disease patches or plaques on <10% of the skin surface, whereas T4 is erythroderma flat and patch-like with diffusely infiltrated skin and thickening and fissuring of the palms and soles of the feet. LN4 nodes are effaced by tumor cells and characterize patients with poor prognosis.

Answer 31.33. **The answer is C.**

The most common presentation of primary central nervous system lymphoma is the frontal lobe and is associated with changes in personality and level of alertness. Headaches and symptoms of increased intracranial pressure are seen frequently. Many lesions are periventricular, allowing tumor cells to gain access to the cerebrospinal fluid.

Answer 31.34. **The answer is B.**

Optic nerve involvement can occur.

Answer 31.35. **The answer is D.**

The risk of multifocal leukoencephalopathy is higher in older patients and when chemotherapy and RT are overlapping. Radiation boost to affected areas should be avoided. Most often chemotherapy is administered before RT in PCNSL to avoid cognitive damage and decrease neurotoxicity. The blood–brain barrier after completion of cranial RT may remain open weeks to for months, thereby increasing the risks of leukoencephalopathy when drugs accumulate in brain tissue.

Answer 31.36. **The answer is D.**

Hodgkin Reed-Sternberg (HRS) cells express many cytokines and chemokines, thereby explaining the inflammatory infiltrates seen in affected lymph nodes. IL-5 is expressed in 95% of HRS cells and 63% of elaborate eotaxin, thereby providing proliferation and chemotactic signals to recruit eosinophils to the site(s) of HL. Genes like IL (IL-13, 6, 12, and 10), interferon-γ, tumor necrosis factor (TNF)-α, and IL-1 are expressed by HRS cells and mediate the B symptoms and immune dysregulation seen in patients with HL at presentation.

Answer 31.37. **The answer is C.**

Mutations of IκBα were found in 15 of 26 primary cHL cases, 11 of which were EBV-negative.

Answer 31.38. **The answer is A.**

HRS cells effectively escape the host immune system by modulating the immune response in the direction of an impaired Th2 response. Surrounding eosinophils inhibit an effective Th1 response in favor of a primarily humoral Th2 response, which helps the growth of malignant cells in cHL.

Answer 31.39. **The answer is C.**

Transformation of NLPHL to DLCBL occurs in 2% to 6% of cases. The complete response rate after initial therapy is more than 90%. The immunophenotype is an important part of the definition of NLPHL. Unlike typical B-cell lymphomas, however, they are usually immunoglobulin-negative by routine techniques.

Answer 31.40. **The answer is D.**

In the German Hodgkin Study Group, the OS of LRCHL was significantly worse than that of NLPHL.

Answer 31.41. **The answer is C.**

Rare cases of B-cell CLL may contain RS cells, and others may evolve into HL (HL variant of Richter's syndrome). These cases may or may not be clonally related to the CLL. Lymphomas are presumed to arise in the setting of immune deficiency (estimated risk 1% to 5%), and cases of MF, lymphomatoid papulosis, and HL have been reported. Recent gene expression profiling data suggest that mediastinal large B-cell lymphoma is closely related to cHL.

Answer 31.42. **The answer is D.**

Patients with nodular sclerosis (NS) and mixed cellularity (MC) most convincingly display contiguous HL spread. The left and right sides of the neck were each involved in >60% of patients with NS and MC histologies. These sites were at least four times more common as other nodal sites above and below the diaphragm. Most patients with NS or MC HL have a central pattern of nodal involvement (cervical, mediastinal, para-aortic). In MC histology, the spleen is more frequently involved, along with adenopathy below the diaphragm and B symptoms.

Answer 31.43. **The answer is C.**

Patients who relapse after RT alone for conventional HL have satisfactory results with conventional combination chemotherapy. Prior RT does not cause drug resistance or a clinically significant compromise of chemotherapy dose intensity. Patients who relapse with stage IV disease or "B" symptoms have a 10-year disease-free survival as high as 34% and should be treated initially with conventional chemotherapy. It does appear that ABVD gives a better disease-free survival when compared with MOPP in patients with recurrence after radiation (81% with ABVD vs. 54% with MOPP).

Answer 31.44. **The answer is C.**

Women also have a high risk of loss of fertility with pelvic irradiation. There is a lower risk of loss of fertility in women aged less than 25 years who are treated with chemotherapy, not RT.

Answer 31.45. **The answer is B.**

HL is the fourth most common cancer diagnosed during pregnancy and has been reported in 1 of every 1000 to 6000 deliveries. Several studies have shown that pregnancy does not worsen the clinical course of HL, and that the long-term survival of pregnant women with HL is not different from that of nonpregnant women. The ABVD regimen may be used when chemotherapy is indicated beyond the first trimester. Because drugs accumulate in the milk, mothers are advised not to breastfeed during treatment.

Answer 31.46. **The answer is A.**

More cases of secondary AML are seen after MOPP chemotherapy because of exposure to alkylating agents. Diffuse large B-cell lymphoma is more often seen after HL treatment.

Answer 31.47. **The answer is B.**

RT, bleomycin, and high-dose BCNU exposure are all associated with a higher risk of late complications, including severe pulmonary fibrosis.

Answer 31.48. **The answer is B.**

The total rate of secondary neoplasms was highest in the COPP/ABVD arm.

Answer 31.49. **The answer is D.**

In the GHSG HD7 trial, the patients who received two cycles of ABVD had a statistically significant improvement in freedom from treatment failure (91% vs. 75% for irradiation alone, $p < .0001$). This study raised several questions. Is the benefit in freedom from treatment failure worth the risk of long-term toxicity from the exposure to doxorubicin and bleomycin? Will it be more difficult to salvage the patients who relapse after the irradiation if they have already received two cycles of ABVD? Only longer follow-up will answer these questions.

Answer 31.50. **The answer is B.**

The CD20 antigen is expressed on all malignant cells in nodular LPHL. Two phase II trials with rituximab showed promising results with high overall response rates (86% to 100%).

John Welch
Amanda F. Cashen

Acute Leukemias

Directions   Each of the numbered items below is followed by lettered answers. Select the ONE lettered answer that is BEST in each case unless instructed otherwise.

QUESTIONS

Question 32.1.   **The favorable cytogenetic rearrangement in acute myeloid leukemia (AML) resulting from the t(8;21) juxtaposes which genes?**

A. AML1-ETO
B. RUNX1-RUNX1T1
C. A core binding factor and a zinc finger protein
D. All of the above

Question 32.2.   **You are caring for a 25-year-old woman with AML-M2 and normal cytogenetics. She receives 7 + 3 induction therapy, and her day-14 bone marrow biopsy is ablated. She returns to clinic and her day-45 bone marrow biopsy shows normal cellularity with 25% blasts. Which of the following likely contributed to her rapid relapse?**

A. FLT3-ITD
B. CEBPA mutation
C. NPM mutation without FLT3-ITD
D. Her age

Question 32.3.   **Your well-read 30-year-old patient with AML asks you how you will follow her disease once she is in remission. She asks which is the most sensitive test for minimal residual disease? In which order are these assays most sensitive (least to most sensitive)?**

A. Cytopathology < fluorescence in situ hybridization (FISH) < polymerase chain reaction (PCR)
B. FISH < cytogenetics < PCR
C. PCR < cytopathology < FISH
D. Cytogenetics < PCR < flow cytometry

Corresponding Chapter in *Cancer: Principles & Practice of Oncology*, Eighth Edition: 52 (Acute Leukemias).

Question 32.4. Mutations in which pair of transcripts would be expected to cooperatively contribute significantly to leukemia?

    A. FLT3 and ABL
    B. A core binding factor and the retinoic acid receptor alpha
    C. FLT3 and the retinoic acid receptor alpha
    D. Tel-PDGFβR and FLT3

Question 32.5. A 52-year-old man presents with AML. On day 2 of induction therapy he develops diffuse alveolar hemorrhage. An expected physical finding on examination would be:

    A. Diffuse ecchymosis
    B. Diffuse intravascular coagulopathy
    C. Swollen gums
    D. Cardiac rub

Questions 32.6.–32.7. You have been following a 75-year-old woman in clinic with mild renal insufficiency and progressive anemia. She presents to clinic with a 3-day history of progressive fatigue and new headaches. Her white blood cell (WBC) count is 53,000 with 50% blasts.

Question 32.6. Given her history, you might expect to find what on her cytogenetics?

    A. t(15;17)
    B. − 7
    C. inv(16)
    D. t(8;21)

Question 32.7. Which of these improves her prognosis?

    A. Probable leukostasis
    B. Her age
    C. Prior myelodysplastic syndrome (MDS)
    D. Good performance status

Question 32.8. You are caring for a 70-year-old man with newly diagnosed AML. According to his cytogenetics you give him an unfavorable prognosis based on which result:

    A. − 7
    B. t(15;17)
    C. inv(16)
    D. t(8;21)

Question 32.9.   A 25-year-old African American woman presents with pre–B-cell acute lymphoblastic leukemia (ALL). Her initial performance status is 0, albumin is 3.5 mg/dL, and WBC is 25,000/μL. Cytogenetics show a t(12;21) rearrangement. She undergoes induction therapy. Her peripheral blasts resolve by day 5, and her day-14 marrow shows no blasts. Her day-45 marrow again shows no blasts and no t(12;21) rearrangement. All of these are standard risk factors, EXCEPT:

A. Ethnicity
B. Time to clinical remission (CR)
C. Cytogenetics
D. WBC count

Question 32.10.   A 70-year-old man presents with newly diagnosed AML-M4 with eosinophilia. Choice of treatment will be based on all, EXCEPT:

A. His age
B. His performance status
C. His cytogenetics
D. Excellent response to $7+3$ induction therapy in the elderly

Question 32.11.   You have been following a 54-year-old woman with acute promyelocytic leukemia (APL) in clinic. After 2 years she returns to clinic with fatigue, an elevated WBC, and increased promyelocytes. Peripheral blood PCR confirms recurrence of her t(15;17) translocation. Before starting arsenic salvage therapy you obtain which test?

A. Liver function test (LFT)
B. Erythrocyte sedimentation rate (ESR)
C. D-dimer
D. Electrocardiogram (EKG)

Question 32.12.   You have been caring for a 65-year-old woman with a distant history of breast cancer treated with adjuvant cyclophosphamide and Adriamycin. During the last year she developed progressive anemia and thrombocytopenia. She also recently developed leukopenia. Her bone marrow biopsy shows decreased cellularity with dysplastic features and 25% blasts. Which of the following cytogenetic changes might you expect to find?

A. t(15;17)
B. t(9;21)
C. Complex cytogenetics
D. Trisomy 21

Question 32.13.   Which of the following treatment options have shown improved survival in patients aged more than 60 years with AML?

A. Subcutaneous ARA-C
B. Decitabine
C. $7+3$ induction followed by intermediate-dose ARA-C (IDAC) consolidation
D. None of the above

Questions
32.14.–32.18.

You are consulted to see a 20-year-old Hispanic woman who presented with progressive fatigue during the last week and then significant epistaxis. Her WBC is 12,000/μL with 40% promyelocytes and a platelet count of 15,000/μL. Her international normalized ratio (INR) is 2.7 with a prothrombin time (PT) of 45 and partial thromboplastin time (PTT) of 65. Her fibrinogen is 82. On review of her peripheral smear, you observe many promyelocytes with large granules and multiple Auer rods.

Question 32.14.

After review of her peripheral smear, you suspect that she has APL. Your initial therapy would include all of the following, EXCEPT:

A. Fresh-frozen plasma
B. Cryoprecipitate
C. All-trans retinoic acid (ATRA)
D. Arsenic trioxide

Question 32.15.

Three days after starting daunorubicin and ATRA, her coagulopathy has improved. She has shortness of breath in the morning and rapidly becomes hypoxic over the course of the day. Which of the following would prove most helpful in treating her hypoxia?

A. High-flow facemask oxygen
B. Lasix
C. Methylprednisolone
D. Albuterol

Question 32.16.

Fifteen days into treatment she develops a severe headache. Her neurologic examination results are normal, as are her funduscopic examination results. Review of her morning laboratory tests reveal a WBC of 0.6/μL, hematocrit (Hct) of 9.8, platelet count of 25,000/μL, INR of 1.4, and fibrinogen of 190. You obtain a noncontrast head computed tomography (CT) scan but are more worried that this is a result of:

A. Relapse
B. ATRA
C. Daunorubicin
D. Transfusion reaction

Question 32.17.

Six months later you are reviewing her chart. Her CBC has normalized, and she has tolerated consolidation therapy. Her most recent PCR showed no sign of residual disease. You are most concerned about relapse because of:

A. Her microgranular variant presentation
B. Her presenting coagulopathy
C. Her presenting WBC
D. Her ethnicity

Question 32.18.   **Three years later she presents to clinic with an elevated leukocyte count. PCR of peripheral blood confirms the presence of her initial t(15;17) translocation. Treatment options at this point include all of the following, EXCEPT:**

A.   Arsenic trioxide
B.   Gemtuzumab ozogamicin
C.   Autologous transplant after achieving CR
D.   Clofarabine

Question 32.19.   **A 30-year-old, otherwise healthy woman is diagnosed with AML. Cytogenetics reveal inv(16). She undergoes induction therapy. Day-14 bone marrow biopsy shows an ablated marrow. Her day-45 marrow shows restored cellularity without evidence of disease. Repeat cytogenetics do not reveal the inv(16) rearrangement. Appropriate consolidation therapy would be:**

A.   Allogeneic transplant if a matched sibling donor is available
B.   High-dose cytarabine (HIDAC) 3 g/m^2 every 12 hours on days 1, 3, and 5 for four 28-day cycles
C.   Intermediate-dose cytarabine (IDAC) 300 mg/m^2 every 12 hours on days 1, 3, and 5 for four 28-day cycles
D.   Arsenic 0.15 mg/kg on days 1 to 5 for four 28-day cycles

Question 32.20.   **Which of the following regimens require graft-versus-tumor effects to remove residual AML blasts?**

A.   Busulfan-cyclophosphamide
B.   Cyclophosphamide-TBI
C.   Busulfan-fludarabine
D.   Busulfan-VP16

Question 32.21.   **High-dose busulfan used in myeloablative preparative regimens for stem cell transplantation may result in all of the following side effects, EXCEPT:**

A.   Seizures
B.   Mucositis
C.   Pancytopenia
D.   MDS

Question 32.22.   **Central nervous system (CNS) prophylaxis should be considered in which of the following patients?**

A.   A 25-year-old Latina woman with APL who presents with a WBC of 2500/µL, an INR of 2.5, and fibrinogen of 100
B.   A 78-year-old man with AML evolved from MDS
C.   A 30-year-old woman with AML who develops headaches while receiving ondansetron for nausea on day 9 of induction therapy
D.   A 20-year-old man with Down's syndrome and ALL who presents with leukocytosis (WBC 120,000/µL)

Question 32.23.   **Dexamethasone has replaced prednisone in ALL induction therapy because of improved penetration in which tissue?**

A.   Testes
B.   Spleen
C.   Bone marrow
D.   Brain

Question 32.24.   **Maintenance therapy for ALL with daily 6-mercaptopurine, weekly methotrexate, and monthly vincristine and prednisone should be continued for how long?**

A.   6 months
B.   12 months
C.   24 to 36 months
D.   Until relapse

Question 32.25.   **Which of the following targeted agents have been shown to be beneficial in adult ALL?**

A.   Imatinib
B.   Alemtuzumab
C.   Gemtuzumab ozogamicin
D.   Sunitinib

Question 32.26.   **For which of the following patients would you consider myeloablative stem cell transplantation in CR1?**

A.   30-year-old woman with inv(16) AML-M4 with eosinophilia
B.   50-year-old man with complex cytogenetics AML-M1
C.   65-year-old man with complex cytogenetics AML-M1
D.   50-year-old woman with t(15;17) AML-M3

ANSWERS

Answer 32.1.   **The answer is D.**

The favorable t(8;21) translocation results in the juxtaposition of the initially named AML1 gene with the ETO gene (the acute myeloid leukemia gene and the eight-twenty-one gene). These two have recently been renamed RUNX1 and RUNX1T1, respectively. RUNX1 is a member of the core binding factor family of transcription factors, which regulate differentiation of normal blasts. This fusion protein creates a dominant negative protein, which results in a differentiation block. Inv(16) and the t(16;16) rearrangements likewise result in dominant negative effects on core binding factors and are associated with a favorable prognosis.

Answer 32.2.   **The answer is A.**

FLT3 is a tyrosine kinase involved signal transduction leading to myeloid proliferation. The internal tandem duplication (ITD) rearrangement results in constitutive kinase activity and an increase in proliferation. Evidence is mounting that the FLT3-ITD is a marker of unfavorable prognosis. CEBP/α is a transcription factor involved in myeloid differentiation thought to be activated by ATRA treatment in APL. Mutations in the CEBPA gene have been noted in other FAB-AML classifications and have been associated with a superior outcome compared with the wild-type transcript. Nucleophosmin (NPM) mutations, in the absence of the FLT3-ITD, have also been associated with improved prognosis. Age is a strong prognostic factor. However, it is patients who are older than 65 years who have a worse prognosis. Her young age would be a marker of a good prognosis.

Answer 32.3.   **The answer is A.**

Cytopathology requires >5% blasts on a bone marrow biopsy to diagnose AML relapse. This results in a sensitivity of 1 in 20. A cytogenetic review of 30 metaphases results in a 1 in 30 sensitivity. FISH has a sensitivity of approximately 1 in 500. PCR techniques allow sensitivity of approximately 1 in 10^4. However, both FISH and PCR require screening for defined cytogenetic changes. Because initial cytogenetic changes typically recur during AML relapse, this is generally not a significant barrier, unless patients present with uncommon cytogenetic changes for which FISH and PCR probes are not commercially available.

Answer 32.4.   **The answer is C.**

Current models of leukemia suggest that two separate classes of mutations are required for leukemogenesis: an activating mutation and a differentiation mutation. Activating mutations result in dysregulation of proliferative signaling pathways and thus lead to hyperproliferation. Important targets of activating mutations in leukemia include FLT3-ITD, RAS, BCR-ABL, TEL-PDGFβR, and PTPN11. Many of these contain tyrosine kinase domains. Leukemogenic mutations often result in constitutive kinase activity and thus constitutive activity in signal transduction pathways leading to growth and proliferation. Important targets of differentiation mutations include core binding factors (RUNX1 or AML1, CBFβ), retinoic acid receptor alpha, HOXA9, and MOZ. Mutations in these transcripts (frequently resulting from balanced chromosomal rearrangements) result in blocks in differentiation. Current paradigms suggest that leukemia requires both a differentiation block and a dysregulated proliferation. Thus, the common combination of FLT3-ITD and the t(15;17) PML-RARα translocation may be involved in APL leukemogenesis, whereas the other combinations are each within the same functional group.

Answer 32.5.   **The answer is C.**

Diffuse alveolar hemorrhage is a rare complication of induction therapy in AML, which carries significant mortality risk. However, it is most commonly reported in patients with AML and myelomonocytic or monocytic features (M4 or M5). These myelomonoblasts and monoblasts display a predilection for tissue invasion, such as in the gums, as well as into the lungs. This is thought to result from their high expression of adhesion molecules: intercellular adhesion molecule (ICAM) and vascular cell adhesion molecule (VCAM). During initial treatment, activation and death of circulating blasts may lead to pulmonary inflammation and alveolar hemorrhage. Because of the rarity of such events, treatment options remain poorly studied. In small series, high-dose steroids have shown benefit.

Answer 32.6.   **The answer is B.**

AML, which has evolved from MDS, is especially recalcitrant to therapy. It may be associated with −5 or −7 cytogenetic abnormalities but is most commonly associated with complex cytogenetics. This patient is presenting with many poor-risk features (age >60 years, symptoms suggestive of leukostasis, and underlying organ insufficiency), which will make response to therapy difficult.

Answer 32.7.   **The answer is D.**

There are many prognostic factors for AML. Of particular note are age, cytogenetics, and performance status. Age greater than 65 years has been associated with worse outcomes independently of cytogenetics. AML evolving from prior MDS also confers a worse prognosis. Leukostasis at presentation presents significant early morbidity and mortality, especially in an older patient. An elevated peripheral blast count, which may be associated with leukostasis, is also associated with a poor long-term prognosis.

Answer 32.8.   **The answer is A.**

AML prognosis is currently separated into three broad categories based on cytogenetic results: favorable (inv[16]; t[8;21] and t[15;17]); intermediate (normal, +8); and unfavorable (−5, −7, complex with ≥5 chromosomes involved). Some studies have also included 11q, +8, del(20q), t(6;9), and 17p abnormalities in the unfavorable risk group.

Answer 32.9.   **The answer is A.**

High-risk ALL prognostic factors include age >50 years, poor performance status, African American ethnicity, low albumin, leukocytosis (>30,000/μL B-lineage or >100,000/μL T-lineage), a late clinical response (continued peripheral blasts at day 7, continued bone marrow blasts on day 14, >4 weeks to CR). Immunophenotypes including early and mature-T ALL and pro-B ALL are considered high risk. Cytogenetics including the Philadelphia chromosome (t[9;22]) and t(4;11) are both high-risk prognostic factors. However, concurrent imatinib therapy appears to abrogate much of the Philadelphia chromosome risk.

Answer 32.10.   **The answer is D.**

Treatment of AML in the elderly (>65 years) is difficult because of the heterogeneous nature of response and the generally high rate of treatment-related mortality. Older patients at MD Anderson with a performance status >2, bilirubin >1.9 mg/dL, or serum creatinine >1.9 mg/dL had a treatment-related mortality of 62% and only a 27% complete remission rate. Thus, decision to undergo standard induction therapy must be based on a careful assessment of the patient's ability to tolerate the therapy and his/her prognosis. The patient's age, performance status, and low-risk cytogenetics might influence a physician to recommend standard therapy.

Answer 32.11.   **The answer is D.**

Arsenic trioxide has demonstrated considerable activity in salvage therapy for APL. Arsenic trioxide has been associated with prolonged QTc syndrome. Because of this, EKGs should be performed before and during therapy. Electrolytes should also be monitored and corrected. Additional medications that may prolong the QTc should be eliminated if possible.

Answer 32.12.   **The answer is C.**

Prior alkylator therapy increases the risk of myelodysplastic syndrome and treatment-related AML. Her recent history of progressive anemia and thrombocytopenia, with dysplastic features seen in her marrow, are all suggestive of an underlying MDS. Her blast count >20% meets criterion for AML under current World Health Organization (WHO) standards. AML evolved from MDS could carry a loss of chromosome 5 or 7 associated with the prior MDS, but most often is associated with complex cytogenetics. It also carries an unfavorable prognosis in multiple studies. t(15;17) is associated with APL but is not associated with prior breast cancer or alkylator therapy. t(9;21) is associated with the Philadelphia chromosome and seen in chronic myelocytic leukemia or acute lymphocytic leukemia, but not acute myeloid leukemia or MDS. Trisomy 21 is associated with AML-M7 with increased megakaryocytes. Recent data suggest this may be associated with the concomitant overexpression of an miRNA carried on chromosome 21.

Answer 32.13.   **The answer is D.**

Treatment of older patients with AML as a group has been difficult. These patients generally present with worse performance status, unfavorable cytogenetics, and organ insufficiency. Older patients as a group do worse than their younger counterparts independently of these poor prognostic factors. Treatments remain unsatisfactory, and no therapy has been shown to be definitively better than another. Choice of therapy thus relies heavily on the oncologist's assessment of the patient and the patient's interest in pursuing aggressive therapy. Although older patients who achieve a CR do better than those without a CR, it is unclear how best to achieve CR in these patients.

Answer 32.14.   **The answer is D.**

Patients with APL are at considerable risk of early morbidity and mortality because of disseminated intravascular coagulation (DIC) and bleeding complications. Aggressive management of coagulopathy is mandatory, with the goal of maintaining the fibrinogen >150, INR <1.5, and platelet count >30,000. Patients with WBC >10,000/μL are at a higher risk of differentiation syndrome once ATRA is started. Typically, ATRA is held while daunorubicin is started until the WBC is <10,000/μL. Arsenic trioxide has demonstrated significant efficacy in the setting of relapsed APL. Ongoing studies are evaluating its efficacy during induction therapy in conjunction with ATRA. However, it is not currently standard of care during induction therapy.

Answer 32.15.   **The answer is C.**

Differentiation syndrome can be a life-threatening complication of APL and ATRA treatment. As the granule-laden promyelocytes differentiate, the granular products stimulate pulmonary edema and fluid retention. Fevers and weight gain are common symptoms of differentiation syndrome. Treatment includes steroids and management of coagulopathy. Differentiation syndrome may affect as many as 10% to 25% of patients with APL.

Answer 32.16.   **The answer is B.**

Headache is a common side effect from ATRA. Treatment options include dose reduction and symptom management with analgesics. Unfortunately, patients occasionally require drug discontinuation because of this side effect.

Answer 32.17.   **The answer is C.**

The greatest risk of relapse in APL is associated with an elevated WBC >10,000/μL on presentation. Patients with presenting WBC <10,000/μL achieve CR approximately 90% of the time.

Answer 32.18.   **The answer is D.**

Clofarabine is being studied in relapsed AML, but it has not been evaluated in APL. Arsenic trioxide has demonstrated significant efficacy in relapsed APL and in consolidation protocols. APL promyelocytes commonly express high levels of CD33, and gemtuzumab ozogamicin (anti-CD33) has demonstrated efficacy in relapsed APL. APL is one of the few cases in AML in which autologous transplantation has demonstrated significant benefit, and it is often used in a salvage consolidation protocol.

Answer 32.19.   **The answer is B.**

Although most patients with AML will relapse without consolidation therapy, the appropriate consolidation therapy remains unclear for the majority of these patients. Young patients with good-risk cytogenetics are one of the few cohorts with AML in whom specific consolidation recommendations are supported by clinical data. A study sponsored by the Cancer and Leukemia Group B (CALGB) found that young patients with inv(16) had a 78% CR rate at 5 years after four cycles of HIDAC therapy, whereas 57% remained in CR in the IDAC arm and only 16% remained in CR with conventional 100 mg/m^2 dosing. Patients with normal cytogenetics fared less well as a group with equivalent outcomes (47% vs. 37% CR at 5 years) in the HIDAC and IDAC arms and worse outcomes with conventional dosing (20%). Patients with unfavorable cytogenetics should be considered for allogeneic transplant in first CR. Arsenic has shown benefit in a consolidation protocol for APL, but it has not been evaluated in general AML consolidation protocols.

Answer 32.20. **The answer is C.**

Nonmyeloablative conditioning regimens require a graft-versus-leukemia effect to improve the clearance of residual AML blasts not eliminated by the conditioning regimen.

Answer 32.21. **The answer is D.**

High-dose busulfan decreases the seizure threshold of patients, and therefore seizure prophylaxis is commonly used. Mucositis commonly follows busulfan therapy, especially during prolonged neutropenia. Pancytopenia naturally follows a myeloablative regimen. Risk for MDS may increase after alkylator and topoisomerase II inhibitor therapy. However, MDS is not a risk of myeloablative preparatory regimens.

Answer 32.22. **The answer is D.**

CNS prophylaxis may consist of intrathecal chemotherapy (methotrexate, cytarabine, corticosteroids), high-dose chemotherapy (methotrexate, cytarabine, L-asparaginase), or CNS irradiation. Patients with ALL with increased risk for CNS disease include those with an elevated WBC count, an elevated lactate dehydrogenase (LDH), a traumatic lumbar puncture, and T-lineage ALL. Although APL may relapse in the CNS, relapse is uncommon in patients with a presenting WBC <10,000/µL. CNS evaluation and prophylaxis are not routinely recommended in patients with APL. There is no role for CNS prophylaxis in elderly patients with AML without neurologic deficits. Although CNS disease must be considered in a patient with AML and headaches, a new headache caused by CNS leukemia on day 9 of induction therapy would be unusual and treatment could be delayed until proper evaluation is completed.

Answer 32.23. **The answer is D.**

Dexamethasone has improved penetration in the CNS. Given the high risk of CNS disease in patients with ALL, dexamethasone is preferred over prednisone.

Answer 32.24. **The answer is C.**

Attempts have been made to shorten maintenance therapy to 12 to 18 months, with inferior results. Current recommendations are for 2 to 3 years.

Answer 32.25. **The answer is A.**

Philadelphia chromosome positive ALL carries a high-risk prognosis, but this has improved with the ABL tyrosine kinase inhibitor imatinib. Second-generation inhibitors such as dasatinib and nilotinib may also prove of value in the future. Alemtuzumab is an anti-CD52 monoclonal antibody that has demonstrated significant efficacy in the treatment of CLL. It has not been evaluated in ALL, which typically does not express CD52. Gemtuzumab ozogamicin is an anti-CD33 monoclonal antibody cross-linked to a cytotoxin, calicheamicin. It has been shown to improve outcomes in relapsed AML. Sunitinib is a nonspecific tyrosine kinase inhibitor. It has significant activity against FLT3 and may prove of value in the treatment of AML with FLT3-ITD.

Answer 32.26. **The answer is B.**

Stem cell transplantation for AML remains a developing field. Current studies and meta-analysis have not found benefit in CR1 for patients with favorable cytogenetics (e.g., inv[16] and t[15;17]). Benefit is uncertain in patients with normal cytogenetics. Future trials may be able to assess the benefit of transplant in CR1 in higher-risk subpopulations of normal cytogenetics (e.g., FLT3-ITD). Patients aged less than 55 years who have unfavorable cytogenetics (e.g., -5, -7, complex cytogenetics) appear to benefit from myeloablative transplantation in CR1. However, older patients tolerate this approach less well, with increased treatment-related morbidity and mortality. Decision-making in older patients must be individualized, and nonmyeloablative transplant approaches are being explored.

James C. Mosley, III
Keith Stockerl-Goldstein

Chronic Leukemias

Directions

Each of the numbered items below is followed by lettered answers. Select the ONE lettered answer that is BEST in each case unless instructed otherwise.

QUESTIONS

Question 33.1.

A 54-year-old white man with chronic-phase chronic myeloid leukemia (CML) has quickly obtained a complete hematologic response while receiving imatinib 400 mg daily. He has been receiving therapy for 5 months, but you have noticed that his neutrophil count has gradually decreased to 0.9×10^9/L and now has a platelet count of 42×10^9/L. What is the MOST appropriate therapeutic intervention?

A. Decrease dose of imatinib to 200 mg by mouth every day.
B. Interrupt therapy until recovery of blood counts.
C. Discontinue therapy with imatinib and initiate therapy with dasatinib.
D. Discontinue therapy with imatinib and initiate therapy with interferon.

Question 33.2.

A 49-year-old woman with recently diagnosed CML presents for an initial consultation from her primary care doctor. You discuss with her that the current standard of care is initiation of imatinib therapy. You counsel her about response rates seen with this therapy. Which of the following is CORRECT?

A. Of patients who achieve a complete cytogenetic response after the first 12 months of treatment, 97% will remain in the chronic phase at 5 years.
B. For patients who obtain a complete cytogenetic response, the Sokal risk score is predictive of disease progression at 5 years.
C. Of patients who have a partial cytogenetic response after 12 months, 81% remain in chronic phase at 5 years.
D. The complete hematologic response rate at 1 year is 85%.

Corresponding Chapter in *Cancer: Principles & Practice of Oncology*, Eighth Edition: 53 (Chronic Leukemias).

Question 33.3.   A 58-year-old man was diagnosed with chronic-phase CML 2 years ago. He was initially treated with imatinib with a rapid induction of a partial cytogenetic response. He was then noted to display an increase in the proportion of Ph+ cells in his bone marrow. His therapy was changed to dasatinib, but after 2 months of therapy, his white blood cell (WBC) count is now 42×10^9/L with 88% of the cells Ph+. What is the MOST likely explanation for his treatment failure?

A. T315I point mutation in the BCR-ABL kinase
B. BCR-ABL gene amplification
C. Clonal evolution
D. Induction of a drug-efflux pump

Question 33.4.   Which of the following is TRUE concerning patients treated with imatinib before autologous stem cell transplantation (ASCT) compared with patients directly proceeding to ASCT in CML?

A. Treatment with imatinib during the chronic phase before transplantation is associated with a worse overall survival after ASCT.
B. Treatment with imatinib before transplantation results in more organ toxicity in the posttransplant setting.
C. Patients treated with imatinib before transplant have no difference in overall survival or progression-free survival.
D. Patients with imatinib-resistance mutations display inferior overall survival compared with cohorts with advanced stages of disease.

Question 33.5.   A 34-year-old man was diagnosed with chronic-phase CML 3 years ago. He was initially treated with imatinib and rapidly obtained a partial cytogenetic response. Unfortunately, the patient was noted to have developed a relapse of disease. The patient has an human leukocyte antigen (HLA)-matched sibling, and the decision was made to undergo a myeloablative stem cell transplant. Six months after transplantation, the patient is noted to have developed evidence of BCR-ABL fusion by qualitative reverse transcriptase polymerase chain reaction (RT-PCR) assessment. Which of the following is the MOST appropriate initial course of action?

A. Continued observation because reemergence of the leukemic clone is common up to 1 year after transplantation
B. Donor lymphocyte infusion
C. Retransplantation from an unrelated donor
D. Initiation of imatinib 400 mg daily

Question 33.6. A 43-year-old man with no medical history is referred for evaluation of recently diagnosed CML. His peripheral blood differential is notable for 20% circulating blasts and 25% basophils, consistent with accelerated-phase disease. Which of the following is the MOST appropriate management?

A. Initiation of imatinib 400 mg daily with immediate HLA typing of the patient and his siblings
B. Initiation of imatinib 600 mg daily with immediate HLA typing of the patient and his siblings
C. Initiation of dasatinib 70 mg daily with immediate HLA typing of the patient and his siblings
D. Initiation of imatinib 400 mg daily with deferral of HLA typing until patient achieves complete hematologic response

Question 33.7. Which of the following is TRUE regarding chronic lymphocytic leukemia (CLL)?

A. ZAP-70 overexpression is correlated with mutated VH genes.
B. Deletion 13q is the most common genetic aberration by fluorescence in situ hybridization (FISH) in CLL.
C. 11q deletion is thought to be associated with Bcl-2 overexpression.
D. Patients with 17p deletions usually present with early-stage disease that follows an indolent course.

Question 33.8. A 71-year-old white woman presents with a WBC of 39 × 10⁹/L, with 78% mature lymphocytes. Flow cytometry is remarkable for the cells being CD5+, CD19+, CD23+, CD10−. The patient has palpable lymphadenopathy in the cervical region, axillary region, and bilateral groins, with no splenomegaly. Her hemoglobin (Hgb) is 13.9g/dL, and her platelet count is 315 × 109/L. Which of the following is the MOST appropriate therapy at this time?

A. Observation with monitoring of complete blood count (CBC) and physical examination every 3 to 6 months
B. Initiation of single-agent chlorambucil
C. Initiation of single-agent fludarabine
D. Initiation of combination fludarabine, cyclophosphamide, and rituximab

Question 33.9. A 54-year-old man with Rai stage 0 CLL has been followed by you for 2 years. He presents for a routine visit. His physical examination reveals no new lymphadenopathy or splenomegaly. Which of the following findings would be an indication for initiation of systemic therapy?

A. Recent hospitalization for pneumococcal pneumonia and diagnosis of hypogammaglobulinemia
B. An increase in his absolute lymphocyte count from 15×10^9/L to 33×10^9/L over the last 2 years
C. An increase in his absolute lymphocyte count from 24×10^9/L to 38×10^9/L in the previous 2 months
D. Fever of 38°C for the last 1 week without evidence of infection

Question 33.10. **Which of the following is NOT true?**

A. In trials comparing fludarabine versus fludarabine with rituximab, grade 3/4 neutropenia was more common with the combination therapy.

B. In patients with previously untreated CLL, complete remission (CR) rates approaching 70% have been seen with combination fludarabine, cyclophosphamide, and rituximab.

C. Combination therapy with fludarabine plus cyclophosphamide has demonstrated superior overall survival compared with fludarabine alone.

D. Patients with 17q and 11q deletions have demonstrated inferior progression-free survival rates when treated with combination regimens including fludarabine and cyclophosphamide.

Question 33.11. **A 71-year-old woman presents with a mature lymphocytosis, diffuse lymphadenopathy, splenomegaly, thrombocytopenia, and an autoimmune hemolytic anemia. Workup is consistent with CLL. Treatment is initiated with four cycles of fludarabine and cyclophosphamide with a partial response (PR). The patient elects to undergo a treatment break for the next 6 months. She is then noted to have return of her lymphocytosis, lymphadenopathy, and thrombocytopenia. Fludarabine and cyclophosphamide are reinitiated, but she demonstrates continued disease progression. What is the MOST appropriate next line of therapy?**

A. Chlorambucil
B. Single-agent rituximab
C. Combination fludarabine, cyclophosphamide, with addition of rituximab
D. Alemtuzumab

ANSWERS

Answer 33.1. **The answer is B.**

Nonhematologic toxicities are the most frequently observed toxicities during treatment with imatinib and include nausea, diarrhea, muscle cramping, edema, rashes, and fatigue. Grade 3 or 4 myelosuppression occurs in a minority of treated patients and is the result of the predominant Ph-chromosome positive stem cell clone that is driving the majority of the hematopoiesis. The appropriate therapy is to interrupt the dose if the absolute neutrophil count decreases to less than 1.0×10^9/L or platelets decrease to less than 50×10^9/L. Dose reductions are not appropriate because the normal hematopoiesis is minimally effected by imatinib and may allow for emergence of resistant clones.

Answer 33.2. **The answer is A.**

Imatinib as initial therapy for chronic phase CML is very effective. A complete hematologic response rate of 96% at 1 year has been noted.

A landmark analysis of 350 patients with chronic-phase CML treated with imatinib revealed that of patients who achieved a complete cytogenetic response within 12 months of therapy, at 60 months, 97% had not progressed to accelerated phase or blast crisis. For patients achieving a partial cytogenetic response within 12 months of initiation of therapy, 93% had not progressed to accelerated phase or blast crisis at 60 months. Some 86% of patients who did not achieve a major cytogenetic response within the first 12 months were without evidence of progression at 60 months. None of the patients who had a complete cytogenetic response and who had a three-log or more reduction in BCR-ABL transcripts at 12 or 18 months went on to progress. In this analysis, patients who had high Sokal scores were noted to be less likely to attain complete cytogenetic responses on imatinib therapy. Sixty-nine percent of patients with high-risk scores obtained complete cytogenetic responses compared with 91% of patients with low-risk scores.

Answer 33.3.   **The answer is A.**

In patients undergoing treatment of chronic-phase CML with imatinib, disease relapse can occur. The most common mechanism mediating this is a point mutation in the kinase domain of the BCR-ABL fusion. Such mutations render the kinase less sensitive to inhibition by imatinib by causing structural alterations that interfere with the binding of imatinib to the kinase. There are many described mutations, some of which demonstrate response to increased doses of imatinib and others that will respond to other kinase inhibitors such as dasatinib or nilotinib. The point mutation T315I results in a clone that is resistant to imatinib, dasatinib, and nilotinib. Patients such as this should be evaluated for a clinical trial or hematopoietic stem cell transplantation. Clonal evolution, drug efflux, and amplification of the BCR-ABL fusion are far less common mechanisms to account for imatinib resistance.

Answer 33.4.   **The answer is C.**

Although allogeneic stem cell transplantation is the only potentially curative therapy in CML, most patients with chronic-phase disease are treated with imatinib therapy initially. Concerns have been raised that exposure to such kinase inhibitors could result in poorer outcomes if patients were to later proceed with stem cell transplantation as was demonstrated with prolonged exposure to interferon. Large observational studies have suggested that there is no detrimental effect to prior imatinib exposure in patients proceeding with stem cell transplantation. These patients do tend to undergo transplant with more advanced stages of disease and higher EBMT scores, but there has been no evidence for inferior overall survival, disease-free survival, transplant-related mortality, acute graft-versus-host disease (GVHD), engraftment kinetics, or organ toxicity compared with patients who were not exposed to imatinib before transplant. Furthermore, in small case studies it appears that patients harboring imatinib-resistant mutations have outcomes that are similar to what would be expected in clinically advanced disease.

Answer 33.5.   **The answer is D.**

Allogeneic hematopoietic stem cell transplantation (HCT) is the only potentially curative therapy in CML. Induction of molecular remission after transplantation is more durable than that obtained with imatinib alone. After allogeneic HCT, evidence of the leukemic clone can be detected in many patients, but will disappear over time, with very few patients continuing to have molecular evidence of CML at 2 years when undergoing transplantation in the chronic phase. The relapse rate after transplantation in the chronic phase is less than 10% in most series with greater than 50% of relapses occurring within the first year and less than 5% occurring after the fifth year.

Early intervention at first documentation of relapse confers the greatest chance of controlling the disease. Initial institution of imatinib 400 mg daily can restore complete molecular remission in 83% of patients with molecular relapse and 56% of patients with cytogenetic relapse. Up to 25% of patients who attain a complete molecular remission can be withdrawn from the imatinib therapy within 6 to 24 months, whereas others may require long-term therapy with imatinib or donor leukocyte infusions (DLIs). Because of the exquisite sensitivity of CML to graft-versus-leukemia effects, patients who relapse into chronic phase by cytogenetics or hematological criteria, 60% to 80% can be treated with DLI alone with 5-year disease-free survival (DFS) rates of 50%. Patients who relapse again after initial DLI can often be retreated with DLI as well. However, DLI carries significant risks with treatment-related mortality of 8% to 20% and adverse effects of acute and chronic GVHD, infectious complications, and others.

Answer 33.6.   **The answer is B.**

Development of accelerated-phase disease is a gradual process in most patients with CML. It can be seen in patients in whom disease was previously well controlled with medical therapy. It appears that in some patients, new cytogenetic and molecular abnormalities occur, including p53 mutations. For patients developing accelerated-phase disease, imatinib has demonstrated significantly improved outcomes with respect to response and survival at 600 mg daily compared with 400 mg daily in a retrospective subgroup analysis. This has led to the recommendation of using a starting dose of 600 mg daily in patients with accelerated-phase disease. Alternate kinase inhibitors, such as nilotinib and dasatinib, have demonstrated significant activity in patients with accelerated-phase disease who have relapsed on imatinib therapy.

Unfortunately, remissions from accelerated-phase disease are usually short-lived. Because of the high relapse rates in this setting, kinase inhibitor therapy should be viewed only as a bridge to allogeneic stem cell transplantation, because the stage of disease at the time of transplantation is one of the most consistent predictors of outcome in the related and unrelated HCT. Survival rates with accelerated-phase disease are approximately half compared with matched cohorts undergoing HCT in chronic phase.

The majority of patients who develop myeloid blast crisis have additional cytogenetic abnormalities detectable. Only 20% of these patients will enter a second chronic phase with combination chemotherapy regimens with short remission durations and survival. Similar results are seen with imatinib or newer kinase inhibitors emphasizing the importance of allogeneic transplant for these patients.

Answer 33.7.   **The answer is B.**

Much insight has been gained into the molecular abnormalities associated with CLL. Various chromosomal abnormalities can be reliably detected by FISH, with greater than 80% of cases demonstrating abnormalities. The most commonly encountered abnormality is a deletion of chromosome 13q, found in approximately 55% of cases. Further investigation of this common abnormality has led to the observation that this is often associated with deletion or downregulation of two microRNA genes (miR15 and miR16), which may downregulate the antiapoptotic protein, bcl-2. Other less common chromosomal abnormalities occur, such as 11q deletion, trisomy 12, and 17p deletion. Of these, 11q and 17p deletions tend to present at more advanced stages and follow more aggressive courses. Early investigations have noted that approximately 50% of patients have unmutated VH genes, which has been associated with a poorer prognosis in retrospective analyses compared with cohorts with mutated VH genes. Further investigation noted that patients with unmutated VH genes had high expression of the T-cell receptor signal transduction protein, ZAP-70.

Answer 33.8.   **The answer is A.**

This patient has Rai stage I CLL as evidenced by her lymphadenopathy, lack of splenomegaly, and lack of anemia or thrombocytopenia, placing her at intermediate risk. Her flow cytometry studies are typical of CLL. Despite the diagnosis of CLL, immediate treatment in this situation is not warranted. It is believed that CLL is not curable with current treatment approaches, so treatment is directed at symptomatic disease or patients who are likely to have poor prognosis. Most patients with CLL will have a prolonged course, and many studies have demonstrated that treatment with combinations of therapies can prolong progression-free survival and increase response rates compared with single-agent therapies, but no survival advantage has been noted in early intervention trials. Continued observation of patients with early-stage disease with attention to prognostic factors, such as lymphocyte doubling time, ZAP-70 expression, and karyotype, is indicated.

Answer 33.9.   **The answer is C.**

Because CLL can be a heterogeneous disease, the National Cancer Institute–sponsored Working Group has established guidelines addressing indications to initiate treatment for patients. These include constitutional symptoms attributable to CLL, including weight loss of greater than 10% of baseline weight within the preceding 6 months, extreme fatigue, Eastern Cooperative Oncology Group performance status of 2 or greater, temperature greater than 38°C or 100.5°F for at least 2 weeks, or night sweats without evidence of infection; evidence of progressive bone marrow failure characterized by the development or progression of anemia or thrombocytopenia, or both; autoimmune hemolytic anemia or autoimmune thrombocytopenia, or both, which are poorly responsive to corticosteroid therapy; massive or progressive splenomegaly; massive or progressive lymphadenopathy; progressive lymphocytosis, defined as an increase in the absolute lymphocyte count by greater than 50% over a 2-month period, or a lymphocyte doubling time predicted to be less than 6 months. Diagnosis of hypogammaglobulinemia is not an indication for initiation of therapy.

Answer 33.10.   **The answer is C.**

Studies of chemotherapy regimens in CLL have repeatedly demonstrated the activity and tolerability of the purine analog fludarabine as the most effective single-agent chemotherapy. Not surprisingly, this agent has been used as the backbone of other combination regimens in clinical trials. With various clinical trials including fludarabine in combination with other agents, CR and overall response rates have been superior with the combination arm. However, because of the usually long duration of disease that most patients experience, no trials have consistently demonstrated superior overall survival rates with one chemotherapy regimen over another. In the CALGB 9712 trial of sequential fludarabine and rituximab versus concurrent therapy, there was a significant increase in the CR rate, but there was also an increase in the incidence of grade 3 and 4 neutropenia. The combination of fludarabine, cyclophosphamide, and rituximab has been evaluated in both treatment-naïve and previously treated patients. In treatment-naïve patients, a CR rate of 70% was observed with a projected failure-free survival at 4 years of 69%; this is the highest response rate reported for any regimen for previously untreated patients in CLL. Unfortunately, patients carrying deletions in 17p or 11q have repeatedly demonstrated inferior outcomes with respect to progression-free survival in these studies.

Answer 33.11.   **The answer is D.**

Alemtuzumab is a humanized monoclonal antibody targeting CD52, which is highly expressed on CLL cells in addition to normal B and T lymphocytes. In a pivotal study of patients who were previously treated with fludarabine, second-line therapy with alemtuzumab was able to induce a CR in 2% of patients and a PR in 31% of patients. Some 59% of patients achieved stable disease as well. This led to the Food and Drug Administration (FDA) approval of single-agent alemtuzumab for patients with fludarabine-refractory CLL. Alemtuzumab is effective at treatment of marrow and peripheral blood disease; however, it is less effective at treating patients with bulky lymphadenopathy. Of note, this agent is associated with an increased risk of cytomegalovirus infections and is also effective in patients with 17p deletion, which has generally been resistant to therapy with other agents.

Another monoclonal antibody, rituximab, directed against CD20 on malignant and normal B cells, has very limited activity as a single agent in CLL. This is likely because CLL cells demonstrate relatively low levels of expression of CD20 compared with normal lymphocytes, as well as the demonstration of increased levels of soluble CD20 in patients with CLL, which may interfere with rituximab's ability to induce antibody-dependent cellular cytotoxicity on target cells. Because this patient has progressed on combination therapy with fludarabine and cyclophosphamide, continuation with this regimen with addition of rituximab is unlikely to be of much clinical benefit.

Plasma Cell Neoplasms

Directions   Each of the numbered items below is followed by lettered answers. Select the ONE lettered answer that is BEST in each case unless instructed otherwise.

QUESTIONS

Question 34.1.   **An 80-year-old woman presents to the emergency department with progressive low back pain for 3 weeks. On examination she has tenderness at multiple levels on her spine but no neurological deficits. She has an Eastern Cooperative Oncology Group (ECOG) performance status of 2. Laboratory testing shows a hemoglobin (Hb) of 7.8 g/dL, creatinine of 2.1 mg/dL, calcium of 8.8 mg/dL, and albumin of 4.1 g/dL. She has a skeletal survey showing multiple osteolytic lesions, including multiple vertebral compression fractures. She has a serum protein electrophoresis (SPEP) showing a monoclonal protein of 6.2 g/dL. Serum immunofixation shows a monoclonal immunoglobulin (Ig)G kappa light chain protein. Her beta-2 microglobulin level is 5.3 mg/L. She has a bone marrow biopsy that shows a hypercellular marrow with 60% plasma cells, and cytogenetic analysis reveals a normal female karyotype. Of the following treatment options, which would be considered the MOST appropriate?**

A. Melphalan and prednisone (MP)
B. Melphalan, prednisone, and thalidomide (MPT)
C. Thalidomide and dexamethasone (TD)
D. Melphalan 100 mg/m^2 followed by autologous stem cell transplantation

Corresponding Chapter in *Cancer: Principles & Practice of Oncology*, Eighth Edition: 54 (Plasma Cell Neoplasms).

444

Question 34.2.   A 59-year-old man is evaluated for anemia with an Hb of 9.2 g/dL. He has no other medical comorbidities and is asymptomatic. His clinical examination reveals no abnormality. He is found to have a high total protein of 12 g/dL and albumin of 3.2 g/dL. His serum creatinine is 1.0 mg/dL and serum calcium is 9.3 mg/dL. He has a serum protein electrophoresis that shows a monoclonal protein level of 8.6 g/dL, and serum immunofixation shows an IgG lambda monoclonal protein. His skeletal survey is normal. His serum beta-2 microglobulin is 4.3 mg/L. He has a bone marrow examination that shows 40% plasma cells, and cytogenetic analysis reveals a normal male karyotype. He is being considered for autologous stem cell transplantation. Which of the following induction regimens would give the best chance of complete remission after autologous stem cell transplantation?

A.   Vincristine, Adriamycin, and dexamethasone (VAD)
B.   Thalidomide and dexamethasone (TD)
C.   Bortezomib and dexamethasone (VD)
D.   Bortezomib, thalidomide, and dexamethasone (VTD)

Question 34.3.   A 52-year-old woman is evaluated for progressive fatigue. Clinical examination is remarkable only for pallor. Further investigation reveals an Hb of 8.2 g/dL with mean corpuscular volume (MCV) of 88 fL. Her iron studies, vitamin B_{12} levels, and folate levels are normal. Her serum creatinine is 0.8 mg/dL. Her SPEP reveals a monoclonal protein level of 3.8 g/dL, and serum immunofixation shows a monoclonal IgG kappa light chain protein. Further investigation reveals a calcium of 8.8 mg/dL, albumin of 4.2 g/dL, and beta-2 microglobulin of 2.1 mg/L. Skeletal survey shows multiple lytic lesions. She has a bone marrow examination that shows 80% cellular marrow with 50% plasma cells. Cytogenetic analysis shows normal female karyotype, and a fluorescence in situ hybridization (FISH) panel is positive for 13q deletion in 50% of plasma cells. Which of the following treatment options would be considered MOST appropriate for the patient?

A.   Bortezomib/dexamethasone induction followed by high-dose melphalan and autologous stem cell transplantation (HDCT)
B.   Bortezomib and dexamethasone with no option for HDCT
C.   Melphalan and prednisone
D.   Melphalan, prednisone, and thalidomide

Question 34.4.   A 58-year-old woman is incidentally found to have a monoclonal protein on SPEP with a monoclonal protein concentration of 1.7 g/dL, and on immunofixation she is found to have monoclonal IgG kappa free light chains. She is asymptomatic, and clinical examination results are normal. Her laboratory investigations show an Hb of 13.1 g/dL, creatinine of 0.7 mg/dL, serum albumin of 4.7 g/dL, calcium of 9.3 mg/dL, and beta-2 microglobulin of 1.7 mg/L. The skeletal survey was negative for any lytic lesions. Bone marrow examination shows 13% plasma cells, and cytogenetics shows normal female karyotype. What is the chance of this patient developing multiple myeloma at 5 years?

A. 5%
B. 10%
C. 30%
D. 50%

ANSWERS

Answer 34.1.   **The answer is B.**

The choice of initial therapy for elderly patients with multiple myeloma has been a subject of several clinical trials. There have been three randomized controlled trials (IFM 99-06: Facon T, Mary JY, Hulin C, et al. Lancet 2007;370[9594]:1209–1218; IFM 01-01: Hulin C, Virion J, Leleu X, et al. Am J Clin Oncol 2007;25[18S]:8001; GIMEMA: Palumbo A, Bringhen S, Caravita T, et al. Lancet 2006;367[9513]:825–831.) comparing MPT and MP regimens. All three studies showed superiority of MPT over MP on the basis of response including complete remission (13% to 16% vs. 2% to 2.4%) and progression-free survival (24 to 27.5 months vs. 17.8 to 19 months). In the IFM studies, the improved response rate of MPT over MP translated into improved overall survival (OS) (45 to 50 months vs. 27 to 33 months). The VISTA trial (San Miguel et al. Blood [ASH Annual Meeting Abstracts] 2007;110[11]:2712) recently showed the melphalan, prednisone, and bortezomib (MPV) combination to be superior to MP (CR rate: 35% vs. 5%, 2-year OS: 83% vs. 70%). There is no study comparing MPV with MPT. The combination of Thalidomide and dexamethasone (TD) has been compared with MP (Ludwig H et al. Hematologica 2007;92[10]: 1411–1414). Although TD showed a better response rate (CR/near CR: 30% vs. 14%), it resulted in inferior survival (OS: 44.6 vs. 57.9 months) secondary to its toxicity. HDCT with melphalan 200 mg/m^2 has emerged as standard of care for transplant-eligible patients. However, patients aged more than 75 years are usually not considered for transplantation because of the toxicity of the treatment in this group. In the IFM 99-06 study, patients who received MPT showed a superior survival compared with reduced-dose melphalan 100 mg/m^2 followed by autologous stem cell transplantation (OS: 51.6 vs. 38.3 months). Thus, the MPT regimen would be the most appropriate for this patient.

Answer 34.2.   **The answer is D.**

The choice of the optimal induction therapy before autologous stem cell transplantation for patients with multiple myeloma has been the subject of several randomized clinical trials. VAD chemotherapy had been the most popular induction chemotherapy regimen in the United States until the 1990s. Several randomized trials have recently compared various regimens for induction therapy before transplantation. Marco et al (Blood [ASH Annual Abstracts] 2007;110[11]) compared TD with VAD as induction regimen before HDCT and reported a good partial response (VGPR) with TD compared with VAD before transplant (35% vs. 12%). However, there was no difference in VGPR at 6 months post-HDCT (44% vs. 41%). Horousseau et al (Blood [AHS Annual Abstracts] 2007;110[11]) reported a higher CR+ near CR postautologous transplantation with VD as induction therapy compared with VAD as induction therapy (41% vs. 29%). In a phase 3 study, Carvo et al (ASH 2007) reported that VTD induction therapy resulted in higher CR+ near CR postautologous transplantation when compared with TD (57% vs. 28%). Phase 2 trials have reported that lenalidomide and dexamethasone are an appropriate induction regimen pretransplant (Lacy et al. Blood [ASH Annual Abstracts] 2006;108[11]). However, there are increasing data on the adverse impact of lenalidomide on stem cell mobilization, and it is recommended that stem cells be collected within the first 4 months of starting a lenalidomide-based regimen. Unfortunately, we do not have any long-term follow-up from these trials showing survival data. However, previous studies such as MRC VII and IFM 90-06 on high-dose chemotherapy reported that patients achieving CR after high-dose chemotherapy had longer progression-free survival and OS compared with those with less than CR. Therefore, the VTD regimen with the highest reported CR rate may be the most appropriate induction regimen.

Answer 34.3. **The answer is A.**

The optimal initial therapy for a young patient with multiple myeloma is currently a subject of controversy. HDCT has been compared with conventional chemotherapy in several randomized controlled trials. The IFM 90-06 and MRCVII established HDCT as standard of care for these patients. The introduction of novel drugs such as thalidomide, lenalidomide, and bortezomib has improved the CR rate in patients with myeloma and led several experts to question the continued role of upfront HDCT for all patients with multiple myeloma. However, regimens containing these novel drugs have not been directly compared with HDCT in randomized trials, and most investigators think that these novel agents should be incorporated with HDCT in the treatment paradigm. Some investigators have suggested delaying the HDCT option for the time of progression. This may be an appropriate strategy because a randomized trial (Fermand JP. Blood 1998;92[9]:3131–3136) showed that HDCT at first progression resulted in OS comparable to patients who underwent HDCT as initial therapy. However, there are no data on delaying HDCT beyond first progression. Other investigators have proposed a risk-stratified approach to HDCT for patients with multiple myeloma. Deletion 13 by conventional cytogenetics was seen in approximately 15% of patients with multiple myeloma and has been shown to be an adverse prognostic factor. Trials with HDCT have reported a median time to progression of 8 to 9 months in this population. However, deletion of chromosome 13 by FISH is detected in 40% to 50% of patients. Individuals with deletion 13 detected by FISH in the absence of deletion 13 by conventional cytogenetics do not seem to have the same adverse impact. Therefore, we think that this patient with deletion 13 detected by FISH alone should be offered HDCT as part of her regimen. Bortezomib has been shown in several studies to negate the adverse impact of deletion 13 detected by conventional cytogenetics. However, because there are no randomized controlled trials comparing bortezomib-based combination regimen alone with HDCT, we think that HDCT cannot be excluded from the treatment paradigm. Melphalan-based regimen should be avoided in a patient eligible for HDCT.

Answer 34.4.   **The answer is D.**

The diagnostic criterion for plasma cell dyscrasias was recently revised. Multiple myeloma is defined as a plasma cell dyscrasia associated with end-organ dysfunction (acronym CRAB: hyperCalcemia, Renal failure, Anemia or Bone lesions). Patients should also have ≥10% clonal plasma cells and a monoclonal protein in serum and/or urine. In the absence of organ involvement, the plasma cell dyscrasia is classified as monoclonal gammopathy of undetermined significance (MGUS) if the monoclonal protein levels are <3 g/dL and the bone marrow contains <10% clonal plasma cells, and as smoldering myeloma if the bone marrow has ≥10% clonal plasma cells and/or monoclonal protein of ≥3 g/dL. On the basis of the above criteria this patient has a smoldering myeloma. Recently, the natural history of these indolent plasma cell dyscrasias have been better defined. MGUS transforms to a clinically significant plasma cell dyscrasia at a constant rate of approximately 1% per year (Kyle et al. N Engl J Med 2002;346[8]:564–569). The serum level of the monoclonal protein and the type of monoclonal protein (IgA and IgM > IgG) were risk factors for progression in the same study. In a subsequent study, Rajkumar et al (Blood 2005;106[3]:812–817) proposed a risk stratification model that included three risk factors (abnormal serum free light chain ratio, non–IgG-type monoclonal protein, and monoclonal protein concentration >1.5 g/dL) to further help predict progression of MGUS to a clinically significant plasma cell dyscrasia. Kyle et al (N Engl J Med 2007;356[25]:2582–2590) reported that the overall risk of progression of smoldering myeloma is approximately 10% per year in the first 5 years, 3% per year in the next 5 years, and decreases to 1% per year thereafter. On the basis of this study, this patient has a 5-year risk of progression of approximately 50%. Kyle et al further classified smoldering myeloma into three risk groups with different rates of progression: group (1) bone marrow plasma cell ≥10%, monoclonal M protein ≥3 g/dL: 15-year progression rate 87%; group (2) bone marrow plasma cells ≥10%, monoclonal M protein ≤3 g/dL: 15-year progression rate 70%; and group (3) bone marrow plasma cells <>10%, monoclonal M protein ≥3 g/dL: 15-year progression rate 39%.

Paraneoplastic Syndromes

Directions   Each of the numbered items below is followed by lettered answers. Select the ONE lettered answer that is BEST in each case unless instructed otherwise.

QUESTIONS

Question 35.1.   **Chronic lymphocytic leukemia (CLL) has been associated with all of the following, EXCEPT:**

A. Pure red cell aplasia
B. Warm antibody hemolytic anemia
C. Microangiopathic hemolytic anemia
D. Paraneoplastic pemphigus

Question 35.2.   **Which of the statements about small cell lung cancer (SCLC) is FALSE?**

A. SCLC is the second-leading cause of ectopic adrenocorticotropic hormone (ACTH) production after bronchial carcinoid.
B. SCLC is the leading cause of syndrome of inappropriate antidiuretic hormone production (SIADH).
C. Subacute sensory neuronopathy and encephalomyeloneuritis (SSN-EMN) is most frequently associated with SCLC, compared with other forms of cancer.
D. Patients with cancer with Lambert-Eaton syndrome most frequently have SCLC as an underlying cause.

Question 35.3.   **Ectopic ACTH production causes all the following, EXCEPT:**

A. Muscle wasting
B. Moon facies
C. Hypokalemia
D. Hyperpigmentation

Corresponding Chapter in *Cancer: Principles & Practice of Oncology,* Eighth Edition: 55 (Paraneoplastic Syndromes).

Question 35.4.   **Many patients with SCLC produce ectopic ACTH, but what percentage develop clinical Cushing's syndrome?**

    A. 3% to 7%
    B. 12% to 15%
    C. 20% to 25%
    D. 33% to 36%

Question 35.5.   **False-positive dexamethasone suppression tests can be seen in patients with all the following problems, EXCEPT:**

    A. Older age
    B. Sleep deprivation
    C. Malabsorption
    D. Weight gain

Question 35.6.   **Which of the following therapies for ectopic ACTH production is considered the therapy of choice?**

    A. Aminoglutethimide
    B. Mitotane
    C. Ketoconazole
    D. Metyrapone

Question 35.7.   **Laboratory findings of SIADH include all of the following, EXCEPT:**

    A. Normal volume status
    B. Plasma osmolality greater than urine osmolality
    C. Elevated renal excretion of sodium
    D. Hyponatremia

Question 35.8.   **Which patient's cancer is more likely to cause hypocalcemia?**

    A. Stage II papillary carcinoma of the kidney
    B. Breast cancer metastatic to the bone
    C. Nodal recurrence of a prior resected melanoma
    D. Locally advanced hepatocellular carcinoma

Question 35.9.   **The two most common tumors causing erythrocytosis are:**

    A. Renal cell carcinoma and Wilms' tumor
    B. Wilms' tumor and uterine fibroids
    C. Hepatoma and sarcomas
    D. Renal cell carcinoma and hepatoma

Question 35.10.   **Which laboratory findings would describe the most common anemia seen in patients with cancer?**

A.   Low serum iron, low ferritin, elevated total iron-binding capacity (TIBC), elevated erythropoietin

B.   Low serum iron, normal ferritin, elevated TIBC, low erythropoietin

C.   Low serum iron, elevated ferritin, low TIBC, low erythropoietin

D.   Normal serum iron, elevated ferritin, low TIBC, elevated erythropoietin

Question 35.11.   **Which of the associations between red cells and disease is FALSE?**

A.   Pure red cell aplasia and thymoma

B.   Microangiopathic hemolytic anemia and adenocarcinoma of the gastrointestinal (GI) tract

C.   Autoimmune hemolytic anemia and CLL

D.   Cold agglutinin disease and ovarian cancer

Question 35.12.   **Independent risk factors for disseminated intravascular coagulation (DIC) include all the following, EXCEPT:**

A.   Female gender

B.   Older age

C.   Advanced stage

D.   Breast cancer

Question 35.13.   **Which of the following renal associations is INCORRECT?**

A.   Minimal change disease and Hodgkin's lymphoma

B.   Immunoglobulin (Ig)A nephropathy and head and neck cancer

C.   Focal and segmental glomerulosclerosis and gastric cancer

D.   Membranous nephropathy and lung cancer

Question 35.14.   **A 54-year-old former smoker develops lung cancer and is noted to have a corrected serum calcium of 11.9. Which histological subtype is most expected?**

A.   Squamous cell

B.   Adenocarcinoma

C.   Small cell

D.   Mesothelioma

Question 35.15.   **Which of the following associations is INCORRECT?**

A.   Sudden appearance of seborrheic keratoses and gastric cancer

B.   Pachydermoperiostosis and SCLC

C.   Acquired ichthyosis and Hodgkin's lymphoma

D.   Necrolytic migratory erythema and glucagonoma

Question 35.16.   **Which of the following associations is INCORRECT?**

A.   Vitiligo and melanoma
B.   Acrokeratosis paraneoplastica and squamous cell carcinoma of the esophagus
C.   Pyoderma gangrenosum and pancreatic cancer
D.   Sweet's syndrome and acute myelogenous leukemia (AML)

Question 35.17.   **A relapsing high-grade fever with fever spikes that are abrupt in onset and resolution should point toward the diagnosis of:**

A.   Diffuse large B-cell lymphoma
B.   Hodgkin's lymphoma
C.   Follicular lymphoma
D.   Renal cell carcinoma

Question 35.18.   **Acquired von Willebrand's disease is seen in all the following, EXCEPT:**

A.   Plasma cell dyscrasias
B.   Lymphoma
C.   Gastric cancer
D.   Hepatocellular carcinoma

Question 35.19.   **Which of the following about clinical thromboembolism is INCORRECT?**

A.   It is the second-leading cause of death in patients with overt malignant disease.
B.   It occurs in as many as 11% of patients with cancer.
C.   Treatment should consist of a heparin product acutely followed by warfarin indefinitely.
D.   Although all cancers can cause venous thromboembolism, pancreatic cancer has the greatest risk.

Question 35.20.   **Which of the following concerning subacute sensory neuronopathy and encephalomyeloneuritis is INCORRECT?**

A.   It is associated with anti-Hu antibodies when SCLC is present.
B.   Treatment does not affect the neurological dysfunction.
C.   Patients can have malignancy and the antibody without neurologic dysfunction.
D.   Dorsal root ganglia show lymphocytic infiltration and loss of neurons.

Question 35.21.   **Which of the following about limbic encephalitis (LE) is INCORRECT?**

A.   Testicular cancers associated with LE have the anti-Hu antibody.
B.   It may be mistaken for herpes simplex encephalitis.
C.   Most cases are associated with SCLC.
D.   It is one of the more treatable forms of central nervous system (CNS) paraneoplastic disorders.

Question 35.22.   **The anti-Yo antibody CNS paraneoplastic disorder has all these in common, EXCEPT:**

    A. It is commonly associated with ovarian and breast cancer.
    B. The antibody is active against the Purkinje cells.
    C. It causes opsoclonus-myoclonus.
    D. The disorder is subacute in onset and usually progressive.

Question 35.23.   **Which of the following about Lambert-Eaton syndrome (LES) is INCORRECT?**

    A. Sixty percent of patients with LES have an underlying cancer.
    B. The malignancy most associated with LES is SCLC.
    C. It is a pure motor syndrome.
    D. Proximal weakness is the common presenting symptom.

Question 35.24.   **Melanoma-associated retinopathy includes all the following, EXCEPT:**

    A. It most commonly appears at the metastatic stage.
    B. It is more common in men.
    C. Only cones are affected, sparing rods.
    D. Progressive blindness is unusual.

ANSWERS

Answer 35.1.   **The answer is C.**

CLL has been described in association with both warm antibody hemolytic anemia and autoimmune hemolytic anemia, but not with microangiopathic hemolytic anemia with its red cell fragmentation.

Answer 35.2.   **The answer is A.**

SCLC is the leading cause of ectopic ACTH production.

Answer 35.3.   **The answer is B.**

Classic hypercortisolism causes moon facies, but ectopic production usually does not.

Answer 35.4.   **The answer is A.**

Some 3% to 7% of patients with SCLC and ectopic ACTH production will develop Cushing's syndrome.

Answer 35.5.   **The answer is D.**

Weight loss, not gain, can contribute to a false-positive dexamethasone suppression test.

Answer 35.6.   **The answer is C.**

Ketoconazole is considered the therapy of choice because of its rapid onset of action and favorable toxicity profile.

Answer 35.7.   **The answer is B.**

Patients have a urine osmolality greater than plasma osmolality.

Answer 35.8.   **The answer is B.**

Osteoblastic metastasis from breast, prostate, and lung all can cause hypocalcemia because of an increased skeletal avidity for calcium.

Answer 35.9.   **The answer is D.**

Although all of the answers listed are associated with erythrocytosis, renal cell carcinoma is the leading cause, with hepatoma being second.

Answer 35.10.   **The answer is C.**

Anemia of chronic disease is the most common anemia seen in patients with cancer and is reflected by a low serum iron, normal or increased ferritin, low TIBC, and low serum erythropoietin.

Answer 35.11.   **The answer is D.**

Cold agglutinin disease is most common in Waldenström's macroglobulinemia.

Answer 35.12.   **The answer is A.**

Male gender is an independent risk factor for DIC.

Answer 35.13.   **The answer is C.**

Focal and segmental glomerulosclerosis is associated with CLL, T-cell receptor lymphomas, and acute myelogenous leukemias, whereas stomach cancer is associated with membranous nephropathy.

Answer 35.14.   **The answer is A.**

Squamous cell cancers of the lung and head and neck are more commonly associated with hypercalcemia than the other subtypes.

Answer 35.15.   **The answer is B.**

Pachydermoperiostosis is most often associated with bronchogenic carcinoma.

Answer 35.16.   **The answer is C.**

Pyoderma gangrenosum is associated with hematological malignancies, as well as gastric carcinoma and other GI abnormalities.

Answer 35.17.   **The answer is B.**

This describes a Pel-Ebstein fever, which although uncommon, should lead one to look for Hodgkin's lymphoma.

Answer 35.18.   **The answer is D.**

Acquired von Willebrand's disease is seen in plasma cell dyscrasias, gastric and adrenal carcinomas, leukemias, and lymphomas.

Answer 35.19.   **The answer is C.**

In patients with malignancy, warfarin is associated with a higher recurrence rate and bleeding complications than long-term low-molecular-weight heparin.

Answer 35.20.   **The answer is B.**

Treatment may ameliorate neurological dysfunction, and immunosuppression may stabilize the disease transiently.

Answer 35.21.   **The answer is A.**

SCLC is associated with the anti-Hu antibody, and testicular cancer is associated with the anti-Ma2 antibody.

Answer 35.22.   **The answer is C.**

Anti-Yo antibody causes progressive cerebellar degeneration, whereas opsoclonus-myoclonus is caused by not one antibody, but several, including anti-Hu, anti-Ri, and antineurofilament.

Answer 35.23.   **The answer is C.**

Lambert-Eaton is not a pure motor disorder because paresthesias are frequently reported, and dry mouth and erectile dysfunction are also reported.

Answer 35.24.   **The answer is C.**

Only rods are affected, and acquired night blindness may occur.

Sunny Wang
Sarita Dubey

Cancer of Unknown Primary Site

Directions   Each of the numbered items below is followed by lettered answers. Select the ONE lettered answer that is BEST in each case unless instructed otherwise.

QUESTIONS

Question 36.1.   **What percentage of unknown primary cancer is adenocarcinoma on light microscopy?**

  A. 15%
  B. 5%
  C. 60%
  D. 30%

Question 36.2.   **On light microscopy, a tumor specimen appears to be a poorly differentiated neoplasm. What is the most common tumor type found among poorly differentiated neoplasms after further specialized pathologic workup?**

  A. Poorly differentiated carcinoma
  B. Non-Hodgkin's lymphoma
  C. Poorly differentiated neuroendocrine tumor
  D. Sarcoma

Question 36.3.   **Which of the following immunohistochemical stains are considered relatively specific for diagnosing the appropriate primary site in the workup of a carcinoma of unknown primary (CUP)?**

  A. Prostate-specific antigen (PSA) and common leukocyte antigen (CLA)
  B. Thyroid transcription factor-1 (TTF-1)
  C. Chromogranin and synaptophysin
  D. Cytokeratin 7 and cytokeratin 20

Corresponding Chapter in *Cancer: Principles & Practice of Oncology,* Eighth Edition: 56 (Cancer of Unknown Primary Site).

Question 36.4. **Which of the following are associated with a favorable outcome in patients with CUP?**

A. Men with tumor in the mediastinum or retroperitoneal lymph nodes
B. Women with peritoneal carcinomatosis
C. Features of lymphoma on detailed pathologic evaluation
D. All of the above

Question 36.5. **A 35-year-old man presents with chest pain, weight loss, and fatigue. Chest radiography and computed tomography (CT) scan reveal a 6-cm mediastinal mass. Biopsy of the mass, on light microscopy, reveals a poorly differentiated carcinoma. Immunohistochemistry is negative for keratin, epithelial membrane antigen (EMA), CLA, TTF-1 stain, serum alpha-fetoprotein (AFP), and beta-human chorionic gonadotropin (β-hCG). Chromosomal analysis was performed and revealed deletion of chromosome 12p. CT scan of the abdomen is negative for any intra-abdominal masses, and testicular ultrasound is negative. Positron emission tomography (PET) scan is only positive for the mediastinal mass. Serum AFP is 3 ng/dL and β-hCG is 92 mIU/mL. He is referred to your oncology clinic for treatment. What is the most appropriate treatment for this patient?**

A. Platinum-based therapy for presumed thymoma
B. Taxane-based therapy for presumed non–small cell lung cancer (NSCLC)
C. Cisplatin-based therapy for presumed extragonadal germ cell tumor
D. Anthracycline-based combination therapy for presumed lymphoma

Question 36.6. **A 65-year-old man with diabetes undergoes renal ultrasound for elevated creatinine 1.8 mg/dL. Multiple hypodense liver lesions are noted, and magnetic resonance imaging (MRI) of the abdomen is ordered to further evaluate. On MRI, there are multiple hypodensities in the right lobe of the liver, ranging in size from 1.7 to 2.5 cm. Biopsy of one of the liver lesions reveals a low-grade neuroendocrine carcinoma. A diagnostic workup, including endoscopies, small bowel follow-through (SBFT), and octreotide scan, does not reveal a primary. Which of the following is the most appropriate treatment option for this patient at the present time?**

A. Immediate right hepatectomy
B. Chemoembolization
C. Liver transplant to improve chances of long-term disease-free survival
D. Observation with close follow-up and serial CT scans; hormonal therapy versus surgery versus chemotherapy at a later date if indicated

Question 36.7.   A 62-year-old woman, smoker, presents with right-sided abdominal discomfort, nausea, and weight loss. CT scan of the abdomen and pelvis
reveals multiple diffuse low-attenuation liver lesions and no biliary ductal
dilatation. CT scan of the chest is also ordered, and no other sites of
disease are identified on CT scan of the chest, as well as abdomen and
pelvis. Mammogram of both breasts is negative. Serum AFP is within
normal limits. Biopsy of one of the liver lesions reveals an adenocarcinoma. Immunohistochemical studies reveal negative results for TTF-1,
estrogen-receptor (ER), and progesterone-receptor (PR) staining. Cytokeratin stains reveal a CK7 negative and CK20 positive tumor. What diagnostic test would you order next?

A.   PET scan
B.   Colonoscopy and upper endoscopy
C.   MRI of breasts
D.   Bronchoscopy

Question 36.8.   A 55-year-old woman presents with right-sided axillary lymphadenopathy.
CT scan of the chest/abdomen/pelvis reveals only right-sided axillary
lymph nodes up to 3 cm in size and is otherwise negative. Mammogram
and ultrasound results of both breasts are negative. Biopsy of the right
axillary lymph nodes reveals moderately differentiated adenocarcinoma.
Immunostaining is negative for TTF-1, ER, PR, and CK20, but positive
for CK7. What is the next diagnostic procedure you would order to ascertain site of origin?

A.   Bronchoscopy
B.   MRI of the breast
C.   Random breast biopsies
D.   PET scan

Question 36.9.   A 55-year-old man, nonsmoker, presents with low back, right hip, and
abdominal pain for 6 weeks. CT scan of the abdomen and pelvis reveals
multiple diffuse liver lesions and lytic lesions in several vertebral bodies
and right iliac wing. CT scan of the chest is negative. PET imaging does
not identify a primary site. Serum PSA is normal. Light microscopy reveals a poorly differentiated carcinoma. Immunohistochemistry is negative for TTF-1, PSA, chromogranin, synaptophysin, CLA, vimentin, and
S-100. Electron microscopy reveals neurosecretory granules. What treatment regimen would you recommend?

A.   Anthracycline-based therapy for presumed lymphoma
B.   Best supportive care
C.   Taxane-based regimen for presumed NSCLC
D.   Platinum-based regimen for presumed poorly differentiated neu-
roendocrine carcinoma

Question 36.10.   A 54-year-old woman presents with an increase in abdominal girth, fatigue, anorexia, and weight loss. CT scan of the abdomen and pelvis reveals peritoneal studding and ascites. The rest of the CT scan is normal. CA-125 is elevated at 438 U/mL. CT-guided biopsy of a peritoneal nodule reveals well-differentiated adenocarcinoma of papillary and serous type. What treatment plan would you recommend?

A. Optimal debulking surgery followed by chemotherapy
B. Surgery alone
C. Radiation
D. Chemotherapy

Question 36.11.   A 52-year-old man has a growing mass in his left neck. He is an active smoker and has a history of heavy alcohol use. CT scan with contrast of the head and neck only reveals a 2-cm lower cervical lymph node. CT scan of the chest is negative. Biopsy of the mass reveals a poorly differentiated squamous cell carcinoma. Direct laryngoscopy and bronchoscopy are negative. What would you order next to help identify a primary site?

A. CT scan of the abdomen and pelvis
B. Esophagoscopy
C. PET scan
D. All of the above

Question 36.12.   A 58-year-old man, active smoker, presents to your office with newly diagnosed metastatic poorly differentiated squamous cell carcinoma. His only site of disease is a 2-cm subdigastric lymph node, based on CT scans of the head, neck, and chest with contrast, as well as PET scan. Direct laryngoscopy and nasopharynx survey reveal no suspicious lesions. Biopsies of inconspicuous sites and ipsilateral tonsillectomy are negative. Pathology of the excised lymph node reveals carcinoma contained within the lymph node without evidence of extracapsular spread. What would be the most appropriate therapy for this patient?

A. Radical neck dissection
B. Watchful waiting
C. Definitive radiation therapy
D. Chemotherapy alone

Question 36.13.   What are the chances of achieving a long-term disease-free state for the patient described in Question 12?

A. 0%
B. 15%
C. 25%
D. 40%

Question 36.14. **A 69-year-old man who retired from working in a shipyard presented with a 2-month history of dyspnea. He has an 80 pack-year history of tobacco use. Imaging reveals a large right-sided pleural effusion. After thoracentesis, a repeat CT scan is performed that reveals no primary lesion in the lung despite significant reduction in the pleural effusion. Cytology reveals malignancy. What following evaluation tests will you perform to identify the site of origin?**

    A. Request further pathological evaluation with TTF-1, CK7, and CK20 on immunoperoxidase staining and electron microscopy

    B. MRI of brain

    C. Serum AFP and hCG levels

    D. ER and PR expression of the malignant cells

Question 36.15. **After thoracentesis, his performance status dramatically improves to an ECOG 0. Final pathological diagnosis reveals adenocarcinoma of pulmonary origin. How would you treat him?**

    A. Observation

    B. Chemotherapy

    C. Surgery

    D. Radiation

ANSWERS

Answer 36.1. **The answer is C.**

Among cancers of unknown primary site, there are five major light microscopic diagnoses. Their distribution is as follows: approximately 60% are adenocarcinoma, 30% are poorly differentiated carcinoma or poorly differentiated adenocarcinoma, 5% are squamous carcinoma, 5% are poorly differentiated malignant neoplasm, and 1% are neuroendocrine carcinoma. Further characterization requires specialized pathologic study and/or assessment of clinical features.

Answer 36.2. **The answer is B.**

Among poorly differentiated neoplasms identified on light microscopy, the most frequent tumor type identified after further specialized pathologic study is lymphoma (i.e., non-Hodgkin's lymphoma). In various case series, it has been reported that 35% to 65% of poorly differentiated neoplasms are lymphomas. Most of the rest of the tumors are carcinomas, including poorly differentiated neuroendocrine tumors. Melanoma and sarcoma make up the rest of the group, approximately 15% of patients.

Answer 36.3. **The answer is A.**

CLA and PSA are specific for the diagnosis of hematologic malignancies and prostate cancer, respectively. However, false-positive and false-negative results can still occur with these stains.

PSA is rarely positive in salivary gland carcinoma. Technical expertise is required for accurately performing and interpreting these stains. TTF-1 is positive in 75% of cases of lung adenocarcinoma, as well as small cell carcinoma. Cytokeratin 7 and 20 staining are increasingly being used and can help guide further diagnostic workup, but are not very specific. S-100 and HMB-45 stains are associated with melanoma. Vimentin, desmin, and Factor VIII antigen are associated with sarcoma. ER and PR positivity suggests breast carcinoma. Chromogranin and synaptophysin staining support the diagnosis of neuroendocrine carcinoma/differentiation.

Answer 36.4. **The answer is D.**

In a large clinical trial of 220 patients, some subsets were identified as having a more favorable prognosis. These subsets include (i) tumors in the retroperitoneum, mediastinum, or peripheral lymph nodes; (ii) two or more features associated with germ cell syndrome; (iii) women with peritoneal carcinomatosis; (iv) poorly differentiated neuroendocrine tumors; (v) poorly differentiated neoplasm not otherwise specified; and (vi) anaplastic lymphoma. Many of these patients were proven to have thymomas, germ cell tumors, primary peritoneal carcinomatosis, lymphomas, and neuroendocrine carcinomas. These tumors are very responsive to chemotherapy with a complete response rate in different clinical trials ranging from 10% to 26%.

Answer 36.5. **The answer is C.**

This patient is a young man with a mediastinal mass diagnosed on pathology as a poorly differentiated CUP. Although his immunohistochemical staining does not specifically reveal a primary site, he has an elevated serum β-hCG and has had chromosomal studies done.

Genetic analyses of these tumors have shown abnormalities of chromosome 12 (i[12]p; del [12p]; multiple copies of 12p), which are diagnostic of germ cell tumors. Even without these chromosomal studies, this young man has a poorly differentiated carcinoma of the mediastinum with elevated hCG and should be treated with a cisplatin-based chemotherapy regimen used to treat a presumed extragonadal germ cell tumor.

Answer 36.6. **The answer is D.**

Low-grade neuroendocrine carcinomas are often indolent for many years, with a very slow rate of progression. The goal of therapy is to treat hormone-related symptoms with somatostatin analogs. This patient is asymptomatic and does not require immediate treatment. Laboratory data, such as urine 5-HIAA and/or serum chromogranin may be elevated and can be followed as markers of disease progression. If he becomes symptomatic, he can be treated with endocrine therapy, such as somatostatin analogs, for hormone-related symptoms. If the symptoms are not well controlled with hormone treatments, or if there is significant local pain secondary to tumor growth, other treatment modalities, including R hepatectomy, chemoembolization, or chemotherapy (e.g., streptozocin, Adriamycin, and 5FU), can be offered.

Answer 36.7.   **The answer is B.**

The patient presents with adenocarcinoma of unknown primary with liver metastasis. TTF-1 staining is approximately 75% positive in cases of lung adenocarcinoma, and negative staining does not rule out a lung primary. ER and PR positivity are suggestive of breast cancer, but up to 15% of patients are negative for ER, PR, and HER2-neu. Cytokeratin staining has been used to help facilitate further diagnostic approaches but is not diagnostic on its own. CK7 negative and CK20 positive staining pattern is suggestive of colorectal carcinoma and is sometimes seen in gastric cancers. CK7 positive and CK20 negative are suggestive of carcinomas of the lung, breast, ovary (nonmucinous), endometrium, and cervix, as well as mesothelioma. Mammogram is routine in the workup of CUP in women and is negative in this patient. The yield of bronchoscopy is low given no pulmonary symptoms and negative CT chest scan. The role of PET scan is helpful as an adjunct in the workup of an unknown primary cancer but is ordered when all other tests are inconclusive. It is of high yield in cases of squamous cell cervical CUP, where an occult primary is identified in 70%. Invasive testing, such as endoscopy, is not indicated routinely. In this case, however, the presentation of liver metastasis and CK7 negative and CK20 positive staining suggests a colorectal primary, and colonoscopy would be indicated in this setting.

Answer 36.8.   **The answer is B.**

Isolated axillary adenopathy in a woman is suggestive of occult breast cancer. The next step, if mammogram and ultrasound are negative, would be an MRI of the breast. In two small studies, an occult breast primary lesion was identified in 70% of cases on MRI using a dedicated breast coil. Even when MRI and PET are negative for a primary lesion, modified radical mastectomy has been recommended in such patients. An occult primary has been identified in 44% to 80% of patients after mastectomy. Radiation therapy after axillary lymph node dissection is a reasonable alternative primary therapy. Women with only isolated axillary adenopathy and no primary identified should be treated as having stage II breast cancer. As a result, they should receive neoadjuvant or adjuvant chemotherapy. To guide therapy, the pathologic tissue is checked for ER, PR, and HER2-neu status.

Answer 36.9.   **The answer is D.**

In 10% of poorly differentiated carcinomas, where immunohistochemistry is inconclusive, electron microscopy reveals neurosecretory granules, diagnostic of poorly differentiated neuroendocrine carcinoma. This group makes up 70% of all neuroendocrine CUP site. Most of these tumors have typical immunohistochemical staining patterns, positive for chromogranin, synaptophysin, and/or neuron-specific enolase (NSE). Electron microscopy is usually the most accurate means of diagnosis. Molecular genetic studies can be done to rule out other causes, such as chromosome 12p abnormalities identifying a germ cell tumor or 11;22 translocation (identifying peripheral neuroepithelioma, Ewing's sarcoma, or desmoplastic small round cell tumor).

Although the origin of poorly differentiated neuroendocrine tumors remains undefined, they are highly responsive to chemotherapy, namely, platinum-based regimens, as given in small cell lung carcinoma.

Answer 36.10.   **The answer is A.**

Adenocarcinoma causing diffuse peritoneal involvement is a typical presentation of ovarian carcinoma. However, it can also be present in cases of gastrointestinal (signet-ring gastric cancer), lung, or breast carcinomas. Women who present with peritoneal carcinomatosis, elevated CA-125, but no identifiable primary on imaging or even laparotomy, are described as having primary peritoneal carcinomatosis. There is an increased incidence of this entity in patients with BRCA-1 mutations. Carcinomas arising from the peritoneal surface often share the same biology and similar lineage with ovarian cancers (i.e., Mullerian derivation). Recent studies have shown that they also share similar gene expression profiles. Therefore, treatment strategies should match that for advanced ovarian cancer. They should receive aggressive surgical cytoreduction followed by postoperative chemotherapy with a taxane in combination with carboplatin.

Answer 36.11.   **The answer is D.**

The patient presents with metastatic squamous cell CUP, with lower cervical node disease. So far he has had CT scans of the head, neck, and chest; direct laryngoscopy; and bronchoscopy. The latter is important, because lower cervical and supraclavicular nodes are associated with occult lung cancer. The patient still needs further diagnostic tests in an attempt to find a primary site. This workup should include esophagoscopy, CT scans of the abdomen and pelvis, and a PET scan. Several series of patients with unknown primary cancers, including head and neck presentations, have demonstrated that PET can detect a primary tumor in 40% of all patients and up to 75% in squamous cell cervical CUP. Identifying a potential site for direct biopsy, as well as determining extent of disease, helps with the planning of radiation therapy.

Answer 36.12.   **The answer is C.**

This patient presents with metastatic poorly differentiated squamous cell CUP, with the only site of disease at a level II node. Radiotherapy is the treatment recommended to control his cervical CUP and any suspected primary mucosal sites. Studies have shown that results with high-dose radiation therapy alone, radical neck dissection, or a combination of the two are similar. Most authorities prefer radiation therapy alone, with good long-term disease-free survival.

Answer 36.13.   **The answer is D.**

The patient in Question 12 should be aggressively treated because he has a very favorable presentation and high chance of a long-term remission. Patients who present with cervical CUP have better prognosis than patients with CUP and disseminated metastases. Their long-term disease-free survival after aggressive local treatment is up to 40%. Moreover, patients with N1 or N2 disease do better than patients with N3 disease or very bulky neck adenopathy. On the other hand, patients with low cervical and supraclavicular node presentation, as in Question 11, may not do as well as those with high cervical node presentation because a substantial number of these patients may have an occult lung primary. Patients who have bulky adenopathy may benefit from a combination of chemotherapy and radiation rather than radiation therapy alone.

Answer 36.14.   **The answer is A.**

An isolated malignant pleural effusion in a man with the above given history could be related to NSCLC or mesothelioma. Immunohistochemistry evaluation of pathology would reveal a NSCLC if positive for TTF-1 and CK7. Electron microscopy is helpful in identifying mesothelioma. In women, such a presentation can also represent the manifestation of an occult abdominal neoplasm, such as ovarian cancer or primary peritoneal carcinomatosis. An exploratory laparotomy may be diagnostic but not therapeutic in this situation.

Answer 36.15.   **The answer is B.**

Patients with good performance status should be offered chemotherapy. In an older series of patients with pleural effusion of unknown primary, 78% symptomatically responded to chemotherapy and their median survival was 12 months. Definitive surgery or radiation is not recommended for patients with malignant pleural effusion.

Peritoneal Carcinomatosis

Directions   Each of the numbered items below is followed by lettered answers. Select the ONE lettered answer that is BEST in each case unless instructed otherwise.

QUESTIONS

Question 37.1.   **Peritoneal carcinomatosis may arise from tumors of which of the following structures?**

    A.   The peritoneal lining
    B.   Intra-abdominal viscera
    C.   Extra-abdominal organs
    D.   All the above

Question 37.2.   **Which is the most common type of cancer presenting with isolated peritoneal carcinomatosis?**

    A.   Ovarian
    B.   Appendiceal
    C.   Colon
    D.   Stomach
    E.   A and B

Question 37.3.   **Unlike high-grade, poorly differentiated tumors, low-grade, well-differentiated tumors disseminate via which of the following mechanisms?**

    A.   Cell shedding
    B.   Hematological spread
    C.   Pressure-burst phenomenon
    D.   Lymphatic spread

Question 37.4.   **The mere presence of free-floating tumor cells within the peritoneal cavity does not universally correlate with peritoneal carcinomatosis. True or False?**

    A.   True
    B.   False

Corresponding Chapter in *Cancer: Principles & Practice of Oncology,* Eighth Edition: 57 (Diagnosis and Treatment of Peritoneal Carcinomatosis).

Question 37.5.   **Which imaging modality is the best tool to detect peritoneal recurrence?**

A. Computed tomography (CT)
B. Magnetic resonance imaging (MRI)
C. Abdominal ultrasonogram
D. Positron emission tomography (PET)

Question 37.6.   **What is the most important adverse prognostic factor associated with pseudomyxoma peritonei?**

A. Presence of malignancy
B. Amount of mucin
C. Abdominal distention
D. Abdominal pain

Question 37.7.   **The features of disseminated peritoneal adenomucinosis (DPAM) include?**

A. Peritoneal tumor
B. Scant cellularity
C. Abundant extracellular mucin
D. Low-grade endothelial cells
E. All of the above

Question 37.8.   **A 63-year-old patient presented with bowel obstruction and underwent exploratory laparotomy that revealed a ruptured appendix with abundant mucin. Scant, atypical cells without obvious malignant histology were reported by the pathologist. What treatment plan results in the best clinical outcome in this patient?**

A. Maximal tumor debulking immediately followed by hyperthermic intraperitoneal mitomycin C with or without 5FU and augmented with adjuvant systemic therapy with 5FU and mitomycin C
B. Maximal tumor debulking followed by adjuvant systemic 5FU and mitomycin C
C. Systemic 5FU and mitomycin C alone without surgical resection
D. Close observation

Question 37.9.   **Which of the following factors predicts the worst outcome in patients with mucinous adenocarcinoma of appendix?**

A. Histologic grade
B. Age
C. Performance status
D. The use of intraperitoneal therapy

Question 37.10. **A 45-year-old woman presented with 3 months' duration of abdominal discomfort and chronic reflux. She underwent an esophagogastroduodenoscopy (EGD) that showed a stomach mass at the antrum. Endoscopic ultrasound (EUS)/fine-needle aspiration (FNA) confirmed an adenocarcinoma with clinical staging of a T3N0 lesion. CT scans did not show any metastatic lesions. The patient is scheduled for curative surgical resection and now wants to discuss the potential use of intraperitoneal chemotherapy.**

    A. Postoperative intraperitoneal chemotherapy provides survival benefit when compared with surgery alone and should be offered as part of the standard of care.

    B. The role of adjuvant intraperitoneal chemotherapy after complete resection of primary tumors remains to be determined.

    C. 5FU and mitomycin C will be used as part of intraperitoneal treatment.

    D. Cisplatin and mitomycin C are the agents of choice for intraperitoneal therapy.

Question 37.11. **A 50-year-old man was found to have a near obstructing adenocarcinoma involving the splenic flexure of his colon. His staging CT scans showed five small nodules associated with the greater omentum. No distant metastases were identified. He underwent surgical resection of the primary mass and debulking of his intraperitoneal carcinomatosis. However, complete cytoreduction was not possible because of the intraoperative discovery of multiple tumor masses firmly adhering to intra-abdominal vital organs. He now wants to know his overall prognosis and treatment plan.**

    A. His prognosis is the same as if he had complete cytoreduction.

    B. Hyperthermic intraperitoneal chemoperfusion does not significantly improve prognosis in incomplete cytoreduction.

    C. His prognosis is much poorer when compared with those with complete cytoreduction, and the need for systemic chemotherapy is inevitable.

    D. Both B and C.

Question 37.12. **What is not a risk factor for malignant peritoneal mesothelioma?**

    A. Asbestos exposure

    B. Abdominal radiation

    C. Simian virus 40 exposure

    D. Cigarette smoking

Question 37.13. **Which of the histologic subtypes of malignant peritoneal mesothelioma has the best prognosis?**

    A. Epithelial

    B. Sarcomatoid

    C. Mixed

Questions
37.14.–37.15.

A 65-year-old man, who is a retired asbestos miner, began developing progressive abdominal bloating approximately 3 months ago. CT scan of his chest and abdomen showed omental caking and diffuse peritoneal implants associated with massive ascites. Analysis of his ascitic fluid showed malignant cells consistent with primary malignant mesothelioma. During the last 2 months, he has required frequent large-volume paracentesis to control his ascites. His performance status concomitantly has significantly deteriorated from an Eastern Cooperative Oncology Group (ECOG) performance status (PS) of 0 to 3.

Question 37.14. What is NOT the frequent cause of death in patients with primary peritoneal mesothelioma?

A. Metabolic effects of the tumor volume
B. Decreased nutritional intake
C. Protein loss and dehydration associated with massive ascites and frequent paracentesis
D. Peritonitis

Question 37.15. What is the median survival in untreated patients with malignant peritoneal mesothelioma?

A. 6 months
B. 1 year
C. 15 months
D. 2 years

Question 37.16. Which of the following factors has no significant impact on overall survival in patients with malignant peritoneal mesothelioma undergoing surgical debulking and hyperthermic chemotherapeutic perfusion?

A. Age <60 years
B. Ability to resect all disease to a volume of <1 cm
C. Agents for perfusion therapy
D. Absence of deep tissue invasion

Question 37.17. A 40-year-old woman presented with abdominal distention and early satiety. On examination, the patient was found to have massive ascites. CT scan showed massive ascites and multiple peritoneal implants. In addition, a single 2-cm deposit was noted on the surface of the right ovary; her bilateral ovaries otherwise appear normal. The patient underwent paracentesis, which revealed malignant serous type cells. A PET scan did not reveal other metastatic sites except what appears on the CT. What is the diagnosis in this patient?

A. Primary peritoneal carcinoma
B. Peritoneal mesothelioma
C. Metastatic ovarian cancer
D. Adenocarcinoma of unknown primary

Question 37.18. A 45-year-old woman presented with lower abdominal pain, and imaging study revealed a moderate amount of ascites with large peritoneal implants and one suspicious 3 × 5-cm heterogeneous mass in the right ovary. The patient also has high CA-125. FNA of the ovarian mass showed a malignant serous type cells. No other lesions were seen. What would be the next step of diagnosis or treatment?

A. Exploratory laparotomy with optimal surgical debulking
B. Systemic chemotherapy with platinum and paclitaxel
C. Surgical debulking and intraperitoneal chemotherapy
D. Surgical debulking and intraperitoneal chemotherapy followed by systemic chemotherapy

Question 37.19. A 50-year-old man with a history of gastric cancer with diffuse peritoneal involvements progressed after two lines of chemotherapy, now with persistent nausea, vomiting, and constipation. An abdominal CT scan showed multiple air fluid levels but no clear obstruction transition points. The patient also has poor performance status. What would you consider to relieve his obstruction?

A. Diverting colostomy
B. Gastrostomy tube placement
C. Surgical exploration to locate the site of obstruction
D. Gastrointestinal (GI) evaluation for possible stent placement

Question 37.20. A 65-year-old man with progressive and refractory pancreatic cancer who presented with a large amount of ascites resulted in shortness of breath at rest. The patient underwent a large-volume paracentesis but returned 1 week later with reaccumulated fluid. What would be the next step to manage his ascites?

A. Repeat paracentesis
B. Initiation of antidiuretics, such as spironolactone
C. Placement of a peritoneovenous shunt
D. Placement of a Denver catheter

ANSWERS

Answer 37.1. **The answer is D.**

Peritoneal carcinomatosis can arise from tumors of all these structures with or without concurrent systemic metastases.

Answer 37.2. **The answer is E.**

Intraperitoneal viscera, including the ovary and appendix, are the most common source of tumors presenting with isolated peritoneal carcinomatosis.

Answer 37.3.   **The answer is C.**

Low-grade, well-differentiated tumors disseminate via a pressure-burst phenomenon, common to slow-growing tumors such as mucinous tumors of the appendix and ovary, where the slow tumor growth permits the sheer volume of tumor cells to rupture through viscera and contaminate the peritoneum with tumor cells. In contrast, high-grade, poorly differentiated tumors spread through primary organ invasion with subsequent cell shedding and distant organ attachment, often with concurrent lymphatic or hematologic metastases.

Answer 37.4.   **The answer is A.**

Identification of free-floating tumor cells within the peritoneal cavity (e.g., after cytological examination of ascitic fluid) does not always mean peritoneal carcinomatosis. Attachment, implantation, and proliferation are all necessary steps in the establishment and growth of intraperitoneal disease.

Answer 37.5.   **The answer is B.**

MRI has been shown to be superior to helical CT in the assessment of bowel and mesenteric thickening. Sensitivity and specificity for MRI were demonstrated to be 84% and 100%, respectively, for the detection of peritoneal recurrence in ovarian carcinoma. PET has gained growing acceptance for assessing intraperitoneal carcinomatosis; however, its major drawback is the lack of efficacy in the evaluation of lesions less than 1 cm in diameter.

Answer 37.6.   **The answer is A.**

The presence of tumor cells in peritoneal washings obtained at the time of surgical resection correlates with increased local recurrence and decreased survival, even in the absence of nodal or systemic metastases. In DPAM, the absence of malignant cells is associated with significantly improved disease-free and overall survival.

Answer 37.7.   **The answer is E.**

DPAM includes peritoneal tumors with scant cellularity in the presence of abundant extracellular mucin. Endothelial cells present are histologically bland with low-grade adenomatous features, minimal cytologic atypia, and low mitotic activity.

Answer 37.8.   **The answer is A.**

In the series of 65 patients from Ronnet et al (Cancer 2001;92) and a review of 62 patients with pseudomyxoma peritonei by van Ruth et al (Eur J Surg Oncol 2003;29), median survival was significantly improved in patients with DPAM who were treated with maximal tumor debulking followed by intraperitoneal mitomycin C alone or in combination with 5FU. Three additional cycles of systemic 5FU/mitomycin C chemotherapy were given to all patients in the Ronnet series but was reserved only for patients with pathological evidence of malignancy in the van Ruth series. Both approaches appear to confer similar survival outcomes.

Answer 37.9.   **The answer is A.**

In mucinous adenocarcinoma of the appendix, histologic grade is the single most important prognostic indicator, with high-grade histologic atypia associated with the poorest outcome. In a series of 94 consecutive patients with adenocarcinoma of the appendix, the presence of high-grade "colonic type" tumors was reported in 45% of patients and was associated with higher grade tumors and higher stage, and ultimately poorer prognosis when compared with benign mucinous tumors (Nitecki et al. Ann Surg 1994;219).

Answer 37.10.   **The answer is B.**

Data regarding adjuvant intraperitoneal chemotherapy for high-risk tumors have been mixed. Yu et al (Ann Surg 1998;64) randomized 248 patients with stage II and III gastric cancer to surgical resection alone versus resection plus postoperative intraperitoneal mitomycin C and 5FU, with an increase in survival seen only in the subset of patients with stage III cancer. Other series of similar patients using intraperitoneal cisplatin or mitomycin C did not show statistically significant improvements in local control or survival, except in patients with serosal invasion by tumors (Sautner et al. J Clin Oncol 1994;12; Ikeguchi et al. Eur J Surg 1995;161).

Answer 37.11.   **The answer is D.**

When complete resection of the primary tumor along with all peritoneal disease is not possible, surgical intervention merely delays the inevitable need for intravenous chemotherapy. Complete surgical cytoreduction was achieved in only 43% of the cases in one series. Compared with patients with complete surgical debulking, those without total resection of the primary and intraperitoneal disease fare much worse regardless of the use of hyperthermic intraperitoneal chemoperfusion.

Answer 37.12.   **The answer is D.**

All of these factors have been associated with increased risks for malignant peritoneal mesothelioma. Reported associations between asbestos and malignant mesothelioma range from 50% to 83%, but the link appears to be less than that seen with pleural mesothelioma.

Answer 37.13.   **The answer is A.**

The epithelial type of malignant peritoneal mesothelioma is the most common and carries the best prognosis, although significant variability in the extent of disease at presentation is common.

Answer 37.14.   **The answer is D.**

The most frequent cause of death in malignant peritoneal mesothelioma is the overall debilitation associated with the metabolic effects of the tumor volume, the decreased nutritional intake from early satiety, and the protein loss and dehydration associated with the massive ascites and frequent therapeutic paracentesis. Diffuse compression of abdominal viscera resulting in early satiety and overall inanition is rare and can occur in rare instances of massive tumor load.

Answer 37.15.   **The answer is B.**

Median survival in untreated patients with malignant peritoneal meso-thelioma is less than 1 year.

Answer 37.16.   **The answer is C.**

In a series of 49 patients with malignant peritoneal mesothelioma reported by Feldman et al. (J Clin Oncol 2003;21), age less than 60 years, presence of previous debulking surgery, absence of deep tissue invasion, and minimal residual disease after resection were associated with improved progression-free and overall survival. Reports from expanded patient groups at other institutions have confirmed these results. Although cisplatin, mitomycin C, and 5FU have been used for continuous hyperthermic peritoneal perfusion postsurgery, to date there have been no randomized trials comparing these agents to determine superiority in long-term disease control.

Answer 37.17.   **The answer is A.**

Primary peritoneal carcinoma is a rare group of tumors of unclear origin arising in the peritoneal cavity. Primary peritoneal carcinoma can be distinguished from ovarian cancer by the following criteria: Both ovaries must be normal in size; the amount of extraovarian tumor must be greater than the involvement on the surface of the ovary; the ovarian component must be less than 5 × 5 mm within the ovary and otherwise confined to the surface of the ovary; and the cytologic characteristics must be of the serous type. Treatment for primary peritoneal carcinoma follows programs established for ovarian carcinoma, including operative debulking and adjuvant chemotherapy.

Answer 37.18.   **The answer is D.**

The differential diagnosis for this patient's cancer is primary peritoneal carcinoma versus ovarian carcinoma versus carcinoma of unknown origin. The elevated CA-125 and the large heterogeneous mass in the right ovary favor ovarian carcinoma, although the serous histology is more consistent with primary peritoneal carcinoma. However, treatment programs for primary peritoneal carcinoma usually follow those established for ovarian carcinoma. These regimens traditionally involve surgical debulking supported by intraperitoneal chemotherapy and followed by systemic chemotherapy with a combination of a platinum and a taxane.

Answer 37.19.   **The answer is B.**

Diffuse carcinomatosis often results in functional, not anatomic, obstruction that may only be effectively palliated through placement of a gastrostomy tube.

Answer 37.20.   **The answer is B.**

Conservative management of recurrent malignant ascites through diuretic therapy is effective in up to 47% of patients and should be initiated first. Spironolactone therapy starting at 150 mg per day may be necessary for prolonged periods to establish and maintain control of the ascites. Direct drainage of ascitic fluid through repeated paracentesis or a surgically placed peritoneovenous shunt provides immediate relief but carries increased risk of infection and protein loss. Peritoneal shunts (Denver catheter) remove ascitic fluid and return it to the systemic circulation. Successful, prolonged control of ascites is possible in up to 70% of patients; however, disseminated intravascular coagulation, pulmonary emboli, pulmonary edema, and rarely tumor emboli are the complications associated with these catheters.

Immunosuppression-Related Malignancies

Directions Each of the numbered items below is followed by lettered answers. Select the ONE lettered answer that is BEST in each case unless instructed otherwise.

QUESTIONS

Question 38.1. **Which of the following forms of lymphoma are NOT significantly increased in human immunodeficiency virus (HIV)-infected patients compared with uninfected patients:**

A. Hodgkin's disease
B. Follicular lymphoma
C. Burkitt's lymphoma
D. Diffuse large B-cell lymphoma (DLBCL)
E. Primary effusion lymphoma

Question 38.2. **Chemotherapy is usually well tolerated with concomitant highly active antiretroviral therapy with which of the following exceptions:**

A. Zidovudine, nucleotide reverse transcriptase inhibitor therapy
B. Protease inhibitors
C. Raltegravir, the new integrase inhibitor
D. Fuzeon, the HIV entry inhibitor

Question 38.3. **Appropriate therapy for a patient with newly diagnosed HIV-associated symptomatic pulmonary Kaposi's sarcoma includes:**

A. Liposomal anthracycline
B. Paclitaxel
C. Highly active antiretroviral therapy
D. Thalidomide
E. A and C or B and C

Corresponding Chapter in *Cancer: Principles & Practice of Oncology*, Eighth Edition: 58 (Immunosuppression-Related Malignancies).

Question 38.4. **Which of the following is true about the combination of rituximab with chemotherapy for acquired immunodeficiency syndrome (AIDS)-associated lymphomas?**

    A. Adding rituximab to cyclophosphamide, doxorubicin, vincristine, and prednisone (CHOP) chemotherapy in patients with CD4 <50/mm^3 may result in higher rate of neutropenic infections.

    B. Rituximab is of no added benefit to CHOP or infusional etoposide, vincristine, and doxorubicin, bolus cyclophosphamide, and daily prednisone (EPOCH) chemotherapy for AIDS-associated DLBCL.

    C. Rituximab with chemotherapy is usually beneficial in plasmablastic lymphoma.

    D. Rituximab with chemotherapy is usually beneficial in primary effusion lymphoma.

Question 38.5. **Which is NOT true concerning primary central nervous system (CNS) lymphoma in AIDS?**

    A. Positive cerebrospinal fluid (CSF) Epstein-Barr virus (EBV) polymerase chain reaction (PCR) test, a consistent radiological picture, and brain biopsy are necessary to diagnose primary CNS AIDS lymphoma.

    B. In patients with CD4 count < 50/mm^3 and poor performance status, cranial radiotherapy alone may be appropriate.

    C. In patients with CD4 count >50/mm^3 and good performance status, the use of high-dose methotrexate with leucovorin rescue may be appropriate.

    D. Addition of highly active antiretroviral therapy may increase the duration of response.

ANSWERS

Answer 38.1. **The answer is B.**

The standard incidence ratio (incidence in HIV vs. noninfected individuals) is approximately 10 for Hodgkin's disease and approximately 50 for diffuse large B-cell lymphoma, Burkitt's lymphoma, and primary effusion lymphoma. In contrast, more indolent lymphomas, such as follicular lymphomas, are not significantly increased in HIV-infected patients.

Answer 38.2. **The answer is A.**

Zidovudine is generally poorly tolerated with chemotherapy because of myelosuppression. Protease inhibitors are generally well tolerated with chemotherapy, although they may affect metabolism of many drugs through effects on cytochrome P450-associated enzymes. Preliminary results with the most recently approved HIV drugs suggest that the integrase inhibitor raltegravir, coreceptor inhibitor maraviroc, and fusion inhibitor fuzeon are also well tolerated with chemotherapy.

Answer 38.3. **The answer is E.**

Lipsomal anthracyclines and paclitaxel each have response rates of 50% to 80%, but highly active antiretroviral therapy (HAART) alone has more limited activity. Thalidomide has activity for cutaneous Kaposi's sarcoma, but its role in symptomatic pulmonary Kaposi's sarcoma is not adequately documented. There are many benefits of combining HAART with chemotherapy, including improved responses, decreased toxicity, and improved survival.

Answer 38.4.   **The answer is A.**

Although the role of rituximab with chemotherapy in non–HIV-infected patients has been documented, its role in AIDS lymphoma is more controversial. Although several studies have suggested that there is a benefit to the addition of rituximab to CHOP or EPOCH chemotherapy, in patients with CD4 <50 to 100/mm^3 there are reports of excess neutropenic fevers and infections. Rituximab is usually not beneficial for treatment of plasmablastic lymphomas and primary effusion lymphomas, because CD20 is usually not expressed on the malignant cells.

Answer 38.5.   **The answer is A.**

CSF EBV PCR is a rather sensitive (~80%) and highly specific test (>95%) for diagnosis of primary CNS lymphoma, and together with a consistent radiological picture, brain biopsy may not be required to establish the diagnosis. In patients with low CD4 counts or poor performance status, cranial radiotherapy is the treatment of choice for primary CNS lymphoma, because opportunistic infections cause much greater morbidity and mortality than recurrent lymphoma. In contrast, for patients with higher CD4 counts and good performance status, high-dose systemic methotrexate therapy with leucovorin rescue may be associated with improved responses, as reported in non–HIV-associated primary CNS lymphoma.

Giridharan Ramsingh
Daniel Morgensztern

Oncologic Emergencies

Directions   Each of the numbered items below is followed by lettered answers. Select the ONE lettered answer that is BEST in each case unless instructed otherwise.

QUESTIONS

Questions 39.1.–39.3.   A 48-year-old white man presents with a history of progressive facial swelling and shortness of breath for 1 month. He has a 40-pack-year smoking history. On examination, the patient has cervical and thoracic venous distention. Laboratory test results revealed normal blood counts, basic metabolic profile, and liver functions. Computed tomography (CT) scan revealed a 6 × 5-cm lung mass with liver metastases.

Question 39.1.   What is the most likely cause of his condition?

A. Small cell lung cancer
B. Non-Hodgkin's lymphoma
C. Non–small cell lung cancer
D. Superior vena cava (SVC) thrombosis

Question 39.2.   Biopsy was performed and showed small cell lung cancer. Which is the best initial modality of treatment for this patient?

A. Surgery
B. Radiation therapy
C. Chemotherapy
D. SVC stent

Question 39.3.   What is the most likely location for the primary tumor?

A. Peripheral left lung
B. Peripheral right lung
C. Central left lung
D. Central right lung

Corresponding Chapter in *Cancer: Principles & Practice of Oncology,* Eighth Edition: 59 (Oncologic Emergencies).

Question 39.4.   Which among the following brain metastases is least likely to undergo hemorrhagic transformation?

A.   Choriocarcinoma
B.   Papillary thyroid carcinoma
C.   Lung cancer
D.   Renal cell carcinoma

Question 39.5.   A 57-year-old man presents with severe back pain and bilateral leg weakness for 3 days. Magnetic resonance imaging (MRI) of the spine reveals metastatic lesion at T10 vertebral body with significant cord compression. What are the most likely primary tumors?

A.   Lung cancer and breast cancer
B.   Lung cancer and lymphoma
C.   Breast cancer and lymphoma
D.   Colon cancer and prostate cancer

Question 39.6.   A 65-year-old man with non–small cell lung cancer presented to the emergency department with an inability to walk for the last 3 days. He had brain metastases at presentation and was treated with whole brain radiation and liver metastases with progressive disease after second-line chemotherapy. On examination, the patient has decreased strength in both legs. MRI of the thoracic spine showed multiple bone metastases with spinal cord compression at T4-T5 and T10. Which of the following does NOT represent a relative contraindication for surgery?

A.   Life expectancy
B.   Multiple bone metastases
C.   Duration of paraplegia
D.   Sites of cord compression

Question 39.7.   Which of the following statements regarding rasburicase is FALSE?

A.   Mechanism of action is inhibition of urate oxidase.
B.   Should be avoided in patients with glucose 6-phosphate deficiency (G6PD).
C.   Antibodies against rasburicase or its epitopes may occur in up to 20% of cases.
D.   None of the above; all answers are correct.

Question 39.8.   A 28-year-old man presents with newly diagnosed with acute myeloid leukemia. He has a white cell count of 140,000/mm^3, glucose of 96 mg/dL, sodium of 138 mEq/L, potassium of 4 mEq/L, creatinine of 1.1 mg/dL, blood urea nitrogen (BUN) of 15 mg/dL, uric acid of 4.8 mg/dL, albumin of 5.2 g/dL, and calcium of 10.2 mg/dL. He is started on induction chemotherapy, aggressive intravenous fluids and allopurinol. Twelve hours later, the patient developed cardiac arrest not responsive to cardiopulmonary resuscitation and died. What is the most likely cause of his death?

A.   Leukostasis
B.   Electrolyte imbalance
C.   Pulmonary embolism
D.   Chemotherapy-induced cardiac arrhythmia

Question 39.9.   A 45-year-old woman with newly diagnosed diffuse large B-cell lymphoma presents with fatigue, weight loss, sweating, tremors, and confusion. Neurological examination showed no focal deficits. Laboratory evaluation showed white blood cell (WBC) count of 12,000/mm^3 with 80% neutrophils, hemoglobin of 9 g/dL, platelets of 70,000/mm^3, glucose of 40 mg/dL, sodium of 145 mEq/L, potassium of 3.8 mEq/L, bicarbonate of 12 mEq/L, chloride of 105 mEq/L, creatinine of 1.2 mg/dL, BUN of 35 mg/dL, total bilirubin of 1.5 mg/dL, direct bilirubin of 1.2 mg/dL , alkaline phosphatase of 410 IU/L, serum glutamic oxaloacetic transaminase (SGOT) of 150 IU/L, serum glutamate pyruvate transaminase (SGPT) of 195 IU/L, uric acid of 8.2 mg/dL, lactate dehydrogenase (LDH) of 2300 U/L, albumin of 3.5 g/dL, prothrombin time of 16 secibds, and activated partial thromboplastin time of 28 seconds. CT scan showed multiple involved lymph node chains in both sides of the diaphragm and extensive liver involvement. What is the most likely diagnosis?

A.   Liver failure
B.   Lymphomatous meningitis
C.   Lactic acidosis
D.   Tumor lysis syndrome

Question 39.10.   A 63-year-old man with metastatic squamous cell carcinoma of the lung presents with worsening confusion, constipation, and nausea for 3 days. Laboratory tests revealed hemoglobin 13.5 d/dL, WBC of 12,500/mm^3, platelets of 155,000/mm^3, sodium of 149 mEq/L, potassium of 4.8 mEq/L, bicarbonate of 28 mEq/L, BUN of 44 mg/dL, creatinine of 1.8 mg/dL, albumin of 2.8 g/dL, and calcium of 13.6 mg/dL. What is the most appropriate initial therapy?

A.   Intravenous fluids and bisphosphonate
B.   Intravenous fluids, bisphosphonate, and calcitonin
C.   Intravenous fluids, bisphosphonate, and gallium nitrate
D.   Intravenous fluids, bisphosphonate, and plicamycin

ANSWERS

Answer 39.1.   **The answer is A.**

Malignant disease is the most common cause of SVC syndrome. Among the malignancies, the most common is small cell lung cancer, followed by squamous cell lung cancer and lymphoma in most series. Diffuse large B-cell lymphoma and lymphoblastic lymphoma are the most common among lymphomas that cause SVC syndrome. Although Hodgkin's disease frequently involves mediastinum, it rarely causes SVC syndrome. Breast cancer is the most common metastatic cancer that causes SVC syndrome. Nonmalignant condition causing SVC syndrome is increasingly becoming more common because of the use of vascular devices, which can result in SVC thrombosis.

Answer 39.2.   **The answer is C.**

Studies have shown that both radiation therapy and chemotherapy are equally effective in relieving symptoms in small cell lung cancer and lymphoma. Surgery is not a good option for this patient with extensive-stage small cell lung cancer, and an SVC stent may be used in case of lack of response or relapsed obstruction after initial therapy. Although radiation could be used for immediate symptomatic relief, combination chemotherapy is also very effective and preferable as initial therapy, avoiding the large radiation field and also addressing the metastatic lesions.

Answer 39.3.   **The answer is D.**

The SVC extends from the junction of the right and left innominate veins to the right atrium and is completely encircled by lymph node chains draining from the right thoracic cavity and lower part of the left thorax. Approximately 80% of the tumors causing SVC syndrome are located in the right lung. In the absence of mediastinal lymph node enlargement, the most likely cause of the SVC is direct extension from the centrally located right-sided tumor.

Answer 39.4.   **The answer is C.**

Because lung cancer is the most common primary tumor in patients with brain metastases, it accounts for most cases of tumor bleeding. However, the probability of cerebral hemorrhage is much higher in patients with melanoma, renal cell carcinoma, choriocarcinoma, and papillary thyroid carcinoma.

Answer 39.5.   **The answer is B.**

Although most patients with malignant spinal cord compression (MSCC) have a history of malignancy, approximately 20% develop this complication at the initial presentation. Breast cancer is a common cause of MSCC during the course of the disease, but this manifestation rarely occurs at presentation. Colon cancer is an uncommon cause of MSCC, and prostate cancer usually affects the lumbosacral spine. The most common causes of MSCC at presentation are lung cancer, non-Hodgkin's lymphoma, and multiple myeloma.

Answer 39.6.   **The answer is B.**

The role of surgical treatment in patients with spinal cord compression remains undefined, and this procedure should be performed only in carefully selected patients. In a prospective trial reported by Patchell and colleagues (Direct decompressive surgical resection in the treatment of spinal cord compression caused by metastatic cancer: a randomized trial. Lancet 2005;366:643–648), surgical decompression followed by radiation was associated with a prolonged ability to walk compared with radiation alone. Inclusion criteria for the study included duration of paraplegia less than 48 hours, spinal cord compression at a single level, and life expectancy beyond 3 months. The number of bone metastases by itself is not a reliable indicator for therapeutic success from surgical decompression.

Answer 39.7.   **The answer is A.**

Urate oxidase catalyzes the conversion of uric acid to allantoin. This enzyme is present in most mammals but not in humans. Rasburicase is a recombinant urate oxidase produced in *Saccharomyces cerevisiae*. This medicine should be avoided in patients with G6PD because it may cause hemolysis as a result of the increase in the byproduct hydrogen peroxidase, and approximately 10% to 20% of patients taking rasburicase may develop antibodies, increasing the risk of allergic reaction with subsequent treatments.

Answer 39.8.   **The answer is B.**

Despite vigorous hydration, the most likely cause of death soon after initiating chemotherapy is tumor lysis syndrome (TLS). Among the metabolic complications of TLS, hyperkalemia caused by the release of intracellular potassium from tumoral cells represents the most important cause of early mortality. Leukostasis, pulmonary embolism, and cardiac arrhythmia are possible causes that are far less likely in this patient.

Answer 39.9.   **The answer is C.**

Despite extensive liver involvement, liver failure is unlikely in this patient because of the slightly abnormal synthetic hepatic function reflected by near normal albumin and prothrombin time. Lymphomatous meningitis is rare and usually associated with focal deficits, generally involving cranial nerve palsies. Elevated LDH and uric acid in a patient with aggressive lymphoma is concerning for TLS. However, although the patient may have some evidence for laboratorial TLS, most of the symptoms suggest an alternative diagnosis.

The high anion-gap metabolic acidosis in a patient with lymphoma and extensive liver involvement is most likely caused by lactic acidosis.

This manifestation occurs when the increased lactic acid production by the malignant cells cannot be used by the liver. Massive liver involvement is the most likely cause for the symptomatic hypoglycemia manifested as tremors, sweating, and confusion. Even with optimal therapy, the mortality is very high, ranging between 60% and 90% according to some studies.

Answer 39.10. **The answer is B.**

This patient has severe hypercalcemia and requires prompt reduction in the calcium levels. Intravenous hydration is the most important initial step, with or without the addition of furosemide, which may enhance the renal calcium excretion. Bisphosphonates are also very effective and well tolerated. However, because the patient is symptomatic and the effect of bisphosphonates may take a few days, he will require an additional short-acting agent. Gallium nitrate is usually given by continuous infusion for 5 days, with a gradual reduction in the calcium during the infusion time. Although plicamycin lowers the calcium levels typically within 12 hours, side effects including thrombocytopenia and nephrotoxicity limit its use to patients with severe and refractory hypercalcemia. Calcitonin is safe and relatively nontoxic, and may result in a rapid decrease in calcium levels within 2 to 6 hours. In this patient, the calcitonin may provide a fast improvement in the hypercalcemia, whereas bisphosphonate can cause a more sustainable effect.

Treatment of Metastatic Cancer

Directions   Each of the numbered items below is followed by lettered answers. Select the ONE lettered answer that is BEST in each case unless instructed otherwise.

QUESTIONS

Question 40.1.   **Which of the following cancers has the highest 5-year cumulative incidence of brain metastasis?**

A. Breast cancer
B. Colorectal cancer
C. Renal cell carcinoma
D. Lung cancer

Question 40.2.   **What is the median interval from diagnosis of cancer to brain metastasis?**

A. 2 months
B. 6 months
C. 24 months
D. 12 months

Question 40.3.   **What is the most common clinical presentation of brain metastases?**

A. Seizures
B. Focal weakness
C. Ataxia
D. Headache

Corresponding Chapter in *Cancer: Principles & Practice of Oncology*, Eighth Edition: 60 (Treatment of Metastatic Cancer).

Question 40.4.   **Which factors are critical in establishing prognosis in patients treated with radiation therapy for brain metastasis?**

    A.   Karnofsky performance score, patient's age, controlled primary tumor, no extracranial metastasis

    B.   Patients receiving stereotactic radiation plus whole brain radiation therapy

    C.   Patients receiving surgery and whole brain radiation therapy

    D.   All of the above

Question 40.5.   **A 54-year-old woman presented to the local emergency department with a seizure and history of worsening headaches that started 2 months before presentation. Physical examination revealed nonfocal neurological evaluation. Brain magnetic resonance imaging (MRI) demonstrated the presence of a single brain lesion in the frontal lobe. Further workup was with computed tomography (CT) scans of the chests and pelvis; mammography and positron emission tomography (PET) scan were negative. What is the MOST optimal management plan for this patient?**

    A.   Biopsy, followed by whole brain radiation therapy

    B.   Biopsy, followed by surgical resection and whole brain radiation therapy

    C.   Biopsy, followed by steroid therapy, best supportive care, and a consultation with hospice

    D.   Whole brain radiation therapy and empiric chemotherapy with temozolomide

Question 40.6.   **A 67-year-old woman presented with a cough and shortness of breath over the last month. In the course of the evaluation, chest radiogram demonstrated a presence of a large left hilar mass, and CT scan indicated the presence of metastatic disease in the liver. Biopsy of the liver led to the diagnosis of small cell lung carcinoma. As part of the staging procedure, brain MRI is performed, which demonstrates multiple brain metastases with an area of brain edema. What would be appropriate brain metastases management for this patient?**

    A.   Whole brain radiotherapy, dexamethasone 10-mg loading dose, followed by 16 mg per day in divided doses with a fast taper, phenytoin for seizure prevention

    B.   Whole brain radiation therapy, dexamethasone 10-mg loading dose, followed by 16 mg per day in divided doses

    C.   Whole brain radiotherapy, low-molecular-weight heparin, and phenytoin

    D.   Dexamethasone followed by whole brain radiation therapy

Question 40.7.   **What are the complete response rates of brain metastases from renal cell carcinoma to whole brain radiation therapy?**

    A.   35%

    B.   14%

    C.   0%

    D.   37%

Question 40.8.   **Which of the following statements related to whole brain radiation therapy is INCORRECT?**

A. Acute side effects after whole brain radiation include ototoxicity, fatigue, skin reaction, and hair loss.
B. Long-term radiation-induced effects include dementia.
C. The most radiation sensitive brain area is the hippocampus.
D. Carbamazepine reduces the risk of symptomatic toxicity in patients receiving whole brain radiation.

Question 40.9.   **Which of the following statements is TRUE?**

A. The use of radiosensitizers has been shown to improve tumor control.
B. Motexafin gadolinium improves the median survival of patients with brain metastasis and median time to neurologic progression.
C. Anemia in patients receiving whole brain radiation therapy may adversely affect survival.
D. RSR13 and supplemental oxygen given to patients with brain metastases from breast cancer do not improve median survival time.

Question 40.10.   **Which one of the following statements is FALSE?**

A. Metastases in thalmic basal ganglia and in the brainstem are not usually considered for resection.
B. The average median survival in patients with resected single brain metastasis from lung cancer is 12 months.
C. Multiple brain metastases are not resectable.
D. Thirty-day surgical mortality rates after surgical resection of single metastases is approximately 0% to 10%.

Question 40.11.   **What is the added benefit of whole brain radiation therapy after surgical resection of a single brain metastasis?**

A. Decreased risk of local and distant recurrence in brain
B. Decreased risk of death as the result of neurologic symptoms
C. Improvement in overall survival
D. All of the above

Question 40.12.   **A 48-year-old man with metastatic renal cell carcinoma controlled on sunitinib therapy develops chronic headaches. On follow-up, his MRI demonstrates a single brain metastasis located close to the motor strip. Gamma-knife radiation therapy is used. His headache symptoms improve. However, symptoms of headache recur 4 months later. The repeat brain MRI shows increased size of the irradiated region and increased brain edema. What is the next MOST optimum management of this patient?**

A. Starting steroid therapy and consultation for resection of the lesion
B. Additional dose of gamma-knife radiation therapy to brain lesion
C. Starting dexamethasone and repeat MRI in 1 month
D. PET-CT scan of the brain

Question 40.13. **Which of the following tumors is LEAST prone to spread to the bronchus?**

  A. Colon
  B. Renal cell carcinoma
  C. Breast carcinoma
  D. Melanoma

Question 40.14. **Which of the following radiologic techniques is the MOST useful with detection of metastasis to the lung?**

  A. Chest radiography
  B. MRI
  C. PET scan
  D. CT

Question 40.15. **What is the MOST commonly used surveillance for lung metastasis recurrence after complete resection of lung metastasis?**

  A. Chest radiogram every 6 months for first 2 years and then once per year for the next 5 years
  B. Chest CT scans every 3 months for the first year and then once every 6 months for the next 4 years
  C. CT scans every 3 months for 2 years and then every 6 months for another 3 years
  D. CT scans of chest once per year for 5 years

Question 40.16. **A 63-year-old woman presents with upper quadrant abdominal pain, and cholecystitis is diagnosed on physical examination. Chest radiogram done during preparation for elective cholecystectomy reveals the presence of a right upper lobe 2.5-cm spiculated nodule. Her medical history is important for a right nephrectomy for stage II renal cell carcinoma 3 years before presentation. The patient has a 40-year smoking history but quit smoking at the time of the kidney cancer diagnosis. What is the BEST management for this patient at this time?**

  A. The patient should be offered sunitinib therapy to improve progression-free survival.
  B. Complete staging with CT scan of chest, abdomen, and pelvis should be performed, followed by transthoracic needle biopsy of pulmonary nodule.
  C. Staging CT scan with chest, abdomen, and pelvis followed by elective right upper lobectomy.
  D. CT scan of chest, abdomen, and pelvis, and treatment with interferon therapy for renal cell carcinoma.

Question 40.17. **In patients with Ewing's sarcoma with five metastatic bilateral pulmonary nodules, what would be the BEST management?**

  A. Radiation therapy to involve the lobes
  B. Stereotactic radiation
  C. Chemotherapy
  D. Surgical resection of all visible metastasis

Question 40.18. **Which of the following is NOT an indication for metastasectomy?**

    A. The lung is the only site of metastasis.
    B. The primary tumor is controlled.
    C. Germ cell tumors.
    D. Breast cell carcinoma with metastasis to the two lobes of the lung.

Question 40.19. **Which of the following primary tumors is the LEAST common source of metastasis to the liver?**

    A. Breast
    B. Gastrointestinal
    C. Urologic
    D. Ocular melanoma

Question 40.20. **Which of the following is the BEST factor associated with survival after hepatic resection?**

    A. Squamous cell histology
    B. Neuroendocrine histology
    C. Extrahepatic disease
    D. Incomplete resection

Question 40.21. **Which of the following local therapies for liver metastasis are LEAST commonly used?**

    A. Hepatic arterial infusion
    B. Radiofrequency ablation
    C. Isolated hepatic perfusion
    D. Chemoembolization

Question 40.22. **In patients with isolated multiple liver metastasis, which of the following radiation therapies has been largely abandoned?**

    A. Whole liver radiation therapy
    B. Yttrium-90 microspheres liver treatment
    C. Stereotactic liver radiation
    D. Cyber-knife radiation treatment

Question 40.23. **Which of the following techniques has the LEAST sensitivity in imaging liver metastasis?**

    A. Ultrasound
    B. CT scan
    C. MRI with superparamagnetic oxide
    D. FDG-PET

Question 40.24. **Which of the following factors predict the BEST outcome of surgical resection of liver metastasis?**

    A. Size of the largest lesion is between 5 to 10 cm
    B. Less than 25% of liver replacement by tumor
    C. Bilobar distribution of disease
    D. Increasing number of lesions

Question 40.25. **What are the risk factors associated with shortened overall and disease-free survival after neoadjuvant chemotherapy followed by resection for patients with colorectal cancer liver metastases?**

A. Preoperative tumor size greater than 10 cm
B. Metastatic celiac lymph nodes
C. More than three metastases at operation
D. All of the above

Question 40.26. **In which of the following primary tumors has chemoembolization been MOST successful?**

A. Colorectal carcinoma
B. Breast cancer
C. Renal cell carcinoma
D. Neuroendocrine tumor

Question 40.27. **What is NOT a cause of hypercalcemia of malignancy?**

A. Excessive osteolysis
B. Parathyroid hormone-related protein
C. Disuse osteolysis
D. Increased osteoblastic function

Question 40.28. **Which of the following is NOT a proven test for diagnosis of bone metastasis?**

A. CT
B. Plain radiograms
C. PET
D. Bone scans

Question 40.29. **Which of the following therapies has NOT shown a proven effect in the treatment of metastatic bone cancer?**

A. Endocrine therapy in bone metastasis caused by breast or prostate cancer
B. Oral bisphosphonate therapy
C. Cytotoxic chemotherapy
D. Intravenous bisphosphonate therapy

Question 40.30. **The use of intravenous bisphosphonates has NOT shown effectiveness in reducing skeletal-related events in which of the following tumors?**

A. Prostate cancer
B. Renal cell carcinoma
C. Breast cancer
D. Small cell lung cancer

Question 40.31. **There is a controversy in adequacy of pain control by single fraction therapy of bone metastasis versus protracted treatments. Which of the following statements are INCORRECT?**

A. The common treatment scheme of palliative radiotherapy for bone metastases is a single 8 Gy dose, 20 Gy in five daily treatments, or 30 Gy in 10 daily treatments.
B. The Dutch Bone Metastasis study showed no difference in pain relief or quality of life after single 8 or 24 Gy dosing in six daily radiation treatments.
C. Grade 2 to 4 acute toxicity can be more frequently seen in single fraction versus multiple fraction treatments.
D. Eight gray is probably the lowest effective dose of the single fraction radiation treatments for painful bone metastasis.

Question 40.32. **Which of the following statements regarding re-irradiation of painful bone metastasis is CORRECT?**

A. Re-irradiation of painful bone metastasis has less than a 20% response rate.
B. The degree of response depends on whether patients receive the single initial dose of radiation or multiple fraction regiments.
C. Patients with lack of response to initial radiation therapy are very likely to respond to re-irradiation therapy.
D. An international trial of single versus multiple fractions for re-irradiation of painful bone metastasis demonstrated superiority of multiple fraction treatment.

Question 40.33. **What type of cancer is the MOST common cause of malignant pleural effusions?**

A. Breast cancer
B. Lymphoma
C. Carcinoma of unknown primary
D. Primary lung cancer

Question 40.34. **Which of the following biochemical and pathological features of malignant plural effusions correlate with advanced disease, poor response to palliative pleurodesis, and minimal survival?**

A. Lactic dehydrogenase (LDH) greater than 200 U/mL
B. Fluid-to-serum LDH ratio greater than 0.6
C. Fluid-to-serum protein ratio greater than 0.5
D. Fluid pH less than 7.3 and glucose to serum ratio less than 0.5

Question 40.35. **Which of the following statements pertaining to tube thoracotomy with pleurodesis is CORRECT?**

A. Pleurodesis can be done when the daily drainage from plural cavity is 250 mL.
B. Chest pain occurs in 40% of patients receiving pleurodesis with doxycycline.
C. Pigtail catheter drainage and pleurodesis are less effective than chest tube pleurodesis.
D. Rotating patients from lateral decubitus, to supine, and to prone position increases the likelihood of successful pleurodesis.

Question 40.36. **Which of the following is the MOST successful pleurodesis agent?**

A. Thiotepa
B. Tetracycline
C. Bleomycin
D. Talc

Question 40.37. **Which of the following statements is TRUE?**

A. Thoracoscopic talc insufflation has resulted in higher success rates than talc slurry in pleurodesis of malignant pleural effusions in patients with primary lung or breast cancer.
B. Respiratory complications are greater in talc slurry group.
C. Quality-of-life measurements demonstrated less fatigue with talc slurry.
D. Most common side effects of talc pleurodesis are respiratory failure and pneumonitis.

Question 40.38. **Which of the following are the advantages of pleural catheter placement over chest tube insertion?**

A. Ease of insertion
B. Minimal or no hospitalization
C. Rapid drainage of recurrent symptomatic effusions
D. All of the above

Question 40.39. **Which of the following statements is INCORRECT?**

A. Stripping of a parietal pleura is 100% effective in controlling malignant pleural effusions.
B. Pleurectomy has a low complication rate.
C. Contraindications to placement of pleuroperitoneal shunt include pleural infection, multiple loculations, short life expectancy, and obliterated peritoneal space.
D. Pleurectomy should be reserved for good-risk patients.

Question 40.40. **Which of the following statements regarding pericardial effusion is IN-CORRECT?**

A. The most common echocardiographic sign of cardiac tamponade is right atrial and ventricular collapse with sensitivity ranging from 38% to 60% and specificity ranging from 50% to 100%.

B. Computed axial tomography (CAT) scan is a preferable method of choice for evaluating pericardial effusion.

C. Signs and symptoms of cardiac tamponade include dyspnea, orthopnea, jugular venous distension, pulsus paradoxus, and narrowed pulse pressure.

D. Some 50% to 60% of pericardial effusions in patients with cancer can be found malignant by cytologic examination.

Question 40.41. **Which of the following statements is INCORRECT?**

A. The rate of pericardial fluid reaccumulation was reported to be as low as 44% and as high as 70%.

B. Doxycycline is a preferable sclerosing agent for the treatment of pericardial effusions.

C. Complications of percutaneous balloon-tube pericardiostomy include fever, pleural effusions, and pneumothorax.

D. The most common procedure for treatment of pericardial effusions is subxyphoid pericardiostomy.

Question 40.42. **What is the MOST common cause of malignant ascites?**

A. Portal hypertension, secondary to massive liver metastasis

B. Lymphatic obstruction, secondary to a metastatic lesion in the lymphatic system

C. Peritoneal carcinomatosis

D. Hepatorenal syndrome

Question 40.43. **What factors contribute to the formation of malignant ascites?**

A. Production and release of vascular endothelial growth factor

B. Decreased capillary oncolytic pressures

C. Lymphatic obstruction

D. All of the above

Question 40.44. **Which from the following findings help in differentiating malignant ascites from ascites from other causes?**

A. Real-time ultrasound showing large amount of ascites with bowel loops fixed to adjacent organs.

B. History of cancer

C. New, rapid onset of increased abdominal girth

D. Serum to ascites albumin gradient value of 1.1 g/dL or greater

Question 40.45. **Which of the following statements is INCORRECT?**

A. The causes for newly diagnosed ascites include cirrhosis, congestive heart failure, nephrosis, pancreatitis, infectious processes, and malignancy.

B. Of patients with known malignancy and ascites, approximately one third will have nonmalignant causes for their ascites.

C. Abdominal paracentesis with ascitic fluid analysis is the most effective way to determine the cause of the ascites.

D. Neutrophil cell count greater than $250/mm^3$ is highly suggestive of malignancy.

Question 40.46. **Which of the following statements is INCORRECT?**

A. Treatment with diuretics in the management of malignant ascites caused by peritoneal carcinomatosis in patients who do not have portal hypertension is unlikely to improve ascites.

B. Frequent drainage procedures with a therapeutic paracentesis can be associated with significant protein loss, electrolyte imbalance, hypotension, septic complications, and visceral or vascular injury.

C. Contraindications to peritoneovenous shunt placement include hemorrhagic ascites and chylous ascites.

D. Intraoperative use of hyperthermic intraperitoneal chemotherapy has been indicated as highly effective in a majority of patients with malignant ascites.

ANSWERS

Answer 40.1. **The answer is D.**

A 2002 population-based study in The Netherlands found that the highest 5-year incidence of brain metastasis was for patients with lung cancer; 16% of patients with this diagnosis develop brain metastasis, compared with 10% of patients with renal cell carcinoma, 7% of patients with melanoma, 5% of patients with breast cancer, and 1% of patients with colorectal cancer.

Answer 40.2. **The answer is D.**

The median interval from diagnosis of cancer to that of brain metastasis is 12 months. In 30% of patients, however, synchronous metastasis brain metastases are diagnosed within 1 month of primary cancer diagnosis.

Answer 40.3. **The answer is D.**

The most common sign of brain metastases is headache (24% to 53%), followed by focal weakness (16% to 40%), altered mental status (24% to 31%), seizures (15% to 16%), and ataxia (9% to 20%).

Answer 40.4. **The answer is D.**

In a study performed by Gasper et al (Recursive partitioning analysis [RPA] of prognostic factors in three Radiation Therapy Oncology Group [RTOG] brain metastases trials. Int J Radiat Oncol Biol Phys 1997;37[4]: 745–751), of more than 1100 patients receiving radiotherapy for brain metastasis, four significant prognostic factors were found to be critical in discerning patients' high risks. Patients aged less than 65 years, with Karnofsky performance scores of 70 or greater, a controlled primary tumor, and no extracranial metastasis had a median survival of 7.1 months. However, the median survival was only 2.3 months in patients with a Karnofsky performance score of less than 70. A study by Kondziolka et al (Stereotactic radiosurgery plus whole brain radiotherapy versus radiotherapy alone for patients with multiple brain metastases. Int J Radiat Oncol Biol Phys 1999;45[2]:427–434) found that survival is substantially greater in patients receiving stereotactic followed by whole brain radiation therapy in comparison with patients receiving only whole brain radiation therapy. In addition, patients receiving local therapy with surgery plus whole brain radiation therapy have a more favorable prognosis than surgery alone.

Answer 40.5. **The answer is B.**

Rudà et al (Brain metastases from unknown primary tumour: a prospective study. Neurol 2001;248[5]:394–398) reported that patients with a biopsy-proven single brain metastasis from unknown primary had a median survival of 13 months. In addition, patients with symptoms related to the lesions had improvement in neurological function. The single brain lesion should be biopsied first. In one study of 54 patients with single brain lesions, 11 had noncancerous lesions, including abscess and inflammatory process; therefore, the biopsy is necessary to guide appropriate treatment. The best answer to this question is B.

Answer 40.6. **The answer is B.**

Use of corticosteroids is especially effective in patients with symptomatic brain metastasis. Whether it is useful in patients without neurologic symptoms remains uncertain; however, it is still an acceptable clinical standard to use dexamethasone with a loading dose of 10 mg followed by 16 mg per day divided dosage. The use of antiseizure medication in patients with brain metastasis should be limited to patients with seizure presentation. In the study presented by Forsyth et al (Prophylactic anticonvulsants in patients with brain tumour. Can J Neurol Sci 2003;30[2]:106–112), 100 newly diagnosed patients with brain tumors were randomized to antiepileptic therapy or observation. Seizure-free survivals were similar in both groups. Patients with brain tumors have an increased risk for thrombosis; however, treatment with anticoagulation is thought to increase the risk of brain hemorrhage. One study suggested that anticoagulation is safe in patients with cancer pathology that is less prone to hemorrhage. At present, however, the benefits and risks of anticoagulation in patients with brain metastases are not well established, and although prophylactic anticoagulation could be considered, it is not routinely used.

Answer 40.7.   **The answer is C.**

The complete response rate for patients with renal cell carcinoma was 0% in a study reported by Nieder et al (Treatment of brain metastases from hypernephroma. Urol Int 1996;57[1]:17–20). The best response was seen in patients with small cell carcinoma (37%), followed by breast cancer (35%), squamous cell carcinoma (25%), and nonbreast adenocarcinoma (14%).

Answer 40.8.   **The answer is D.**

Acute side effects shortly after whole brain radiation therapy include hair loss, mild skin reaction, fatigue, and, in some patients, ototoxicity. Hair regrows in 6 to 12 months after radiation therapy. The issue of dementia was evaluated in one study involving 47 patients; dementia was seen in 11% of patients with nonrecurrent brain metastasis. The hippocampus has very low radiation tolerance, and new efforts are being made to spare this brain structure from radiation therapy. A recent study by Nieder et al used carbamazepine to decrease the risk of symptomatic lay toxicities in patients receiving whole brain radiation therapy and found an increased rate of toxicities in patients receiving carbamazepine (50% vs. 18% in those who did not receive carbamazepine).

Answer 40.9.   **The answer is C.**

Recent evaluation of the impact of anemia on the effectiveness of whole brain radiation therapy demonstrated its adverse effect on survival. The radiosensitizer effect in patients receiving whole brain radiation therapy is currently under evaluation. In one study patients were randomized to motexafin gadolinium with whole brain radiation or whole brain radiation therapy alone. In this study there was no significant difference in median survival or median time to neurologic progression in both arms. A study of RSR13 (allosteric modifier of hemoglobin that reduces hemoglobin O2 binding affinity) resulted in a greater median survival in patients in the RSR13 arm of the study compared with the control arm, especially in patients with breast cancer, in whom the median survival was 8.7 months (vs. 4.6 months in the control arm).

Answer 40.10.   **The answer is C.**

Patients with tumor brain metastases located in the thalamic basal ganglia or brainstem are not usually considered for resection because of excessive risk of morbidity after surgery. The median survival time is 12 months for patients with a single brain metastasis from lung cancer, 7 months for patients with melanoma, 10 months for patients with renal cell carcinoma, 12 months for patients with breast cancer, and 9 months for patients with colon cancer, and is also dependent on whether patients have controlled or uncontrolled systemic disease. A small retrospective analysis of patients with a resected single brain metastasis or multiple brain metastases and patients with at least one unresected lesion demonstrated a significantly better survival in patients who had all multiple metastases resected that was equal to that of patients with a single metastatic lesion. The general mortality of more than 30 days after surgical resection of a single metastasis is approximately 0% to 10%.

Answer 40.11.   **The answer is D.**

In one study patients were randomized to have observation after single brain metastasis resection or surgery followed by whole brain radiation therapy. The addition of whole brain radiation significantly decreased the risk of local recurrence (10% vs. 46%), distant brain metastases (14% vs. 37%), and any brain failure (18% vs. 70%). In another study, survival and overall local brain metastases control were superior in patients receiving additional whole brain radiation therapy after single brain metastasis resection.

Answer 40.12.   **The answer is C.**

Radiation-induced necrosis can be seen in up to 17% of cases of gamma-knife radiation therapy and has to be differentiated from tumor regrowth. Starting steroid therapy is helpful to decrease edema, and that should be considered in the case of radiation necrosis or suspected tumor growth. To differentiate between necrosis and tumor growth, PET scan of the brain may be useful in making that distinction. Repeating MRI in 1 month may also be an alternative.

Answer 40.13.   **The answer is D.**

Melanoma. Although melanoma metastases are frequent to the lung parenchyma, the bronchial metastasis for melanoma is less frequent compared with colon, renal cell carcinoma, or breast carcinoma.

Answer 40.14.   **The answer is D.**

CT scan is the most effective method of imaging lung metastases. It is superior to chest radiography for imaging hilar, mediastinal, and pleural structures. It has a sensitivity of 82% and can detect pulmonary nodules 6 mm or greater with 95% sensitivity and nodules less than 6 mm with a 69% sensitivity. In contrast, MRI has limited use in patients because of motion artifact and lower spatial resolution. PET scan has 87% sensitivity but is unable to detect subcentimeter nodules.

Answer 40.15.   **The answer is C.**

Most cancer centers perform chest CT scans every 3 months for the first 2 years and then every 6 months for another 3 years after complete resection of lung metastasis.

Answer 40.16.   **The answer is B.**

Although this patient has a history of renal cell carcinoma, and now presents with a new pulmonary nodule, the assumption cannot be made that she has recurrent metastatic disease to lung from kidney cancer primary. In young patients with a history of osteosarcoma, new pulmonary nodules generally do not need to be biopsied before treatment. In this clinical scenario, the patient may have primary lung cancer. Suspicion for this diagnosis is raised by her 40-year tobacco smoking history. Therefore, a biopsy is needed to make appropriate management of primary lung cancer.

Answer 40.17.   **The answer is C.**

Chemotherapy is the best first-line approach in treating Ewing's sarcoma metastatic to lung. The value of radiation therapy to involved sites has been studied in a randomized trial that demonstrated superiority in survival favoring the chemotherapy group. Stereotactic radiation to multiple pulmonary nodules is at present considered experimental. Accurate survival data for lung metastasis radiated with this technique are lacking. Although surgical resection even for multiple pulmonary metastasis may have a role in treatment of osteosarcoma, chemotherapy remains the best first-line treatment for patients with Ewing's sarcoma.

Answer 40.18.   **The answer is D.**

Chemosensitive tumors, such as breast cell carcinoma and germ cell tumors, should be treated with chemotherapy as a primary option. If there is a persisting pulmonary tumor mass after chemotherapy for germ cell tumor, it should be resected.

Answer 40.19.   **The answer is D.**

Ocular melanoma. In a review of 1452 patients, the most common primary tumors metastatic to liver were of breast, gastrointestinal, or urologic origin.

Answer 40.20.   **The answer is B.**

Patients with neuroendocrine tumors have the best survival. The factors associated with poor survival after liver resection are melanoma or squamous cell histology, age greater than 60 years, short disease-free interval between treatment of the primary tumor and diagnosis of liver metastasis, extrahepatic disease, and incomplete resection.

Answer 40.21.   **The answer is C.**

Isolated hepatic perfusion has been performed for many years, but only in limited centers. Because of its technical complexity and lack of documented efficacy, isolated hepatic perfusion has not gained widespread and consistent clinical evaluation.

Answer 40.22.   **The answer is A.**

Whole liver radiation therapy has largely been abandoned in favor of modern techniques. The major problem with whole liver radiation therapy is the relatively low tolerance of liver tissue and relatively frequent induction of radiation-induced hepatitis.

Answer 40.23. **The answer is A.**

The least sensitive technique to detect liver metastasis is the ultrasound, which has a sensitivity of 55% compared with 72% for CT scan, 76% for MRI, and 90% for FDG PET. The MRI performed with superparamagnetic oxide increases sensitivity; however, it is not commonly used at present.

Answer 40.24. **The answer is B.**

Patients with less than 25% liver involvement by tumor have better survival. All other factors mentioned prognosticate poor outcome.

Answer 40.25. **The answer is D.**

All of the above are predictors of shortened overall and disease-free survival after neoadjuvant chemotherapy; in addition, a diagnosis of rectal primary, preoperative CA 19-9 more than 100 IU/L, disease progression on therapy, noncurative liver metastases resection, and history of two hepatic tumor resections are also associated with this poor outcome.

Answer 40.26. **The answer is D.**

Hepatic artery chemoembolization using doxorubicin or streptozotocin showed an overall response rate of 37% in patients with neuroendocrine tumors, and the 5-year survival rate was 50%. In one study (Bloomston M, Al-Saif O, Klemanski D, et al. Hepatic artery chemoembolization in 122 patients with metastatic carcinoid tumor: lessons learned. J Gastrointest Surg. 2007;11[3]:264–271) of 122 patients with carcinoid tumor, significant palliation of symptoms occurred in more than 90% of patients with an overall survival of 33 months. In contrast, in patients with other malignancies, hepatic artery chemoembolization has been less effective with objective response rates of less than 30%.

Answer 40.27. **The answer is D.**

Hypercalcemia is caused by excessive osteolysis, secretion of parathyroid hormone-related protein, and disuse osteolysis. Although osteoblastic lesions may be a cause of increased levels of calcium in serum, this results from the activation of bone resorption by osteoclasts.

Answer 40.28. **The answer is C.**

Plain radiography, CT, MRI, and bone scans have established value in diagnosis of metastatic disease to bone. The value of PET in diagnosis of bone metastasis is currently under research investigation.

Answer 40.29. **The answer is B.**

Oral bisphosphonate therapy, although effective in treatment of osteopenia, has not been shown to be an effective strategy in treatment of metastatic disease to bone. Hormonal therapy of breast or prostate cancer, and cytotoxic therapy have activity against metastatic disease to bone.

Answer 40.30.   **The answer is D.**

The use of intravenous bisphosphonates in patients with bone metastasis caused by breast cancer, prostate cancer, renal cell carcinoma, and non–small cell lung cancer reduces skeletal-related events. Intravenous bisphosphonates reduced the severity of pain and decreased levels of bone turnover markers. The use of bisphosphonate in small cell lung cancer has not yet been fully evaluated.

Answer 40.31.   **The answer is C.**

Acute grade 2 to 4 toxicity was more frequent in a multiple fraction arm (17%) than in a single arm fraction (10%) in the Radiation Therapy Oncology Group (RTOG) study of patients with breast and prostate cancer treated for painful bone metastasis. The other statements are correct.

Answer 40.32.   **The answer is B.**

In one study, the overall response rates of initial irradiation were 80% in patients who had a prior single fraction dose and 66% in patients who had a single fraction, versus 33% who had multiple fraction treatments. All other statements are correct.

Answer 40.33.   **The answer is D.**

Some 35% of malignant pleural effusions are attributable to primary lung cancer, 23% are attributable to breast cancer, 12% are attributable to carcinoma of unknown primary, and 10% are attributable to lymphoma.

Answer 40.34.   **The answer is D.**

Fluid pH less than 7.3 and glucose to serum ratio less than 0.5 are associated with poor response to palliative pleurodesis and minimal survival. Other answers indicate exudative nature of malignant pleural effusions.

Answer 40.35.   **The answer is B.**

Chest pain occurs in 40% of patients receiving pleurodesis with doxycycline and in 7% of patients receiving talc pleurodesis. Rotating patients is not necessary for successful pleurodesis. The pleurodesis procedure should be done once complete drainage of the pleural cavity is obtained (confirmed radiologically or by <150 mL of fluid drainage per day). Pigtail catheter is as effective as a chest tube and associated with less discomfort.

Answer 40.36.   **The answer is D.**

Talc pleurodesis is highly effective with the overall response rates ranging from 80% to 100%. In a large study of 327 evaluable patients, pleurodesis was successful in 90% at 1 month, and 82% had lifelong success. In contrast, in a study comparing talc and bleomycin, successful pleurodesis was obtained in only 67% of patients treated with bleomycin. Tetracycline has an overall efficacy of 70% for successful pleurodesis.

Answer 40.37.   **The answer is A.**

Thoracoscopic talc insufflation in patients with breast or lung cancer had a higher success rate of pleurodesis than talc slurry (82% vs. 67%; $p = .022$), and talc insufflation resulted in less fatigue; however, the incidence of respiratory complications was greater in the talc insufflation group. The most commonly reported adverse events of talc pleurodesis are fever and pain. Respiratory failure, pneumonitis, and empyema are infrequent complications of talc pleurodesis.

Answer 40.38.   **The answer is D.**

Pleural catheter placement has a higher success rate in pleural fluid drainage than chest tube with spontaneous pleurodesis, occurring in 46% of patients. Ease of insertion, minimal discomfort, little or no hospitalization, and rapid drainage of recurrent symptomatic effusions are the advantages of pleural catheter placement.

Answer 40.39.   **The answer is B.**

Pleurectomy has high morbidity (23%) and mortality (10%) rates and should be reserved only for good-risk patients who are refractory to other approaches for treatment of malignant pleural effusions. This procedure is highly effective (100%). Contraindications to placement of pleuroperitoneal shunt include pleural infection, multiple loculations, short life expectancy, and obliterated peritoneal space.

Answer 40.40.   **The answer is B.**

Echocardiogram is a preferable test for pericardial effusion diagnosis. Only 50% to 60% of pericardial effusions in patients with cancer are found to be malignant by cytologic evaluation. Signs and symptoms of cardiac tamponade include dyspnea, orthopnea, jugular venous distension, pulsus paradoxus, narrowed pulse pressure, and distant heart sounds. Electrocardiogram shows low voltage complexes. The most common echocardiographic finding of cardiac tamponade is right atrial and ventricular collapse.

Answer 40.41.   **The answer is B.**

Bleomycin is the preferable sclerosing agent in the treatment of malignant pericardial effusions. It is as effective as doxycycline but creates less retrosternal pain. The rate of pericardial fluid reaccumulation was reported to be as low as 44% and as high as 70%. Complications of percutaneous balloon-tube pericardiostomy include fever, pleural effusions, pneumothorax, and myocardial injury. The most common procedure for treatment of pericardial effusions is subxyphoid pericardiostomy.

Answer 40.42.   **The answer is C.**

Two thirds of patients with malignancy-related ascites have peritoneal carcinomatosis with cytologic evidence of tumor cells in the ascitic fluid.

Answer 40.43.   **The answer is D.**

The proposed pathophysiology involves the production by tumor cells of vascular endothelial growth factor, which leads to increased peritoneal neovascularization and capillary permeability, which in turn causes decreased capillary oncotic pressures and increased net capillary filtration that leads to the increased peritoneal cavity fluid production. At the same time, peritoneal tumors can cause lymphatic obstruction, which leads to decreased fluid efflux from the peritoneal cavity, which contributes to formation of malignant ascites.

Answer 40.44.   **The answer is D.**

Serum to ascites albumin gradient value of 1.1 g/dL or greater is diagnostic of portal hypertension as a cause of ascites.

Answer 40.45.   **The answer is D.**

Neutrophil count greater than $250/mm^3$ is highly suggestive of intraabdominal infection and not malignancy. Malignant ascites accounts for 10% of all cases of ascites. Approximately one third of patients with known malignancy have ascites from nonmalignant causes. Abdominal paracentesis with ascitic fluid analysis is the most effective way of diagnosing the cause of the ascites.

Answer 40.46.   **The answer is D.**

The use of hyperthermic therapy in patients with malignant ascites is reserved only for patients in whom an aggressive combined approach can be performed. At this time, this approach is still considered experimental, and there are no data supporting the superiority of this approach versus other therapeutic options. Diuretics can be especially effective in patients with ascites caused by liver cirrhosis; however, the use of diuretics is not likely to be successful in patients with peritoneal carcinomatosis.

41

Stem Cell Transplantation

Directions   Each of the numbered items below is followed by lettered answers. Select the ONE lettered answer that is BEST in each case unless instructed otherwise.

QUESTIONS

Question 41.1.   **The curative potential of allogeneic hematopoietic stem cell transplantation (HSCT) may be derived from which of the following:**

A. High-dose chemotherapy
B. Graft-versus-leukemia (GVL) effect
C. Graft-versus-host effect
D. A and B

Question 41.2.   **The allogeneic transplant conditioning regimen serves to achieve which of the following:**

A. Provide immunosuppression to prevent rejection
B. Provide immunosuppression to prevent graft-versus-host disease
C. Eradicate malignant cells
D. A and C

Question 41.3.   **Which of the following regimens is considered myeloablative?**

A. Cyclophosphamide 60 mg/kg/d intravenously (IV) × 2 days plus 1200 cGy total body irradiation (TBI)
B. Cyclophosphamide 60 mg/kg/d IV × 2 days plus busulfan 3.2 mg/kg/d IV × 4 days
C. Fludarabine 30 mg/kg/d IV × 5 plus busulfan 3.2 mg/kg/d IV × 2 plus antithymocyte globulin (ATG) 2.5 mg/kg/d IV × 4
D. A and B

Corresponding Chapter in *Cancer: Principles & Practice of Oncology*, Eighth Edition: 61 (Stem Cell Transplantation).

Question 41.4.   **Which conditioning regimen leads to improved disease-free survival in chronic myeloid leukemia (CML)?**

A. Cyclophosphamide 60 mg/kg/d IV × 2 days plus busulfan 3.2 mg/kg/d IV × 4 days
B. 1200 cGy TBI and cyclophosphamide 60 mg/kg/d IV × 2 days
C. Chemotherapy and radiation-based conditioning are equivalent
D. Fludarabine 30 mg/kg/d IV × 5 plus busulfan 3.2 mg/kg/d IV × 2 plus ATG 2.5 mg/kg/d IV × 4

Question 41.5.   **Which of the following myeloablative conditioning regimens results in the BEST relapse-free survival in patients with acute lymphoblastic leukemia (ALL)?**

A. TBI-based regimen
B. Busulfan plus etoposide
C. Busulfan plus cyclophosphamide
D. Imatinib plus busulfan and etoposide

Question 41.6.   **TBI-based conditioning is associated with an increased risk of all the following, EXCEPT:**

A. Cataracts
B. Growth retardation
C. Veno-occlusive disease (VOD)
D. Secondary malignancies

Question 41.7.   **The GVL effect after transplant is MOST pronounced in which of the following malignancies?**

A. Acute myelogenous leukemia (AML)
B. ALL
C. Chronic-phase CML
D. Accelerated-phase CML

Question 41.8.   **Which of the following increases the risk of relapse after transplant?**

A. Human leukocyte antigen (HLA)-mismatched transplant
B. CD34 cell dose >2 × 106 but <5 × 106/kg recipient body weight
C. Acute and chronic graft-versus-host disease (GVHD)
D. T-cell–depleted graft

Question 41.9.   **Each of the following measures is effective at reducing the indicated regimen-related toxicities, EXCEPT:**

A. Hydration, Mesna (sodium 2-sulfanylethanesulfonate), and forced diuresis during cyclophosphamide for prevention of hemorrhagic cystitis
B. Phenytoin before and during busulfan infusion for prevention of seizures
C. Dexamethasone and ondansetron before conditioning for nausea prophylaxis
D. Granulocyte colony-stimulating factor (G-CSF) growth factor support to decrease infection-related mortality

Question 41.10.   **VOD of the liver is associated with:**

A. Myeloablative versus reduced-intensity conditioning
B. Oral busulfan conditioning
C. Prior treatment with gemtuzumab
D. All of the above

Question 41.11.   **All of the following are part of the clinical syndrome of VOD, EXCEPT:**

A. Jaundice
B. Tender hepatomegaly
C. Weight gain and ascites
D. Diarrhea

Question 41.12.   **A 50-year-old man presents to the hospital with shortness of breath and fevers 2 months after an unrelated donor HSCT for AML (M5). He is found to be hypoxic on presentation. Chest radiography shows diffuse pulmonary infiltrates. He is placed on broad-spectrum antibiotics and has been compliant with antifungal and anti-*Pneumocystis jirovecii* pneumonia (PCP) prophylaxis since his transplant. Sputum culture is negative. Peripheral blood cytomegalovirus (CMV) polymerase chain reaction (PCR) shows an unquantifiable number of viral DNA copies. A bronchoscopy is performed with lavage showing bloody secretions with negative aerobic, anaerobic, fungal, and viral cultures. Bronchoalveolar lavage (BAL) is tested for galactomannan, which is negative, and the tumor necrosis factor (TNF)-α level is found to be elevated. His condition fails to improve with antibiotics. What is the most likely diagnosis?**

A. CMV pneumonitis
B. Idiopathic pneumonitis
C. Pneumocystis pneumonia
D. Relapsed leukemia

Question 41.13.   **All of the following are risk factors for developing acute GVHD post-transplant, EXCEPT:**

A. T-cell replete graft
B. Mismatch at HLA DP
C. Older age of recipient
D. Unrelated donor

Question 41.14.   **Each of the following are appropriate as infection prophylaxis in a patient with chronic GVHD on corticosteroids, EXCEPT:**

A. Dapsone
B. Fluconazole
C. Penicillin VK
D. Ganciclovir

Question 41.15. **The risk for graft failure is increased by all of the following, EXCEPT:**

    A. T-cell depletion of the product
    B. Less than 1×106 CD34+ cells/kg recipient body weight
    C. Matched sibling stem cell product
    D. Umbilical cord blood transplant

Question 41.16. **In which setting is the risk of CMV reactivation the highest after allogeneic HCT?**

    A. CMV-positive donor to a CMV-negative recipient
    B. CMV-negative donor to a CMV-positive recipient
    C. CMV-negative donor to a CMV-negative recipient
    D. CMV-positive donor to a CMV-positive recipient

Question 41.17. **Peripheral blood mobilized stem cell allografts, compared with bone marrow, are associated with which of the following:**

    A. Shorter period of neutropenia
    B. Shorter period to platelet recovery
    C. Equivalent T-cell numbers
    D. Equivalent incidence of acute GVHD
    E. A, B, and D

Question 41.18. **For which of the following patients with an HLA-matched donor is allogeneic stem cell transplantation MOST appropriate?**

    A. 35-year-old man with AML with inversion 16 in CR1 after $7+3$
    B. 40-year-old woman with AML and complex cytogenetics in first clinical remission (CR)
    C. 48-year-old woman with diffuse large B-cell lymphoma (DLCL) with chemosensitive relapse after initial remission of 18 months
    D. 55-year-old man with Rai stage III chronic lymphocytic leukemia (CLL) in first remission

Question 41.19. **All of the following are potential complications of donor lymphocyte infusion (DLI), EXCEPT:**

    A. Bone marrow aplasia
    B. GVHD flare
    C. VOD
    D. A and B

Question 41.20. **Common manifestations of CMV reactivation after allogeneic stem cell transplant (SCT) include each of the following, EXCEPT:**

    A. Pneumonitis
    B. Colitis
    C. Retinitis
    D. Bone marrow suppression

Question 41.21. **Limitations of autologous SCT, compared with allogeneic SCT, include all of the following, EXCEPT:**

A. Lack of potential graft-versus-tumor effect
B. Higher treatment-related mortality
C. Potential graft contamination with tumor cells
D. Higher relapse risk

Question 41.22. **Factors that influence the choice of conditioning regimen include:**

A. Underlying malignancy and prior treatment
B. Patient age and comorbidity
C. Donor:recipient HLA compatibility
D. All of the above

Question 41.23. **Potential benefits of reduced-intensity conditioning regimens for allogeneic SCT include all of the following, EXCEPT:**

A. Decreased period of neutropenia
B. Improved tumor cytoreduction
C. Decreased regimen-related toxicity
D. Appropriate for older patients or with significant comorbidity

Question 41.24. **Evidence supporting the existence of the graft-versus-tumor effect includes the following, EXCEPT:**

A. Decreased relapse risk among patients with acute and chronic GVHD
B. Increased relapse risk among recipients of identical twin donor grafts
C. Decreased relapse risk among recipients of T-depleted grafts
D. Spontaneous remission after posttransplant relapse on tapering of immunosuppression

Question 41.25. **Late complications after allogeneic SCT include:**

A. Skeletal complications, including osteoporosis and avascular necrosis
B. Secondary malignancies
C. Endocrine failure
D. All of the above

Question 41.26. **Risk factors for acute GVHD includes the following, EXCEPT:**

A. Increased age
B. Graft T-cell depletion
C. Donor:recipient HLA disparity
D. Inadequate GVHD prophylaxis

Question 41.27. **Which of the following statements regarding the use of corticosteroids for the prevention or treatment of acute GVHD is TRUE?**

A. Response to initial steroid treatment correlates with improved survival.

B. Anti–T-cell antibodies represent effective salvage therapy for patients with steroid-refractory acute GVHD and improve overall survival.

C. Corticosteroid doses of up to 10 mg/kg/d result in improved response rates compared with 2 mg/kg/d.

D. Prednisone plus cyclosporine plus methotrexate is superior to cyclosporine plus methotrexate alone for acute GVHD prophylaxis.

Question 41.28. **The type and duration of prior antineoplastic therapy are strong predictors of success in autologous stem cell mobilization.**

A. True

B. False

Question 41.29. **Graft manipulation ex vivo to purge contaminating tumor cells is a strategy that has been successful in reducing the rate of relapse after autologous stem cell transplantation.**

A. True

B. False

Question 41.30. **Autologous HCT is considered potentially curative in which of the following clinical scenarios?**

A. Intermediate-grade non-Hodgkin's lymphoma in chemotherapy-sensitive first relapse

B. Multiple myeloma after complete response to initial therapy

C. Small lymphocytic lymphoma in second CR

D. Chemotherapy-sensitive metastatic breast carcinoma

Question 41.31. **The chemotherapy agents and doses used in conditioning regimens for autologous HSCT are chosen with the primary goal of achieving complete ablation in the normal recipient marrow.**

A. True

B. False

Question 41.32. **Which of the following is NOT a complication associated with autologous HSCT?**

A. Late incidence of myelodysplastic syndrome

B. Varicella zoster reactivation

C. *Pneumocystis carinii* pneumonia

D. Pericarditis

ANSWERS

Answer 41.1. **The answer is D.**

High-dose chemotherapy (and/or radiation) conditioning regimens have significant antitumor activity and are typically used in younger patients with aggressive hematologic malignancies. Historically it was believed that the curative potential of allogeneic HCT was derived entirely from the conditioning regimen, and that the donor graft served only as hematopoietic "rescue." It is now known that the graft can mediate a powerful immunologic "GVL effect" that can contribute significantly to the curative potential of the transplant. GVHD represents the deleterious reverse of GVL, an immunologic attack on normal tissue.

Answer 41.2. **The answer is D.**

The primary objectives of allogeneic transplant conditioning are to provide sufficient immunosuppression of the host immune system to permit donor engraftment, and particularly with fully myeloablative regimens, to achieve significant cytoreduction of tumor cells by incorporating agents with known activity against the underlying malignancy. The conditioning regimen, administered before infusion of donor cells, does not exert a significant impact on the risk of GVHD.

Answer 41.3. **The answer is D.**

High-dose cyclophosphamide in combination with 1200 to 1350 cGy TBI or busulfan 13.8 mg/m^2 IV constitute the two most commonly used myeloablative conditioning regimens for allogeneic transplantation. Fludarabine and ATG, although significantly lymphosuppressive, have minimal myelosuppressive effects.

Answer 41.4. **The answer is C.**

Two randomized clinical trials have failed to demonstrate differences in disease-free survival among patients with CML conditioned with either cyclophosphamide and busulfan or cyclophosphamide and TBI. Although the use of reduced-intensity conditioning regimens (answer D) has shown promise in older patients with CML, there are insufficient data comparing such approaches with traditional myeloablative regimens to recommend their routine use in younger patients who are candidates for myeloablative conditioning.

Answer 41.5. **The answer is A.**

TBI-containing regimens have been shown in two randomized trials of patients with ALL to be superior to chemotherapy-based regimens. The routine use of imatinib in the allogeneic transplant setting is not justified by published data.

Answer 41.6. **The answer is C.**

TBI-containing regimens are associated with an increased risk of several regimen-related toxicities, including cataracts, growth retardation, and secondary malignancies. The incidence of VOD, however, is higher among patients receiving busulfan conditioning, particularly among those with high busulfan area under the concentration-time curve. The use of intravenous busulfan has been shown to lower the incidence of VOD because of its more predictable pharmacokinetics than the traditional oral formulation.

Answer 41.7. **The answer is C.**

It was primarily on the basis of retrospective studies of outcomes among patients with chronic-phase CML that the GVL effect was first recognized, and a majority of patients treated with donor lymphocyte infusion (DLI) for posttransplant relapse of CML achieve a durable molecular remission. In contrast with CML, only a minority of patients with relapsed acute leukemias or more advanced CML are rendered long-term disease-free survivors after donor lymphocyte infusion.

Answer 41.8. **The answer is D.**

Posttransplant disease relapse risk is inversely related to the incidence of acute and chronic GVHD. HLA-mismatched transplants, with a correspondingly higher risk of GVHD, also confer a lower risk of relapse. T-cell depletion, although an effective strategy for lowering the risk of GVHD, confers an increased risk of disease relapse.

Answer 41.9. **The answer is D.**

G-CSF administration after stem cell infusion has been shown in randomized studies to shorten the time to sustained myeloid engraftment but has not been shown to affect treatment-related mortality. Hemorrhagic cystitis, resulting from urinary secretion of acrolein, a metabolite of cyclophosphamide, can be prevented by its inactivation with concurrent Mesna administration or by dilution through hyperhydration with intravenous fluids. High-dose busulfan is known to lower the threshold for developing seizures, which can be effectively prevented by the prophylactic use of phenytoin. Concurrent ondansetron and dexamethasone is an effective and widely used regimen for nausea prophylaxis during highly emetogenic conditioning.

Answer 41.10. **The answer is D.**

The incidence of VOD, thought to result from chemotherapy or radiation-induced injury to the small venules in the liver, is associated with increased conditioning regimen intensity, prior exposure to gemtuzumab, oral busulfan conditioning, and preexisting liver disease.

Answer 41.11. **The answer is D.**

The typical presentation of VOD includes isolated hyperbilirubinemia in the context of tender liver enlargement, ascites, and weight gain during the first 2 to 3 weeks posttransplant. Diarrhea is not typically associated with VOD but may be present concurrently because of other causes in the immediate posttransplant period. The diagnosis of VOD can often be reliably made solely on the basis of clinical grounds, although in complicated clinical scenarios, a liver biopsy may be helpful, demonstrating sinusoidal congestion, fibrin deposition, fibrosis, and surrounding hepatocyte damage.

Answer 41.12. **The answer is B.**

This scenario, with pulmonary infiltrates, hypoxia, and culture-negative hemorrhagic lavage, is most consistent with idiopathic pneumonitis with diffuse alveolar hemorrhage, a complication of allogeneic HCT generally observed in the first several weeks posttransplant. High-dose corticosteroids, and more recently recombinant Factor VII, have been used with some success, although mortality remains high.

Answer 41.13. **The answer is B.**

Whereas HLA-A, B, C, and DR mismatches have been associated with an increased risk of GVHD, the impact of mismatches at HLA-DP (and -DQ) is minimal. Compared with T cell-depleted grafts, T cell-replete grafts confer a higher risk of GVHD. Older recipient age is also associated with an increased risk of acute GVHD.

Answer 41.14. **The answer is D.**

Knowledge of the types of opportunistic infections that patients with allogeneic HCT are at risk for at various time points allows for a rational, targeted strategy for prophylaxis. Patients with chronic GVHD requiring ongoing immunosuppression remain at increased risk for a variety of opportunistic infections, including pneumocystis, fungal, and viral infections, as well as CMV. The routine use of ganciclovir as prophylaxis is not indicated, however, because of its significant myelosuppression, and instead a more rational approach to preventing CMV disease involves periodic monitoring of peripheral blood with CMV PCR and reserving ganciclovir for preemptive use in the event of detectable CMV viremia.

Answer 41.15. **The answer is C.**

Graft failure remains a relatively uncommon complication (2% to 3%) of matched sibling allogeneic HSC, although the risk is increased in the setting of an HLA-mismatched or unrelated donor, marginal CD34+ cell dose, or T depletion. Cell doses are often limiting in cord blood products, particularly for adult recipients, which are associated with a higher risk of graft failure.

Answer 41.16. **The answer is B.**

The risk of developing CMV infection with a CMV-negative donor and recipient is negligible. Among CMV-positive recipients, a CMV-positive donor confers a lower risk of reactivation because of the transfer of preexisting CMV immunity to the recipient, compared with a CMV-naïve donor.

Answer 41.17. **The answer is E.**

Mobilization and harvest of hematopoietic stem cells from peripheral blood with G-CSF leads to significantly higher numbers of CD34+ cells and results in a shorter time to engraftment of both neutrophils and platelets, compared with bone marrow. Despite significantly higher numbers of T cells, there was no evidence of a significant increase in the incidence of acute GVHD in a randomized trial of peripheral blood mononuclear cell (PBMC) versus bone marrow (BM), although a trend toward increased chronic GVHD in PBMC recipients was observed.

Answer 41.18. **The answer is B.**

Because of its substantial treatment-related morbidity and mortality, allogeneic stem cell transplantation is generally reserved for patients with hematologic malignancies with a low likelihood of cure with lower risk alternatives, including conventional chemotherapy and/or autologous HCT. Patients with AML with inversion 16 and translocation (8;22) in remission have a favorable prognosis for cure with high-dose cytarabine consolidation and are generally only considered for allogeneic HCT in the event of relapse. In contrast, patients with AML with high-risk cytogenetics, including deletions of chromosomes 5 and 7, and complex karyotypes, are rarely cured with conventional chemotherapy or autologous HCT, and should be referred for consideration of allogeneic HCT when in remission. Relapsed patients with intermediate-grade non-Hodgkin's lymphoma who respond to salvage chemotherapy may be cured with autologous stem cell transplantation with a relatively low risk of treatment-related morbidity and mortality. Because of the generally indolent nature of CLL, initial remissions may persist for years. Although potentially curative for CLL, the early mortality risk associated with allogeneic HCT is generally not justified in this scenario, although it may be appropriate in selected patients with more advanced, multiply relapsed disease.

Answer 41.19. **The answer is D.**

Donor lymphocyte infusions by design result in the infusion of large numbers of effector T cells with the goal of augmenting an alloimmune response directed against residual host-derived tumor cells. An unintended negative consequence, however, is the simultaneous infusion of alloreactive T-cell clones directed at normal tissue that may result in a significant flare in GVHD. In the case of relapsed CML, a substantial percentage of host hematopoiesis may be derived from the residual leukemic clone at relapse, in which case the development of the desired GVL effect may be associated with transient marrow aplasia. VOD is typically observed during the first 2 to 3 weeks posttransplant and is thought to result from endothelial damage caused by the conditioning regimen.

Answer 41.20. **The answer is C.**

Some 40% to 60% of CMV-seropositive allogeneic HCT recipients undergo CMV reactivation posttransplant. Asymptomatic CMV viremia is often detected by regular PCR monitoring of peripheral blood, although it may be heralded by an unexplained decline in white blood cell (WBC) or platelet counts. Pneumonitis is the most common manifestation of CMV-mediated disease after allogeneic HCT and is associated with a significant mortality rate. CMV colitis may mimic gastrointestinal (GI) GVHD and usually requires colonoscopic biopsy to distinguish. CMV retinitis, a common manifestation of CMV reactivation among patients with acquired immunodeficiency syndrome (AIDS), is relatively uncommon among allogeneic HCT recipients.

Answer 41.21. **The answer is B.**

Autologous HCT is associated with a higher risk of relapse than allogeneic HCT, likely resulting from a combination of the potential for tumor cell contamination of the autologous graft and the absence of an immune-mediated graft-versus-tumor effect associated with the latter. The major advantage of autologous HCT is its relatively low treatment-related morbidity and mortality (3% to 5% in most cases).

Answer 41.22. **The answer is D.**

The choice of conditioning regimen is driven by multiple factors, including, for both autologous and allogeneic HCT recipients, the underlying malignancy and its predicted responsiveness to various therapeutic agents. Similarly, the age and comorbidities of the recipient may dictate the use of a regimen with a lower predicted toxicity profile. For recipients of allogeneic HCT, donor:recipient HLA mismatching may influence the use of a more immunosuppressive conditioning regimen to lower the risk of graft rejection.

Answer 41.23. **The answer is B.**

Reduced-intensity conditioning regimens for allogeneic HCT were developed to exploit the curative potential of the GVL effect with reduced toxicity among older, sicker patients who might not otherwise be candidates for traditional myeloablative conditioning. Because reduced-intensity regimens are generally less myelosuppressive, a period of mixed myeloid chimerism often persists during the peritransplant period that may attenuate the period of absolute neutropenia. A potential limitation of these regimens is that their reduced cytotoxicity limits the tumor cell kill, rendering them less effective in the setting of refractory disease with significant tumor burdens.

Answer 41.24. **The answer is C.**

Retrospective studies of allogeneic transplant recipients has demonstrated that the highest incidence of relapse is among patients who experienced either acute or chronic GVHD, were the recipients of T-depleted grafts, or received grafts from identical twin donors. In some patients, discontinuation of immunosuppression may be sufficient to induce regression of the leukemic clone. Each of these observations provides indirect evidence of the existence of the GVL effect. Definitive evidence, however, is derived from the ability of donor lymphocyte infusions to reinduce complete remissions in the absence of any additional cytotoxic therapy.

Answer 41.25.   **The answer is D.**

Allogeneic HCT recipients remain at risk for a variety of long-term complications, including skeletal complications (especially with chronic steroids), infertility, secondary malignancies, and endocrine failure, for which ongoing follow-up and monitoring are indicated.

Answer 41.26.   **The answer is B.**

Several factors are associated with an increased risk of acute GVHD, including recipient age, HLA disparity, and inadequate prophylaxis. T-cell depletion of the graft decreases the incidence of GVHD.

Answer 41.27.   **The answer is A.**

GVHD represents the most significant obstacle to a successful outcome after allogeneic HCT. Corticosteroids remain the standard of care for up-front therapy for acute GVHD, and response to therapy correlates with overall survival. Corticosteroid dosages more than methylprednisolone 2 mg/kg/d offer no additional benefit. Therapy for steroid-refractory acute GVHD remains unsatisfactory, and there is no clearly superior second-line therapy that exerts a significant impact on the high mortality rates associated with steroid-refractory GVHD. The addition of prednisone to cyclosporine and methotrexate as GVHD prophylaxis provides no additional benefit to these agents alone.

Answer 41.28.   **The answer is A.**

Alkylating agents (e.g., melphalan and nitrogen mustard), multiple cycles of intensive combination chemotherapy regimens, and wide-field radiation are associated with a decreased likelihood of success in collecting sufficient hematopoietic stem cell numbers (1.5 to 2 million CD34+ cells/kg) to proceed with autologous stem cell transplantation.

Answer 41.29.   **The answer is B.**

Attempts to purge tumor cells from autologous hematopoietic stem cell grafts, using either negative or positive selection strategies, have not been proven to reduce the risk of relapse or prolong overall survival.

Answer 41.30.   **The answer is A.**

Autologous HCT is curative in approximately 40% to 50% of relapsed diffuse large cell non-Hodgkin's lymphoma cases but has not been shown to be curative in the case of low-grade lymphoproliferative disorders, multiple myeloma, or breast carcinoma.

Answer 41.31. **The answer is B.**

Autologous stem cell transplantation is a strategy for bypassing the dose-limiting marrow suppression of commonly used chemotherapy drugs to potentially increase tumor cell kill of chemosensitive tumors. The choice of drugs used in various conditioning regimens is usually driven by knowledge of the relative sensitivity of various tumors to different agents.

Answer 41.32. **The answer is C.**

Myelodysplastic syndrome occurs in 10% to 20% of long-term survivors of autologous stem cell transplantation, although it may be impossible to dismiss the potential contribution of pretransplant chemotherapy regimens to its development. *Varicella zoster* outbreaks are commonly observed up to 6 to 12 months posttransplant and form the basis for the widespread practice of posttransplant antiviral prophylaxis. Pericarditis and myocarditis are observed in association with high-dose cyclophosphamide, usually in the immediate peritransplant period. Pneumocystis pneumonia is a frequent complication of allogeneic stem cell transplantation, because of prolonged systemic immunosuppression, but is rarely observed in the autologous transplant setting except in patients treated with chronic corticosteroids before transplant.

Alex E. Denes

Infections in Cancer Patients

Directions Each of the numbered items below is followed by lettered answers. Select the ONE lettered answer that is BEST in each case unless instructed otherwise.

QUESTIONS

Question 42.1. **A patient with Hodgkin's disease who undergoes splenectomy should be immunized against which of the following organisms?**

    A. *Streptococcus pneumoniae*
    B. *Hemophilus influenzae*
    C. *Neisseria meningitidis*
    D. All of the above

Question 42.2. **Randomized controlled trials of antibacterial prophylaxis in patients with neutropenia have shown which of the following?**

    A. No difference in fever, infection, or mortality rates
    B. Decreased episodes of fever but no difference in infection or mortality rates
    C. Decreased episodes of fever and infections but no difference in mortality rates
    D. Decreased episodes of fever and infections, and lower mortality rates

Question 42.3. **A 32-year-old man who has received allogeneic bone marrow transplantation for acute myelogenous leukemia is now receiving immune-suppressing medications for the prevention of graft-versus-host disease. The MOST effective prophylaxis for *Pneumocystis jiroveci* (formerly carinii) is which of the following?**

    A. Atovaquone
    B. Dapsone
    C. Inhaled pentamidine
    D. Trimethoprim-sulfamethoxazole (TMP/SMX)

Corresponding Chapter in *Cancer: Principles & Practice of Oncology*, Eighth Edition: 62 (Infections in the Cancer Patient).

Question 42.4.   A cytomegalovirus (CMV)-seronegative patient is about to receive an allogeneic hematopoietic stem cell transplant (HSCT) from a CMV-seropositive donor. Which of the following strategies are acceptable for the prevention of CMV disease?

A. Prophylaxis with an antiviral agent such as ganciclovir.
B. Treatment when CMV antigen is detected by highly sensitive polymerase chain reaction (PCR).
C. Both A and B. Both are acceptable strategies.
D. Neither A nor B. The transplantation should not be performed.

Question 42.5.   A 54-year-old male patient with stage IV diffuse large B-cell lymphoma (DLBCL) calls with fevers and chills 9 days after receiving his third cycle of R-CHOP chemotherapy. Which of the following is the Infectious Diseases Society of America (IDSA) definition of fever in a patient with severe neutropenia?

A. Single oral temperature >38.0°C
B. Single oral temperature >38.3°C or >38.0°C for more than 1 hour
C. Oral temperature >38.3°C for more than 1 hour
D. Oral temperature >37.0°C for any duration

Question 42.6.   A 56-year-old patient with breast cancer receives chemotherapy and 1 week later experiences a fever of 39.1°C (102°F). She has a complete blood count drawn that reveals a total white blood count of 1000/μL and an absolute neutrophil count of 200/μL. She has an indwelling central venous catheter that appears normal and has no localizing symptoms. Appropriate antibiotic therapy could consist of which of the following options?

A. Cefepime or ceftazidime
B. Choice A plus vancomycin
C. Choice A plus an aminoglycoside
D. Choice A plus ciprofloxacin

Question 42.7.   This patient is started on appropriate empiric antibiotics and remains clinically stable but with persistent fever after 4 days. The addition of what agent would be indicated at this time?

A. Caspofungin
B. Liposomal amphotericin B
C. Voriconazole
D. Any of the above

Question 42.8. A 70-year-old man with metastatic non–small cell lung cancer presents with fever and neutropenia 1 week after chemotherapy. He is admitted and started on appropriate empiric antibiotics, and his fevers resolve after his first dose. For how long should his antibiotic therapy be continued?

    A. Discontinue immediately
    B. Until 24 to 48 hours after the last fever
    C. For a total of 7 days
    D. Until resolution of neutropenia

Question 42.9. A 68-year-old man with metastatic colon cancer receiving FOLFOX chemotherapy has a fever to 102.5°F. Examination reveals tenderness and warmth at the infusion port site of his surgically implanted catheter. Blood cultures are positive for *Staphylococcus aureus*, and sensitivities are pending. What is the MOST appropriate management strategy?

    A. Vancomycin
    B. Vancomycin and imipenem
    C. Vancomycin and removal of catheter
    D. Await drug sensitivity testing for the isolated organism

Question 42.10. A 52-year-old man with acute myelogenous leukemia who has received an allogeneic hematopoietic stem cell transplant presents with sinus congestion, fever, and headaches. Sinus computed tomography (CT) reveals a maxillary sinus mass with bone erosion. Zygomycosis (or mucormycosis) is isolated on fungal culture. What is the MOST appropriate management?

    A. Amphotericin B, with surgical debridement as salvage therapy, if necessary
    B. Amphotericin B and early surgical debridement
    C. Voriconazole and early surgical debridement
    D. Voriconazole, with surgical debridement as salvage therapy, if necessary

Question 42.11. A 61-year-old woman with non-Hodgkin's lymphoma presents with fever, cough, and prolonged neutropenia. A chest CT reveals bilateral lung nodules with the "halo sign." A serum galactomannan assay is positive. What is the MOST likely causative agent?

    A. Aspergillus species
    B. *Pseudomonas aeruginosa*
    C. *S. aureus*
    D. Zygomycetes

Question 42.12.   A 56-year-old man with stage III non–small cell lung cancer is being treated with concurrent chemotherapy and radiation therapy. He has odynophagia and retrosternal chest pain that have gradually worsened over the past few weeks. He has an absolute neutrophil count of 800/μL. Which of the following causes is the LEAST likely cause of his symptoms?

    A. Candida
    B. Herpes simplex virus (HSV)
    C. CMV
    D. Radiation esophagitis

Question 42.13.   A 34-year-old woman diagnosed with acute myelogenous leukemia receives induction chemotherapy. Ten days later, she experiences severe right-sided abdominal pain with nausea, vomiting, and diarrhea. On examination, she has a fever to 101°F and her abdomen is tender without rebound or guarding. Absolute neutrophil count is 0/μL. Lactic acid is not elevated, and stool *Clostridium difficile* toxin assay is negative on three separate samples. What is the MOST likely diagnosis?

    A. CMV colitis
    B. Typhlitis
    C. Bowel ischemia
    D. Bowel perforation

Question 42.14.   A 64-year-old man with pancreatic cancer is diagnosed with *C. difficile* colitis. He is treated with a course of oral metronidazole 500 mg three times per day, but he continues to have diarrhea and stool *C. difficile* toxin remains positive. What is the MOST appropriate treatment at this time?

    A. Intravenous metronidazole
    B. Oral vancomycin
    C. Intravenous vancomycin
    D. Probiotic agents

Question 42.15.   A 47-year-old woman with metastatic colorectal cancer is treated with systemic chemotherapy. She develops pain on defecation along with low-grade fevers. Laboratory tests are obtained, and her white blood cell count is 1000/μL (20% neutrophils). Visual inspection reveals a perianal fissure with erythema and induration. What should you do next?

    A. Digital rectal examination to rule out rectal abscess
    B. Recommend stool softeners, sitz baths, and analgesics
    C. Administer broad-spectrum antibiotics without anaerobic coverage
    D. Administer broad-spectrum antibiotics with anaerobic coverage

Question 42.16.   A 68-year-old man with a retroperitoneal soft tissue sarcoma receiving chemotherapy presents with fever and headache. A lumbar puncture reveals cerebrospinal fluid (CSF) pleocytosis (mostly neutrophils), along with decreased glucose and elevated protein levels in the CSF. Gram stain does not reveal any organisms, and cultures and further microbiology tests are pending. Empiric therapy should consist of which agents?

   A.   Ceftriaxone and vancomycin
   B.   Ceftriaxone, ampicillin, and vancomycin
   C.   Acyclovir, ceftriaxone, and vancomycin
   D.   Acyclovir and ceftriaxone

Question 42.17.   A 62-year old man with squamous cell carcinoma of the oral cavity in remission presents with headaches, diplopia, and low-grade fevers. Brain magnetic resonance imaging (MRI) reveals a ring-enhancing lesion within the brain parenchyma. You suspect a brain abscess and call the neurosurgeon for needle aspiration. Pending cultures, which of the following empiric regimens should be recommended?

   A.   Ceftriaxone
   B.   Vancomycin and metronidazole
   C.   Ceftriaxone and metronidazole
   D.   Voriconazole

Question 42.18.   A 45-year-old woman with hepatocellular carcinoma undergoes chemoembolization. What is the rate of infection associated with this procedure?

   A.   1%
   B.   10%
   C.   20%
   D.   30%

Question 42.19.   Vancomycin-resistant enterococcus faecium (VRE) is isolated from blood culture in a patient with cancer and normal hepatic and renal function. Which of the following choices is acceptable first-line antibiotic therapy?

   A.   Linezolid
   B.   Daptomycin
   C.   Quinupristin-dalfopristin
   D.   Any of the above

Question 42.20.   A 44-year-old man with refractory acute myelogenous leukemia has multiple painful sores in his mouth, and oral swab culture is positive for HSV. He has lost 15 lbs with decreased food intake because of his painful lesions. He also has lightheadedness on standing but denies other symptoms. What is the preferred treatment?

   A.   Oral acyclovir 400 mg three times daily
   B.   Intravenous acyclovir 5 mg/kg every 8 hours
   C.   Intravenous acyclovir 10 mg/kg every 8 hours
   D.   Oral valacyclovir 1 g twice daily

Question 42.21.   **Posttransplant lymphoproliferative disorder (PTLD) is induced by which pathogen?**

A.   Epstein-Barr virus (EBV)
B.   Human herpes virus-6 (HHV-6)
C.   CMV
D.   Varicella-zoster virus (VZV)

ANSWERS

Answer 42.1.   **The answer is D.**

Patients without a functional spleen are at risk for overwhelming sepsis by encapsulated bacteria. The most common causative pathogens include *S. pneumoniae, H. influenzae,* and *N. meningitides.* Asplenic patients should receive the pneumococcal polysaccharide vaccine. The conjugated meningococcal vaccine is preferred over the polysaccharide version because it provides longer lasting immunity. Immunization is ideally performed at least 2 weeks before scheduled splenectomy, but may still be administered after surgery if unable to administer prior to surgery.

Answer 42.2.   **The answer is C.**

Antibiotic prophylaxis in neutropenic patients has led to decreased episodes of fever and decreased infections, but has demonstrated no difference in mortality in randomized controlled trials. This has primarily been evaluated with oral fluoroquinolones such as levofloxacin. The benefit is more pronounced in patients with prolonged neutropenia, and prophylaxis is not routinely recommended in patients expected to have neutropenia lasting 7 days or less.

Answer 42.3.   **The answer is D.**

The most effective prophylaxis is trimethoprim/sulfamethoxazole (TMP/SMX). Numerous dosing schedules, including one double-strength tablet daily, one single-strength tablet daily, and one double-strength tablet 3 days per week, appear to be effective. Second-line agents, including dapsone, inhaled pentamidine, and atovaquone, may be administered in patients unable to receive TMP/SMX because of marrow intolerance or hypersensitivity reaction, but appear to be less effective.

Answer 42.4.   **The answer is C.**

CMV disease may be prevented in the setting of preexisting infection through one of two equally acceptable approaches: prophylaxis with antiviral agents or preemptive therapy. In the latter strategy, active surveillance with highly sensitive methods of detection such as CMV DNA by PCR may be used to trigger preemptive antiviral therapy in asymptomatic patients with CMV reactivation. Both strategies are considered appropriate in guidelines published by the Centers for Disease Control and Prevention (CDC), although the preemptive approach is more widely adopted.

Answer 42.5. **The answer is B.**

According to Infectious Diseases Society of America (IDSA) guidelines, fever is defined as a single oral temperature of >38.3°C or a temperature of >38.0°C for 1 hour or more. Severe neutropenia is defined as a neutrophil count of <500 cells/μL or a count of <1000 cells/μL with a predicted decrease to <500 cells/μL.

Answer 42.6. **The answer is A.**

Neutropenic patients with fever require prompt empiric administration of a broad-spectrum B-lactam antibiotic with activity against *P. aeruginosa,* such as ceftazidime, cefepime, imipenem, or meropenem. The addition of an aminoglycoside or ciprofloxacin is warranted for patients with hemodynamic compromise. The empiric addition of vancomycin has not been shown to improve outcomes and is not indicated for initial empiric therapy in hemodynamically stable patients in the absence of clinically apparent catheter-related infections. Vancomycin should also be considered in patients with severe mucositis, previous use of fluoroquinolone antibiotic prophylaxis, and history of methicillin-resistant *S. aureus* (MRSA) infection.

Answer 42.7. **The answer is D.**

In patients with persistent neutropenic fever, the addition of antifungal agents after 4 to 7 days is standard practice. Randomized prospective studies have shown decreased invasive fungal infections with this strategy. Liposomal amphotericin B, itraconazole, voriconazole, and caspofungin are all acceptable alternatives, with no agent demonstrating higher overall efficacy than the others. Some authorities feel that fluconazole or anidulafungin are acceptable alternatives.

Answer 42.8. **The answer is D.**

Antibiotic treatment for neutropenic fever that resolves after initiation of empiric therapy should be continued until resolution of neutropenia. For patients with prolonged neutropenia, 2 weeks of antibiotics may be sufficient. In clinically stable patients, it may be acceptable to switch initial intravenous antibiotics to an oral regimen, such as ciprofloxacin with amoxicillin/clavulanate. Some authors have also suggested that select patients can be treated on an outpatient basis with close monitoring.

Answer 42.9. **The answer is C.**

Intravascular catheter-associated infections are common given the widespread use of central venous catheters in patients with cancer. These consist of exit-site infections, tunnel or pocket infections, and catheter-related bacteremia. Tunnel (or port) catheter infections typically require catheter removal. Although catheter salvage may be attempted with certain pathogens, IDSA guidelines suggest routine removal of catheters for infections with *S. aureus,* fungi, and mycobacteria. Attempts at catheter salvage may be considered with *S. epidermidis,* with removal of catheter should bacteremia not be resolved with antibiotics.

Answer 42.10. **The answer is B.**

Zygomycosis (or mucormycosis) is seen most commonly in patients with prolonged neutropenia or corticosteroid use, including those with hematologic malignancies and allogeneic hematopoietic stem cell transplant recipients. Sinus or pulmonary involvement is typical. Therapy should consist of lipid formulation amphotericin B along with early and aggressive surgical debridement in those with sinus or localized skin disease. Voriconazole and echinocandins are not active. Posaconazole has shown promising results as salvage therapy.

Answer 42.11. **The answer is A.**

Neutropenic patients with persistent fever are at risk for fungal pneumonia. CT imaging of the chest may disclose characteristic signs, such as the nodules, masses, or the "halo sign." This latter finding is highly suggestive of invasive aspergillosis but may also be seen with *P. aeruginosa* or other molds. The serum galactomannan assay is specific (although not highly sensitive) for aspergillus species, because invasive zygomycosis does not cause positive results. Prompt treatment with voriconazole or amphotericin B is indicated.

Answer 41.12. **The answer is C.**

The causative agents in esophagitis include candida, HSV, CMV, bacteria, and aspergillus. Erosive esophagitis caused by radiation therapy or chemotherapy-induced mucositis may also produce a similar clinical picture. CMV infections occur mainly in patients with prolonged immunosuppression, such as patients who have undergone hematopoietic stem cell transplantation.

Answer 42.13. **The answer is B.**

Typhlitis, or neutropenic enterocolitis, occurs in patients receiving chemotherapy toxic to the bowel mucosa, most commonly during treatment for acute leukemia. CT findings include bowel wall thickening, mucosa edema, pericecal fluid, and a right lower quadrant inflammatory mass. Treatment should consist of broad-spectrum antibiotics including coverage against gram-negative and anaerobic organisms. CMV infection is uncommon in patients with cancer without prior allogeneic stem cell transplantation.

Answer 42.14. **The answer is B.**

C. difficile colitis is common in those with cancer because of the frequent use of broad-spectrum antibiotics and often prolonged hospitalizations that facilitate transmission. Treatment options for *C. difficile* colitis include oral metronidazole (or intravenous administration in those unable to receive oral medications) and oral vancomycin. The latter option may be considered in patients with severe diarrhea, significant comorbidities, or persistent infections. Intravenous vancomycin is not effective because it is not transported through the bowel wall. Studies regarding the efficacy and safety of probiotics have been inconclusive to date.

Answer 42.15. **The answer is D.**

Anorectal infections are most commonly caused by organisms commonly found in the gastrointestinal tract, such as Enterobacter species, Enterococcus, *P. aeruginosa,* or anaerobes, and are often polymicrobial. Digital rectal examination should be avoided in patients with neutropenia. Broad-spectrum antibiotics are required in anorectal infections, and anaerobic coverage is also indicated in the presence of fistula formation, induration, or cellulitis. Local comfort measures may also be used, but antibiotic treatment should be initiated without delay. Pelvic CT to rule out perirectal abscess requiring surgical management should also be considered.

Answer 42.16. **The answer is B.**

These findings are suggestive of bacterial meningitis. Empiric therapy should consist of ceftriaxone, ampicillin, and vancomycin, which would provide coverage for typical pathogens (*S. pneumoniae, N. meningitides, H. influenzae*) along with Listeria and penicillin-resistant *S. pneumoniae*. If HSV meningoencephalitis is clinically suspected, such as with mental status changes or CSF findings typical of viral meningitis, acyclovir should also be administered.

Answer 42.17. **The answer is C.**

Brain abscesses may present with symptoms including headache, neurologic deficits, or seizures, and appear as ring-enhancing lesions on MRI. In immunocompetent patients, bacterial brain abscess is frequently caused by dental flora. Third-generation cephalosporins, such as ceftriaxone and metronidazole, are recommended for empiric therapy, particularly in a patient with a suspected oral source. Voriconazole may be added to broad-spectrum antibacterial coverage in immunocompromised patients, who are more likely to have a fungal cause.

Answer 42.18. **The answer is A.**

Liver-directed therapies, such as chemoembolization and radiofrequency ablation, are effective palliative measures in selected patients with hepatic tumors. Resultant tumor necrosis may serve as a nidus for infection, with an incidence of approximately 1% after these procedures. Prior biliary enteric anastomosis is the primary risk factor for liver abscess after chemoembolization, with an incidence of approximately 5% in these patients.

Answer 42.19.   **The answer is D.**

Enterococcus species are common pathogens in bacteremia. Colonization with VRE is frequently detected in patients with cancer with repeated hospitalizations. VRE bacteremia typically occurs in severely debilitated patients and is associated with high mortality. First-line agents include linezolid and daptomycin. Quinupristin-dalfopristin is effective in *E. faecium* infections, but not E. *faecalis,* and has moderate efficacy comparable to linezolid. Unfortunately, refractory bacteremia is not rare in this disease.

Answer 42.20.   **The answer is B.**

Oropharyngeal HSV is commonly seen in patients with prolonged chemotherapy-induced neutropenia and may lead to significant morbidity in these patients. Oral acyclovir (400 mg given five times daily) or valacyclovir for 7 to 10 days may be considered in some patients, but intravenous acyclovir (5 mg/kg every 8 hours) is preferred for patients with significant mucosal disease causing impaired oral intake. Disseminated HSV should be treated with intravenous acyclovir (10 mg/kg every 8 hours).

Answer 42.21.   **The answer is A.**

Solid-organ and hematopoietic stem cell transplant recipients are at risk for PTLD, which is an abnormal proliferation of EBV-infected B cells. There are varied clinical manifestations, including a mononucleosis-like syndrome, generalized adenopathy, and extranodal organ involvement. Treatment strategies include reduction of immune suppression, rituximab, and adoptive transfer of EBV-specific cytotoxic T lymphocytes. For those with a more aggressive clinical course, combination chemotherapy may also be warranted.

Management of Adverse Effects of Treatment

Directions   Each of the numbered items below is followed by lettered answers. Select the ONE lettered answer that is BEST in each case unless instructed otherwise.

QUESTIONS

Question 43.1.   **Rare, serious adverse events associated with the rHu granulocyte colony-stimulating factor (G-CSF) include all of the following, EXCEPT:**

A. Allergic-type reactions
B. Splenic rupture
C. Adult respiratory distress syndrome
D. Moderate bone pain

Question 43.2.   **Primary prophylactic G-CSF administration is recommended in which cases?**

A. Chemotherapy regimens in which the expected incidence of febrile neutropenia is 20% or greater.
B. A decrease of dose intensity would compromise long-term outcomes, such as survival or cure.
C. The patient is at increased risk for serious complications or death from febrile neutropenia.
D. All of the above are true.

Question 43.3.   **Which is NOT a risk factor for cancer-associated thrombosis?**

A. African American race
B. Younger age
C. Inherited prothrombotic mutations
D. Metastatic disease

Corresponding Chapter in *Cancer: Principles & Practice of Oncology*, Eighth Edition: 63 (Management of Adverse Effects of Treatment).

Question 43.4.   **Regarding the use of prophylactic anticoagulation for central venous catheters, which of the following statements is TRUE?**

A. Fixed-dose warfarin is more effective than low-molecular-weight heparin.

B. Symptomatic catheter-related thrombosis rates of 15% were reported without the use of prophylaxis.

C. The American College of Chest Physicians (ACCP) 2004 guidelines recommend against the use of routine prophylaxis using low-molecular-weight heparin and fixed-dose warfarin.

D. The use of fixed-dose warfarin (1 mg daily) is not associated with increased bleeding risk.

Question 43.5.   **Chemotherapy-induced nausea and vomiting (CINV) include which of the following types?**

A. Acute CINV

B. Delayed CINV

C. Anticipatory CINV

D. All of the above

Question 43.6.   **Patient-related factors important in increased risk of chemotherapy-induced nausea and vomiting include all of the following, EXCEPT:**

A. Female gender

B. Younger age

C. History of chronic alcohol consumption

D. History of motion sickness

Question 43.7.   **Recommended antiemetic therapy for the prevention of acute emesis with high emetic risk chemotherapy include all of the following, EXCEPT:**

A. $5\text{-}HT_3$ receptor antagonist

B. Phenothiazine

C. Aprepitant

D. Dexamethasone

Question 43.8.   **Delayed chemotherapy-induced nausea and vomiting appear to be mostly related to which mechanism?**

A. Substance P

B. Dopamine

C. 5HT

D. All of the above

Question 43.9.   **Agents commonly causing chemotherapy-induced diarrhea include all of the following, EXCEPT:**

A. Fluoropyrimidines

B. Platinum agents

C. Irinotecan

D. Taxanes

Question 43.10.   Other causes of treatment-related diarrhea include which of the following?

A. Radiation
B. Enteral feedings
C. Celiac plexus block
D. All of the above

Question 43.11.   The somatostatin analog octreotide has all of the following actions, EXCEPT:

A. Suppresses inflammatory bowel disease
B. Suppresses release of insulin and vasoactive intestinal peptide
C. Reduces motility
D. Alters increased gastrointestinal absorption of water and electrolytes

Question 43.12.   Agents commonly causing constipation in patients with cancer include all of the following, EXCEPT:

A. Opioid analgesics
B. Antidepressants
C. Phenothiazine antiemetics
D. Diuretics

Question 43.13.   Patient-related risk factors for stomatitis include which of the following?

A. Age more than 65 years or less than 20 years
B. Inadequate nutritional status
C. Exposure to oral stressors, including alcohol and smoking
D. All of the above

Question 43.14.   Common prophylactic measures for the prevention of chemotherapy- and radiation-induced stomatitis include all of the following, EXCEPT:

A. Chlorhexidine gluconate
B. Viscous lidocaine
C. Sodium bicarbonate rinses
D. Ice

Question 43.15.   Regarding the treatment of xerostomia, which is NOT true?

A. Xerostomia is related to radiation dosage, location, and volume of exposed salivary glands.
B. Pilocarpine is commonly used as a stimulant for saliva production because of its low toxicity.
C. Amifostine was shown to decrease acute and late xerostomia.
D. The consumption of sugarless gum and hard candy increases patient comfort.

Question 43.16. **Regarding radiation pneumonitis, which is FALSE?**

A. It develops in 5% to 15% of patients receiving external beam radiation for lung cancer.
B. It can be divided into early, intermediate, and late stages.
C. The use of corticosteroids can prevent the onset of radiation pneumonitis.
D. Dyspnea is the main presenting symptom.

Question 43.17. **Some factors that are associated with increased risk of chemotherapy-induced pulmonary toxicity include which of the following?**

A. Total dose of chemotherapy
B. Simultaneous or prior radiation to the lungs
C. Renal function
D. All of the above

Question 43.18. **Cardiac irradiation can induce which symptoms of heart disease?**

A. Pericarditis and pericardial effusion
B. Ischemic heart disease
C. Electrical conduction abnormalities
D. All of the above

Question 43.19. **Regarding early detection of cardiac dysfunction, which is NOT used?**

A. Electrocardiograms
B. Measurement of left ventricular ejection fraction by echocardiography
C. Serum cardiac troponin T levels
D. Serum brain natriuretic peptide levels

Question 43.20. **All of the factors below are associated with alopecia, EXCEPT:**

A. Thyroid disease
B. Malignancy
C. Malnutrition
D. All of the above

Question 43.21. **All of the following antitumor agents cause prolonged azoospermia in men, EXCEPT:**

A. Radiation to the testis
B. Carboplatin
C. Cyclophosphamide
D. Melphalan

Question 43.22. **Regarding interventions for cancer-related fatigue, which of the following did NOT show improvement in fatigue?**

A. Massage therapy
B. L-carnitine supplementation
C. Stress-reduction intervention
D. Omega-3 fatty acid supplementation

ANSWERS

Answer 43.1. **The answer is D.**

Allergic-type reactions, splenic rupture, and adult respiratory distress syndrome have been reported as rare, serious adverse events associated with the administration of rHu G-CSF. Mild-to-moderate bone pain is the most common side effect from rHu G-CSF.

Answer 43.2. **The answer is D.**

Primary prophylactic use of G-CSF is recommended in all of the above scenarios as per the American Society of Clinical Oncology 2006 Guidelines.

Answer 43.3. **The answer is B.**

There are many risk factors for cancer-associated thrombosis. They can be divided into four categories: patient demographics, patient comorbidities, cancer-related factors, and treatment-related factors. Demographic risk factors include older age and African American race. Patient comorbidity risk factors include obesity, infection, renal disease, pulmonary disease, arterial thromboembolism, history of venous thromboembolism, and inherited prothrombotic mutations (e.g., factor V Leiden and prothrombin gene mutation). Cancer-related factors include primary site of cancer (gastrointestinal, brain, lung, gynecologic, renal, hematologic), initial period of diagnosis, and metastatic disease. Treatment-related factors include major surgery, hospitalization, chemotherapy, hormonal therapy, antiangiogenic therapy, erythropoiesis-stimulating agents, and central venous catheters.

Answer 43.4. **The answer is C.**

Multiple trials have shown that the prophylactic use of either warfarin or low-molecular-weight heparin is effective in reducing symptomatic catheter-related thrombosis. These rates are approximately 4% with some possible increased bleeding complications in those on anticoagulation. Current ACCP guidelines recommend against the use of routine anticoagulation prophylaxis.

Answer 43.5. **The answer is D.**

Acute, delayed, and anticipatory nausea and vomiting make up the three clinical syndromes of CINV. Acute CINV occurs within the first 24 hours of chemotherapy administration, whereas delayed CINV occurs more than 24 hours after chemotherapy administration. Anticipatory CINV occurs as a conditioned response to stimuli that reminds patients of previous episodes of nausea and vomiting.

Answer 43.6. **The answer is C.**

Patient-related factors that increase the risk of chemotherapy-induced nausea and vomiting include female gender, younger age, CINV with previous chemotherapy treatment, history of pregnancy-associated nausea and vomiting, and history of motion sickness. A history of chronic alcohol consumption is associated with a decrease in risk of CINV. Treatment-related factors that increase the risk of chemotherapy-induced nausea and vomiting include the agent, dose, rate, and route of administration.

Answer 43.7.   **The answer is B.**

With high emetic-risk chemotherapy, recommended antiemetic therapy includes medications from the following classes: 5-HT$_3$ receptor antagonist (dolasetron, granisetron, ondansetron, tropisetron, palonosetron), corticosteroids (dexamethasone), and NK1 receptor antagonist (aprepitant). Phenothiazines, such as prochlorperazine, have a lower therapeutic index.

Answer 43.8.   **The answer is A.**

The pathophysiology of delayed CINV may be more dependent on Substance P as seen by the efficacy of NK1 antagonists in the delayed emesis setting. Because 5-HT3 receptor antagonists and dopamine D2 antagonists have less efficacy in this setting, 5-HT and dopamine appear to have a less important role in delayed CINV.

Answer 43.9.   **The answer is B.**

Agents such as 5-fluorouracil, capecitabine, and irinotecan are chemotherapy agents that commonly cause diarrhea. Docetaxel is also associated with a mild diarrhea but can also cause severe enteritis and colitis.

Answer 43.10.   **The answer is D.**

Targeted therapy, radiation, clostridium difficile, enteral feedings, and celiac plexus block are all causes of treatment-related diarrhea.

Answer 43.11.   **The answer is A.**

Octreotide has multiple methods of activity in the reduction of diarrhea. It can suppress the release of insulin, glucagon, vasoactive intestinal peptide, and gastric acid; reduce gastrointestinal motility and decrease pancreatic exocrine function; and alter the increased absorption of water, electrolytes, and nutrients from the gastrointestinal tract.

Answer 43.12.   **The answer is C.**

Drugs that commonly cause constipation in patients with cancer include opioid analgesics, serotonin 5HT3 receptor antagonists, vinca alkaloids, thalidomide, antidepressants, aluminum- or calcium-containing antacids, iron supplements, and diuretics.

Answer 43.13.   **The answer is D.**

Study results of chemotherapy-related stomatitis are conflicting, but some patient-related factors include age more than 65 years or less than

20 years, female gender, inadequate nutritional status, herpes simplex infection, and decreased chemotherapy metabolism. Oral factors such as periodontal disease, microbial flora, chronic low-grade mouth infection, salivary gland secretory dysfunction, ill-fitting dental prostheses, and exposure to oral stressors including alcohol and tobacco can also contribute to risk of stomatitis.

Answer 43.14. **The answer is B.**

Chlorhexidine gluconate, saline rinses, sodium bicarbonate rinses, acyclovir, amphotericin B, and ice are common prophylactic measures used in the prevention of stomatitis. Viscous lidocaine and Carafate suspension, dicyclomine hydrochloride, opioids, and mixtures (including ingredients such as diphenhydramine, Maalox, viscous lidocaine, and nystatin) are commonly used in the treatment of stomatitis-related pain.

Answer 43.15. **The answer is B.**

Because of toxicity related to glaucoma and cardiac issues, pilocarpine is used with caution in patients with xerostomia. Although patients have reported increased oral comfort with gum and hard candy, the use of artificial saliva has not demonstrated the same.

Answer 43.16. **The answer is C.**

Patients with radiation pneumonitis typically present with dyspnea, self-limited or progressive. They can also present with cough, fever, chest pain, tachypnea, and cyanosis. Corticosteroids are not used as a prophylactic measure or in the treatment of radiation fibrosis; however, prednisone is commonly used in the treatment of radiation pneumonitis, but data are mixed.

Answer 43.17. **The answer is D.**

Many factors are associated with increased risk of chemotherapy-induced pulmonary toxicity. Bleomycin, for example, is associated with increased risk of pulmonary toxicity in terms of total dose, advanced age, oxygen therapy, simultaneous or prior radiation therapy to the lungs, combination with other drugs, and renal dysfunction.

Answer 43.18. **The answer is D.**

Radiation-induced heart disease covers a wide clinical spectrum, including pericardial disease, acute pericarditis, pericardial effusion, constrictive pericarditis, myocardial dysfunction, valvular heart disease, electrical conduction abnormalities, and congestive heart disease.

Answer 43.19. **The answer is A.**

Early detection of cardiac dysfunction is important in the prevention of overt cardiomyopathy during the administration of chemotherapy. Echocardiograms or radionuclide imaging can directly measure left ventricular ejection fraction. Other measures of cardiac dysfunction include measuring serial diastolic pressures, serum cardiac troponin T levels, and brain natriuretic peptide levels. Electrocardiograms have little value in early detection of cardiac dysfunction because changes tend to occur late.

Answer 43.20. **The answer is D.**

Alopecia is associated with many chronic diseases, including thyroid disease, malnutrition, iron-deficiency anemia, pancreatic disease, and zinc deficiency. Some malignancies (acute myeloid leukemia, lung cancer, breast cancer, gastric cancer, squamous cell cancer of the tongue) have been linked to alopecia. Systemic chemotherapy tends to induce hair follicle dystrophy leading to chemically induced alopecia.

Answer 43.21. **The answer is B.**

Prolonged azoospermia is often seen with radiation to the testis, chlorambucil, cyclophosphamide, procarbazine, melphalan, and cisplatin. Carboplatin does not often cause prolonged azoospermia. Other agents (doxorubicin, cytosine arabinoside, vinblastine, vincristine) can be additive in causing prolonged azoospermia when combined with other agents that affect sperm production but cause only temporary reductions in sperm when used alone.

Answer 43.22. **The answer is D.**

Several interventions have been shown to improve cancer-related fatigue. These include supplementation with mistletoe extract, L-carnitine, and high-dose vitamin C, as well as massage therapy, stress-reduction intervention, polarity therapy, and relaxation breathing. Data are mixed for progressive muscle relaxation, psychoeducation, virtual reality distraction, and yoga. The use of music therapy, omega-3 fatty acid supplementation, and reiki did not show an improvement in fatigue symptoms.

44

Supportive Care and Quality of Life

Directions   Each of the numbered items below is followed by lettered answers. Select the ONE lettered answer that is BEST in each case unless instructed otherwise.

QUESTIONS

Question 44.1.   **ATAC trial results suggested that women taking aromatase inhibitors have less sexual problems compared with those taking tamoxifen.**

A. True
B. False

Question 44.2.   **Christine is a 45-year-old woman with newly diagnosed triple negative metastatic breast cancer. She and her husband have two school-aged children. She is beginning chemotherapy and asks you, "How much should we share with the kids?" Your advice is:**

A. I am sorry, this is out of my area of expertise, but I will be glad to refer you to a social worker.
B. Talk as little as possible about the cancer to preserve the sense of normalcy in the children's lives.
C. Sit the children down and explain her disease process, including eventual death from cancer.
D. Try to let the children initiate the discussion, and then answer all of their questions in an age-appropriate manner, including fears and concerns about their mother dying.

Corresponding Chapter in *Cancer: Principles & Practice of Oncology*, Eighth Edition: 64 (Supportive Care and Quality of Life).

Question 44.3. Christine is treated with Abraxane and bevacizumab and achieves a very good partial response. However, she has numbness, tingling, and aching in her hands. You diagnose her as having treatment-related grade 2 peripheral neuropathy. In addition to giving her a chemotherapy holiday, you will also recommend:

    A. Oxycodone 5 mg every 6 hours as needed
    B. Gabapentin 300 mg three times per day
    C. Dexamethasone 4 mg every 6 hours
    D. Refer her to neurologist for electromyography (EMG)

Question 44.4. Two years have passed. On her most recent visit, she reports headaches and nausea. Brain magnetic resonance imaging (MRI) shows multiple metastases. You treat her with dexamethasone and refer her for whole brain radiation therapy. On her next follow-up visit, she reports difficulty sleeping at night. The following medications are implicated in causing insomnia:

    A. Corticosteroids
    B. Prochlorperazine
    C. Zofran
    D. All of the above

Question 44.5. Christine completed whole brain radiation, which she tolerated poorly with worsening fatigue. Unfortunately, 2 months later, she is more short of breath. Her CT scan shows worsening pulmonary and liver metastases. Her Eastern Cooperative Oncology Group (ECOG) performance status (PS) is 3. You are convinced that there is no further standard therapy that would be of benefit to her. She is not eligible for any clinical trials available at your institution. After discussing her latest scan results, you say:

    A. I am sorry, but there is nothing more I can offer you.
    B. There are no other treatments against the cancer, but I will continue taking care of you and make sure your comfort remains a priority.
    C. Unfortunately, you have only 2 months to live, but we will make sure you have as much quality time as possible.
    D. I can offer you other chemotherapy, but it is unlikely that it will provide any benefit.

Question 44.6. Palliative care is:

    A. A growing specialty with more than 100 fellowship positions and is now a board-certified subspecialty of internal medicine.
    B. Same as hospice.
    C. Proven to improve patient satisfaction, decrease hospital stays, and decrease total cost of care in patients with life-threatening illness and prognosis of less than 1 year.
    D. B and C.

Question 44.7.   **Which of the following is TRUE about palliative care services?**

A. Patients need to abandon other forms of therapy, such as chemo-therapy, to receive palliative care.
B. Palliative care has no role in management of patients with curable cancers.
C. Total costs of care are higher for patients who died in the palliative care unit, compared with those who died outside the unit.
D. Palliative care teams can assist oncology patients and their doctors with symptom management, as well as other forms of pain, at any point along the disease trajectory, beginning from diagnosis.

Question 44.8.   **The MOST common symptom experienced by patients in the last days to week before death is:**

A. Fatigue and/or pain
B. Restlessness/delirium
C. Dyspnea
D. Nausea and vomiting

Question 44.9.   **Christine enters a home hospice program. She has been taking 90 mg of MS-Contin every 8 hours for pain from liver metastases. Her pain is well controlled, but she develops hallucinations and is unable to take pills. The hospice nurse recommends replacing oral morphine with a fentanyl patch. What is the appropriate equivalent dose of transdermal fentanyl?**

A. 25 μg/h
B. 50 μg/h
C. 200 μg/h
D. 100 μg/h

Question 44.10.   **Which statement(s) is/are TRUE regarding nausea and vomiting that occurs during treatment with opioid analgesics:**

A. It is produced through chemoreceptor trigger zone.
B. Tolerance rarely develops to these side effects.
C. Switching to alternative opioid often results in improvement.
D. A and C.

Question 44.11.   **Which of the following can be a cause of depression in terminally ill patients?**

A. Hypercalcemia
B. Uncontrolled pain
C. Steroid treatment
D. All of the above

Question 44.12. **Which of the following factors have been shown to be associated with high rates of primary caregiver burnout?**

A. Lower socioeconomic status
B. Race
C. Caring for a patient for more than 6 months
D. All of the above

Question 44.13. **Professional barriers to cancer pain management include:**

A. Inadequate knowledge of pain mechanisms
B. Fear of producing iatrogenic complications
C. Time and reimbursement pressures
D. All of the above

Question 44.14. **Lisa, a 45-year-old woman with locally advanced right-sided breast cancer, undergoes neoadjuvant chemotherapy, followed by modified radical mastectomy and axillary dissection. She achieves partial response and undergoes adjuvant irradiation to total dose of 55 GY. Five years later, she has no evidence of disease recurrence. However, on routine visit she reports right shoulder ache, arm/hand numbness, and weakness. There is mild arm edema. Her symptoms have been slowly progressive during the last year. The best test to determine the cause of her symptoms is:**

A. Brachial plexus magnetic resonance imaging (MRI)
B. Cervical spine MRI
C. Bone scan
D. EMG

Question 44.15. **Lisa is very relieved that her symptoms are not related to progressive disease. However, she is distressed by her pain and decreased ability to function. On her recent office visit she is tearful. Treatment approaches to this patient's problem may include:**

A. Physical therapy
B. Support group
C. Antidepressants and anticonvulsants
D. All of the above

Question 44.16. **John is an 80-year-old man with ECOG PS 2 and metastatic hormone refractory prostate cancer (HRPC) to the bones. He is treated with Taxotere, bisphosphonates, and ibuprofen. His pain is initially controlled well on 60 mg twice per day of long-acting morphine with short-acting morphine 15 mg every 6 to 8 hours as needed. If his pain is increased, all of these approaches may be reasonable, EXCEPT:**

A. Increase morphine by 50% to 100%
B. Add corticosteroids
C. Treatment with strontium-89 or samarium-153
D. Change to methadone 60 mg by mouth twice per day

Question 44.17.   **In this patient, anticipated adverse effects of morphine include all of the following, EXCEPT:**

A. Sedation
B. Respiratory depression
C. Nausea and vomiting
D. Constipation

Question 44.18.   **You eventually increase John's morphine to 120 mg twice per day with 30 mg as needed, which he takes every 3 hours, and add corticosteroids. Unfortunately, the patient's pain is still poorly controlled, and he develops increasing sedation and drowsiness. Further evaluation shows normal electrolytes and no evidence of further disease progression. You refer him to a palliative care specialist who recommends switching to methadone at a dose ratio of 6:1. Properties of methadone that make it somewhat difficult to use include:**

A. Cost
B. QT prolongation
C. Requires up to 1 week to achieve steady state
D. C and B

Question 44.19.   **John achieves good pain control on methadone 40 mg/d and enjoys a good quality of life with his family. Which of the following best explains his response to methadone?**

A. He reached a maximum tolerated dose of morphine.
B. He developed tolerance to morphine.
C. NMDA receptor plays a critical role in opioid tolerance and may explain the dramatic reduction of dosage when his medication is switched from morphine to methadone.
D. Both B and C.

Question 44.20.   **Which of the following medications are effective as adjuvants in treating neuropathic pain?**

A. Tricyclic antidepressants
B. Anticonvulsants
C. Local anesthetics
D. All of the above

Question 44.21.   **Which of the following is TRUE about using anesthetic and neurosurgical approaches to treat cancer pain?**

A. Celiac ganglion block is effective in 50% of patients treated.
B. Peripheral nerve blocks are most useful in patients with somatic pain.
C. Cordotomy is almost always complicated by motor paresis.
D. Epidural local anesthetics delivered by continuous low-dose infusion are useful long term for cancer pain.

Question 44.22. John eventually develops liver metastases and enters hospice care. His elderly wife is unable to manage him at home, and he is transferred to inpatient hospice after a few weeks. Eventually he becomes bed-bound and mostly unresponsive. In the last 24 hours, his respirations are becoming irregular, and he appears agitated, moaning, and restless. No recent changes to his medications have been made. Appropriate management of his condition include:

A. Lorazepam 1 mg every 2 hours
B. Opioid drip to control dyspnea
C. Haldol 1 mg intravenously (IV) administered every 2 hours
D. All of the above

Question 44.23. Despite appropriate medications, the patient continues to be restless and uncomfortable. You discuss his condition with his wife and explain to her that he most likely has terminal delirium and dyspnea and suggest further treatment with IV barbiturates. Which of the following best describes use of IV thiopental in the management of imminently dying patients:

A. It should never be used.
B. It should be considered only if opioid analgesics and adjuvant drugs fail to control symptoms or produce intolerable side effects.
C. It can relieve both physical and psychological pain.
D. B and C.

Question 44.24. What threshold is used to define critical weight loss in patients with cancer?

A. 10% of baseline body weight in 6 months
B. 10% of lean body mass in 6 months
C. 10% of baseline body weight in 3 months
D. 10 lbs in 1 month

Question 44.25. Which of the following metabolic abnormalities is/are present in cancer cachexia?

A. Increased gluconeogenesis
B. Decreased lipoprotein lipase activity
C. Decreased body glucose consumption
D. A and B

Question 44.26. All of the following have been implicated in development of cancer cachexia, EXCEPT:

A. Tumor necrosis factor (TNF)-α
B. Interleukin (IL)-6
C. Proteolysis-inducing factor
D. Direct cytotoxic effects of chemotherapy

Question 44.27. **Which of the following patients is NOT a good candidate for total parenteral nutrition?**

A. A 50-year-old man with colon cancer who undergoes surgical resection and develops enterocutaneous fistula.

B. A 75-year-old woman with ECOG PS 2, stage IIIC ovarian cancer who develops small bowel obstruction because of multiple adhesions. She is receiving single-agent paclitaxel, and her abdominal computed tomography (CT) shows stable disease. She is not a surgical candidate because of a recent myocardial infarction (MI).

C. A 32-year-old woman with rapidly progressing metastatic gastric cancer, not responding to chemotherapy.

D. A 62-year-old man with stage IVA head and neck cancer, receiving chemoradiation, who develops a 10% weight loss in the last 3 months as the result of mucositis and is unable to tolerate G-tube feedings because of diarrhea.

Question 44.28. **Which of the following is NOT true about the National Comprehensive Cancer Network (NCCN) Distress Thermometer?**

A. It includes a visual analog tool.

B. It includes a problem list of possible causes of distress.

C. A score of 5 of 10 provides a validated indication of distress.

D. It only addresses physical causes of distress.

Question 44.29. **All of the following outcomes have been consistently documented in clinical trials of psychosocial interventions aimed at patients with metastatic breast cancer, EXCEPT:**

A. Improved survival

B. Reduced depression

C. Reduced pain

D. Reduced overall distress scores

Question 44.30. **Which of the following antidepressants can also be used for neuropathic pain?**

A. Venlafaxine (Effexor)

B. Mirtazapine (Remeron)

C. Desipramine (Norpramin)

D. A and C

Question 44.31. **Your patient with newly diagnosed early-stage breast cancer asks your opinion about complementary and alternative medicine (CAM). She has not selected any specific modality yet. She makes it clear that she wants to combine CAM with her adjuvant therapy. You advise her:**

A. Not to use any modalities, because there are no data, and they are likely to be harmful.

B. She can use herbal preparations as long as she has no adverse effects.

C. She needs to select a licensed professional to administer her CAM.

D. To inform you if she decides to use CAM, so you can help her avoid unfavorable adverse effects and interactions with chemotherapy, and devise an integrated treatment plan, if possible.

ANSWERS

Answer 44.1. **The answer is B.**

The ATAC trial included a subprotocol evaluating quality of life. After 2 years on the study, more women taking Arimidex developed vaginal dryness, dyspareunia, and loss of libido, compared with those taking tamoxifen.

Answer 44.2. **The answer is D.**

In addition to other professionals, such as social workers and school counselors, the oncology team plays an important role in helping patients explain to their children about their illness and prognosis. In 2002, Rauch et al. (Rauch PK, Muriel AC, Cassem NH. Parents with cancer: who's looking after the children? J Clin Oncol 2002;20(21):4399–4402) published recommendations that addressed this difficult issue. For school-aged children, the guidelines include sharing information honestly, avoiding euphemisms, encouraging the children to ask questions, and letting them initiate the discussions.

Answer 44.3. **The answer is B.**

This patient has neuropathic pain, in this case related to her treatment. Although corticosteroids have a role in treating refractory neuropathic pain, they are generally not used first line. Likewise, opioid drugs can be useful, especially methadone, in more refractory settings and for severe pain. However, neuropathic pain has a variable responsiveness to opioids and may be less responsive than other types of pain. Most common drug classes used as first line for mild to moderate neuropathic pain include antidepressants and anticonvulsants. Controlled trials of gabapentin show 30% to 50% response rates in neuropathic pain. The major adverse effect is sedation.

Answer 44.4. **The answer is D.**

Although corticosteroids are commonly implicated in inducing insomnia in patients with cancer, other medications, such as antiemetics, can also cause this troubling problem. Several antiemetic classes, including 5HT3 receptor antagonists, have been linked to insomnia.

Answer 44.5.   **The answer is B.**

Dealing with situations when the oncologist believes treatment will do more harm than good is very challenging for both the physician and the patient. The key is in the words used and their implications, not just their literal meanings. The goal is to convey a caring attitude and hope that her quality of life will remain as good as possible, without making the patient feel abandoned or unsure in regard to goals of therapy.

Answer 44.6.   **The answer is A.**

Palliative care is a growing subspecialty of medicine, with the broad focus that includes symptom management; emotional, spiritual, and existential suffering; advanced care planning; care at the end of life; and closure and legacy. Palliative care teams take care of patients at all stages of their illness, from diagnosis to dying. Hospice and Palliative Care Medicine was accepted as specialty by the American Board of Medical Specialties (ABMS) in 2006. There are currently 125 fellowship positions in the United States.

Answer 44.7.   **The answer is D.**

There are still many misconceptions regarding palliative care programs. Unlike entering hospice care, patients do not need to change or abandon their current treatment program to benefit from additional services provided by palliative care specialists. Several studies in the United States, Canada, and England demonstrated that hospital-based palliative care programs are generally cost-saving for the hospitals. For example, studies done in palliative care units demonstrated significantly decreased daily charges and decreased total costs for patients who died in the unit, compared with age and diagnosis-matched patients who died outside the unit.

Answer 44.8.   **The answer is B.**

Delirium is present is up to 80% of dying patients. Delirious patients may appear agitated or hypoactive, or may alternate between these states. Frequent symptoms of delirium include insomnia, restlessness, or agitation (which can mimic uncontrolled pain), irritability, anxiety, and hallucinations.

Answer 44.9.   **The answer is D.**

The patient's total daily dose of IV morphine is 90 mg (ratio of 1:3). This equates to approximately 4 mg/h, and 4 mg/h of IV administered morphine is equal to approximately 100 µg/h of transdermal fentanyl.

Answer 44.10.   **The answer is D.**

Although the exact mechanism is unclear, it is accepted that opioid analgesics produce nausea and vomiting by action limited to the medullary chemoreceptor trigger zone. Fortunately, tolerance frequently develops to these side effects. Rotating opioids and adding antiemetics, such as Compazine, are both effective in reducing or obviating this effect.

Answer 44.11. **The answer is D.**

Although there are many existential reasons that depression is common in the terminally ill, physical factors can also produce symptoms of depression or mimic it. Corticosteroids can trigger psychosis, as well as depressive symptoms. Hypercalcemia can result in an altered, depressed mood. Uncontrolled pain, especially if prolonged, induces a sense of helplessness and depression.

Answer 44.12. **The answer is D.**

Race, low socioeconomic status, and prolonged time in caring for the patient have all been demonstrated to independently predict high rates of primary caregiver burnout.

Answer 44.13. **The answer is D.**

Several studies have addressed the issue of professional barriers to effective cancer pain management. Surveys of oncologists demonstrated that both inadequate knowledge and regulatory pressures contribute to inadequate analgesia in patients with cancer.

Answer 44.14. **The answer is A.**

The patient has chronic post-radiation brachial plexopathy. It is important to recognize and effectively manage treatment-related chronic pain syndromes, because these patients frequently need integrated approach to treatment. Brachial plexus MRI is able to distinguish between tumor infiltration and radiation fibrosis. Radiation fibrosis injury typically produces low signal intensity on T2-weighted images, generally not enhancing with gadolinium.

Answer 44.15. **The answer is D.**

Although it is consoling to the patient to realize that her symptoms are not related to recurrent cancer, the persistence of pain is a constant remainder of the previous cancer diagnosis. Psychological factors play a significant role in how these patients adapt to and function with chronic pain. A multidisciplinary approach combining a wide range of therapies is usually needed. It is also very important to select appropriate analgesics for neuropathic pain. Antidepressants and anticonvulsants will likely be most effective. Antidepressant drugs should be first-line agents, given her tearfulness and anxiety.

Answer 44.16. **The answer is D.**

Approaches A to C are both reasonable options when dealing with a patient with uncontrolled bone pain from prostate cancer. Opioid rotation can also be attempted if tolerance to morphine is suspected. Methadone can be considered, although conversion can be more challenging than for other opioids because of prolonged plasma half-life but relatively short duration of anesthesia. When converting from another opioid to methadone, marked reduction of equianalgesic dose often results. A reasonable starting methadone daily dose for this patient would be approximately 30 mg of methadone divided into three doses (6:1 ratio for oral morphine, based on 180 mg of oral morphine per day).

Answer 44.17.   **The answer is B.**

All listed adverse effects can occur with opioids, but respiratory depression is unlikely is this setting. This adverse effect most commonly occurs after a short course of intravenous administration of an opioid. Tolerance to this effect develops rapidly with repeat drug doses, which allows prolonged use without significant risk of respiratory depression.

Answer 44.18.   **The answer is D.**

Cost is one of the biggest advantages of methadone, which is relatively inexpensive, compared with other opioids. Because of prolonged half-life, it requires careful titration and may take up to 1 week to achieve steady state. QT prolongation syndrome can occur with methadone and is a cause for concern in those with cancer, who might be taking other agents known to prolong QT interval.

Answer 44.19.   **The answer is D.**

Development of tolerance to opioids is not well understood but is generally suspected when patients on a previously stable dosage begin to require more frequent doses. Often, there is simultaneous disease progression, complicating the issue of tolerance. However, incomplete cross-resistance among opioids often allows for "opioid rotation" and achievement of effective analgesia. Methadone is known to bind to NMDA receptors in the brain, in addition to opioid receptors. This may be one of the mechanisms that explains dramatic dose reductions when a patient's medication is switched from morphine or hydromorphone to methadone.

Answer 44.20.   **The answer is D.**

In addition to commonly used classes, such as antidepressants and anticonvulsants, the use of local anesthetics has demonstrated some efficacy in the management of chronic neuropathic pain. Mexiletine is the oral local anesthetic for which there are pilot data to support analgesic efficacy. The starting dose is low, at 150 mg/d, with gradual titration. Epidural local anesthetics (lidocaine and bupivacaine) have been widely used to manage refractory neuropathic pain, either alone or with opioid.

Answer 44.21.   **The answer is B.**

Continuous epidural low-dose infusion of local anesthetic via a pump is associated with development of tolerance within days to weeks, limiting long-term use. It is most useful in patients who experience acute pain crisis or in patients in whom the use of spinal opioids is considered but who have developed tolerance from large doses of systemic opiates. Temporary use of this technique allows for reducing systemic opioids doses, therefore partially reversing tolerance. Celiac ganglion block is reported to be effective in 70% to 85% of appropriately selected patients. Cordotomy is associated with a 10% to 20% risk of ipsilateral motor weakness, which results from inadvertent extension of the lesion anteriorly to involve corticospinal tract.

Answer 44.22.   **The answer is D.**

This patient is nearing the end of life. The goal is to control any symptoms that he is experiencing. Possible causes of his dyspnea include anxiety, tumor infiltration, and other cardiac and pulmonary conditions. Patients with continuous dyspnea benefit from opioids; if the patient is no longer able to take pills, opioid drips can be very effective. For patients with perceived anxiety, anxiolytics should be added. Haldol can also be useful to control symptoms of agitated delirium.

Answer 44.23.   **The answer is D.**

Despite appropriate medications, a small number of dying patients (<5%) continue to experience intolerable physical, psychological, or spiritual/existential symptoms. For these patients, palliative sedation can be used. The goal of palliative sedation is to relieve intractable distress but not hasten death. Palliative sedation is legal throughout the United States and should not be confused with euthanasia. Expert palliative care and pastoral consultation, evaluation by a psychiatrist, and discussions with family members, the patient (if feasible), and among the healthcare team should always be undertaken before palliative sedation is administered.

Answer 44.24.   **The answer is A.**

Loss of excess of 10% of baseline body weight over 6 months is defined as critical weight loss.

Answer 44.25.   **The answer is D.**

Cancer cachexia is a complex process, mediated by the induction of inflammatory response to the tumor. The hallmark of cancer cachexia is increased catabolism and limited anabolism. This includes an increase in hepatic gluconeogenesis to compensate for increased body glucose consumption. Lipoprotein lipase activity is decreased, and fat breakdown is increased. Muscle proteolysis and hepatic protein synthesis are both increased as well.

Answer 44.26.   **The answer is D.**

There is no evidence that chemotherapy itself is contributing to the mechanism of cancer cachexia. Chemotherapy frequently produces anorexia and dysgeusia, which contribute to cancer-associated weight loss. Cancer cachexia is thought to be primarily mediated by inflammatory cytokines and tumor-related peptides, including proteolysis-inducing factor and lipid-mobilizing factor.

Answer 44.27. **The answer is C.**

Total parenteral nutrition (TPN) is not indicated in patients with rapidly progressive tumor growth that is unresponsive to therapy. Brief, in-hospital TPN is indicated in severely malnourished patients who are responding to chemotherapy and in whom gastrointestinal or other toxicities preclude adequate enteral intake for 7 to 10 days or longer. Prolonged in-hospital or home TPN is indicated in those patients in whom treatment-related toxicities preclude the use of enteral nutrition and represent the primary impediment to the restoration of performance status. TPN can also be considered in select malnourished patients with cancer in whom the natural history of the disease can be expected to permit a period of good performance status. Such patients should be receiving antitumor therapy with a reasonable expectation of response, or the natural history of an untreated tumor is such that a reasonable quality of life is expected, with survival of 6 to 12 months.

Answer 44.28. **The answer is D.**

The NCCN "distress thermometer" is a visual analog self-report tool that also includes a list of possible sources of distress, including practical problems, family problems, emotional problems, and a comprehensive list of physical problems. Using a cutoff of 4 to 5 of a score of 10 provides an indication of distress that has been validated against other screening tools for psychological distress.

Answer 44.29. **The answer is A.**

Even though a few small studies, including a well-known study by Spiegel in 1989, reported improved survival, more recent studies, including a large multicenter trial, did not confirm these results. However, every well-conducted study of psychotherapy in patients with cancer improved quality of life or reduced stress. A study by Goodwin in patients with metastatic breast cancer showed decreased pain scores, reduced depression, and overall reduced distress.

Answer 44.30. **The answer is D.**

Remeron (mirtazapine) is most useful when agitation, anxiety, and anorexia are present, in addition to depressive symptoms. Selective serotonin reuptake inhibitors and tricyclic antidepressants have been demonstrated to be useful adjuncts in treatment of neuropathic pain.

Answer 44.31. **The answer is D.**

Use of CAM among patients with cancer is frequent and growing. There is also expanding body of knowledge regarding different forms of CAM and several completed and ongoing large-scale clinical trials of various modalities. These include herbal preparations, energy-based approaches, manipulative and body-based approaches, and mind–body medicine. It is extremely important to ask patients about their use of CAM therapies and monitor side effects that may occur, as well as incorporate knowledge into the treatment plan. Several websites have been developed to aid clinicians in identifying purported mechanisms and possible adverse effects and drug interactions of various forms of CAM, especially herbal-derived preparations.

Janakiraman Subramanian

Rehabilitation of the Cancer Patient

Directions   Each of the numbered items below is followed by lettered answers. Select the ONE lettered answer that is BEST in each case unless instructed otherwise.

QUESTIONS

Question 45.1.   **Which chemotherapy is commonly associated with peripheral neuropathy resulting in sensory ataxia and pain, usually without weakness?**

A.   Platinum analogs
B.   Vinca alkaloids
C.   Taxanes
D.   Methotrexate

Question 45.2.   **In which of the following settings is exercise NOT recommended in a patient with cancer?**

A.   Platelets 30,000 to 50,000/m^3
B.   Bony metastases with 25% to 50% cortex involvement
C.   Hematocrit <25%
D.   Sodium of 127 mmol/L

Question 45.3.   **Therapy that is specifically directed toward helping the patient's ability to perform activities of daily living is:**

A.   Occupational therapy
B.   Physical therapy
C.   Recreational therapy
D.   Speech therapy

Corresponding Chapter in *Cancer: Principles & Practice of Oncology*, Eighth Edition: 65 (Rehabilitation of the Cancer Patient).

Question 45.4.   **The treatments for radiation therapy-induced hyposalivation include all of the following, EXCEPT:**

    A. Bromhexine
    B. Pilocarpine
    C. Moist and soft foods
    D. Anticholinergic agents

Question 45.5.   **A 56-year-old Caucasian woman has recently been diagnosed with extensive-stage small cell carcinoma of the lung. She is currently undergoing chemotherapy and is having severe pain caused by metastases to her ribs. Which of the following is contraindicated?**

    A. Oxycodone
    B. Deep heat application over the ribs
    C. Rib belt
    D. Topical lidocaine

Question 45.6.   **The following therapies are approved for the management of lymphedema, EXCEPT:**

    A. Manual lymphatic drainage
    B. Compression bandaging
    C. Resistance exercises
    D. Benzopyrones

Question 45.7.   **Treatment modalities for patients with cancer who are at risk for fracture of the spine include all of the following, EXCEPT:**

    A. Surgery
    B. Thoracolumbar corset
    C. Bed rest
    D. Walker

Question 45.8.   **In patients with cancer with foot drop who have severe pain from ankle motion, the preferred ankle orthotic device is:**

    A. Solid ankle-foot orthosis
    B. Posterior leaf spring orthosis
    C. Hinged ankle foot orthosis
    D. None of the above

Question 45.9.   **The employment rights of patients with cancer are mainly protected by the:**

    A. Americans with Disabilities Act of 1990
    B. Family and Medical Leave Act of 1993
    C. Federal Rehabilitation Act of 1973
    D. Employee Retirement Income Security Act of 1974

Question 45.10.   **Of the following choices, the MOST common cause of spinal cord injury is:**

A. Leptomeningeal tumor
B. Epidural tumor
C. Intramedullary tumor
D. Paraneoplastic phenomenon

Question 45.11.   **The MOST common indication for rehabilitation care in patients with cancer undergoing treatment for their malignancy is:**

A. Deconditioning
B. Impaired mobility
C. Impaired activities of daily living
D. Reduced range of motion

Question 45.12.   **All of the following are associated with improved rehabilitation gains in patients with brain tumors, EXCEPT:**

A. Meningioma
B. Presenting at initial diagnosis
C. Left-sided brain tumor
D. Receiving radiation therapy

Question 45.13.   **The MOST common functional limitation reported by cancer survivors returning to work is:**

A. Performing physical tasks
B. Analyzing data
C. Prolonged mental concentration
D. Lifting heavy loads

ANSWERS

Answer 45.1.   **The answer is A.**

Taxanes and vinca alkaloids cause a predominately length-dependent motor and sensory axonal polyneuropathy in a distal symmetric distribution. Resulting in paresthesias, pain, sensory ataxia, and potentially weakness, this condition usually improves when the treatment is stopped. The platinum analogs damage the cell body of the sensory nerves in the dorsal root ganglion and at higher doses can damage the anterior horn cell within the spinal cord. As a result, it is more likely for patients treated with platinum analogs to have sensory neuropathy without motor weakness. The clinical manifestations include severe sensory ataxia and pain, usually without weakness. Peripheral neuropathy is not a commonly reported toxicity of methotrexate.

Answer 45.2.   **The answer is D.**

For platelets 30,000 to 50,000/m^3, the recommended activities are range of motion (ROM) exercises, aerobic activity, light weights, and ambulation. If hematocrit is <25%, ROM exercise and isometric exercises are recommended. However, aerobic exercises should be avoided. For bone metastasis involving 25% to 50% of the cortex, mild aerobic and weight-bearing exercises are recommended. In patients with sodium <130 mmol/L and potassium <3 mmol/L, no exercises are recommended until evaluated by a physician.

Answer 45.3. **The answer is A.**

Occupational therapy is directed toward helping patients perform their activities of daily living. It involves assessing their activity level, living environment, and interventions, such as exercises for strengthening, improvement in dexterity, proper posture, energy conservation, and instruction in the use of adaptive equipment. Physical therapy involves the development of strength, promotion of mobility, and pain-control techniques. Recreational therapists provide treatment services and recreation activities for individuals with disabilities or illnesses. Speech therapists address people's speech production, vocal production, swallowing difficulties, and language needs.

Answer 45.4. **The answer is D.**

Anticholinergic drugs are a well-known cause of hyposalivation, and as a result, they should not be used in patients with radiation-induced hyposalivation. Pilocarpine is a sialogogue that promotes saliva secretion by muscarinic stimulation of the salivary glands. Bromhexine promotes increased salivary secretion and reduces the viscosity.

Answer 45.5. **The answer is B.**

Cancer pain control includes both pharmacologic and nonpharmacologic treatment modalities. Both opioid medications and topical anesthetics are recommended for cancer pain control. Rib belts help with pain control in patients with rib metastasis but should not be used continuously because they can affect respiratory effort. Deep-heat modalities are recommended for cancer pain control but should not be applied directly over the malignant tumor because they can cause significant tissue damage.

Answer 45.6. **The answer is D.**

The mainstay for the management of lymphedema is complex decongestive therapy (CDT). This consists of manual lymphatic drainage by gentle massaging and compression bandaging. Resistance exercises can be performed safely by patients with lymphedema wearing compression garments. Benzopyrones are not approved in the United States in the management of lymphedema.

Answer 45.7. **The answer is C.**

Both surgical and nonsurgical treatments are recommended for impending fracture of spine caused by metastasis. In patients who are not surgical candidates or refuse surgery, alternatives include thoracolumbar corset and gait aids such as walkers. However, bed rest is not recommended, because this can result in further functional loss and increased risk for deep vein thrombosis.

Answer 45.8. **The answer is A.**

In most patients with foot drop, a ready-made or custom-made posterior leaf spring orthosis is sufficient. In patients with severe pain caused by ankle movements, an immobilizing solid ankle-foot orthosis may be more helpful.

Answer 45.9. **The answer is A.**

The Americans with Disabilities Act of 1990 protects the employment rights of patients with cancer. Additional protections are provided in the Family and Medical Leave Act of 1993, Federal Rehabilitation Act of 1973, and Employee Retirement Income Security Act of 1974.

Answer 45.10. **The answer is B.**

Epidural-based tumors are the most common cause of spinal cord injury, whereas leptomeningeal involvement occurs in only 3% to 8% of all spinal metastasis. The incidence of intramedullary tumors is less than both epidural and leptomeningeal tumors.

Answer 45.11. **The answer is A.**

In one study, the frequency of indications for rehabilitation in patients with cancer were as follows: 76% with deconditioning, 58% with mobility impairment, 43% with reduced range of motion, and 22% with impaired activities of daily living.

Answer 45.12. **The answer is D.**

Left-sided brain lesion and meningioma are associated with favorable rehabilitation outcomes. Patients with recurrence or relapse of tumor have poor outcomes when compared with patients at initial presentation. In the case of radiation therapy, there is no clear evidence regarding whether this has an adverse or favorable impact on rehabilitation.

Answer 45.13. **The answer is D.**

According to a study with 253 cancer survivors, the most common functional limitation reported was difficulty lifting heavy objects (26%), followed by performing physical tasks (18%), prolonged mental concentration (12%), and analyzing data (11%).

Societal Issues in Oncology

Directions   Each of the numbered items below is followed by lettered answers. Select the ONE lettered answer that is BEST in each case unless instructed otherwise.

QUESTIONS

Question 46.1.   **Which of the following is NOT an element of valid informed consent?**

A.   Competence or mental capacity
B.   Disclosure of information relevant to the decision
C.   Assurance of favorable outcome from treatment
D.   Voluntariness of choice, free from excessive pressure

Question 46.2.   **Surrogates should decide which interventions to provide a patient who cannot give informed consent for himself/herself according to what standards?**

A.   Substituted judgment (predicting patient's treatment preference, if competent)
B.   Best interest of the patient
C.   Best interest of the patient's family
D.   Both A and B

Question 46.3.   **Institutional review boards (IRBs) review proposed clinical trials to ensure that research trials with human beings meet all of the following requirements EXCEPT which one?**

A.   Financial incentive for subject
B.   Scientific validity
C.   Favorable risk–benefit ratio
D.   Fair subject selection

Corresponding Chapter in *Cancer: Principles & Practice of Oncology*, Eighth Edition: 66 (Societal Issues in Oncology).

Question 46.4. **Randomized controlled trials provide the highest level evidence for the efficacy and safety of a medical intervention. The ethical justification for these includes the concept of clinical equipoise, which is best defined in what manner?**

A. Determination of physician to give best treatment irrespective of trial mandates

B. Uncertainty about the merit of a treatment versus the current standard of care

C. Valuation of societal benefit over individual patient outcome by the clinician

D. Ability of study subjects to withdraw from a clinical trial whenever desired

Question 46.5. **Conflict of interest is a potential risk when industry sponsors a clinical trial. Research shows that one of the most significant impacts of industry funding is which of the following?**

A. Less rigorous methodology compared with non–industry-sponsored research

B. Data interpretation that is favorable to the company instead of objective

C. Controlled reporting and dissemination of study results

D. Frequent ownership of stock by investigators of industry-funded trials

Question 46.6. **In Cruzan v. Director of Missouri Department of Health, a case involving a 33-year-old woman in a permanent vegetative state sustained by J-tube feedings, the U.S. Supreme Court decision upheld which principle?**

A. The state has a vested interest in maintaining life regardless of circumstance.

B. Patients have a right to refuse medical treatments, including artificial nutrition.

C. Patients have a right to refuse "extraordinary means," but not basic life-sustaining interventions such as nutrition and hydration.

D. Patients may refuse all medical interventions, but surrogates must act to uphold life if the patients' wishes were not explicitly documented.

Question 46.7. **The 1976 Quinlan case supported the right to refuse life-sustaining treatments, such as respirators, and led to the establishment by several state laws authorizing the use of living wills. A living will is an example of what type of legal document?**

A. Durable power of attorney

B. Advanced healthcare directive

C. Healthcare proxy form

D. Euthanasia directive

Question 46.8. **A patient with terminal cancer asks for your assistance in hastening her death (through physician-assisted suicide or active euthanasia). The most appropriate response to this request is which of the following?**

    A. Provide active euthanasia, but not physician-assisted suicide

    B. Provide physician-assisted suicide, but not active euthanasia

    C. Intensify palliative care

    D. Refer the patient to a psychiatrist

Question 46.9. **A 41-year-old woman is diagnosed with early-stage breast cancer. Genetic testing reveals that she is BRCA1 mutation positive. She has two younger sisters who are in their late 30s. What is the most appropriate action?**

    A. Call her sisters and request that they be tested for BRCA1 status.

    B. Offer referral to a genetic counselor and provide informed consent for testing.

    C. Order mammograms for her sisters.

    D. Recommend prophylactic mastectomy for her sisters.

Question 46.10. **A study is undertaken to determine the timeliness of administration of intravenous antibiotics for patients with cancer with fever and neutropenia. This is an example of which type of quality measurement?**

    A. Process measure

    B. Structural measure

    C. Outcome measure

    D. Technical measure

Question 46.11. **What sources of data may be used for quality assessment?**

    A. Medical records

    B. Administrative databases

    C. Cancer registries

    D. All of the above

Question 46.12. **Strategies for implementing quality improvement include which of the following?**

    A. Use of evidence-based guideline recommendations in clinical practice

    B. Improvement in documentation of cancer care

    C. Implementation of health information technology

    D. All of the above

Question 46.13. **Investigational New Drug (IND) applications are submitted to the Food and Drug Administration (FDA) for review at which phase of development?**

    A. Before phase I trials

    B. Before phase II trials

    C. Before phase III trials

    D. After completion of a phase III trial demonstrating clear evidence of efficacy

Question 46.14.   **Pharmaceutical companies submit a New Drug Applications (NDA) to the FDA for approval of the sales and marketing of a new drug. These sponsors must provide evidence that the drug is safe and effective based on "adequate and well-controlled clinical investigations." Oncology drugs have been approved by the FDA on the basis of supporting clinical trials with which of the following primary endpoints?**

    A. Overall survival or disease-free survival
    B. Tumor response rate
    C. Palliation
    D. All of the above

Question 46.15.   **Expanded access protocols are designed with what goal in mind?**

    A. Increasing the size of a clinical protocol for statistical robustness
    B. Enabling access to investigational drugs when no viable alternative is available
    C. Providing medications to patients unable to afford prescribed drugs
    D. Increasing market share of a newly approved medication

Question 46.16.   **Which of the following statements is NOT true?**

    A. Black Americans have higher cancer-specific mortality than white Americans.
    B. Black Americans have lower survival than white Americans.
    C. Black Americans have higher cancer incidence rates than white Americans.
    D. None of the above; all are true.

ANSWERS

Answer 46.1.   **The answer is C.**

Legal rulings have clarified that essential components of informed consent include competence (the mental capacity of a person to make healthcare decisions), disclosure (information on the diagnosis, proposed intervention, potential risks and benefits, and alternative treatments), understanding (patient's grasp of information disclosed), and voluntariness (choice that is free from interference by others, such as coercion or excessive pressure).

Answer 46.2.   **The answer is D.**

There are two standard principles to guide surrogate decision-makers for patients who cannot give informed consent: substituted judgment and best interests. Substituted judgment refers to the attempt to determine the incompetent person's preferences regarding a decision if that person were to be competent. The best interest standard refers to an objective evaluation of benefits and risks, and selection of the treatment in which benefit maximally outweighs the burdens of treatment for the individual patient.

Answer 46.3.   **The answer is A.**

Ethical requirements of clinical trials on human subjects are meant to minimize exploitation of research participants. These ethical principles, stated in guidelines issued by multiple agencies, include the principles of collaborative partnership, social value, scientific validity, fair subject selection, favorable risk–benefit ratio, independent review, informed consent, and respect for potential and enrolled subjects.

Answer 46.4.   **The answer is B.**

Clinical equipoise is present when there is a legitimate disagreement among clinicians about optimal treatment, particularly when there is lack of reliable data and genuine uncertainty about which treatment is best for a patient. When this principle is met, there is no violation of the physician–patient relationship, in which the physician is acting on behalf of the patient's best interest.

Answer 46.5.   **The answer is C.**

Studies sponsored by industry have been found to be at least as methodologically rigorous, if not more so, than non-industry sponsored trials. Financial incentive for companies to avoid methodologic flaws that discredit study results has been suggested as the reason for this finding. There is little evidence to suggest that interpretation of data is frequently biased by financial considerations. Several studies point to the impact of industry funding on dissemination of trial results, including suppression of adverse findings, delayed or lack of publishing negative results, and multiple publications of results favorable to industry. Although personal stock ownership by clinical investigators is a common concern, this is rare in actual practice.

Answer 45.6.   **The answer is B.**

The U.S. Supreme Court affirmed patients' right to refuse medical treatments in its Cruzan decision. The rationale was that patients have a right to determine which treatments are acceptable and that any medical interventions including medications, respirator care, and gastric tubes may be refused by competent patients or their surrogates. The ruling also upheld that in the absence of "clear and convincing evidence" of a patient's wishes, states may regulate how families exercise a patient's "right to die."

Answer 46.7.   **The answer is B.**

The Quinlan case, involving a 21-year-old New Jersey woman in a persistent vegetative state dependent on a respirator, upheld the right to refuse life-sustaining treatments. The 1976 case led to the passage of the first living will law in California, and nearly all states now have similar legislation. Living wills, which specify a patient's preferences regarding specific care decisions, and durable power of attorney documents, which authorize an individual selected by the patient to act as a proxy regarding healthcare decisions, are both forms of advanced healthcare directives.

Answer 46.8.   **The answer is C.**

The most appropriate response to a patient's request for hastened death is to intensify palliative care. Exploration of a patient's request often results in identifying unmet needs and new palliative care interventions that may be helpful, as stated in the National Comprehensive Cancer Network guidelines. Active euthanasia, in which a physician intentionally ends a patient's life at his/her request and with his/her consent, is not legal anywhere in the United States. Physician-assisted suicide, in which a physician provides a medication or other intervention to a patient with the understanding that the patient intends to use them to commit suicide, is legal only in the states of Oregon and Washington.

Answer 46.9.   **The answer is B.**

Genetic testing may be advisable for people with increased susceptibility to cancer because of family history or other predisposing factors. Such information may provide useful information to patients and their families to seek further interventions, such as early mammography or prophylactic mastectomy in patients with BRCA1 mutations. Testing may be associated with potential psychological, social, or economic harm, and a proper informed consent process should include discussion about the pros and cons. Genetic counselors may provide help in this process.

Answer 46.10.   **The answer is A.**

Quality measurement refers to the practice of evaluating care processes to bring about improvement and include structural, process, and outcome measures. Structural measures evaluate characteristics of providers or the care system, such as rates of board certification or volume of procedures. Process measures examine the actions taken by providers, such as delivery of a specific care component that has been demonstrated to be favorable for patient outcomes based on clinical trials or guideline recommendations. Outcome measures refer to patient results, including measures of quality of life, disease-free survival, and overall survival.

Answer 46.11.   **The answer is D.**

Quality data sources include medical records, patient surveys, administrative databases (e.g., Medicare claims), and registries. The National Cancer Data Base (NCDB) and the Surveillance Epidemiology and End Results (SEER) program of the National Cancer Institute (NCI) are examples of cancer registry programs in the United States. Each of these data sources may provide useful information for quality research.

Answer 46.12.   **The answer is D.**

All of the above measures are examples of strategies to improve quality of care delivered to patients with cancer. Guideline recommendations, such as the National Comprehensive Cancer Network (NCCN), may help to integrate evidence-based medicine into clinical practice. Improved documentation of cancer care can facilitate better care coordination, safety, and efficiency. Health information technologies, when implemented in the context of an overall process design, may improve efficiency and quality of care through measures such as point-of-service reminders or standardized order sets.

Answer 46.13.   **The answer is A.**

Investigational drugs must be administered under an IND application that is submitted to the FDA. The initial IND application typically consists of a proposed phase I clinical protocol and supporting data regarding safety. These data may include in vitro, animal, or human evidence describing drug toxicity and a predicted safe starting dose, as well as manufacturing data regarding the drug product. A panel of scientific reviewers from the FDA then determines if such data are sufficient to proceed with the proposed study without unreasonable risk of injury or harm.

Answer 46.14.   **The answer is D.**

From 1990 to 2006, 94 oncology drug marketing applications were approved by the FDA. End points supporting FDA approval included overall survival and disease-free survival, tumor response rates, response rate supported by additional data, and palliation or amelioration of symptoms (e.g., Neulasta, Leukine, and Ethyol approvals).

Answer 46.15.   **The answer is B.**

Expanded access protocols are designed to facilitate availability of investigational drugs when certain conditions are met: No satisfactory alternative treatment is available, the drug sponsor is pursuing marketing approval with due diligence, the drug is nearing the end of its development, and data support efficacy for use in the intended population. The National Cancer Institute (NCI) has provided expanded access to investigational drugs through an agreement with the FDA in these situations.

Answer 46.16.   **The answer is D.**

Research based on the SEER database has consistently shown that compared with white Americans, black Americans have higher cancer incidence rates, cancer-specific mortality rates, and all-cause mortality rates. These racial disparities have been attributed to inadequate access to financial and healthcare resources, risk-promoting lifestyles and behavior, and social inequities.

Information Systems in Oncology

Directions: Each of the numbered items below is followed by lettered answers. Select the ONE lettered answer that is BEST in each case unless instructed otherwise.

QUESTIONS

Question 47.1.   **Which of the following is NOT a criterion for being defined as an electronic health record (EHR) according to the Institute of Medicine (2003 report)?**

A.   It includes a longitudinal collection of information about individuals pertaining to the health of or healthcare provided to that individual.

B.   It offers immediate electronic access to information about individuals and populations by authorized users.

C.   It is accessible to the patient to facilitate compilation of records in case of a need to transfer medical care.

D.   It incorporates knowledge and decision support to enhance quality, safety, and patient care efficiency.

E.   It improves the efficiency of healthcare delivery.

Question 47.2.   **Of the many terms used to describe electronic health information, which is MOST commonly used and describes an electronic method of storing and integrating patient information in an organized, clinically pertinent, and legal format that assists in the care of patients?**

A.   EHR

B.   Electronic medical record (EMR)

C.   Electronic patient record (EPR)

D.   Computer-based patient record (CPR)

Corresponding Chapter in *Cancer: Principles & Practice of Oncology*, Eighth Edition: 67 (Information Systems in Oncology).

Question 47.3.   **All of the following are commonly accepted advantages of an EMR over paper charts, EXCEPT:**

A. Smaller space requirements
B. Improved provider accessibility
C. Traceable record of provider access
D. Greater cost-effectiveness
E. None of the above

Question 47.4.   **Which of the following does NOT help to improve efficiency of documentation in EMRs?**

A. The ability to "cut and paste" or use shortcuts to facilitate quick repetition of pertinent data
B. The ability to "pull" information from defined data fields into notes
C. Electronic proofreading functions to ensure uniform note structure
D. Ability to dictate and have notes transcribed into electronic chart records
E. None of the above

Question 47.5.   **All of the following mechanisms enhance patient safety with EMRs, EXCEPT:**

A. Removal of variable of physician handwriting
B. Notification about relevant allergies
C. Alerts about limitations in standard dose ranges
D. Notifications about potentially harmful medication interactions
E. None of the above

Question 47.6.   **How are outside records MOST commonly integrated into EMRs?**

A. Results are summarized into a separate document that is typed into the electronic record.
B. Outside documents are scanned into the EMR.
C. Results are dictated into the electronic record.
D. Note is made of off-site storage of paper records available as needed.

Question 47.7.   **Which of the following statements is TRUE about the state of EMR implementation (as of 2006)?**

A. The United States is among the world leaders in adopting this technology.
B. The majority of current hospitals use EMRs.
C. Errors and unforeseen technical problems rarely occur.
D. It is often recommended that clinics decrease their planned workflow by 50% in the first week after implementation.

Question 47.8.   **All of the following are reasons that computerized order entry functions must be accessible from within the patient chart, EXCEPT:**

A. Automated billing can be facilitated by linking orders to patient records in real time.
B. The system should link the orders with the correct patient.
C. The healthcare provider can have access to current clinical data.
D. "Rules engines" can generate alerts if needed on the basis of allergies or laboratory results.

Question 47.9.   **Which of the following is NOT a component of computerized provider order entry systems in general?**

A. Order sets
B. Electronic prescribing (outpatient)
C. Outpatient scheduling
D. Approval by supervising physicians or with pharmacy approval before implementation

Question 47.10.   **Which of the following is NOT a feature of oncology-based EMRs systems?**

A. Schedules of treatment cycle administration
B. Dose therapy calculations
C. Adverse event monitoring
D. Automated calculation of tumor sizing on follow-up imaging

Question 47.11.   **Advantages of patient portals to EMRs commonly include all of the following, EXCEPT:**

A. Patient access to view clinic schedules
B. Ability to have unlimited access to their patient record and imaging
C. Ability to request prescription refills
D. Secure messaging communication, with a means of asking questions to their physicians

Question 47.12.   **Which of the following statements about Internet use is INCORRECT?**

A. Use for gathering information about healthcare has been rapidly increasing over the past several years.
B. Seekers of health information generally restrict their focus to needs for their personal medical issues.
C. Access is largely correlated with higher household income.
D. It often has an impact on treatment decisions.

Question 47.13.   **Which of the following topics is typically the subject of a search for information on cancer management on the Internet?**

A. Diagnostic tests
B. Common treatment approaches
C. Clinical trials
D. Physicians
E. All of the above

Question 47.14.   **All of the following statements about Internet-based searching for medical information are true, EXCEPT:**

A. More people seek medical information from a search engine than a health-related website.
B. Content retrieved from different search engines is largely redundant.
C. Significant amounts of valuable information are often not available via search engine because it is too "deep" and not "crawled" by automated search engine cataloguing software.
D. Much of the medical information available on the Internet is available only by paid subscription.

Question 47.15.   **Which of the following is NOT a principle of the Health on the Net code of conduct?**

A. Financial disclosure of funding sources
B. Justifiability of conclusions about the efficacy of approaches by evidence
C. Interactivity to allow healthcare information seekers to reach information providers
D. Authority, specifically conveying the qualifications of authors

Question 47.16.   **Saved searches can be sent as e-mail alerts with the following application:**

A. Pubmed's "My NCBI"
B. Google Scholar
C. Wikipedia
D. Blogsearch

Question 47.17.   **Which of the following is NOT a social networking site?**

A. Wikipedia
B. Healtheva
C. Medicine blogs
D. American Society of Clinical Oncology (ASCO) site

ANSWERS

Answer 47.1.   **The answer is C.**

The four main characteristics of an EHR according to the 2003 Institute of Medicine report are that it (a) includes a longitudinal collection of information about individuals pertaining to the health of an individual; (b) offers immediate electronic access to information about individuals and populations solely by authorized users; (c) incorporates knowledge and decision support to enhance quality, safety, and patient care efficiency; and (d) improves the efficiency of healthcare delivery. Limited accessibility of information directly to the patient is sometimes a feature but is not considered a central characteristic of an EHR.

Answer 47.2.   **The answer is B.**

EHR is the broadest term and refers to all records of a patient's care across multiple institutions, sites, and providers, with integration of that documentation to other information technology. EPR and CPR are both synonymous with the term "electronic medical record" (EMR), which is the most commonly used term that is applicable to the discussion of a particular patient's computerized medical record at a specific institution.

Answer 47.3.   **The answer is D.**

There are many advantages of an EMR with paper charting, including smaller space requirements, improved provider accessibility such as synchronous use by more than one provider, a traceable record of provider access, and other factors, but an EMR clearly requires a significant initial cost outlay and training time. Although there is some debate that an EMR may be cost-effective compared with paper over time, it is widely accepted that the initial costs of an EMR are a significant disadvantage.

Answer 47.4.   **The answer is C.**

There are many time-saving features commonly incorporated into the documentation process for EMR systems. These typically include an ability to cut and paste content from one document into another, as well as the ability to automatically populate data fields in a note with information available in the system. Moreover, providers can enter content via direct typing, dictation/transcription, and sometimes "drop-down" menus of common text options for text fields. However, EMR systems do not typically offer electronic proofreading functions at this time.

Answer 47.5.   **The answer is E.**

Patient safety is enhanced using an EMR by all of the noted factors, including improved legibility of documentation and orders, notification of medicine and other relevant allergies, alerts about limitations in medicine dosing, notifications about potentially harmful medication interactions, and alerts about abnormal laboratory values and other issues that may change therapeutic decisions.

Answer 47.6.   **The answer is B.**

Currently, the most common solution for integrating paper records, such as informed consents, outside medical records, and other documentation that is not available in electronic form, is to scan this information and incorporate it into a patient's electronic record. This typically limits the ability to find and search for information within outside records. Ideally, relevant reports are placed in the appropriate area of the EMR and can be retrieved directly by clicking within the EMR to view scanned documents.

Answer 47.7.   **The answer is D.**

Implementation of EMR solutions is still in the early stages and not yet prevalent in the United States, compared with countries such as Sweden and The Netherlands, among others. As of 2006, only a small minority of U.S.-based inpatient and outpatient facilities have a comprehensive EMR system, although the majority of healthcare systems view laboratory data electronically. Despite planning, it is very typical for bugs and glitches in work flow to occur as a new EMR system "goes live," leading to the typical recommendation for healthcare providers to significantly reduce their planned schedules, both inpatient and outpatient, in the first few days after a new EMR is implemented.

Answer 47.8.   **The answer is A.**

Computerized provider order entry (CPOE) is conducted from within a specific patient's electronic record to ensure association of new orders with the correct patient, to provide access to the most recent laboratory and other clinical results for the patient, and to generate any indicated alerts based on laboratory values, concurrent medications, allergies, and other relevant clinical data. Although some systems may include features that help facilitate billing, this has been complex and associated with practical problems that limit the utility of automated in this setting, and it is not a common aspect of CPOE at the present time.

Answer 47.9.   **The answer is C.**

CPOE adds convenience in many respects, including the ability to develop customized order sets for commonly repeated activities, prescriptions for outpatient medications, and preliminary orders that can be activated later on the basis of defined laboratory parameters or the co-signature of an attending physician. Outpatient scheduling is not generally integrated into CPOE functions.

Answer 47.10.   **The answer is D.**

EMR systems can offer several benefits related to organization and documentation specific to the practice of medical oncology. These include easier tracking of the schedule of treatment with chemotherapy or other approaches, automated calculations of medication dosing that incorporates relevant patient data, and cataloguing of adverse events that includes timing and severity. Although measurement of tumor size on serial body imaging is a necessary component of oncology practice, this remains outside of the technical capabilities of current automated systems and is not included among the anticipated features of an EMR system.

Answer 47.11.   **The answer is B.**

Patient portals offer many advantages for patients that may improve reported satisfaction with their care. The most common include the ability for patients to log in securely and view their appointment and test schedules, to request refills of outpatient medications, to communicate via a secure channel with their health team and ask clinical questions, and sometimes to review limited portions of the EMR for their care. Patient portals do not routinely include unlimited access to all documentation and imaging results.

Answer 47.12.   **The answer is B.**

It is true that use of the Internet for the collection of healthcare information has been rapidly increasing in recent years, and that this information commonly has an impact on patient management? Users of the Internet tend to have higher household incomes and are most typically in the younger age range compared with the general population. The healthcare information collected is not typically limited to applicability for the individual seeking information, but rather is often for the benefit of family or friends.

Answer 47.13.   **The answer is E.**

Searches for information on cancer management commonly focus on diagnostic tests, common treatment strategies, available clinical trial options, and recommendations for and background of relevant physicians.

Answer 47.14.   **The answer is B.**

Searches for medical information more commonly begin from general search engines than a website providing specific medical information. However, much of the data-rich medical content is not indexed by automated webcrawler applications and may require users to register to see this information, and a significant subset of this information may only be available with a paid subscription. Interestingly, results obtained from different search engines while using the same search terms are largely nonoverlapping.

Answer 47.15.   **The answer is C.**

The Health on the Net Foundation's "HONcode" notes that health and medical websites should be authoritative, should attribute sources of published information, and should demonstrate complementarily, privacy, justifiability, transparency, financial disclosure of funding sources, and sponsorship by clearly distinguishing advertising from editorial content. Interactivity is a feature that is uncommonly incorporated into a medical website but is not a component of the HONcode.

Answer 47.16.   **The answer is A.**

PubMed includes a feature for those who register for a free My NCBI account in which searches can be saved and sent as-mail alerts. Google Scholar does not include e-mail alerts, but it is possible to generate these using Google Alerts (http://www.google.com/alerts) to receive notification of news articles about medical topics. Wikipedia and Blogsearch both include medically relevant information but do not incorporate searches that are saved and e-mailed.

Answer 47.17. **The answer is D.**

Social networking websites allow groups of individuals to converge and share information, and such sites include weblogs ("blogs"), wikis (communal, collaborative authoring of information at a central website), and physician-oriented social websites such as Healtheva (http://www.healtheve.com) to exchange thoughts and network. The ASCO website includes a vast array of oncology information, but it is not currently designed for the interactivity typical of what would be considered a social networking site.

Complementary, Alternative, and Integrative Therapies in Cancer Care

Directions   Each of the numbered items below is followed by lettered answers. Select the ONE lettered answer that is BEST in each case unless instructed otherwise.

QUESTIONS

Question 48.1.   **A 55-year-old African American woman recently diagnosed with metastatic carcinoma of the colon has been scheduled for first-line chemotherapy with irinotecan (CPT-11) and 5-fluorouracil and leucovorin. She was advised by her aunt to take an herbal potion containing St. John's Wort (*Hypericum perforatum*) for anxiety relief. She tells her that it helped her deal with anxiety before her breast cancer surgery. Which one of these responses is appropriate regarding the use of this herbal supplement during chemotherapy with irinotecan?**

A.   There is no scientific evidence supporting its anxiolytic effects.
B.   St. John's Wort increases the side effects from treatment with irinotecan.
C.   St. John's Wort results in more than 50% reduction in serum levels of the active metabolite of irinotecan.
D.   There is an increased risk of bleeding when used concomitantly with irinotecan.

Question 48.2.   **Which of the following commonly used herbal supplements inhibit the hepatic cytochrome P450 system?**

A.   St. John's wort (*Hypericum perforatum*)
B.   Oregano (*Origanum vulgare*)
C.   Psyllium (*Plantago ispaghula*)
D.   Grapefruit juice

Corresponding Chapter in *Cancer: Principles & Practice of Oncology*, Eighth Edition: 68 (Complementary, Alternative, and Integrative Therapies in Cancer Care).

Question 48.3.   **Which of the following herbal medicine products has significant effects on the antitumor properties of tamoxifen?**

    A. Tea tree oil
    B. Fish oil (omega-3)
    C. Soy supplements
    D. Kava

Question 48.4.   **A 70-year-old Caucasian man with refractory multiple myeloma was treated with lenalidomide plus dexamethasone. After two cycles the patient developed pulmonary embolism and deep vein thrombosis of the right leg. Chemotherapy was discontinued, and the patient was started on anticoagulation with home enoxaparin injections. He comes to your office for a scheduled visit and reports taking an herbal remedy containing Ginkgo extracts to help his memory and cognitive function. Which of the following statement is TRUE regarding the effects of Ginkgo?**

    A. Increases the risk of serious bleeds
    B. Will increase the metabolism of enoxaparin
    C. Decreases the responsiveness of myeloma to further chemotherapy
    D. May increase risk of infection from immunosuppression

Question 48.5.   **Radiation-induced oral mucositis is common among patients with cancer being treated with radiation, particularly in patients with head and neck carcinoma. Which of the following interventions may decrease the incidence of symptomatic oral radiation-induced oral mucositis?**

    A. α-tocopherol (vitamin E) rinse before and after therapy
    B. Yucca extracts
    C. Saw palmetto
    D. Aloe vera

Question 48.6.   **Which of the following statements regarding the relation between diet and prostate cancer risk is/are TRUE?**

    A. High lycopene-containing diet is associated with reduced risk for developing prostate cancer.
    B. Fish oil (omega-3) supplements can reduce the risk for prostate cancer.
    C. Diet rich in lycopene and fish oil may offer meaningful protection against prostate cancer progression.
    D. All the above.

Question 48.7.   A 60-year-old Hispanic man with early-stage squamous cell carcinoma of the lung has recently undergone surgical resection. He comes to your office for recommendations on adjuvant chemotherapy. He tells you that after his surgery he has been taking some herbal supplements "to fight his cancer," sent by his friend from Mexico. He has felt weak and anorectic for the past few weeks and experienced mild intermittent pain in the right upper quadrant of his abdomen. He takes no other medications, including over-the-counter medications. He does not use alcohol regularly and had no other known medical disorders. On examination of the patient, jaundice was noted, but no other significant findings were present. His initial laboratory test results revealed abnormal liver function tests, with total bilirubin 5.9 mg/dL, direct bilirubin 4.4 mg/dL, aspartate aminotransferase 52 U/L, alanine aminotransferase 272 U/L, total alkaline phosphatase 153 U/L, and γ-glutamyltransferase 226 U/L (0 to 45 U/L). The prothrombin time was normal. Which of the following herbal supplements has been associated with severe hepatotoxicity?

A. Mistletoe
B. Chaparral
C. Green Tea
D. Maitake

Question 48.8.   Which of the following herbal remedies has been widely used for treatment of prostate cancer?

A. Kava (*Piper methysticum*)
B. Ginger (*Zingiber officinale*)
C. PC-SPES
D. Alfalfa (*Medicago sativa*)

Question 48.9.   A 45-year-old African American man with locally advanced adenocarcinoma of the lung is currently undergoing concurrent chemotherapy with radiation. On one regular office visit, the patient reports taking Kava extracts (60 mg/d) to relieve his anxiety and insomnia. He tells you that it helped his symptoms very well and asks you if it is safe to continue taking this medicine. Which of the following responses is TRUE regarding Kava extracts?

A. There is no scientific evidence supporting the efficacy of Kava extracts in relieving anxiety and insomnia in patients with cancer.
B. Significantly reduces chemotherapy agents in the blood levels.
C. Increases the toxicity of chemotherapy.
D. Kava extracts may cause severe hepatotoxicity.

Question 48.10. **A 50-year-old woman with metastatic breast cancer completed her fourth cycle of single-agent docetaxel 4 days ago. She now presents to the emergency department with severe nausea, vomiting, and diarrhea. Her laboratory test results reveal severe neutropenia with a total white blood cell (WBC) count of 400 cells/mm^3 and severe thrombocytopenia with a platelet count of 30,000 mm^3. She is admitted to the hospital, and with appropriate supportive care she recovers well from the episode and presents to your clinic for further chemotherapy. On careful history taking, she reveals that after her last cycle of chemotherapy she started taking grapefruit juice to relieve her heartburn symptoms from chemotherapy. Which of the following is the appropriate next step in her care?**

A. Discontinue grapefruit juice and continue chemotherapy at scheduled dose.

B. Discontinue grapefruit juice and delay the next dose of chemotherapy.

C. Continue taking grapefruit juice and resume chemotherapy with a 25% dose reduction.

D. Resume chemotherapy at the current dose as scheduled.

ANSWERS

Answer 48.1. **The answer is C.**

St. John's wort has been extensively studied in the treatment of mild to moderate depression and was found to be more effective than placebo and equally effective as tricyclic antidepressants (TCAs) in the treatment of mild-to-moderate major depression. However, because of multiple well-documented drug interactions, its use has been discouraged in patients. Hyperforin, a principal constituent of St John's wort, appears to induce the hepatic enzyme cytochrome P-4503A4 with repeated administration. Irinotecan is metabolized via this pathway, and patients receiving irinotecan (CPT-11) have a greater than 50% reduction in serum levels of the active metabolite SN-38 after concomitant administration of St. John's wort. St John's wort may increase CYP3A4 activity to a greater extent in women than in men. Thus, use of such herbal supplements that interact with the P450 system is of particular concern to patients with cancer, because many chemotherapeutic agents (e.g., cyclophosphamide, ifosfamide, docetaxel, paclitaxel, vincristine, vinblastine, vinorelbine, irinotecan, and etoposide) are CYP3A4 and/or p-glycoprotein substrates.

Answer 48.2. **The answer is D.**

Several herbal remedies inhibit cytochrome P-450 and increase the blood levels of drugs metabolized by the P-450 system. Common agents in this category include grapefruit juice, milk thistle, goldenseal, cat's claw, wild cherry, cannabinoids, chamomile, and licorice.

Answer 48.3.   **The answer is C.**

Some women experience menopause-like symptoms with tamoxifen, including hot flashes and emotional changes. Phytoestrogens, such as genistein, are the major constituents of soy and exhibit selective estrogen receptor modulator activity. Soy products are popular among women experiencing perimenopausal symptoms. However, in patients with breast cancer, genistein might antagonize the effects of tamoxifen, making it less effective and possibly helping proliferation of the breast cancer cells.

Answer 48.4.   **The answer is A.**

Herbs such as ginkgo, feverfew, ginger, and garlic have anticoagulant effects and should be avoided by patients using warfarin, heparin, aspirin, and related agents.

Answer 48.5.   **The answer is A.**

Patients undergoing radiation for head and neck cancers have a high incidence of radiation-induced mucositis. Acute severe oral mucositis is associated with significant discomfort and impairment of the patient's ability to eat and swallow. Oral rinses with vitamin E before and after radiation therapy appear to decrease the incidence of symptomatic oral radiation-induced mucositis.

Answer 48.6.   **The answer is D.**

Several case control studies have reported reduced risk of developing prostate cancer with a diet rich in lycopene and fish oil (omega-3 fatty acids). Some studies have also shown that a diet including lycopene and fish oil reduces disease progression in patients with prostate cancer.

Answer 48.7.   **The answer is B.**

Chaparral is a Native American herb that has purported anti-inflammatory and anticancer effects. There is no scientific evidence supporting the anticancer effects of chaparral. Numerous reports indicate hepatotoxicity after the use of chaparral and often severe fulminant hepatic failure requiring transplantation. Other common herbal supplements with significant hepatic toxicity include birch oil, blessed thistle, kava, germander, dehydroepiandrosterone (DHEA), and turmeric.

Answer 48.8.   **The answer is C.**

PC-SPES is an herbal product that is a mixture of eight herbs: reishi mushroom, baikal skullcap, Rabdosia, Dyer's woad, chrysanthemum, saw palmetto, Panax ginseng, and licorice. PC-SPES was a very popular herbal supplement to treat prostate cancer. Use of PC-SPES has demonstrated significant decreases in androgen and prostate-specific antigen (PSA) levels in humans. In vitro experiments revealed inhibition of growth and proliferation of human tumor cell lines, including androgen-sensitive and insensitive prostate cancer.

Answer 48.9.   **The answer is D.**

Kava extracts are commonly used by patients with cancer for anxiety and insomnia. Several randomized, controlled clinical trials have reported relief of anxiety and insomnia. However, numerous reports of severe hepatotoxicity have been reported. The use of Kava extracts has not been approved by the Food and Drug administration for the above indication.

Answer 48.10.   **The answer is B.**

Grapefruit extracts inhibit cytochrome P450 isoenzymes and therefore affect serum concentrations of drugs metabolized by the cytochrome P450 3A4 system. Several chemotherapy agents, including docetaxel, paclitaxel, vincristine, vinblastine, vinorelbine, irinotecan, etoposide, and tamoxifen, are metabolized by the cytochrome P450 3A4 system, and concomitant use of grapefruit juice would decrease the clearance of these drugs and thus increase the toxicity from these drugs. Patients should discontinue grapefruit consumption for at least 96 hours before resuming chemotherapy.

Nithya Ramnath
Anubha Bharthuar
Krishnan Raghavendran

Newer Approaches in Cancer Treatment

Directions   Each of the numbered items below is followed by lettered answers. Select the ONE lettered answer that is BEST in each case unless instructed otherwise.

QUESTIONS

Question 49.1.   **Nonviral methods of gene transfer include all the following, EXCEPT:**

A. Introduction of DNA- or RNA-coated microscopic gold beads into target cells by firing them under high pressure and velocity
B. Use of pulsed electric field to temporarily open microscopic pores in cell membranes allowing entry of nucleic acid into the target cell
C. Formation of DNA and cationic lipid or polymer complexes with uptake by target cell via endocytosis or phagocytosis
D. Use of mobile functional DNA elements with the ability to randomly integrate into target cell genome
E. Polyethylene glycol-bound DNA/RNA, introduced into target cell by ligand binding

Question 49.2.   **Which of the following is essential for viral gene therapy?**

A. Replication defective viral vector
B. Actively dividing host cells
C. Large viral genome
D. Transcription defective viral genome
E. Ability to induce immune response

Corresponding Chapters in *Cancer: Principles & Practice of Oncology,* Eighth Edition: 69 (Gene Therapy), 70 (Cancer Immunotherapy), 71 (Focused Ultrasound), 72 (RNA Inhibition), 73 (Charged Particle Therapy), 74 (Robotic Surgery), and 75 (Nanotechnology).

Question 49.3.   **Adenovirus with E1B gene deletion tested in head and neck cancers uses which principle of gene therapy?**

A. Suicide gene therapy
B. Tumor suppressor gene therapy
C. Oncolytic virus gene therapy
D. Adoptive cell therapy
E. None of the above

Question 49.4.   **A 53-year-old woman underwent resection of a 2.5-mm metastatic melanoma Clark level IV with ulceration on her right forearm. Axillary lymph node dissection revealed one lymph node positive for melanoma. She received adjuvant therapy with interferon-alpha. Two years later she developed chronic cough, and chest computed tomography (CT) revealed multiple lung nodules and bilateral axillary lymphadenopathy. Biopsy of right axillary lymph node was consistent with metastatic melanoma. The patient is enrolled in a clinical trial and scheduled to receive autologous tumor-infiltrating lymphocytes (TILs). Which of the following immunosuppressive regimens will provide her with the BEST chance of being alive at 2 years?**

A. Cyclophosphamide 60 mg/m^2 for 2 days followed by fludarabine 25 mg/m^2 for 5 days
B. Cyclophosphamide 60 mg/m^2 for 2 days and fludarabine 25 mg/m^2 for 5 days, followed by total body irradiation (TBI) 200 cGy
C. Cyclophosphamide 60 mg/m^2 for 2 days followed by TBI 1200 cGy, given over 3 days
D. No immunosuppressive therapy

Question 49.5.   **A 44-year-old patient underwent allogeneic peripheral blood stem cell transplant from a matched unrelated donor for acute meyloid leukemia (AML) FABM5 in first remission. He developed chronic graft-versus-host disease (GVHD) and immunosuppression with mycophenolate, and tacrolimus is continued beyond day 100. Six months after the transplant he reported symptoms of numbness and soreness of the gums. An initial diagnosis of gingivitis was made, but he then developed low-grade fevers, sore throat, bilateral cervical lymphadenopathy, and hepatosplenomegaly. Biopsy of the right cervical lymph node demonstrated B-cell hyperplasia. Immunoperoxidase stain demonstrated Epstein-Barr virus (EBV)-positive B cells, confirming a diagnosis of posttransplant lymphoproliferative disorder (PTLD). Which of the following treatments may have prevented the occurrence of PTLD?**

A. Intravenous gammaglobulin
B. Acyclovir
C. Interferon-alpha
D. EBV-specific donor T-cell lymphocyte infusion

Question 49.6.   A 32-year-old African American woman underwent human leukocyte antigen (HLA)-matched sibling allogeneic bone marrow transplant for Philadelphia chromosome–positive chronic myeloid leukemia (CML) in blast
crisis. Conditioning regimen consisted of TBI and cyclophosphamide.
She received tacrolimus and methotrexate for prevention of GVHD. She
achieved a complete hematologic and molecular remission, as documented by a negative result of reverse transcriptase polymerase chain
reaction (RT-PCR) analysis of the bcr-abl gene product. Seven years later
she developed symptoms of fever, night sweats, early satiety, and weight
loss. Peripheral blood white blood cell (WBC) count was 45,000 with
8% blasts, and immunophenotype was consistent with her pretransplant
CML with 9:22 translocation. What should be done next?

A.   Donor lymphocyte infusion
B.   Imatinib
C.   Induction chemotherapy with high-dose cytarabine and idarubicin
D.   Second allogeneic transplant

Question 49.7.   Please arrange the steps involved in adoptive cell immunotherapy for
patients of metastatic myeloma in the correct sequence.

a.   Infusion of autologous TILs
b.   Selection of culture with antitumor activity for expansion
c.   Generation of multiple cultures of TILs
d.   Interleukin (IL)-2 therapy and CD 34+ autologous cell infusion
e.   Resection of tumor
f.   Lymphodepletion with cyclophosphamide, fludarabine, and total
     body radiation
A.   e, b, c, d, a, f
B.   e, c, b, a, f, d
C.   e, c, b, f, a, d
D.   e, b, c, a, f, d

Question 49.8.   A 59-year-old Hispanic woman is evaluated for postmenopausal bleeding.
Transvaginal ultrasound reveals a 4.5-cm uterine fibroid. The patient
has poorly controlled diabetes and a history of coronary artery disease.
She refuses hysterectomy but is willing to undergo a noninvasive proce-
dure. You are considering performing focused ultrasound surgery.
Which of the following would be a contraindication for this procedure?

A.   History of von Willebrand's disease
B.   Presence of a pacemaker
C.   Weight >300 lbs
D.   History of myocardial infarction 2 weeks ago

Question 49.9.   **In which of the following cases has focused ultrasound been approved by the Food and Drug Administration (FDA)?**

A. A 67-year-old African American man with a history of hepatitis C was recently diagnosed with hepatocellular carcinoma. The patient has Child-Pugh class B with one neoplastic lesion in the right lobe measuring 3.7 cm and two lesions in the left lobe measuring 1.7 and 2.6 cm.

B. A 38-year-old Caucasian woman has a history of uterine leiomyomas. She has been unable to carry a pregnancy to full term and recently started to develop severe lower abdominal and pelvic cramps.

C. A 43-year-old Caucasian woman has a 5-cm breast fibroadenoma. Her Gail model risk score is 1.8. She has two maternal aunts who were diagnosed with breast cancer in their early 50s.

D. A 56-year-old Asian woman was found to have a 2-cm lesion in the upper-outer quadrant of her right breast on mammogram. Biopsy was consistent with estrogen receptor (ER) + /progesterone receptor (PR) + well-differentiated adenocarcinoma.

Question 49.10.   **Focused ultrasound involves all of the following, EXCEPT:**

A. Implosion of microbubbles generating high pressures and propagating shock waves

B. Real-time temperature sensitive imaging

C. Conversion of acoustic energy to thermal energy causing irreversible thermal coagulation necrosis

D. Hyperthermia and tumor killing at a narrow temperature range maintained for a longer time within a large volume

Question 49.11.   **Which of the following is NOT a potential application for focused ultrasound?**

A. Targeted drug delivery and gene therapy

B. Adhesiolysis

C. Tumor ablation

D. Hemostasis and occlusion of blood vessels

Question 49.12.   **True or False:**

A. Genetic alterations in cancer are seen only in the protein coding areas.

B. Inactivation of tumor-suppressing protein coding genes and activation of oncogenic microRNA (miRNA) have the same molecular consequences.

C. It is possible to target the mRNA specifically coding for the protein and thus affect suppression of both the wild-type and mutated protein.

Question 49.13.   **Match the following:**

A. Antisense oligonucleotide
B. Ribozymes
C. miRNA
D. siRNA
1. Single-stranded 19–24nt produced by cleavage of hairpin structure
2. Single-stranded DNA-like molecule
3. RNA molecule that can catalyze a reaction
4. Double-stranded structure homologous to mRNA of a target gene

Question 49.14.   **Major advantages of the use of siRNA in cancer therapeutics include all of the following, EXCEPT:**

A. Well-defined mechanism of action
B. Can be expressed from a vector
C. Immunologically inert
D. Chemical modifications are available

Question 49.15.   **The rationale of using miRNAs as anticancer drugs is based on many observations that include:**

A. Relatively large size.
B. Their natural antisense interactions.
C. Dysregulated expression profiles do not contribute to initiation of cancer.
D. Overexpression of miRNA in cancer cells has no pathogenic effect.

Question 49.16.   **A 65-year-old man was recently diagnosed with a T2N0 prostate cancer with a Gleason score of 4. He does not want to undergo radical prostatectomy and is exploring radiation options. He is presented with a clinical trial that is comparing fast neutron radiotherapy with hormonal blockade versus photon intensity-modulated radiation therapy (IMRT) with hormonal blockade. The following statements are true regarding use of neutrons as charged particle therapy, EXCEPT:**

A. They have high linear energy transfer (LET) properties.
B. They exhibit poor physical dose localization.
C. Their efficacy is less influenced by fractionation compared with standard photon therapy.
D. There are negligible late toxicity rates with neutron therapy.
E. The locoregional failure rates at 5 years are lower with neutrons compared with photons for localized prostate cancer.

Question 49.17.   A 25-year-old man presented with shooting pain along the T7 dermatome. He reported an increase in pain on coughing and bending. CT scans showed a paraspinal mass measuring 6 cm. Magnetic resonance imaging (MRI) showed infiltration into the spinal nerve root. Neurosurgical exploration was undertaken, and the mass was resected. Pathology revealed a poorly differentiated chondrosarcoma. Postoperative adjuvant radiation is recommended. There is concern about achieving the required doses of 60 Gy because of proximity to the spinal cord. The patient is recommended to travel to a facility that offers proton beam therapy. The following considerations regarding protons are true, EXCEPT:

A.   Protons have higher LET properties compared with photons.
B.   Proton therapy requires installation of large synchrotrons or cyclotrons to accelerate protons to energy levels required for deep-seated tumors.
C.   The disadvantage of using a traditional passive delivery system is that a significant amount of dose is delivered in the entrance channel to normal nontarget tissue.
D.   Local regional control at 5 years is low compared with traditional photon-IMRT.

Question 49.18.   A 36-year-old woman is diagnosed with a uveal melanoma. In view of the proximity to the optic nerve, brachytherapy with charged particles is recommended. The use of helium ion radiotherapy (RT) has been associated all of the following, EXCEPT:

A.   Improved local control compared with brachytherapy with I 125 plaques.
B.   Increased rates of surgical nucleation.
C.   Higher anterior segment complication rates, such as angle closure glaucoma compared with I125 plaque therapy.
D.   Improved local control with subsequent addition of proton beam therapy and reduction of original intended dose of helium ion RT.
E.   There are no data on long-term (>10 years) follow-up on patients treated with helium ion RT.

Question 49.19.   A 70-year-old man, otherwise healthy, has been given a recent diagnosis of stage I prostate cancer. He leads a busy life and wants to consider a surgical option that would be least disruptive to his work schedule. The following are true regarding robot-assisted surgery when compared with open and laparoscopic prostatectomy, EXCEPT:

A.   Robotic prostatectomy is associated with less blood loss.
B.   Short-term complications, including continence and erectile function, are much lower.
C.   Pathologic and surgical margins are similar.
D.   Shorter hospital stays.

Question 49.20.   **Nanodevices pertain to size 100 nm or less. Of the following nanode-vices, the ONLY one presently in human trials is:**

A. Dendrimers
B. Liposomes
C. Buckyballs/nanotubes
D. Quantum dots
E. Nanoshells

ANSWERS

Answer 49.1.   **The answer is E.**

Nonviral methods include both physical and chemical methods of gene transfer. Biolistic (gene gun transfer) involves coating of DNA or RNA on an inert microscopic carrier particle, which are then "fired" at high velocity/acceleration under high gas pressure. Electroporation is a process that involves use of pulsed electric field to temporarily open microscopic pores in cell membranes, allowing nucleic acid to enter the cell. Chemical methods include formation of complexes between DNA and cationic lipid or cationic polymer by condensation and uptake by target cell via endocytosis or phagocytosis. This is an extremely inefficient process. Transposons are mobile DNA elements that have the ability to move in the genome. Adenovirus vectors may be bound to polyethylene glycol to blunt immune recognition and are therefore used in retroviral gene therapy.

Answer 49.2.   **The answer is A.**

Replication defective viral vectors are essential for safe use of viral genomes in gene therapy. This involves deletion or modification of genes required for wild-type viral multiplication creation of recombinant virus by the addition of transgenes to prevent active replication of virus inside the host cell. To overcome the inability to replicate, packaging cell lines are used that supply the structural and replication proteins that are necessary to produce genetic elements. Although gamma retroviruses require actively dividing cells for transfection, other viruses, such as lenti virus, adenovirus, and herpes simplex virus, do not. Large viral genomes allow larger size of transgene for transfer into the host cell; however, it is not essential for replication. Removal of other genes, such as those for transcription, also allows for integration of more genomes in the same carrier viral genome; however, it is not an absolute requirement for viral gene therapy. The use of viral vector systems (e.g., adenovirus) may be limited by pre-existing immunity in humans, because they may give rise to cytotoxic T-cell or antibody-induced immune response leading to destruction of the recombinant virus. The immune recognition can be blunted by attaching innate polymers to the recombinant virus or transiently suppressing the immune system at the time of administration.

Answer 49.3.   **The answer is C.**

Adenovirus dl1520/ ONYX-15 is an oncolytic virus with deletion of EB1 gene that prevents its replication in cells with wild-type p53 function, such as normal tissues, but allows it to replicate in p53 deficient cells, which are tumor cells, with subsequent lysis of the tumor cell. Oncolytic viruses can work via two different mechanisms. A gene can be deleted whose function is not essential in a transformed cell, but with this gene the virus does not replicate in normal cells, or an essential gene can be put under the control of a promoter that is highly expressed in transformed cells, which permits efficient growth in the transformed cell. In both cases the virus does not replicate in normal cells but has unchecked growth in the transformed or tumor cells, which leads to cell death. Suicide gene therapy involves delivery of a gene to the tumor mass, which codes for an enzyme that has the potential to activate a prodrug to its toxic derivative, leading to cell lyses and death. Tumor suppressor gene therapy requires administration of a viral vector with intact tumor suppressor gene, which is deficient or mutated in cancer cells, thereby decreasing tumor growth, when used with chemotherapy. Adoptive cell transfer therapy (ACT) requires isolation of highly active antitumor reactive T cells (i.e., TILs). Expansion of these cells in vitro followed by reinfusion of TILs in lymphocyte-depleted host.

Answer 49.4.   **The answer is B.**

Adding TBI to preparative chemotherapy before infusion of TIL and IL-2 has been shown to improve actuarial 2-year survival. In patients receiving ACT after chemotherapy alone, the 2-year survival was 32% compared with 43% in patients who received 200 cGy TBI in conjunction with the chemotherapy regimen. This compares with 9% overall 2-year survival in patients who received ACT in the absence of lymphodepletion in prior trials. Clinical trial with cyclophosphamide, fludarabine, and 1200 cGy of TBI is ongoing.

Answer 49.5.   **The answer is D.**

Reactivation of EBV after bone marrow transplantation can result in EBV-associated lymphoproliferative disease. EBV-specific donor T-cell lymphocyte infusion can produce a virus-specific immune response to EBV that persists for up to 2 years. In a clinical trial with patients at high risk for PTLD who received prophylactic donor T-cell lymphocyte infusion, none of the 36 patients who received prophylaxis developed PTLD, compared with a cumulative risk of 14% in patients who did not receive this treatment. Interferon-alpha has been effective in the treatment of B-cell PTLD, as has been acyclovir, in addition to reduction of immunosuppression. Intravenous immunoglobulin has also been used as adjunctive therapy in the management of PTLD.

Answer 49.6.   **The answer is A.**

Relapse is the main cause of treatment failure after stem cell transplantation for blast phase chronic myeloid leukemia. Donor lymphocyte infusion can mediate complete molecular remissions in up to 80% of patients with relapsed CML and in up to 30% of patients in blast crisis. Induction therapy followed by a second allogeneic transplant is a reasonable option but is associated with higher toxicity and increased mortality, and therefore should be pursued if donor lymphocyte infusion does not produce remission. Imatinib therapy results in a higher incidence of relapse and inferior leukemia-free survival and therefore should not be used alone for treatment of CML relapse after stem cell transplantation.

Answer 49.7.   **The answer is C.**

The adoptive cell cancer immunotherapy approach involves infusion of tumor-bearing host cells with antitumor activity that can recognize cancer antigens and result in destruction of cancer cells. This approach has been successfully applied in clinical trials in the treatment of metastatic melanoma. Metastatic melanoma deposits (minimum of 1 to 2 cm^3) are resected and used to generate multiple cultures of TILs in 24-well tissue culture plates. Each well is individually expanded for several weeks and tested for antitumor activity against either shared melanoma antigens or the autologous tumor. Cultures with antitumor activity are then selected for rapid expansion using IL-2 and OKT3-stimulated feeder cells that provide the necessary components for lymphocyte growth. When cultures reach 1 to 5 $\times$ 10^{10} cells, they are infused into patients after an immunosuppressive preparative regimen consisting of chemotherapy (e.g., cyclophosphamide and fludarabine) and TBI. This is followed by infusion of autologous tumor-infiltrating lymphocytes and then high-dose intravenous IL-2 therapy for 2 to 3 days. CD34+ stem cells harvested after granulocyte cell stimulating factor administration are also infused at this time.

Answer 49.8.   **The answer is B.**

Focused ultrasound surgery requires MRI-based monitoring because integration of MRI with thermal ablation provides "closed-loop" feedback as a means of planning, targeting, guiding, monitoring, and controlling therapy. Therefore, any contraindication to MRI, such as intracranial aneurysm clips and intraorbital metal fragments; any electrically, magnetically, or mechanically activated implants (including cardiac pacemakers, biostimulators, neurostimulators, cochlear implants, and hearing aids); allergy to contrast dye; and claustrophobia, would prevent a patient from undergoing focused ultrasound surgery.

Answer 49.9.   **The answer is B.**

The use of focused ultrasound for treatment of uterine leiomyomas was FDA approved in October 2004. It is a safe, effective, noninvasive, outpatient procedure with fewer complications and rapid recoveries compared with standard treatment (i.e., hysterectomy). In addition, ablation of fibroids via ultrasound enables preservation of fertility. Although focused ultrasound has been used successfully in the setting of clinical trials for treatment of liver neoplasms, breast cancer and fibroadenomas, brain tumors, and prostate cancer, it has not yet been approved for widespread clinical use.

Answer 49.10. **The answer is D.**

Focused ultrasound involves delivery of acoustic energy of concentrated ultrasound waves to a focal point with conversion to thermal energy resulting in local tissue heating and irreversible thermal coagulation necrosis. The temperature in the focal zone is increased to more than 56°C and held for a few seconds until coagulation is achieved. It requires real-time temperature-sensitive imaging to calculate the total thermal dose delivered to target tissues and prevent unwanted heating of normal surrounding tissue. Another mechanism of ultrasound tissue interaction is cavitation or implosion of rapidly developed gas microbubbles at the focal zone, generating high pressures and temperatures and propagating shock waves. This mechanism can influence cell membrane and blood–brain barrier permeability.

Answer 49.11. **The answer is B.**

Focused ultrasound energy delivered above the cavitation threshold can induce focal blood–brain barrier opening without causing thermal effects or damaging neurons. This controlled opening of the blood–brain barrier at a desired location can be exploited to provide access for drugs, chemotherapeutic agents, and gene therapy. It can also be used for hemostasis and occlusion of blood vessels. It can effectively interrupt blood flow to a tumor and may serve as an adjunct to chemotherapy or radiation therapy. It has not been used or tested for adhesiolysis.

Answer 49.12. **The answer is A-False, B-True, C-True.**

Recent advances in the understanding of molecular oncology have suggested that noncoding genes (genes without a significant open reading frame) are also implicated in tumorigenesis. Among these nc-RNAs, the miRNA is most consistently linked to human cancers. In a specific tumor, abnormalities in protein coding genes and miRNA can both be seen. Inactivation of tumor suppressor genes and activation of oncogenic miRNA have the same molecular consequence of reducing apoptosis and increased tumor growth because of reduced levels of protein that block proliferation. Targeting of proteins represents a major focus of molecular therapy in cancer. The malignant cell can produce mutated proteins that can be one of the mechanisms in drug resistance. By targeting the messenger RNA, expression of both the wild-type and mutated protein is affected.

Answer 49.13. **The answer is A-2, B-3, C-1, D-4.**

Antisense oligonucleotides (ASO) are single-stranded, chemically modified DNA-like molecules 7 to 22 nt in length and specifically designed to be complementary to a selected messenger RNA, thus inhibiting specific protein expression. These compounds also inhibit transcription, splicing, and messenger RNA maturation. ASOs were first used in clinical practice. The major disadvantage of ASOs is the induction of immune response. In addition, they cannot be expressed from a vector, and thus continuous stable expression is not possible.

Ribozymes are RNA molecules that can catalyze a chemical reaction. Through base pairing, they cleave the substrate to release the latter. They can target both the nuclear RNA and introns in addition to protein coding sequences. Because of their effectiveness in low concentrations, side effects are few. Because they require specific cleavage sequence, the choice of targets is limited. siRNA is a double-stranded RNA that is homologous to messenger RNA of a target gene. It can be incorporated into a multiprotein RNA-induced silencing complex, leaving the antisense strand to guide the complex to homologous messenger RNA. Its main advantages are the availability of chemical modifications and expressability from a vector. Similar to ASO, it can induce an immune systemic response. It cannot be used to target nuclear RNAs or introns. miRNA is a single-stranded small (19–24nt) RNA produced by cleavage of a hairpin structure by RNases. It inhibits specific proteins by inducing a transcriptional/translational block. Preclinical studies are currently under way in leukemia and lymphomas.

Answer 49.14. **The answer is C.**

Oncogenes expressed at abnormally high levels are the main targets for si-RNA therapy. Their main advantages are the availability of chemical modifications and expressability from a vector. A major mechanism by which siRNA duplexes can induce adverse reactions is the stimulation of the innate immune system and production of interferon. The molecular mechanism may be related to Toll-like receptors located on the plasmacytoid dendritic cells.

Answer 49.15. **The answer is B.**

During the past few years miRNAs have been identified and cloned in many species, including humans. Their main mechanism is based on the imperfect miRNA: messenger RNA interaction. The major reason for the development of miRNA for therapy in cancer is related to the fact that miRNA overexpression in cancer cells have a pathogenic effect. In addition, there are many other advantages to their use in cancer therapeutics. These include their small size and intracellular presence that is not viewed as "nonself," thereby exhibiting natural antisense interaction. This property appears to be a unique feature of this form of RNA inhibition. Dysregulated miRNA expression contributes to the development of carcinogenesis. Thus, miRNA expression profiles can be used to diagnose cancers. Several genome-wide profiling studies, including those in chronic lymphocytic leukemia, papillary carcinoma of the thyroid, and lung cancer, have been performed.

Answer 49.16. **The answer is D.**

Neutron beam therapy has the advantage of high LET that can be used for deep-seated tumors; the high LET properties allow them to render lethal DNA damage. This DNA damage can seldom be repaired. This is in contrast with sublethal DNA damage induced by traditional photons, necessitating frequent fractionation. However, neutrons have poor physical tissue localization giving rise to frequent and significant delayed local side effects.

Answer 49.17.   **The answer is D.**

Protons are highly charged particles that require significant investment in a synchrotron or cyclotron to accelerate protons to energy levels high enough to be delivered to deep-seated tumors. They may also require newer active beam delivery systems to prevent entry channel damage to normal tissue. They have been successfully used in the treatment of uveal melanomas, some early prostate cancers, deep-seated chordomas, and now in early non–small cell lung cancers. The local-regional control at 5 years for paraspinal tumors approaches 100% for chondrosarcoma.

Answer 49.18.   **The answer is B.**

Uveal melanomas in the posterior segment may be treated with I-125 plaque brachytherapy; however, this modality may not be sufficient for melanomas that are larger or close to the optic nerve. Either helium ion RT or proton beam therapy may be used in this situation. Helium ion RT has higher local control and eye retention rates compared with I-125 brachytherapy. However, at high doses of cobalt gray equivalents, there were higher anterior segment complications, including glaucoma, requiring secondary enucleation. These complications decreased by reducing the dose delivered to 48 CGE and following helium ion RT with proton beam therapy.

Answer 49.19.   **The answer is B.**

Robot-assisted surgery is gaining in popularity. Robot-assisted prostatectomy is presently the most common robot-assisted surgery performed in the United States. The steps of robot-assisted prostatectomy are similar to open surgery. However, there is greater ease of dissection and enhanced ability by the surgeon to perform a watertight bladder-neck urethral anastomosis. There is less blood loss and therefore less transfusion requirement. Short-term complications, including incontinence and impotence, are comparable to those of open and laparoscopic prostatectomies.

Answer 49.20.   **The answer is B.**

Nanodevices are being studied for a variety of applications in cancer, including prevention, targeted drug delivery, imaging, and multifunctional therapeutics. Of the nanodevices listed, only liposomes are in human clinical trials. Liposomes are spherical vesicles with a membrane composed of a phospholipid and cholesterol bilayer, usually with an aqueous solution at its core. They have been used to deliver a wide variety of therapeutic and imaging agents.

Index